U0288247

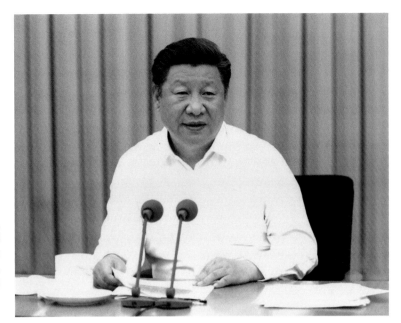

Chinese President Xi Jinping, also general secretary of the CPC Central Committee and chairman of the Central Military Commission, made remarks at the National Health Assembly, Aug. 19th, 2016.

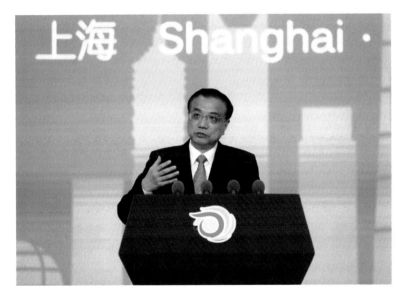

The 9th Global Conference on Health Promotion opened in Shanghai, China's largest city, Nov. 21st, 2016. Li Keqiang, member of the Politburo Standing Committee (PSC) of the CPC Central Committee and Premier of the State Council, addressed the opening ceremony.

Premier Li Keqiang met with Director-General of WHO Dr. Margaret Chan and the senior officials of the United Nations Population Fund (UNFPA) and the United Nations Environment Program (UNEP), in Shanghai, Nov. 21st, 2016.

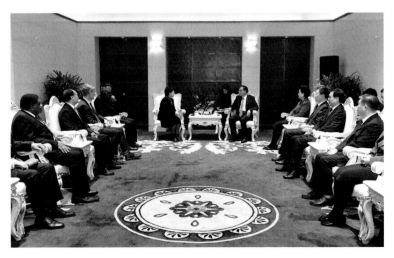

# The 9th Global Conference on Health Promotion

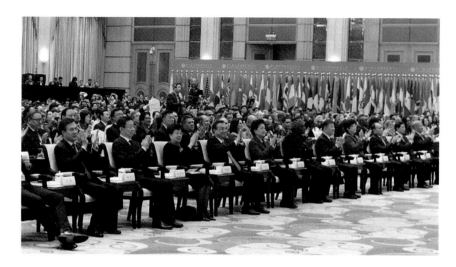

The 9th Global Conference on Health Promotion was held in Shanghai, Nov. 21st-24th, 2016. One hundred and thirty-one countries, 19 international organizations and over 1,200 delegates attended the highest-level international event in the field of health promotion. Premier Li Keqiang and Vice-Premier Liu Yandong announced China's experience, strategies and propositions in their important addresses. With the theme of "health promotion in sustainable development", the Conference hosted some events, such as International Healthy City Mayors' Forum, nine plenary sessions, 30 meetings and China's National Day. The Shanghai Declaration and Shanghai Consensus on Healthy Cities were issued to start a new era of global health promotion.

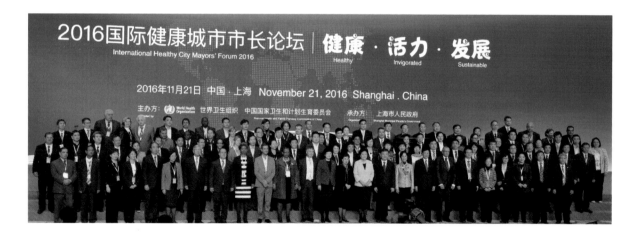

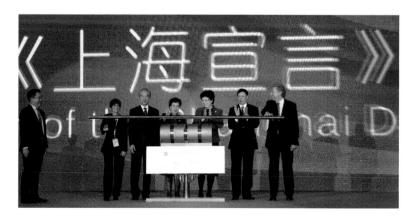

# Conferences and Events

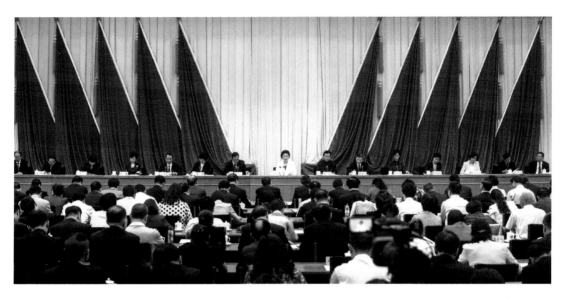

The 8th National Assembly of China Family Planning Association was held in Beijing, May 18th, 2016.

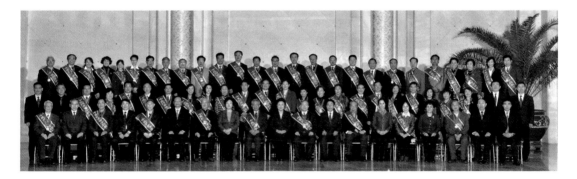

The Forum on the Reform and Development of Higher Education in Traditional Chinese Medicine (TCM) and the Commendation Conference for the Outstanding Teachers of Universities and Colleges of TCM was held in Beijing, Dec. 29th, 2016. Liu Yandong, member of the Politburo of the CPC Central Committee, attended the Forum and took a group photo with the Teachers.

Peng Liyuan, Chinese President Xi Jinping's wife, attended the event of "Publicity of HIV/AIDS Prevention and Control on Campus" at Zhejiang University with the wives of leaders attending the G20 Hangzhou Summit, Sept. 5th, 2016.

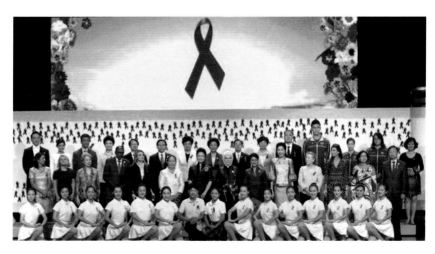

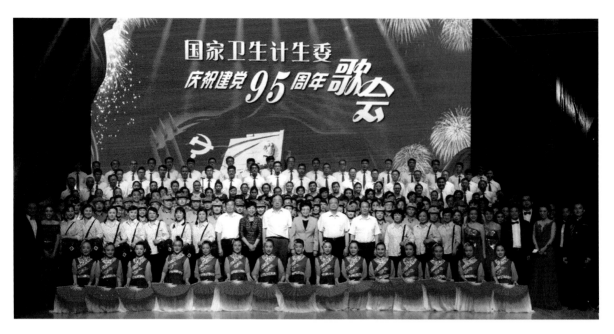

The National Health and Family Planning Commission held a concert marking the 95th anniversary of the founding of the Communist Party of China (CPC), June 27th, 2016.

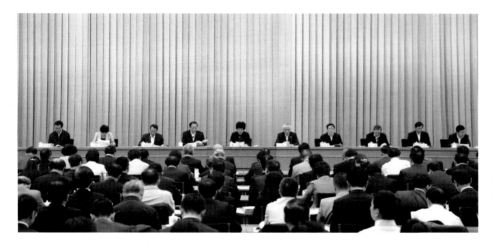

The National Conference on Scientific Innovation of Health was held in Beijing, Oct. 13th-14th, 2016.

The National Health and Family Planning Commission held the televised conference on the start and promotion of the national pilot project for the big data center of healthcare and the construction of industrial park, Oct. 21st, 2016. Minister of the National Health and Family Planning Commission Li Bin and some other officials attended the launch ceremony.

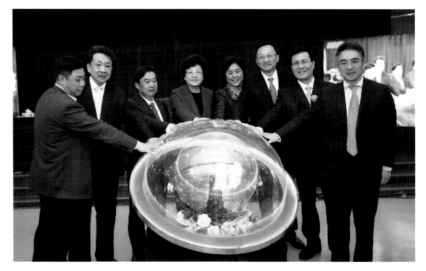

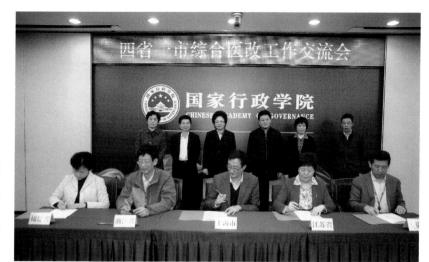

The agreement on the joint conference system of comprehensive healthcare reform among Jiangsu, Zhejiang, Anhui, Fujian and Shanghai was signed, Nov. 13th, 2016.

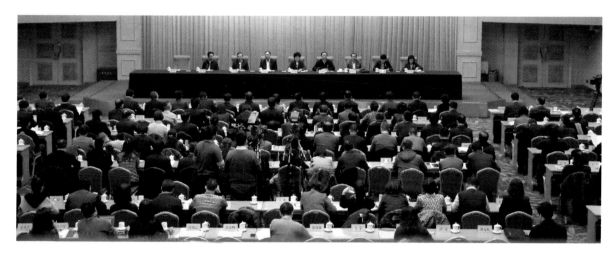

The Party Leadership Group of the National Health and Family Planning Commission held tho televised conference on the experience exchange of ideological and political work within the national health and family planning system, Dec. 12th, 2016.

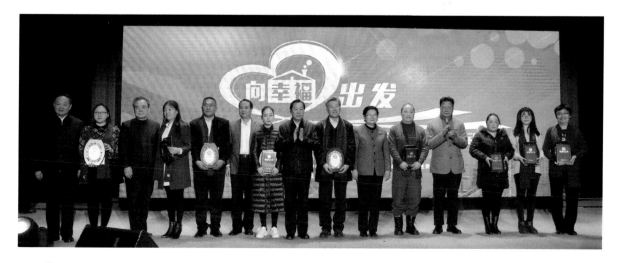

The representatives of the national first batch of happy families received trophies and medals at the event of the Publicity for the Creation of Happy Families Nationwide, Dec. 29th, 2016.

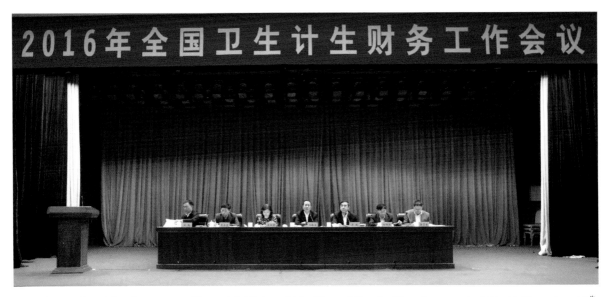

The National Conference on Financial Affairs of Health and Family Planning was held in Beijing, Jan. 20th, 2016.

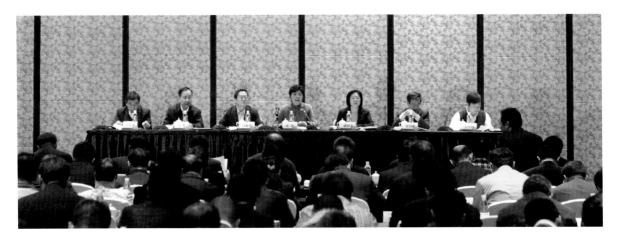

The National Conference on Health Emergency was held in Chongqing, a metropolis of more than 30 million people in Southwest China's Sichuan province, Jan. 28th, 2016.

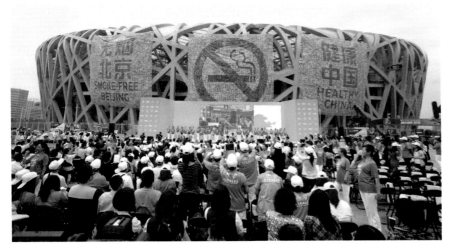

The publicity campaign for World No-Tobacco Day and the 1st anniversary of the implementation of the Beijing Regulations on Smoking Control was launched in Beijing, May 31st, 2016.

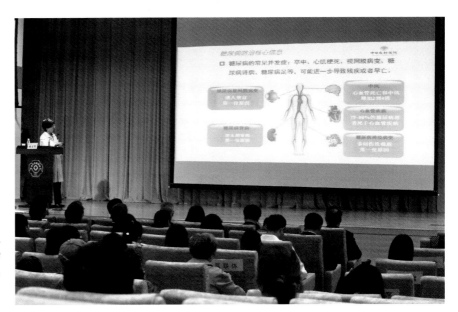

The publicity campaign for World Health Day was launched in Beijing, April 6th, 2016.

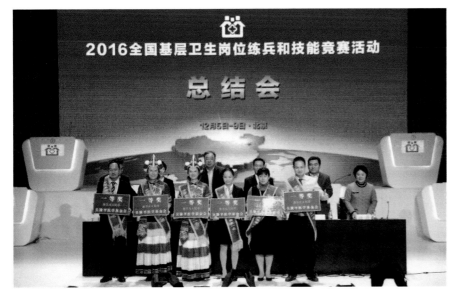

The job training and skill competitions of the national healthcare at the primary level were held in Beijing, Dec. 5th-9th, 2016.

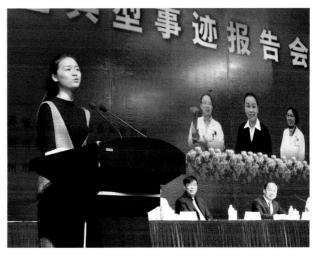

The report meeting on the exemplary deeds of the national health and family planning system was held in Taizhou of East China's Jiangsu province, Dec. 16th, 2016.

# Officials' Surveys and Researches

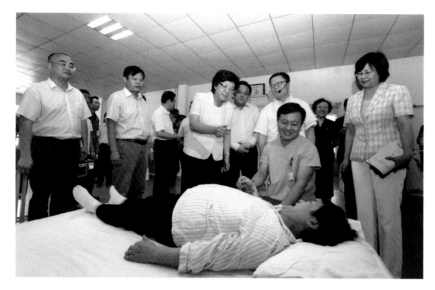

Li Bin, Minister of the National Health and Family Planning Commission, carried out an inspection of community rehabilitation at Mingshui Community Health Service Center in Zhangqiu, Shandong province, Sept. 7th, 2016.

Wang Guoqiang, Vice Minister of the National Health and Family Planning Commission, conducted survey and research on the prevention and control of echinococcosis in Shiqu county, Sichuan province, in July 2016.

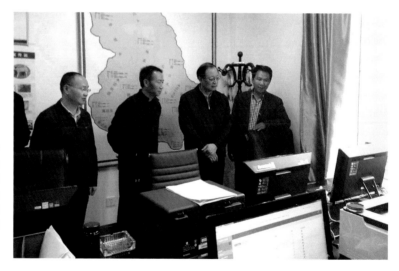

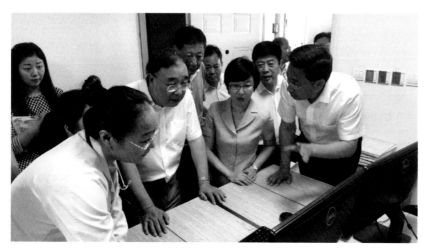

Ma Xiaowei, Vice Minister of the National Health and Family Planning Commission, conducted survey and research on out-of-town settlement and reimbursement of healthcare expenditures under the New Rural Cooperative Medical System (NRCMS) in Henan province, in September 2016.

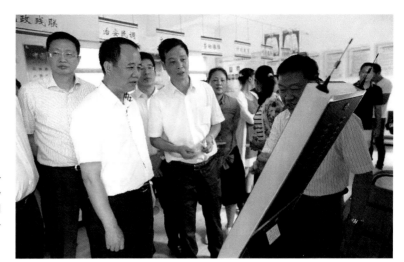

Wang Peian, Vice Minister of the National Health and Family Planning Commission, conducted survey and research at the primary-level healthcare institutions in 2016.

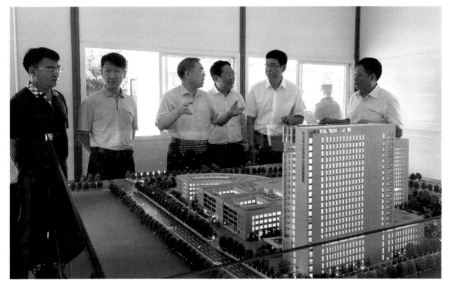

Liu Qian, Vice Minister of the National Health and Family Planning Commission, conducted survey and research on the project construction of Fuwai Hospital of Yunnan province, Aug. 26th, 2016.

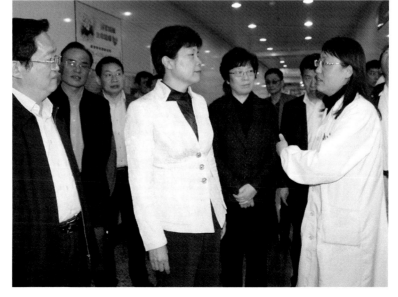

Cui Li, Vice Minister of the National Health and Family Planning Commission, conducted survey and research on health emergency at the First Affiliated Hospital of Anhui Medical University, April 28th, 2016.

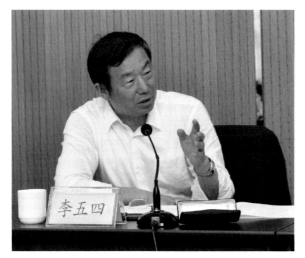

Li Wusi, head of the Discipline Inspection Team of the Central Commission for Discipline Inspection in the National Health and Family Planning Commission, made a speech at the symposium for the heads of the discipline inspection teams in the provincial departments of health and family planning, which was held in Zhejiang province, May 27th, 2016.

Jin Xiaotao, Vice Minister of the National Health and Family Planning Commission, conducted survey and research on information construction in Taiyuan, capital of Shanxi province, May 12th, 2016.

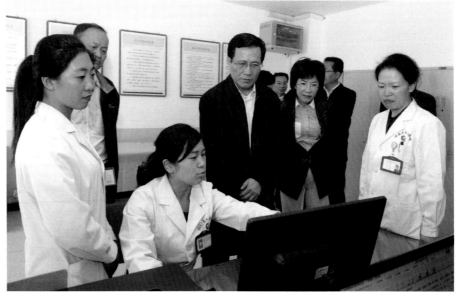

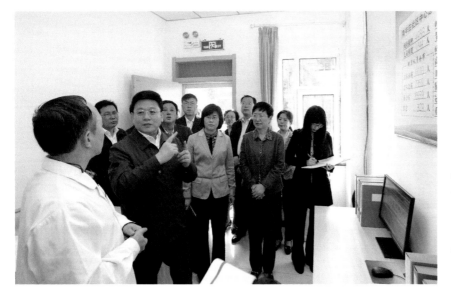

Wang Hesheng, Vice Minister of the National Health and Family Planning Commission, conducted survey and research at Nanxinzhuang Community Health Service Center in Huaiyin district, Jinan, capital of Shandong province, Oct. 11th, 2016.

# Professional Work

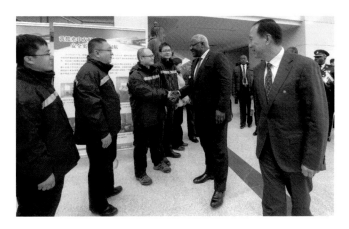

President of the Republic of Sierra Leone visited the Chinese Center for Disease Control and Prevention (China CDC), Dec. 1st, 2016.

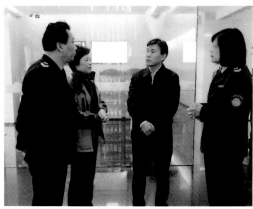

The Center of Inspection and Supervision under the National Health and Family Planning Commission conducted survey and research on the supervision of law enforcement at the Institute of Inspection and Supervision under Shanghai Municipal Commission of Health and Family Planning, Nov. 24th, 2016.

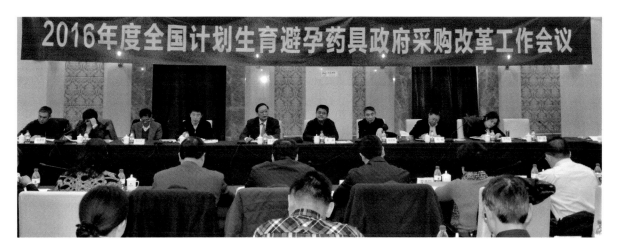

The National Conference on the Reform of Government Procurement for Birth Control Contraceptives was held in Beijing, Feb. 2nd, 2016.

The Logistics Service Bureau under the National Health and Family Planning Commission studied the maintenance and reconstruction of No. 1 Office Building of the Commission in April 2016.

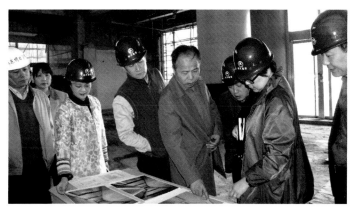

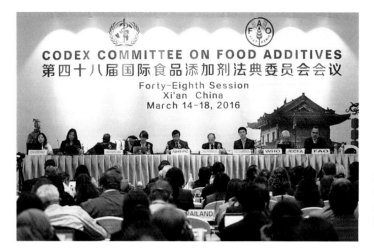

The Forty-Eighth Session of Codex Committee on Food Additives hosted by China National Center for Food Safety Risk Assessment was held in Xi'an, capital of Shaanxi province, Mar. 14th, 2016.

Peking Union Medical College Hospital launched a post-doctoral training program in clinical medicine to implement the elite talent strategy in April 2016. A total of 20 postdocs in clinical medicine were selected during the year.

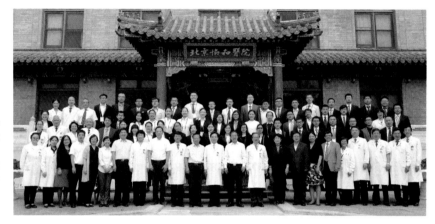

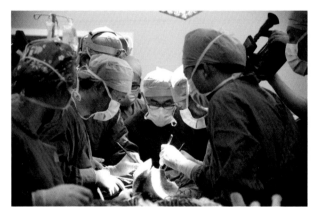

Multiple lung transplantations were performed successfully in China-Japan Friendship Hospital in 2016.

The 9th Conference on China Health Education and Health Promotion was held in Beijing, Sept. 21st-22nd, 2016.

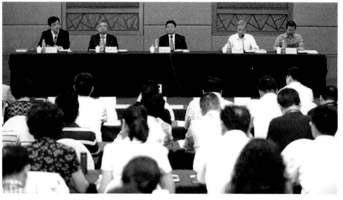

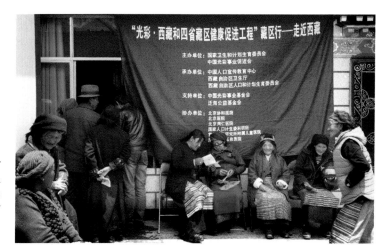

Pictured here is the free clinic for the tour of Tibetan areas for "Honor & Tibet and Maternal & Child Health Initiative in the Tibetan Areas of the Four Provinces" in 2016.

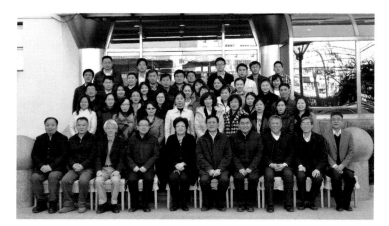

Li Bin and Jin Xiaotao, Minister and Vice Minister of the National Health and Family Planning Commission, took a group photo with the officials and staff of the Cadres' Training Center (Party School of the CPC), Jan. 11$^{th}$, 2016.

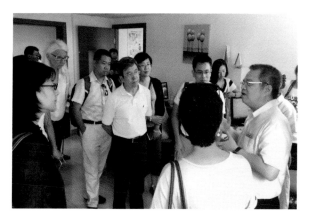

The picture shows the scene of the technical review meeting on the World Bank loan project for China's healthcare reform in 2016.

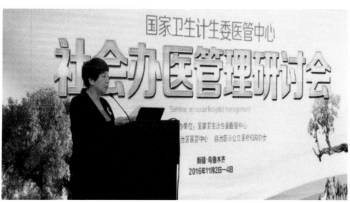

The Symposium on the Management of Nongovernmental Hospitals was held in Urumqi, capital of Xinjiang Uygur Autonomous Region, Jan. 2$^{nd}$-4$^{th}$, 2016.

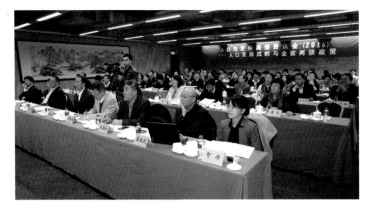

China Population and Development Research Center held 2016 High-level Information Meeting on Population and Development themed with "Population Development Strategy and Universal Two-Child Policy", Nov. 26th, 2016.

The officials and staff of China Population and Development Research Center carried out the activity of thematic Party day in Yan'an, former Chinese revolutionary base in the Northwest China's Shaanxi province, June 17th, 2016.

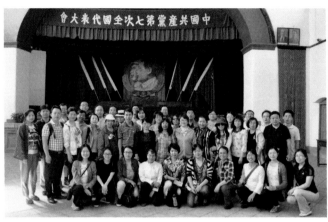

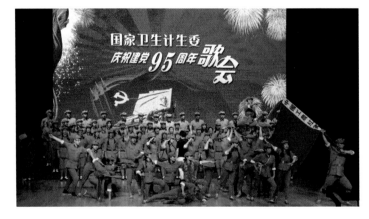

The staff of China Population and Development Research Center acted out "Crossing the Snow Mountains and Marshy Grasslands," at the concert marking the 95th anniversary of the founding of the Chinese Communist Party held by the National Health and Family Planning Commission, June 27th, 2016.

The delegation of China Population and Development Research Center visited Oxford University and the University of Southampton, Dec. 6th-7th, 2016.

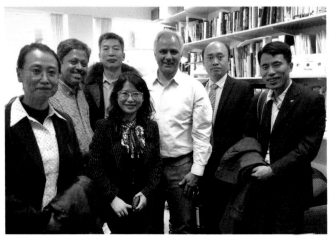

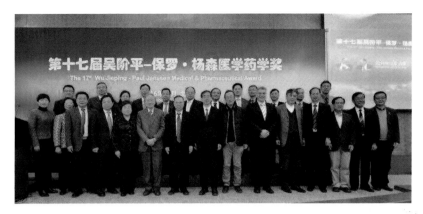

The 17th Wu Jieping-Paul Janssen Medical & Pharmaceutical Award was held in Beijing, Dec. 13th, 2016.

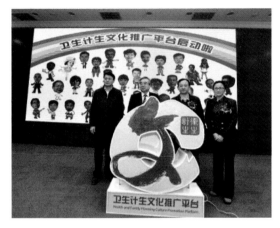

The cultural promotion platform for health and family was officially launched, Jan. 14th, 2016.

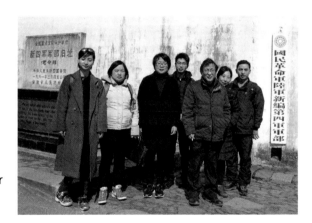

Nanjing Training Center carried out the activity for the Party members in 2016.

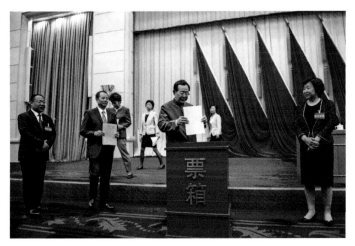

The 3rd Plenary Session of the 8th Congress of China Family Planning Association voted for a new council, May 20, 2016.

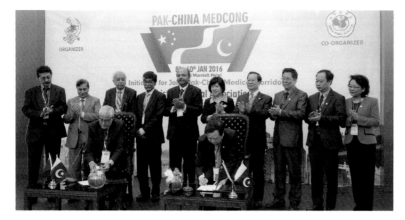

The 1st Pak-China Medical Congress & Belt and Road Forum of Medical Associations was held in Karachi, capital of Pakistan, Jan. 10th, 2016, during which China Medical Association and Pakistan Medical Association signed the Memorandum of Understanding on the Cooperation of the Congress and the Forum to co-build Pak-China Medical Corridor.

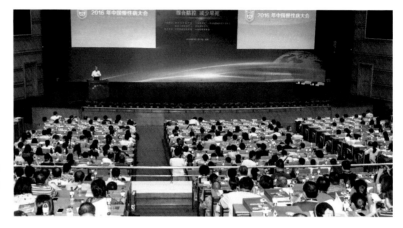

2016 China NCDs Conference was held in Beijing, Sept. 2nd-3rd, 2016.

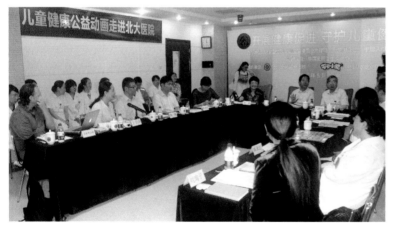

China Population Culture Promotion Association actively carried out grass-roots activities on population culture in 2016.

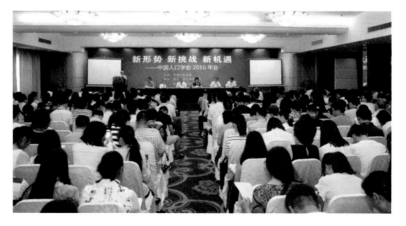

2016 Annual Meeting of China Population Association was held in Xiamen, a beautiful seaside city in Southeast China's Fujian province, July 21st-22nd, 2016.

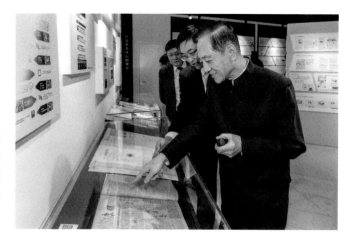

Health News held the symposium marking its 85th anniversary, Oct. 26th, 2016. Han Qide, Vice Chairman of Chinese People's Political Consultative Conference (CPPCC), attended the symposium and visited the museum of the newspaper history.

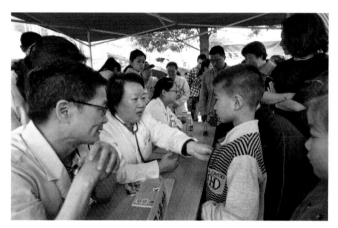

The specialists gave the sick children an on-site free medical consultation at the public welfare lecture on maternal and child health in May 2016. The lecture was given by China Population News.

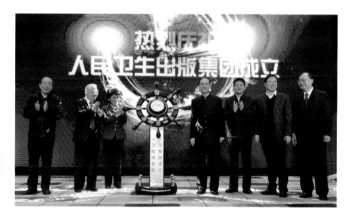

The inauguration ceremony for the People's Medical Publishing Group was held in Beijing, Oct. 30th, 2016.

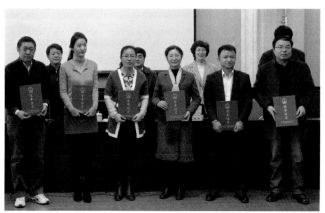

The bilingual book series on nationality population, published by China Population Publishing House, was selected into "the 3rd Session of Nationwide Recommendation for Hundreds of Outstanding Nationality Books."

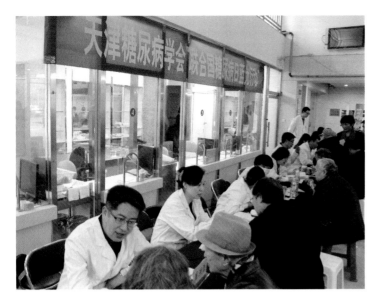

A free medical consultation for World Diabetes Day (WDD) was given in Tianjin, Nov. 12ᵗʰ, 2016.

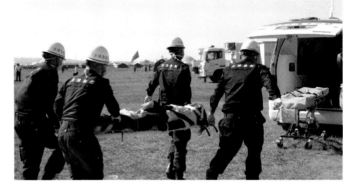

2016 comprehensive health emergency drill for major natural disasters in the greater Beijing-Tianjin-Hebei region was held in Zhangbei county, Hebei province, Sept. 13ᵗʰ, 2016.

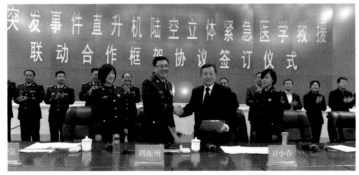

Shanxi Provincial Health and Family Planning Commission and Shanxi Armed Police Corps signed the cooperation framework agreement on helicopter's land-air emergency medical rescue linkage to construct a land-air emergency medical rescue network, April 1ˢᵗ, 2016.

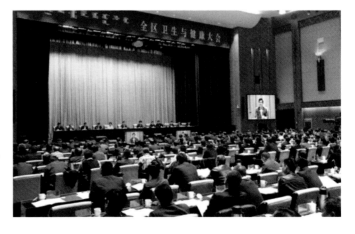

The Health Assembly of Inner Mongolia Autonomous Region was held in Huhhot, capital of the Autonomous Region, Nov. 6ᵗʰ, 2016.

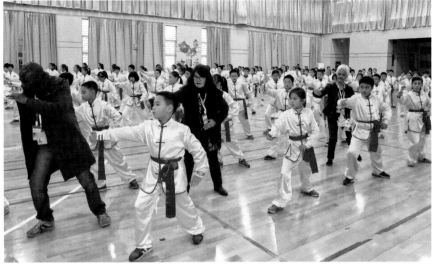

During the event of China's National Day of the 9th Global Conference on Health Promotion, the delegates were practicing martial arts with the school children while inspecting the health promotion at Chengzhonglu Primary School in Jiading district, Nov. 23rd, 2016.

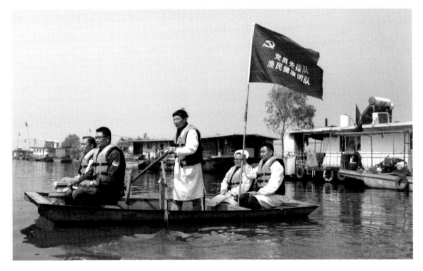

The service team of family doctors of Jiangsu province provided the fishermen with contract signing service in 2016.

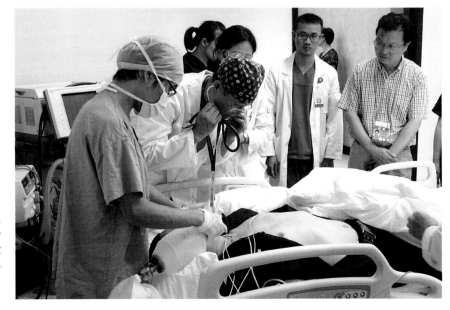

Zhejiang Provincial Health and Family Planning Commission made efforts to provide health emergency protection for the G20 Summit in 2016. Pictured here is the site of emergency drill.

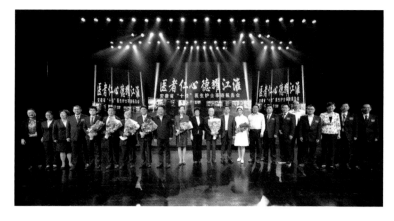

The Report Meeting on the Exemplary Deeds of the Top Ten Doctors and Nurses in Anhui province was held, June 2nd, 2016. TCM master Xu Jingshi, Doctor Liu Hongtao who slept in the ward and some other "angels in while" arose resonance in the audience with their deeds and heartfelt wishes.

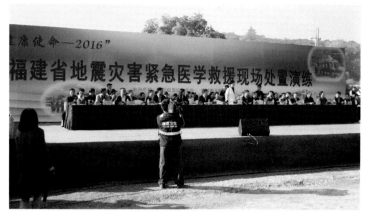

The on-site disposal drill of emergency medical rescue for earthquakes of Fujian province, themed with Health Mission——2016, was held in Changtai county in the city of Zhangzhou, Fujian province, Dec. 1st-3rd, 2016.

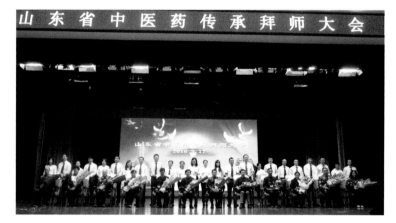

Shandong Provincial Health and Family Planning Commission held the apprenticeship ceremony for the 4th batch of inheritors of academic experience in traditional Chinese medicine, May 17th, 2016.

Picture here is the site of group operation skill examination of the job training and skill competition of the national healthcare at the primary level (Hubei division), Oct. 13th, 2016.

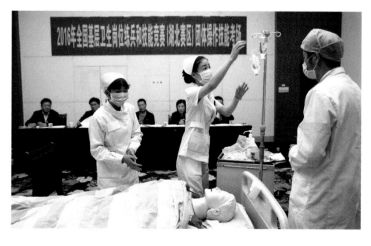

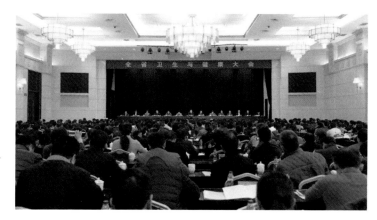

Hunan Provincial Health Assembly was held in Changsha, capital of Hunan province, Dec. 29th, 2016.

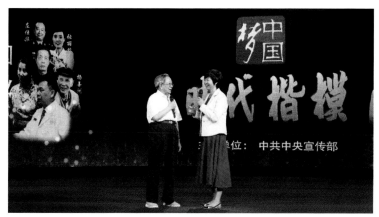

The Propaganda Department of the CPC Central Committee and CCTV made public the exemplary deeds of Luo Kangxian (Left), known as "Model of the Times," July 14th, 2016. As a chief physician of the department of infectious diseases in Nanfang Hospital of Southern Medical University, Luo Kangxian has always put medical ethics first and adhered to the primacy of patients over the past 62 years of medical practice. He has also successfully given treatment to hundreds of thousands of hepatitis B patients, which has been an outstanding achievement to the prevention and control of hepatitis B.

The People's Government of Guangxi Zhuang Autonomous Region, the National Health and Family Planning Commission and the State Administration of Traditional Chinese Medicine co-hosted the 1st China-Asean Health Forum, Oct. 26th-29th, 2016. Pictured here is the site of the opening ceremony.

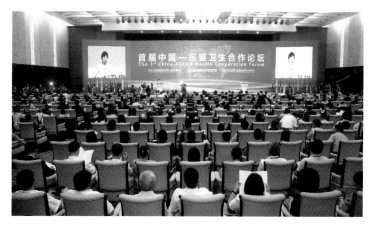

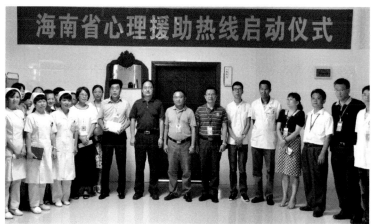

The first Hainan provincial free psychological assistance hotline 96363 used as a public service went into official operation, Aug. 10th, 2016.

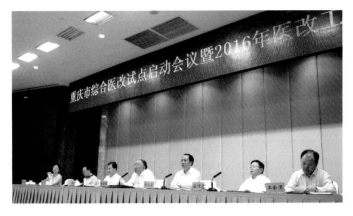

The launching meeting on Chongqing pilot comprehensive healthcare reform and the meeting on 2016 healthcare reform was held, May 30th, 2016.

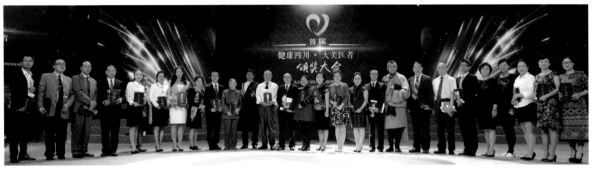

The First Award-Giving Meeting for Healthy Sichuan · Doctors of Great Beauty was held, Sept. 28th, 2016. Pictured here is that some "doctors of great beauty and winners of award nomination had a group photo taken with the presenters.

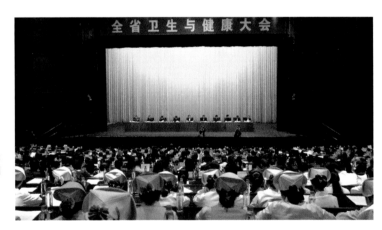

Guizhou Provincial Health Assembly was held in Guiyang, capital of Guizhou province in Southwest China, Nov. 14th, 2016.

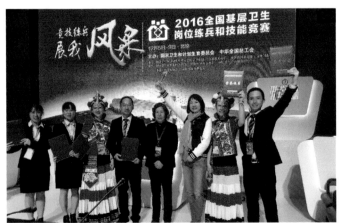

In the national finals of the job training and skill competitions of the national healthcare at the primary level held on Dec. 9th, 2016, Yunnan province won first place in the community teams, second place in the units of general practitioners of urban communities, second place in the units of general practitioners in rural areas, second place in the community care units, special contribution award and outstanding organization award.

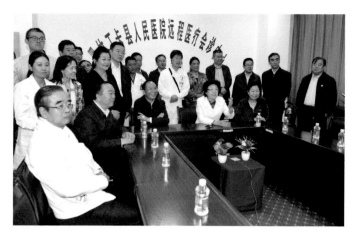

Li Bin, Minister of the National Health and Family Planning Commission, inspected and gave guidance to the telemedicine consultation in the People's Hospital of Maizhokunggar county, July 31st, 2016.

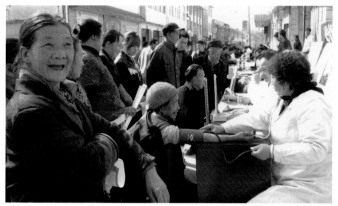

The on-site service of the free clinic provided by the hospital of Foping Hospital in Shaanxi province was very popular among the local people in 2016.

The Signing Ceremony for the 1st International Forum on Traditional Chinese Medicine Culture and Health Industry was held in Dunhuang, a county-level city in Northwest China's Gansu province and well-known for its Mogao Grottoes, Aug. 19th, 2016.

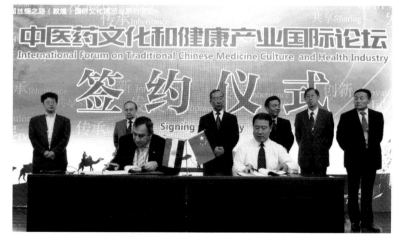

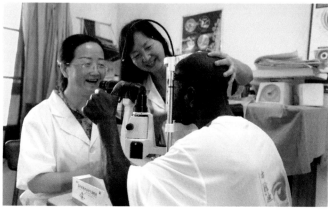

Qinghai Medical Team went to Burundi for the campaign of Light Tour to help 182 Burundian patients with eye problems see again in October 2016.

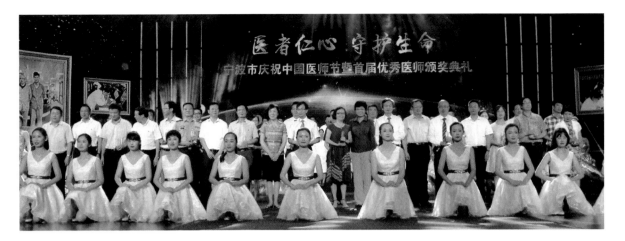

The Conference Celebrating Chinese Doctor's Day and the 1st Commendation Meeting for Ningbo Outstanding Doctors was held, June 24<sup>th</sup>, 2016.

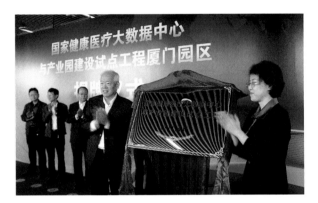

Xiamen zone of the national pilot project for the big data center of healthcare and the construction of industrial park was inaugurated, Nov. 29<sup>th</sup>, 2016.

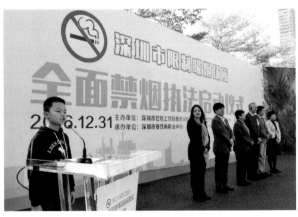

The Launch Ceremony for Comprehensive Anti-smoking Law-Enforcement for Smoking Restrictions in Public Spaces was held in Shenzhen, Dec. 31<sup>st</sup>, 2016.

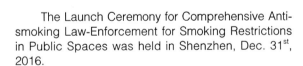
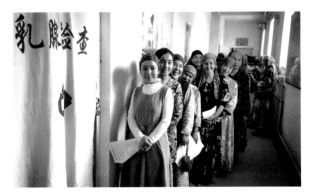

The service and guidance center of family planning of the 1st Division of Xinjiang Production and Construction Corps carried out free comprehensive investigation and comprehensive treatment for women of child-bearing age in minority ethnic groups, May 31<sup>st</sup>, 2016.

**(Shan Yongxiang)**

# *2017*
# HEALTH
## in
## CHINA

Translator-in-Chief

Chen Ying

Qu Yang

Associate Translator-in-Chief

Shan Yongxiang

Translators

Ji Chenglian, Jing Ran, Tong Yanlong, Wang Guimin,
Wang Qinghua, Wang Ruisi, Zhang Nan, Zhao Xuemei,
Zhao Yinghong, Zhao Yueting, Zhou Dan

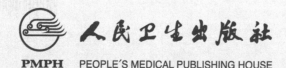

**PMPH**  PEOPLE'S MEDICAL PUBLISHING HOUSE

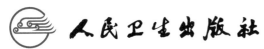

PMPH    PEOPLE'S MEDICAL PUBLISHING HOUSE

http:// www.pmph.com

Book Title: 2017 Health in China
2017 卷中国卫生和计划生育年鉴（英文版）

Contact address: No.19 Pan Jia Yuan Nan Li, Chaoyang District, Beijing 100021, P. R. China
phone/fax: 86 10 5978 7386, E-mail: pmph@pmph.com

---

### Disclaimer

This book is for educational and reference purposes only. In view of the possibility of human errors or changes in medical science, neither the author, editor nor the publisher nor any other party who has been involved in the preparation or publication of this work guarantees that the information contained herein is in every respect accurate or complete. The medicinal therapy and treatment techniques presented in this book are provided for the purpose of reference only. If readers wish to attempt any of the techniques or utilize any of the medicinal therapies contained in this book, the publisher assumes no responsibility for any of such actions.

It is the responsibility of the readers to understand and adhere to local laws and regulations concerning the practice of these techniques and methods. The authors, editors and publishers disclaim all responsibility for any liability, loss, injury, or damage incurred as a consequence, directly or indirectly, of the use and application of any of the contents of this book.

---

First published:
ISBN: 978-7-117-27985-7

**Cataloguing in Publication Data:**
A catalog record for this book is available from the
CIP-Database China.

Printed in P. R. China

ISBN 978-7-117-27985-7

9 787117 279857 >

# Contents

## Chapter II  Speeches by the Leaders of the National Health and Family Planning Commission

## Part III  Deepening the Reform of the Medical and Health System  365

# Part I
# Overview

**Overview of National Health and Family Planning Development in 2016**
**—General Office of the National Health and Family Planning Commission**

**I. We focused on four major tasks, completed the work satisfactorily and made a good start for the 13th Five-year Plan period**

The National Conference on Health and Sanitation was held. The CPC Central Committee and the State Council convened the first national health and hygiene conference since the new century. General Secretary Xi Jinping made an important speech and, from strategic and global heights, profoundly expounded the major policies and basic strategies for building healthy China. Premier Li Keqiang made a systematic deployment on deepening medical reform in an all-round way and speeding up the development of health industry. Vice Premier Liu Yandong made a summary of the conference. The conference opened a new journey for the construction of healthy China.

The *Outline of the Healthy China 2030 Plan* was issued and implemented. Under the direct leadership of the State Council, a drafting group of multi-sector participation was established and the *Outline of the Healthy China 2030 Plan* was compiled and, as the document of the CPC Central Committee and the State Council, was issued and implemented. Based on this *Outline*, the compiling work of the 13th Five-Year Plan on Hygiene and Health and the 13th Five-Year Plan on deepening medical reform was organized. The compiling work of "One Outline and Two Plans" was successfully completed, marking the formation of top-level design for building healthy China, defining the development goals, directions, tasks and paths for the next five to fifteen years and establishing the basic rules of the reform and development of the cause.

The Ninth Global Health Promotion Conference was convened. During November 21st-24th, 2016, the Conference was convened in Shanghai and, as the highest level international event in the field of health promotion, 131 countries, 19 international organizations and over 1,200 representatives attended this conference. Premier Li Keqiang and Vice Premier Liu Yandong delivered important speeches, declaring

China's experience, strategy and advocacy of health promotion. Centering on the theme of "health promotion in sustainable development", mayor forum of Healthy Cities, 9 plenary meetings, 30 sessions and the activities like "China Day" were held, and the *Shanghai Declaration* and the *Shanghai Consensus of Healthy Cities* were issued in this conference, which opened the new era of global health promotion.

The *Law of the People's Republic of China on Traditional Chinese Medicine* was promulgated. With active cooperation with the NPC, the drafting, modification and argumentation of the legislative bill were conducted. The twenty-second plenary meeting of the Standing Committee of the NPC adopted and published the *Law of the People's Republic of China on Traditional Chinese Medicine*, which would be implemented officially on July 1st, 2017. The *Law of the People's Republic of China on Traditional Chinese Medicine* is the first special law in the field of traditional Chinese medicine, which will have a far-reaching impact on maintaining and carrying forward the characteristic advantages of traditional Chinese medicine and promoting the revitalization and development of traditional Chinese medicine.

In 2016, the whole system prioritized the work of the people's health, highlighted the dual directions of needs and problems and promoted the reform and development of health and family planning to get new results.

### II. Breakthroughs were made in deepening the reform of the medical and health system

The reform of public hospitals was solidly advanced. The number of pilot provinces of comprehensive medical reform was expanded from 4 to 11 and the number of pilot cities for comprehensive reform of public hospitals increased from 100 to 200. Four model counties (county-level cities) were established, on-the-spot meeting on comprehensive reform of public hospitals at the county level was held to strengthen the classified guidance and demonstration guidance. The *Opinions on Promoting the Reform of Medical Service Prices* was jointly issued with 4 departments of the Development and Reform Commission and others to steadily adjust prices according to the steps of "clearing space, adjusting structure and ensuring convergence". More than 1,560 urban public hospitals abolished drug markups and eliminated the mechanism of compensating medical cost with drug sale. The national public hospital income structure was continuously optimized, the growth of medical expenses was effectively controlled and the medical burden was continuously reduced.

Preliminary results were achieved in the pilot tiered medical service. Pilot projects were started in 4 municipalities and 266 prefecture level cities to promote Shanghai

"1+1+1" family doctor (team) signing service mechanism and the health management model of " co-management of specialists of large hospitals, primary family physicians and health managers" in Xiamen and Fujian. The resources of family doctors were strengthened, the mechanism of coordination and distribution of responsibilities was perfected, the models of tiered medical service, like medical treatment alliance, were explored and the guarantee mechanism was improved. The coverage rate of contract service of family doctors reached more than 22% with more than 38% for key population, over-fulfilling the annual objectives.

The basic medical insurance function was more perfect. The per capita financial subsidy standard for basic medical insurance of urban and rural residents was increased to 420 *yuan*, major disease insurance was added 10 *yuan* and the reimbursement rate of outpatient and inpatient expenses within the policy scope was stable at around 50% and 75%. According to the requirements of "Six Unifications", the integration of basic medical insurance system for urban and rural residents was speeded up all around the country. The national information technology standard for the New Rural Cooperative Medical Scheme (NRCMS) was unified, realizing the direct settlement of basic medical insurance for medical treatment in different places within a province and carrying out the pilot work of medical settlement for medical treatment in different provinces. More than 500 new clinical pathways were set up, with the total number of clinical pathways up to 1,010 and basically covering common diseases and frequently-occurring diseases. More than 7,700 medical institutions implemented clinical pathway management. Commercial insurance institutions were actively supported to participate in the basic medical insurance and major disease insurance business.

The reform of the drug supply guarantee system was deeply advanced. Centralized quantity procurement of medicines in public hospitals was promoted and the "two-invoice system" for drug purchase and sale was implemented in the pilot provinces of comprehensive health care reform. The negotiation of state drug prices was pushed forward, with the average price drop of negotiated drugs by more than 50% and network procurement in 29 provinces (autonomous regions and municipalities directly under the Central Government). Military medical institutions implemented the results of the national negotiations. The early warning and supply guarantee for drugs in short supply was strengthened, with 9 new varieties of fixed-point production of low-cost drugs in short supply. In conjunction with the relevant departments, the first batch of list of children's medicines encouraged to research, develop and declare was released so as to promote the supply of medicines for children.

The development environment for socially-run medical services was further optimized. The establishment examination and approval of for-profit medical institutions was changed into post-examination and approval. Private hospitals accounted for more than 55.3% of the total number of hospitals, with 2,038 newly-built private hospitals, and nonpublic medical institutions accounted for more than 22% of the rate of diagnosis and treatment. The policy of "License Granted before Certificate" was implemented, regional registration was explored and orderly migration was promoted. By the end of 2016, there were 61,000 doctors registered for multi-point practice across the country, with 43.4% in socially-run medical institutions and 66.3% in primary-level medical and health institutions. Basic standards and norms were speculated for independently setting up institutions of examination and inspection, hospice care and others. With the cooperation of the Ministry of Finance, 36 demonstration projects of governmental and social capital cooperation were promoted in the health field, with the total investment of 21.8 billion *yuan*.

### III. The quality and satisfaction of medical and health services were further improved

The actions to improve medical services were carried out in-depth, with a notice of State Council's commendation. Self-service registration, expert team interview, combined consultation, appointment for referral and many others were adopted in tertiary hospitals and the medical order was obviously improved. Scheduled appointment and treatment was carried out in more than 3,300 medical institutions, with the average rate of appointment and treatment up to 38.6%. High quality nursing service was developed in all tertiary hospitals and over 6,000 secondary hospitals and day-surgery was carried out in more than 2,000 medical institutions, accounting for 11% of elective surgery and obviously benefiting people. Telemedicine service was developed in more than 6,800 medical institutions, covering 1,330 counties. The inter-ministerial mechanism was established for joint prevention and control of bacterial drug resistance to implement the national action plan to curb bacterial resistance, with the results of 37.5% reduction in the utilization rate of antibiotics in nationwide inpatients and 8.7% reduction in the proportion of antibiotics used in outpatient prescriptions. The management and evaluation of rational blood use in clinic was strengthened, with the average blood consumption at the operating table decreasing by 5.7% compared with the same period last year. The nationwide large-scale voluntary consultation activities were continuously organized with over 19.6 million people visiting the clinics. The green channels for donation of human organs were established with the number of donations increasing by more than 50% over the same period last year.

Primary health care services were strengthened. The staffing standard was issued all over the country, deciding staffing according to the service population of 1 per thousand. Totally 3,370 township health centers that were satisfactory to the public were selected and a batch of community health service demonstration institutions was elected. United with the national federation of trade unions, we carried out "National Primary-level Health Post Training and Skills Competition" activities, with 340 thousand primary institutions and 1.5 million medical staff engaged, which further increased primary-level service capability and level.

Working together with 15 departments, we implemented health poverty relief projects. The nationwide household survey of poor households due to illness was completed and, by making clear the true number, treatment schemes for 9 major diseases such as acute lymphocytic leukemia in children were developed. By setting clinical pathways, treatment hospitals, single disease expenses and rates of reimbursement and relief, centralized classification treatment was carried out in Guizhou, Shanxi and other 8 provinces (autonomous regions), with the scope of disease treatment further expanded in some provinces. The "group type" medical assistance was conducted to aid Tibet and Xinjiang, 889 tertiary hospitals assisted 1,149 county hospitals in all poverty-stricken counties and nearly 10,000 doctors at city tertiary hospitals were stationed to offer help at county level hospitals in poor counties. The construction of "Safe Hospitals" was promoted, medical dispute mediation work covered 2,300 county-level hospitals and medical liability insurance and mutual fund for medical risks covered nearly 30,000 medical institutions, so that the long-acting mechanism gradually emerged.

**IV. The overall public health and health emergency response capacity were raised to a new level and major disease prevention and control strategies were constantly improved**

The first plenary session of the inter-ministerial joint conference of the State Council on the prevention and control of major diseases was convened and the special programs to prevent and control major diseases such as AIDS, tuberculosis and chronic diseases were reviewed and approved. The pilot project of graded TB diagnosis and treatment and comprehensive prevention and treatment services was carried out. The pilot program for comprehensive prevention and treatment of echinococcosis in Shiqu County of Sichuan Province was done well and the situation of high incidence of the disease was initially curbed. Poliomyelitis inactivated vaccines and bivalent live attenuated vaccines were incorporated into the national immunization plan and the *Regulations on the Management of Vaccine Circulation and*

*Preventive Vaccination* was revised. The per capita subsidy standard for basic public health services was raised from 40 *yuan* to 45 *yuan* and the service connotation continued to deepen. The measures for the construction and management of the demonstration zone for national comprehensive prevention and control of chronic diseases were issued. The responsibility of guardianship of patients with severe mental disorders was implemented by replacing subsidies with the awards. Together with nine departments, we issued the guideline on strengthening health promotion and education, carried out "Healthy China" activities and did a good job in popularizing health science. The construction of healthy cities and villages and towns was started and the first batch of 38 pilot cities was decided.

Food safety was continuously strengthened. The clean-up and integration of nearly 5,000 food safety standards was completed, and 530 new national food safety standards were issued. The food safety risk monitoring network covered 94% of the counties. Four types of catering service license were integrated and adjusted. A new edition of dietary guidelines for Chinese residents was released to monitor the iodine nutrition of the population in one-third of the counties in the country and to propose a precise iodine supplement strategy.

Solid progress was made in building the core capacity for health emergency response. The imported epidemic situations like Zika virus, yellow fever and other cases were successfully managed, the epidemic situations like human avian influenza and others were effectively controlled, and every effort was made in the post-disaster health and epidemic prevention work during flood prevention and flood fighting. The temporary work subsidies were established for infectious disease prevention and control personnel. China International Emergency Medical Team (Shanghai) was certified by the World Health Organization and became one of the first international emergency medical teams in the world. The medical and health security tasks were successfully completed for the major conferences and activities of our party and country, like G20 summit and others.

### V. The universal two-child policy was smoothly implemented

The *Decision of the CPC Central Committee and the State Council on Implementing Universal Two-child Policy, Reforming and Improving Family Planning Service Management* was carried out. Twenty-nine provinces (autonomous regions and municipalities directly under the Central Government) issued implementation measures and the number of births all year round was in line with policy adjustments. We improved the responsibility system for the object management of family planning, implemented the birth registration service system in an all-round way, and promoted online processing and "Integration of Multiple Certificates into One". We did a good job of family planning special family support care, and raised the assistance standards for rural families with the only child who were wounded, disabled or dead to the same level as that in cities and towns. The "Two Illegal Acts" behaviors were resolutely cracked down on and the sex ratio of the birth population was reduced seven times in a row. The action plan of health promotion for the floating population and left-behind children was implemented and the dynamic monitoring investigation was well conducted. General Secretary Xi Jinping and Premier Li Keqiang issued important instructions at the Eighth Congress of the Chinese Family Planning Association.

In view of the new situation that since the implementation of the universal two-child policy, the cumulative childbearing needs had been centrally released, the number of births had increased significantly, and the proportion of older pregnant women had increased, five ministries and commissions jointly issued *Some Opinions on Strengthening Basic Medical and Health Care Services Throughout Childbirth*, to integrate the resources of maternal and child health services at the prefectural, county and township levels, with an integration rate of 76%. The pregnancy risk assessment of pregnant women was carried out, the green channels were ensured to open for pregnant women and newborns in critical and severe cases, the comprehensive prevention and treatment of birth defects was promoted to ensure the safety of mothers and infants. "Health of Women and Child in China" activities were launched, the demonstration bases of early childhood development were established, the pilot application of maternal and child health manual was carried out in 11 provinces (autonomous regions, municipalities directly under the Central Government), and full course services for eugenics and prenatal care were provided systemically and rationally. Eight colleges and universities re-established undergraduate specialty of pediatrics, improved incentive policy and increased the attraction of pediatrics posts. The hospitals actively deployed their strength to ease the tension of children's medical services.

### VI. Solid steps were made forward in the revitalization and development of traditional Chinese medicine

The State Council issued and implemented the *Outline of the Strategic Planning for the Development of Traditional Chinese Medicine (2016-2030)*, established the system of the joint ministerial meeting on traditional Chinese medicine, and strengthened the organizational leadership and overall coordination. The construction of the national experimental areas of comprehensive reform of traditional Chinese medicine was deepened, the comprehensive reform of public hospitals of traditional Chinese medicine was promoted, and the pilot projects of traditional Chinese medicine participating in the contract service of family doctors were carried out in 270 cities. The standardization project of traditional Chinese medicine was started to promote the development of healthy old-age care and healthy tourism demonstration areas (bases and projects) of traditional Chinese medicine. For the first time, the White Paper "Traditional Chinese Medicine in China" was issued in this field, and the Fifth International Science and Technology Conference on the Modernization of Traditional Chinese Medicine was successfully convened. A recognition conference for famous teachers in teaching of traditional Chinese medicine colleges and universities was held. Ten traditional Chinese medicine centers were built in the countries along the "Belt and Road", and the overseas influence was continuously expanded.

### VII. The development of the health industry entered the fast lane

In conjunction with relevant departments, we issued the second selection catalogue of excellent domestic medical equipment and organized 10 demonstration projects for the use of domestic medical equipment. The project of healthy aging was carried out, and 90 demonstration areas of combining medicine with nursing and 6 demonstration cities of intelligent health care for the aged were selected. A model base for health and medical tourism was established. The construction of the informatization standard system for population health was promoted, and the standardized writing of the first page of the medical record, the coding of disease classifications, the coding of surgical operations, and the "Four Unifications" of medical terminology were initially completed, which laid a foundation for the realization of information interconnection and mutual recognition of examination results. In four cities of two provinces, the construction pilot of the National Health Care Big Data Center and Industrial Park was launched, and the sub-forum of the 3rd World Internet Congress "Internet + Smart Medicine" was successfully held.

### VIII. The supporting role of talent and science and technology was even more prominent

The standardized training for resident doctors recruited 70,000 persons throughout the year, 10,000 of them in general practice and 5,000 in pediatrics. Full coverage of standardized training base at provincial level was realized and dynamic management was strengthened. Focusing on the central and western regions, we started training pilots for rural general practice assistant doctors and enrolled more than 5,600 medical students in targeted medical orders. The nurse training was strengthened and the number of registered nurses was up to 3.56 million, with the rate of doctors to nurses increasing from 1: 0.85 in 2010 to 1: 1.17. Two guiding opinions on comprehensively promoting the development of health and health science and technology innovation and accelerating the transfer and transformation of scientific and technological achievements were issued to promote the establishment and improvement of the mechanism for the benefit distribution and incentives for scientific and technological innovation in health care institutions. The "Science and Technology Innovation Project of Medicine and Health" of the Chinese Medical Academy was launched and implemented. The synergetic mechanism of stem cell clinical research management was established and 32 national clinical medical research centers were brought into the management system of national scientific research base.

**IX. The government's responsibility for running medical services was further implemented**

Under the guidance of "One Outline and Two Plans", 26 special plans for the whole industry were considered and adopted and the *Beijing-Tianjin-Hebei Medical and Health Coordination Development Plan* was implemented. The central government invested 22.2 billion *yuan* in supporting the construction of 3,297 health and family planning projects. The central financial transfer fund reached 261.8 billion *yuan* (excluding capital construction), with an increase of 12.3 percent over the same period last year. Local finance also increased investment in health and family planning. The total health expenditure was expected to reach 4.5805 trillion *yuan* in 2016, with an increase of 10.9% over the same period last year. 136 departmental rules and regulations were comprehensively cleaned up to improve the legitimacy review of normative documents. The supervision and inspection on the implementation of the *Law on Prevention and Control of Occupational Diseases* and the *Law on Population and Family Planning* was carried out, as well as special supervision and inspection on the practice in accordance with the law and the vaccination of medical institutions. In conjunction with the eight departments like the Central Office of Comprehensive Management, a special campaign concentrating on cracking down on the "Scalpers" and "Network Hospital Scalpers" was carried out and achieved results.

**X. The Party building and work style construction were comprehensively strengthened**

The study of the central groups of party committees (party groups) at all levels was strengthened, the spirit of the Sixth Plenary Session of the 18th CPC Central

Committee and General Secretary Xi Jinping's series of important speeches were thoroughly studied and implemented, the study and education of "Two Learnings, One Doing" was carried out in a down-to-earth manner, so that the primary-level organizations and party members were fully covered. We held a system-wide exchange of experience in ideological and political work to consolidate the ideological basis for the common struggle of leaders and workers. The Party's rules and regulations, such as *Some Guidelines on Political Life within the Party in the New Situation* and *CPC Regulations on Internal Supervision*, were comprehensively implemented to conscientiously strengthen the building of party organizations at primary level and seriously enforce political life with the Party. The "Nine Prohibitions" regulations in the medical and health industry were implemented, and the inspections and the "Looking Back" in 27 affiliated hospitals were carried out. The propaganda work was strengthened to organize the major policy interpretation in time, respond to the public opinion's concern in time, and release the progress and effect of the key work in time such as the construction of healthy China, universal two-child policy and deepening the medical reform. Thirteen advanced typical deeds report groups were organized to 19 provinces to hold the report meetings.

At the same time, by serving the national diplomatic strategy, we continued to deepen the international exchanges and cooperation in health and family planning and promoted the integration of health and family planning cooperation into the high-level human exchange mechanism. We actively participated in the multilateral cooperation mechanisms, such as the World Health Organization, UNAIDS and UNFPA, and deepened the regional cooperation mechanisms, such as China, Japan and South Korea, ASEAN, etc. The 1st China-ASEAN Health Cooperation Forum and the 2nd China-Central and Eastern European Health Ministers Forum were successfully held. A seminar on the accessibility of medical products of China and Africa was held, the free cataract surgery projects were implemented, and the first "Maternal and Child Health Project" was launched in Cambodia to show the image of China as a responsible country.

(Chen Ying)

# Part II
# Literature

## Chapter I   Important Documents

**1. Speech of Xi Jinping, General Secretary of the Communist Party of China (CPC) Central Committee, President of the People´s Republic of China (PRC) and Chairman of the PRC Central Military Commission (CMC), Delivered at the 2016 National Health Conference (Excerpt)**

(August 19th, 2016, Beijing)

Health is a must for the overall development of human beings. It is the foundation for the economic and social development and an important token for the national wealth and prosperity, representing the common wishes of people of all ethnic groups in the country. Ever since the founding of the Communist Party of China, the Party has always linked the health of people closely with the national independence and people's liberation. Since the reform and opening-up, the development of health undertaking has been accelerated, the healthcare system has been continuously optimized, the fair accessibility to primary medical and health service has been steadily enhanced, and the overall ability for public health and disease control and prevention has been greatly improved. With the long-tern efforts, we have not only bettered the health of the people, but also explored a health development road that suits China's conditions.

Over a long period of time, the health workers in our country have carried forward the spirits of "cherishing every life, saving the wounded and the dying, being willing to sacrifice and showing boundless love" and served the people whole-heartedly. Especially when facing the threats of major infectious diseases and major natural disasters, all the health workers have been very brave, proceed without hesitation, charged forward without fear, sacrificed themselves to save the patients and won the acclaim of the society. General Secretary Xi Jinping, on behalf of the CPC Central Committee, has expressed the highest respect and heartfelt gratitude to all the officials and health professionals who have worked dedicatedly for a long time in the health care system.

At present, with the industrialization, urbanization and aging population, the disease spectrum, ecological environment and life style are changing constantly, and China is still being threatened by many diseases and affected by multiple health impacting factors. We are faced not only with the health problems existing in the developed countries but also with the health problems existing in the developing countries. If these problems cannot be effectively solved, they will definitely have profound impact on the people's health, hinder the economic development and affect the harmony and stability of the society.

During the construction of a healthy China, we should stick to the health development road with Chinese characteristics and handle well some major issues. We should uphold the correct working policy for health and wellness, lay emphasis on work at the community level, take reform and innovation as the drive, put prevention first, pay equal attention to traditional Chinese medicine and Western medicine, incorporate health into all the policies and make people contribute to and share the benefit. We should uphold the non-profit nature of basic medical care and health services, continue to optimize the institutional arrangements, expand the range of services and improve the quality to ensure that the people can enjoy fair, accessible, comprehensive and continuous health care services in prevention, treatment, rehabilitation, health promotion and so on. The quality and capacity of health care service should be continuously elevated so the people can have equal access. The relation between the government and the market should be correctly handled. In the area of basic medical care and health services, the government must exercise its role and in the area of non-basic medical care and health services, the vitality of market must be shown.

We will stick to the principle of "prevention first", combine prevention with treatment, conduct joint control & prevention and co-governance, mobilize the people to participate in the prevention and control, and strive to provide the cradle-to-grave medical care and health services for the people. We will pay attention to the prevention and control of major diseases, improve the strategy for prevention and control and minimize the incidence of crowd diseases. Emphasis will be laid on promoting health of children and the health management in kindergartens, primary schools and middle schools will be comprehensively enhanced. The dissemination of the health knowledge will be intensified to increase the students' awareness of voluntary prevention of diseases. The target project of providing nutritional meals and packs for students' in the poor areas will be carried out to guarantee their growth and development. We will focus on the healthcare services for priority groups, ensure the health of women and children, provide continuous health management and medical services for the elderly, strive to realize the goal that all the disabled can enjoy the rehabilitative service, attach importance to health of migrant population and further advance the medical programs for poverty reduction. We will advocate the healthy lifestyles, uphold the concepts of holistic health and comprehensive wellbeing, turn our focus from treatment of diseases to maintenance of the people's health, establish and improve the health education system, elevate the health literacy of the people and promote the deep fusion of public fitness with public health. The basic studies of psychological problems will be intensified, the dissemination of knowledge and science on psychological health and diseases should be done well, and the psychological health services like psychological therapy and counseling will be standardized.

A good ecological environment is the foundation for the survival and health of the mankind. We will stick to the concept of green development, implement the strictest ecological and environmental protection institutions, establish and improve the systems for surveillance, survey and risk assessment over environmental and health issues, do well the prevention and management of air, land and water pollution, accelerate the land greening, and actually solve the prominent environmental problems that affect people's health. We will inherit and carry forward the good tradition of patriotic health campaign, continue to enhance the urban and rural environment and sanitation, strengthen the management over the rural residential environment, and construct a healthy, livable and beautiful home. We will implement the food safety law, improve the food safety system, enhance the supervision over food safety, and closely controlled every procedure from farm to table. The concept of safe development will be upheld, the public safety system shall be optimized, and the threats to the life and health of people caused by public safety issues will be minimized. At present, the reform of the healthcare system has entered into the "deep water" and we need to conquer the difficult barriers. We will quicken our pace to accomplish the tasks determined by the Third Plenary Session of the 18th CPC Central Committee. We will put emphasis on advancing the construction of the basic healthcare systems and make breakthroughs in the following five basic medical systems, i.e. the hierarchical diagnosis and treatment system, universal health insurance system, medicine supply and security system and comprehensive supervisory system. We will promote the development and prosperity of traditional Chinese medicine, stick to the principle of attaching equal emphasis on traditional Chinese medicine and Western medicine, boost the complementary development of both traditional Chinese medicine (TCM) and Western medicine and make efforts to innovate and develop TCM-based health care. The health workers will be fully mobilized, starting from the issues like salary, benefit, development space, practicing environment and social status. In addition, the physical and psychological health of the medical workers will be cared, efforts will be made to make the medical workers feel pride of their profession and a social atmosphere of respecting doctors will be created. All the health and medical workers in China will carry forward and stick to the core socialist values, strengthen construction of medical ethics and professional self-discipline, and provide the best medical and health service for the people. The criminal offences involving doctors, especially the violent cases that hurt the medical workers will be strictly cracked down on to protect the personal safety of professional workers.

Promoting the construction of a healthy China is a solemn commitment of the Party to the people. All Party committees and government departments will prioritize this livelihood project on the agenda, shoulder the responsibility and make great efforts to push forward the implementation. The reform of the healthcare system will be incorporated into the course of comprehensively deepening the reform and be deployed, required and assessed at the same time. The localities will be supported to act on the local conditions and make differentiated exploration. Evaluation system for conducting health impact assessment will be established to systemically assess the health impact of economic and social development plans and policies, as well as major projects. Population health information service will be optimized and use of big data in health will be promoted.

Over a long period of time, China has made major breakthroughs in fulfilling the international commitments and engaging in the global health governance, showed the image as a humanistic and responsible country, and won the acclaim of the international society. We will actively participate in the studies and negotiations over the international health standards and norms, improve the emergent foreign assistance mechanism for response to the major international public health events, and enhance the health cooperation with countries along the Belt and Road.

(Qu Yang)

## 2. Xi Jinping, General Secretary of the CPC Central Committee, President of the People's Republic of China (PRC) and Chairman of the PRC Central Military Commission (CMC), Delivered Instructions for the Eighth National Congress of the Family Planning Association of China and the Distinguished Commendation Conference (Excerpt)

(May 18<sup>th</sup>, 2016)

Population issue is always a global, long-term and strategic issue that our country faces. For a long time to come, the basic situation of China's large population will not change fundamentally, the population pressure on economic and social development will not change fundamentally, the tension between population and resource environment will not change fundamentally and the basic national policy of family planning must be adhered to for a long time.

Over the years, the China Family Planning Association has carried out fruitful work and made positive contributions to the cause of family planning in China. I hope that the Chinese Family Planning Association earnestly fulfill its responsibilities, guide the public to correctly understand the great significance of the adjustment and perfection of China's fertility policy at present, and conscientiously do a good job in publicity and education, reproductive health counseling services, guidance for eugenics and good childbearing, family assistance for family planning, rights and interests protection and services for the mobile population. I hope that the committees and governments at all levels will play the organizing role of the Family Planning Association, push forward the implementation of the basic national policy of family planning, promote long-term balanced development of population and family harmony and happiness, and make new and greater contributions to achieving the goal of building a well-off society in an all-round way and realizing the Chinese dream of national rejuvenation.

**(Chen Ying)**

### 3. Congratulatory Letter of Xi Jinping, General Secretary of the CPC Central Committee, President of the People's Republic of China (PRC) and Chairman of the PRC Central Military Commission (CMC), to the Nineteenth International Leprosy Conference

(September 17th, 2016)

On the occasion of the opening of the 19th International Leprosy Conference, on behalf of the Chinese government and people, and in my own name, I would like to express my sincere congratulations on the convening of the Conference, to extend a warm welcome to experts, scholars and guests who are attending the Conference and to pay high tribute to all the people of the international and domestic leprosy circles who have made contributions to human health.

"Creating a World without Leprosy" is the ultimate goal of global leprosy control. The theme of the Conference is "Unfinished Business—Stopping Transmission, Preventing Disability and Promoting Integration", which is of positive significance to the early realization of this goal. The world leprosy control has made great achievements, but there is still a long way to go and we still need the international community to work together to tackle the difficulties and problems. China will increase the investment and safeguard measures, continue to work together with other countries to promote the progress and innovation of leprology, promote the early realization of the goal of eradicating leprosy in China and contribute to the global efforts to eradicate leprosy.

I wish the conference a complete success!

(Chen Ying)

## 4. Congratulatory Letter of Xi Jinping, General Secretary of the CPC Central Committee, President of the People's Republic of China (PRC) and Chairman of the PRC Central Military Commission (CMC), to the 60th anniversary of the Founding of the Chinese Academy of Medical Sciences

(October 27th, 2016)

On the occasion of the 60th anniversary of the founding of the Chinese Academy of Medical Sciences, on behalf of the Central Committee of the Communist Party of China, I would like to extend my warm congratulations and sincere greetings to the vast numbers of scientific and technological workers and staff in China's medical and health system.

Over the past 60 years, the Chinese Academy of Medical Sciences, as the national team and leading soldier in the field of medical and health care, has been pioneering and enterprising in its efforts to overcome difficulties. It has made rich achievements in the prevention and treatment of major diseases, the development and innovation of medical science and technology, the cultivation of high-level medical personnel, the transformation of medical scientific and technological achievements, and the study of medical and health strategies and made important contributions to the development of medical and health services and the improvement of people's health. I hope that you will take the 60th anniversary of the Chinese Academy of Medical Sciences as a new starting point, seize the opportunity to meet the difficulties, and strive to build the Chinese Academy of Medical Sciences into the core base of China's medical science and technology innovation system, and continue to write a new chapter.

(Chen Ying)

**5. Report on the Work of the Government (Excerpt)**

**Delivered at the Fourth Session of the Twelfth National People's Congress by Li Keqiang, Member of the Standing Committee of the Political Bureau of CPC Central Committee and Premier of the State Council**

(March 5$^{th}$, 2016)

### I. Review of the work we did in 2015

Comprehensive reform was carried out in all public hospitals at the county level, the coverage of the serious disease insurance scheme was extended to more rural and non-working urban residents, a system of assistance for treating major and serious diseases was put in place, and a system for providing living allowances for people with disabilities who are in need and for granting nursing care subsidies to persons with severe disabilities was established.

Efforts were stepped up to ensure workplace safety; as a result, we have seen a continued reduction in the number of total accidents, including the number of accidents of a serious or large-scale nature as well as those in industries where accidents tend to be more common. We moved ahead with the demonstration initiative to ensure food safety.

There are many problems in medical care, education, elderly care, food and medicine safety, income distribution, and urban management that are of concern to the people. The situation remains grave when it comes to environmental pollution, and some regions are frequently hit by severe smog. Particularly distressing, last year saw the sinking of the cruise ship Oriental Star on the Yangtze and the massive explosion in Tianjin Port. The deaths and injuries and the damage and loss of property from these incidents were devastating, and the profound lessons these incidents have taught us should never be forgotten.

Basic health insurance was expanded to achieve complete coverage, and participation in basic pension plans exceeded 80% of the whole population.

### II. The main targets, tasks, and measures for the period of the 13th Five-Year Plan from 2016 through 2020

We should make progress in new urbanization and agricultural modernization as well as in balancing development between urban and rural areas and between regions. Narrowing the gap between urban and rural areas and between regions is not only a key part of economic structural adjustment; it is also crucial for unleashing developmental potential. We should advance the new, people-centered urbanization. This will mean granting urban residency to around 100 million people with rural household registration living in urban areas and other permanent urban residents, completing the rebuilding of both rundown areas and "villages" in cities involving about 100 million people, and enabling around 100 million rural residents to live in local towns and cities in the central and western regions. By 2020, permanent urban residents should account for 60% of China's population, and 45% of the Chinese people should be registered as permanent urban residents.

We need to work for progress in building a Healthy China and achieve a one-year increase in average life expectancy.

### III. The major areas of work for 2016

We will advance new urbanization. Urbanization is the path we need to take to develop a modern China. It is where we will find the greatest potential for domestic demand and the most powerful force for sustaining economic development. This year, we will take the following three major steps regarding urbanization. First, we will move faster to see that urban residency is granted to more people with rural household registration living in urban areas. We will deepen reform of the household registration system and relax restrictions on eligibility for urban residency. We will introduce policies for making both the transfer payments and the land designated for urban development granted to the government of a local jurisdiction conditional upon the number of people with rural household registration who are granted permanent urban residency in that jurisdiction. The full range of trials for developing new urbanization will be extended to more areas. Residence cards are important assets for their holders. We must move faster to ensure that permanent urban residents without urban residency are issued residence cards, thus enabling them to enjoy, as provided for by law, the right to access compulsory education, employment, medical care, and other basic public services. We will promote the development of small towns and small and medium-sized cities in the central and western regions to help more rural migrant workers find employment or start businesses in urban areas closer to home so that they do not have to choose between earning money and taking care of the families they leave behind.

We will advance the coordinated reform of medical services, medical insurance, and the medicine industry. Health is at the root of happiness. This year, we aim to realize full coverage of the serious disease insurance scheme, and government funding for the scheme will be increased to reduce the financial burdens of more people suffering from serious diseases. The central government will allocate 16 billion *yuan* to be used in both rural and urban areas for medical assistance and subsidies, an increase of 9.6% over last year. We will merge the basic medical insurance systems for rural and non-working urban residents and raise government subsidies for the scheme from 380 to 420 *yuan* per capita per annum. We will reform the ways for making medical insurance payouts and expedite the building of a nationwide network for basic medical insurance so that medical expenses can be settled where they are incurred via basic medical insurance accounts. We will see that more cities participate in piloting comprehensive public hospital reform; move forward in a coordinated way with medical service pricing reform and reform in medicine distribution; and deepen the reform of the evaluation and approval systems for medicines and medical equipment. We will move faster to train general practitioners and pediatricians. We will carry out trials for tiered medical services in around 70% of prefecture-level cities, increase basic annual per capita government subsidies for public health services from 40 to 45 *yuan*, and see that more medical resources are channeled toward the community level in urban areas and toward rural areas. We will encourage the development of privately run hospitals. We will promote the development of traditional Chinese medicine and the medical traditions of ethnic minorities. We will establish HR and remuneration systems suited to the medical sector to motivate medical practitioners and protect their enthusiasm. We will work to ensure harmony in the relationship between doctor and patient. We will improve the supporting policies to complement the decision to allow all couples to have two children. To see that the health of our people is protected, we will speed up the development of unified and authoritative safety monitoring systems for food and pharmaceuticals and reinforce every line of defense from the farm to the dining table, and from the enterprise to the hospital. This should ensure that people have access to safe food and medicine and can have confidence in what they are eating and taking.

### 6. Speech by Li Keqiang, Member of the Standing Committee of the Political Bureau of CPC Central Committee and Premier of the State Council, Delivered at Opening Ceremony of 9th Global Conference on Health Promotion

(Shanghai, 21$^{st}$ November, 2016)

Health is a cornerstone for the comprehensive development and well-being of the people and a hallmark of national prosperity and social progress. On the occasion of the 9th Global Conference on Health Promotion, I wish to extend, on behalf of the Chinese government, warm congratulations on the opening of the conference and sincere welcome to all the distinguished guests.

This conference coincides with the 30th anniversary of the first International

Conference on Health Promotion. Three decades ago, the Ottawa Charter introduced the concept of "Health Promotion", which has since guided the development of the health cause worldwide. Three decades on, thanks to the joint efforts of countries around the world and the hard work of the World Health Organization (WHO), the world average life expectancy has increased by over eight years. Maternal and infant mortality rate and that of children under five have been lowered by 50% on average, which is a big milestone in the history of human health.

At the same time, we should be aware that we are still confronted with daunting global health challenges. While traditional diseases, health issues and inequality in health remain acute, faster aging of the population, greater trans-border flows of people, the evolving spectrum of disease and changing environment and lifestyles are creating new problems. The threat of multiple diseases and our vulnerability to health risks have both increased. The sluggish world economic recovery and divergent trends of economic growth have added to the difficulty of ensuring the effective supply and the balanced and reasonable allocation of health resources. Promoting health remains an arduous task and nothing short of concerted international efforts is required for truly delivering the goal of "health for all".

This year marks the start of the implementation of the 2030 Agenda for Sustainable Development. The theme of this conference, "health promotion in the sustainable development goals", highlights the important role of health promotion in global sustainable development endeavor. Discussions around this theme will go a long way to promoting consensus building and synergy for the full implementation of the Sustainable Development Goals (SDGs). In this connection, I would like to put forward the following suggestions.

We should enhance policy dialogue and build a platform for health governance cooperation. Health promotion is the common endeavor of mankind. We should build a community of shared future and take concrete actions to advance cooperation. We need to build a multilevel and wide-ranging institutional platform for dialogue and cooperation and support the WHO's efforts to lead, coordinate and implement global health programs. Efforts should also be made to improve health legislation in our respective countries and tighten regulation on health-impairing investment and trading activities through fiscal, taxation and financial policy tools.

At the same time, we need to uphold the principle of common but differentiated responsibilities and increase the representation and voice of developing countries. Developed countries should shoulder more responsibility and support developing countries. We should work together to make global health governance fairer and more reasonable.

We should put in place an inclusive and interconnected system for prevention and control of global public health hazards. No country can stay immune to major public health challenges. Countries need to better coordinate health emergency practices, improve global mechanisms for disease surveillance, early-warning and emergency response, strengthen notification, information sharing and personnel training, and further improve global capacity to address public health emergencies. The Chinese government supports the WHO in putting together its global health emergency task force and contingency fund. We urge developed countries to step up support to developing countries in improving their public health systems, and together build up stronger lines of defense for global health.

We should enhance the capacity for health supply and services through cooperation on innovation. Scientific and technological innovation is the golden key to health. Countries need to enhance research and development of health technologies, actively conduct bilateral and multilateral cooperation, including joint research on frontier and innovative technologies, and tackle common health hazards facing mankind together. We need to expand the network for exchange and cooperation in such areas as the prevention and control of antimicrobial resistance (AMR), advanced health technologies, drug research and development, energy-saving, emissions reduction and the treatment of pollution, and build platforms for entrepreneurship and innovation. There should be wider application and sharing of scientific and technological progress to bring greater benefits to more people.

We should encourage mutual learning and promote greater integration between traditional and modern medical sciences. Throughout history, different countries and nations have developed their own views of health and acquired distinct strengths in the form of traditional medicine. Differences in medical practices should be embraced with equality and open-mindedness, and cultural exchanges be encouraged as a useful way to promote health cooperation. We should encourage mutual learning on the views and culture of health. We need to better promote traditional medicine, make better use of their strengths in preventing and treating diseases, and actively develop services trade in traditional medicine. By leveraging the complementarity between traditional and modern medical sciences, we will make new contribution to human health.

China has been a strong advocate and firm practitioner of health promotion. Since the founding of the People's Republic of China, in particular since reform and opening-up, China has vigorously expanded health care services despite a relatively underdeveloped economy. We have significantly improved the health of our people, and found a path of health development consistent with China's national conditions. In 2009, China started a new round of health care reform. We identified a core objective, which is to offer basic health care services to all people as a public good, and outlined the principle of ensuring basic levels of health care, strengthening community health services and building up health care networks.

Important progress has been made in this direction. We put in place a system of basic medical insurance that covers the entire population of over 1.3 billion people, offering institutional guarantee for universal access. We improved basic rural health service network at county, township and village levels and the system of urban community health services, making such services more convenient and accessible for our people. We took vigorous measures to promote equal access to public health services and offered basic public health services for all urban and rural residents for free. Our spending on public health services has been growing year by year and will continue to grow. We worked out a Chinese solution to advance health care reform, which is a world-wide challenge.

China's average life expectancy now stands at 76.3 years. Maternal mortality rate was reduced to 20.1 per 100,000 and infant mortality rate 8.1 per 1,000, generally better than the average level in middle and high income countries. For the largest developing country with over 1.3 billion people, such accomplishments are no mean feat.

China is at a decisive stage for building a moderately prosperous society in all respects. At the recently held National Health Conference, the first in the new century, President Xi Jinping outlined in an important speech the overall guidelines, targets and tasks for building a healthy China from a strategic and overarching perspective and proposed principles for health-related work. We will focus on work at the community level, pursue reform and innovation as a driving force and disease prevention as the priority, give importance to both traditional Chinese medicine and western medicine, incorporate health into all policy-making, and strive for participation by all and benefits to all. We promulgated the *Outline of Healthy China 2030 Plan* with the aim to provide all-dimensional, whole-of-the-life-cycle health services for all by 2030, increase average life expectancy to 79 years, and reach high-income countries' level in main health indicators. With this in mind, we will make relentless efforts in the following areas:

We will take health as a strategic priority to advance health in tandem with economic and social progress. We will prioritize health in development planning, highlight health targets in economic and social programs, give more weight to health in drafting and implementing public policies, and meet health demand in fiscal spending, with a view to providing basic health services for all.

We will build a whole-process health promotion system to protect people's health throughout the life cycle. There are many factors affecting people's health from the beginning to the end of life. We need to provide whole-of-the-life-cycle health services for the people. Effective measures will be taken for prevention, health care and greater intervention to make people healthier and less vulnerable. We will enhance health education, spread health knowledge and skills, deepen fitness campaigns for all, raise people's health awareness and sense of responsibility, and foster a new health system in which all people will participate, contribute and benefit. We will strengthen prevention and control of major diseases, improve prevention and treatment practices, enforce cross-agency holistic measures at all levels, and reduce damage on people's health from major diseases. We will intensify pollution treatment and foster a sound environment for people's health.

We will work hard to improve community-level health care and strengthen weak links to increase fairness and accessibility of health services. The biggest weakness in China's health system lies at the community level, in rural and poor areas in particular. We will coordinate urban and rural development and pursue a new type of urbanization, make more resources available for community-level health programs. Communities must be equipped with greater capacity of disease prevention and control through cultivating general physicians and providing long-distance medical treatment and paired-up assistance. The advantages of traditional Chinese medicine must be harnessed to widen the availability of medical care and health services. We will implement health-related poverty-alleviation programs, intensify support for poor areas in insurance for major diseases and medical assistance, prevent disease-induced poverty, and narrow the gap in basic health services between urban and rural areas and among different regions and groups of people.

We will continue to deepen health care reform and set up basic health care systems that cover urban and rural areas. Our reform in this area is now in a deep-water zone, which calls for greater courage and wisdom. We will further deepen public hospital reform, quicken the development of tiered medical services, cut red tapes and enhance coordination among medical and health care institutions at various levels and of different categories. This way, we hope to provide high-quality medical services to our people, and help community-level medical institutions improve their performance. Progress has been made in encouraging big, medium-sized and small hospitals and township hospitals to establish the Health Care Alliance (HCA), which would make medical services more accessible and affordable for the people.

We will build up a nationwide basic medical insurance system, reform the way of making medical insurance payouts, merge the basic medical insurance systems for rural and non-working urban residents, and establish a nationwide information network for medical insurances to improve quality and efficiency. We will also reform the supply system of pharmaceuticals to deliver safe and effective medicine to our people. We will advance coordinated reform of medical services, medical insurance and the medicine industry, motivate medical practitioners, including by making their jobs even more dignified, and enhance the vitality and sustainability of medical and health care systems.

We will vigorously develop the health sector to better meet people's increasingly diverse health needs. With higher standards of living and greater awareness about health, our people expect more multi-tiered, diversified and individualized products and services. To respond to their demands, governments and markets both have a role to play. The government needs to ensure basic supply, especially for the most vulnerable groups, while the market can be more active in providing non-basic and more diversified health services. We will encourage increased supply of health products and services from non-governmental sources, and the setting-up of privately run hospitals, thus making it easier for people to get more affordable medical treatment. We will support innovation in medical science and boost integrated development between the health sector and old-age care, tourism, the Internet, fitness and recreation and food industries. We will also promote mass innovation and entrepreneurship in the health sector and practice the "Internet + Health" action plan, so that new industries, new businesses and new models will thrive in this sector.

China has been actively calling for and contributing to global health cooperation, and has fulfilled its due international responsibilities and obligations. During the past half a century, China has sent over 20,000 medical staff to 67 countries and regions, treating patients for over 260 million times. China has contributed its share to the fight against the Ebola epidemic that broke out in West Africa in 2014. China moved promptly to dispatch over 1,200 medical staff and public health experts, who fought against the disease side by side with the people in the affected countries. China highly appreciates the prominent role that the WHO has played over the years in curbing communicable diseases and coordinating global health affairs. Under the framework of the UN and the WHO, China will continue to actively participate in global health promotion efforts and do its best to provide assistance to other developing countries.

Health is an eternal pursuit of mankind, and health promotion is the shared responsibility of the international community. Let us work together to make our world a better and healthier place!

**7. Speech by Liu Yandong, Member of the Political Bureau of the CPC Central Committee and Vice Premier of the State Council at the 60th Anniversary Symposium on the Reform and Development of the Higher Education of Traditional Chinese Medicine (Excerpt)**

(December 29th, 2016, Beijing)

### I. Enormous achievements gained in the development of the higher education of traditional Chinese medicine

Since the 18th National Congress of the Communist Party of China (CPC), the CPC Central Committee with Comrade Xi Jinping as the core has attached more importance to the work of traditional Chinese medicine and General Secretary Xi Jinping has made several important instructions. Last year, General Secretary sent a congratulatory message for the 60th anniversary of the China Academy of Chinese Medical Sciences, in which he extended his sincere wishes to TCM workers, hoping that they would enhance national self-confidence, strive to scale new heights in medicine, mine deeply the essences in the treasure of traditional Chinese medicine, fully play its unique advantages, promote modernization of traditional Chinese medicine, and make traditional Chinese medicine acceptable and popular throughout the world. At this year's National Health Conference, General Secretary Xi Jingping emphasized again that we should protect, inherit and develop traditional Chinese medicine since it is a valued treasure passed down from our ancestors, and endeavor to realize the creative transformation and innovative development of TCM-based health maintenance culture so that traditional Chinese medicine would be integrated with modern outlook on health and serve the people. Premier Li Keqiang has also paid high attention to the work of traditional Chinese medicine and emphasized that we should pay equal attention to the development of traditional Chinese medicine and Western medicine, fully play the role of the characteristics and advantages of traditional Chinese medicine, and make greater contributions in deepening the reform of the medical care and health system and promoting our country's economic and social development. General Secretary Xi Jinping and Premier Li Keqiang point out the direction for TCM work and the higher education.

With unremitting efforts of generation after generation of TCM workers for about 60 years, leapfrog development has been achieved in our country's TCM higher education.

(1) TCM higher education system has improved. The scale of TCM higher education system has been expanding and  a multidimensional education network

covering multiple disciplines at different levels has been formed, including traditional Chinese medicine, traditional Chinese pharmacology, integrated Chinese and Western medicine and ethnic minority medicine at secondary and higher vocational schools, colleges, postgraduate and doctoral studies. Currently, there are throughout the country 42 institutions of higher learning in traditional Chinese medicine, 238 Western medicine institutions of higher learning or nonmedical higher learning institutions offering programs in traditional Chinese medicine, and 46 and 17 higher learning institutions offering TCM master and doctor programs respectively, enrolling in total as many as 752,000 students. TCM basic, classic and clinical courses have been strengthened and structure of academic disciplines has been perfecting. Disciplines have also kept increasing from only traditional Chinese medicine and traditional Chinese pharmacology at the beginning of the founding of institutions of higher learning to acupuncture and moxibustion, integrated Chinese and Western medicine and many others now. A batch of disciplines in ethnic minority medicine has also been established to promote the protection and development of the education of ethnic minority medicine.

(2) The mode of TCM higher education has been innovated. With a focus on the basic ideology of sticking to the characteristics of traditional Chinese medicine and bringing its advantages into play, an overall higher education system has been established, with master-apprenticeship training running through, which attaches importance to humanities, TCM classic treasures, clinical teaching and practical ability, and efforts have also been made to energetically explore the ways of integrating master-apprenticeship training with the education of higher learning institutions. So far 1,016 studios have been set up for carrying forward country-level prominent TCM masters' expertise; 64 studios have been established for promoting various schools of traditional Chinese medicine, and a new pattern of the higher education in traditional Chinese medicine has initially taken shape, with institutions of higher learning as the main body and master-apprenticeship as the characteristic.

(3) A great number of TCM professionals have been cultivated. Over the past 60 years, nearly 2 million TCM professionals have been cultivated by the institutions of higher learning in traditional Chinese medicine and distributed to all areas of traditional Chinese medicine, such as TCM clinical practice, healthcare, research and development, education, industry, culture, and international exchange and cooperation, among whom a batch of academicians, country-level prominent TCM masters and teaching experts have come to the fore, which provides a forceful guarantee for the construction of our country's characteristic health and healthcare service systems.

(4) The internationalization of traditional Chinese medicine has been boosted.

The institutions of higher learning in traditional Chinese medicine have been active in promoting traditional Chinese medicine acceptable and popular in the world and in the strategy of the Belt and Road Initiative. They have established TCM Confucius Institutes, TCM centers and other exchange and cooperation agencies overseas; currently traditional Chinese medicine has spread to 183 countries and regions around the world and some 30 countries and regions have opened a couple of hundred schools of traditional Chinese medicine to train native TCM workers. Every year, in addition to those overseas students who come to China to learn Chinese, more and more come to China to learn traditional Chinese medicine. After their graduation, they will become important ambassadors to promote traditional Chinese medicine to develop throughout the world.

## II. New situations that the reform and development of higher education of tradition Chinese medicine are faced with (Omitted)

## III. New prospects that shall be opened up for the reform and development of the higher education of traditional Chinese medicine

(1) With people's health as the orientation, new momentum shall be provided for deepening the reform of the medical care and health system. Traditional Chinese medicine is a treasure of our country's ancient science and has deep richness in humanities and philosophy. Applying such principles as "man should observe the law of the nature and seek for the unity of the heaven and humanity", "Yin and Yang should be balanced to obtain the golden mean", traditional Chinese medicine displays distinctive characteristics and advantages in the treatment of common diseases, frequently occurring diseases, and difficult and complicated diseases, which is very popular with people and plays an indispensable role in deepening the reform of the medical care and health system and improving the effectiveness of medical and health care. Reform of TCM higher education shall be closely integrated with the goals of the medical and health services so as to improve TCM service capacity, better work for people's wellbeing, more energetically deepen the reform of the medical care and health system, and promote the establishment of the basic medical care system with Chinese characteristics. The first is to develop the concept of "all-round health" and optimize the structure and layout of professional training. In the new era, working focus shall be at the community-level TCM services; reform and innovation shall be taken as the momentum and efforts shall be made to lay great emphasis on prevention, attach equal importance to traditional Chinese medicine and Western medicine, incorporate health into every policy, stick to the policy of everyone's

contribution and sharing of health, promote the transformation of professional training from "medical-care-centered" to "health-centered", scientifically adjust and control the disciplinary structure and the scale of enrollment of TCM colleges and universities, and improve the systems for balancing supply and demand of TCM professionals. More support shall be offered to the development of the TCM colleges and universities in the central and western regions to narrow the gap between regions, institutions and disciplines. The second is to establish the tiered medical care delivery system and strengthen the construction of the taskforce of TCM general practitioners. College graduates majoring in traditional Chinese medicine shall be encouraged to attend standardized training for the general practitioners of traditional Chinese medicine and the taskforce of TCM general practitioners shall be expanded by various ways such as the standardized training for the general practitioners of traditional Chinese medicine, the training for assistant general practitioners, the job-transfer training, and the free targeted cultivation. The role of the general practitioners of traditional Chinese medicine shall be brought into full play in family doctors' contract-based services and the general practitioners of traditional Chinese medicine shall be encouraged to lead the teams of family doctors. The third is to strengthen the training for the professionals of traditional Chinese medicine at the community level. Traditional Chinese medicine serves people and roots deep among the public and the philosophies it contains are easy to understand. The prominent veteran TCM masters and the TCM experts at the community level shall be encouraged to cultivate a batch of outstanding community-level TCM professionals by master-apprenticeship training and endeavors shall be made to set up studios for passing on the expertise of prominent TCM experts at the community level in every county by the end of the "13th Five-Year Plan" period in a bid to dramatically improve the service capacity of traditional Chinese medicine at the community level. Evaluation and incentive systems for the talents of traditional Chinese medicine and evaluation measures for their professional titles shall be optimized to fully arouse TCM workers' enthusiasm and initiatives for serving the people.

(2) The quality of cultivating the professionals of traditional Chinese medicine shall be improved to cultivate modern TCM talents with noble medical ethics and proficient medical skills. Collaboration of medical and teaching institutions is the key to improving cultivation quality. Joint efforts shall be made to eliminate barriers among higher education institutions, disciplines and hospitals, incorporate academic innovation into education, and actively satisfy demands of the development of TCM industry and the development of TCM health services. Structure and layout of the higher education of traditional Chinese medicine shall be optimized and construction of a high-quality, collaborative and effective TCM higher education system shall be

accelerated that suits the growing laws of the professionals of traditional Chinese medicine and satisfies the development demands. The first is to deepen the reform in the curriculum setting of higher education institutions, observe the laws of acquisition of the knowledge on traditional Chinese medicine and the growing laws of TCM professionals, and energetically promote the education reform that highlights inheritance, innovation and characteristics of traditional Chinese medicine. Textbooks on traditional Chinese medicine shall be perfected and a batch of model textbooks conforming to the laws of TCM education and meeting the demands of the reform and development shall be published. Efforts shall be made to improve TCM-related courses, strengthen the link between basic courses and clinical courses so as to make students majoring in traditional Chinese medicine effectively apply theories of traditional Chinese medicine to clinical practices, and give priority to the teaching of Chinese traditional culture and classic connotation of traditional Chinese medicine, and the development of the ways of thinking in accordance with the laws of traditional Chinese medicine and the science. Exploration shall be conducted in extending the length of schooling; the number of colleges and universities that are entitled to offer integrated 5+3 programs (5-year study for bachelor degree and 3-year study for master degree) shall further increase and the linkup between formal schooling and standardized training for the residents of traditional Chinese medicine shall be enhanced. The second is to perfect the master-apprenticeship training system, and in accordance with the laws of traditional Chinese medicine, promote an organic linkup of college, post-graduate and continuing education. Laws of master-apprenticeship training shall be summed up; standards, policies and measures relevant to master-apprenticeship training shall be formulated and master-apprenticeship training shall run through the whole process of cultivating the professionals of traditional Chinese medicine. TCM colleges and universities able to offer master-apprenticeship training shall be encouraged to launch such training in every TCM-related majors; an organic linkup between postgraduate education and master-apprenticeship training shall be pushed forward and master-apprenticeship training shall be incorporated into the standardized training for physicians  of traditional Chinese medicine as a vital part. The conservation and dissemination of the academic ideas and practical experience of prominent veteran TCM masters and various schools of traditional Chinese medicine and the training of outstanding clinical talents shall be continued and the linkup between TCM master-apprenticeship training and academic degrees shall be strengthened. The third is to improve the teaching capacity of TCM colleges and universities for clinical practice. Relationship between colleges and universities of traditional Chinese medicine and their affiliated hospitals and teaching hospitals shall well develop; a number of national bases for TCM teaching, clinical practice, standardized training and continuing education shall be constructed and the leading role of affiliated hospitals in clinical teaching and standardized training shall be fully played. The fourth is to strengthen the construction of teaching faculty in the colleges and universities of traditional Chinese medicine. Cultivation of the masters in master-apprenticeship training, the academic leaders and the young and the middle-aged outstanding teachers shall be enhanced to bring forth a batch of prominent teaching masters and leading scientific researchers. All the colleges and universities of traditional Chinese medicine shall build teaching teams, with prominent veteran TCM experts and teaching masters as the core, to promote the cultivation of the faculty for teaching TCM classic theories and clinical courses, and encourage prominent veteran TCM experts to teach in classroom, young and middle-aged teachers to do clinical work, and clinical practitioners to teach the classics of traditional Chinese medicine. The fifth is to intensify education on medical humanities. "To be a moral person before learning how to be a medical practitioner" is a policy that shall be adhered to. Traditional Chinese medicine represents profound humanities and philosophical ideas of the Chinese nation and highlights "practice of medicine should aim to help people". Colleges and universities of traditional Chinese medicine shall implement such ideology in cultivating that "moral education comes first; importance shall be attached to professional proficiency; instructions on integrating general and specialized knowledge shall be provided", offer moral education through students' whole course of learning, educate students to learn great TCM masters' proficient medical skills and lofty medical ethics, and make them have the ambition to be both experts in traditional Chinese medicine and moral models .

(3) Scientific research on traditional Chinese medicine shall be strengthened to promote the close integration of traditional Chinese medicine and modern science and technology. Modern science and technology propel traditional Chinese medicine to develop and spurt. Efforts shall be made to research science and technology, establish and perfect evaluation methods and standards that conform to the characteristics of the research on traditional Chinese medicine, construct systems of technological innovation, and carry out systematic research on TCM fundamental theories, clinical diagnosis, treatment and therapeutic evaluation to advance progress in traditional Chinese medicine and lay a solid foundation for introduction of traditional Chinese medicine to the rest of the world. Efforts shall also be made to closely integrate the research on traditional Chinese medicine and the research on biology, physics, chemistry, life science, material science, information science and other branches of science and strengthen preservation, rescue and application of the ancient books on traditional Chinese medicine and the traditional knowledge and techniques of diagnosis and treatment. Joint research shall be conducted particularly on the

mechanisms of traditional Chinese medicine and the formulas of traditional Chinese medicinal materials, and innovative achievements shall be gained as soon as possible to improve the capacity and level of the treatment and control of major difficult and complicated diseases. The great number of TCM experts in the colleges and universities of traditional Chinese medicine shall strengthen the research on the policies concerning the major theoretical and practical issues in the development of health and healthcare services, promote the construction of think tanks and provide counseling for the decision making of the Party and the government.

(4) The cultural quintessence of traditional Chinese medicine shall be rediscovered further to make contribution for inheritance and spread of Chinese traditional culture. Traditional Chinese medicine, a key component of the splendid Chinese culture, originated in Chinese nation and has become an important carrier to spread the excellent Chinese traditional culture. Efforts shall be made to systematically research the culture of traditional Chinese medicine, rediscover and categorize TCM cultural connotation and original thinking, summarize Chinese nation's cognition and understanding of life, health and diseases, refine the cultural core and spiritual essence of traditional Chinese medicine, and construct a core value system of TCM culture that features the characteristics of China, traditional Chinese medicine and TCM industry and also embodies the spirit of the time. Spread of the culture of traditional Chinese medicine shall be promoted; in accordance with the strategy of "building a culturally strong country", knowledge on traditional Chinese medicine shall be popularized and spread, and such professionals shall be cultivated. High-quality cultural works shall be produced and effective integration of traditional Chinese medicine with radio, film & television, press & publication, digital publishing, tourism & catering, and sports & fitness shall be promoted to build excellent cultural brands of traditional Chinese medicine.

(5) Diversified social services of traditional Chinese medicine shall be further expanded to better meet people' health needs. Traditional Chinese medicine, combining healthcare services and disease prevention and treatment together, is green and healthy, and more and more people hope to get access to the diversified healthcare services and the treatment of traditional Chinese medicine at their different stages of life. TCM higher education shall meet the new requirements of the supply-side reform, and bring into full play the advantage of the great number of TCM experts and their talent for research in the colleges and universities of traditional Chinese medicine. Active involvement shall be made in the development of products of TCM healthcare, culture and tourism and in the development of new drugs, medical machines, techniques, equipment and health products to foster new types of healthcare services and further develop the industry of traditional Chinese medicine

to satisfy people's needs for diversified TCM healthcare services. Systems shall be established to guide TCM professionals' innovation and development and efforts shall be made to work out supporting policies and perfect the mechanisms for the transformation of research achievements, the division of intellectual property and the collaborative innovation of industry, universities and research institutions and users, accelerate the pace of transformation, and provide continuing momentum for the development of the industry of traditional Chinese medicine. Meanwhile, universities and enterprises shall be promoted to jointly run schools to cultivate interdisciplinary professionals specializing in TCM-based healthcare for the elderly, health tourism and health culture and provide talented professionals for promoting the industrial development of traditional Chinese medicine.

(6) Traditional Chinese medicine shall be introduced to the rest of the world to benefit more people with Chinese wisdom. It has been long time since traditional Chinese medicine spread among people. As early as the Qin and Han dynasties, traditional Chinese medicine was popular in many neighboring countries; the smallpox vaccination technique in traditional Chinese medicine spread outside of China to the rest of the world during the Ming and Qing dynasties; the Ben Cao Gang Mu (Compendium of Materia Medica) was translated into various languages and widely read and Charles Darwin, the British biologist, hailed the book as an "ancient Chinese encyclopedia". Now with China's more and more important role in the world, efforts shall be made to further play the distinctive role of traditional Chinese medicine in deepening people-to-people exchange between China and the rest of the world, develop TCM higher education into a new area of the exchange, and make traditional Chinese medicine have increasingly more say and dominance in the field of traditional medicines. In accordance with the strategy of the "Belt and Road Initiative", exchange and cooperation with the countries concerned shall be enhanced and efforts shall be made to offer services of traditional Chinese medicine and cultivation of TCM professionals and spread stories of China and legends of traditional Chinese medicine to the rest of the world to display the charm of Chinese traditional culture and the vigor of contemporary China. Cooperation with international organizations and foreign governments and regions shall be strengthened and higher learning institutions of traditional Chinese medicine shall be encouraged to establish TCM Confucius institutes and TCM centers overseas and open up new channels for further cooperation. Education for international students shall be promoted more energetically and training of knowledge and techniques concerning traditional Chinese medicine in foreign countries shall be organized actively to improve the quality of education for foreign students and make China the ideal country for foreign students' higher learning of traditional Chinese medicine.

Reform and development of the higher education of traditional Chinese medicine is a significantly fundamental and strategic project as well as a complicated systematic project. All the colleges and universities of traditional Chinese medicine shall earnestly strengthen and improve Party building and ideological work. The Party's leadership is of vital importance in running socialist colleges and universities with Chinese distinctive characteristics and the Party shall play a leading role in the work in every field. The Party's leadership and socialist orientation in education shall be upheld firmly and unswervingly. "Four Consciousness" shall be further strengthened and efforts shall be made to keep in line with the leadership of the Central Committee of the Communist Party of China with Comrade Xi Jinping as the core in ideology, politics and action and implement the Party' policies on education and on traditional Chinese medicine. Inter-sector coordination and cooperation shall be improved and the role of the system for the joint inter-ministerial meeting of the State Council for traditional Chinese medicine shall be fully played. All the member sectors shall closely collaborate to form a joint force for reform. Departments of reform and development, finance and other departments shall provide more support to safeguard a healthy development of the higher education and the services of traditional Chinese medicine.

(Zhao Yinghong)

## 8. *Law of the People's Republic of China on Traditional Chinese Medicine*

Adopted at the 25th Session of the Standing Committee of the Twelfth National Conference of the People's Republic of China on December 25th, 2016

## Chapter I    General Provisions

【Article 1】 The law is enacted for the purpose of inheriting and carrying forward traditional Chinese medicine, ensuring and promoting the development of traditional Chinese medicine for the health of the people.

【Article 2】 Traditional Chinese medicine (hereinafter referred to as TCM) in this law is a general term for the medicine of all ethnic groups including the Han nationality and ethnic minorities in China. It is a medical and pharmacological science system that reflects Chinese people's understanding of life, health and disease, with a long history and unique theories and techniques.

【Article 3】 TCM undertaking is an important part of medicine and healthcare fields in China. The state shall vigorously develop TCM undertaking, carrying out the principle of balance between Chinese and Western medicine, establishing an administrative system that conforms to TCM features and giving TCM full play in the medical and healthcare affairs in China.

In the development of the TCM undertaking, the core value and laws of TCM development shall be followed; the integration of inheritances and innovation adhered to, TCM features and advantages preserved and maximized, and modern scientific technologies utilized, so as to promote the development of TCM theories and practice.

The state shall encourage Chinese and Western medicines to learn and complement one another, develop with coordination, and maximize their own advantages so as to promote the integration of Chinese and Western medicines.

【 Article 4 】 The people's governments at or above the county level shall incorporate TCM into their national economic and social development plans, establish a sound TCM management system and make overall plans for the promotion and development of TCM.

【 Article 5 】 The competent TCM administration department under the State Council shall take charge of the nationwide administration for TCM within its administrative region. Other relevant departments under the State Council shall take charge of other affairs related to TCM administration within their respective authority.

The competent TCM department under the local people's government at or above the county level shall be responsible for the administration of TCM in their respective administrative regions. Other relevant departments of the local people's governments at or above the county level shall be responsible for the affairs related to TCM administration within the scope of their respective functions.

【 Article 6 】 The state shall strengthen the construction of TCM service system, rationally plan and allocate TCM service resources and guarantee available access for citizens to TCM services.

China encourages social sectors to invest in the TCM undertaking and supports organizations and individuals to make donation and provide fund for TCM undertaking.

【 Article 7 】 The state shall promote TCM education to establish a TCM education system satisfying the needs during the developmental progress of TCM undertaking with proper scale, rational structure and different forms to cultivate TCM talents.

【 Article 8 】 The state shall support the scientific research and technological development of TCM, encouraging innovation in TCM science and technologies, promoting the application of scientific and technological achievements of TC, protecting TCM intellectual property and promoting scientific and technological level of TCM.

【 Article 9 】 The state shall support international exchange and cooperation to promote international transmission and application of TCM.

【 Article 10 】 Organizations and individuals that have made outstanding contributions to the TCM undertaking shall be commended and rewarded in accordance with relevant provisions of China.

## Chapter II  TCM Service

【Article 11】 The people's governments at or above the county level shall include the launch of TCM medical institutions into the plan on the setup of medical institutions, launching proper scaled TCM medical institutions, and supporting the development of medical institutions with distinct TCM features and advantages.

To merge or cancel a TCM medical institution launched by the government or convert it into a TCM institution, opinions shall be solicited from the competent TCM department under the people's government at the next higher level.

【Article 12】 The comprehensive hospitals and maternal and child care institutions and qualified specialized hospitals, community health service centers and township health centers launched by the government should set up TCM departments and clinics.

【Article 13】 The state supports non-governmental investment to launch Chinese medical institutions.

Chinese medical institutions launched by non-governmental investment shall enjoy the same rights as those organized by the government related to permission, practice, basic medical insurance, scientific research and teaching, the evaluation of titles for medical personnel, etc.

【Article 14】 To launch a TCM medical institution, the approval formalities shall be undergone according to the provisions of the state on the administration of medical institutions, and the provisions on the administration of medical institutions shall be observed.

To launch a TCM clinic, name, address, scope of service and staffing of the clinic shall be reported to the competent TCM department under the local people's government at the county level and registered before starting medical practice. The TCM clinic shall publicize its medical treatment scope and names of TCM practitioners and their practice scope in a visible position of the clinic. The clinic shall not conduct medical activities beyond the registered scope. The specific provisions shall be formulated by the competent TCM department under the State Council and be submitted to the administrative department of public health under the State Council for review and issuance.

【Article 15】 Personnel engaged in medical activities of TCM shall, in accordance with the provisions of the *Law of the People's Republic of China on Medical Practitioners*, obtain the qualification as a TCM physician through the TCM medical qualification examination, and conduct practice registration. The content of the qualification examination for TCM physicians shall reflect TCM features.

A person who has been learning TCM from a teacher in form of apprenticeship, or indeed has specialty in medical skills through many years of practice shall be recommended by at least two TCM physicians, and may be qualified as a TCM physician after passing the appraisal and examination for the qualification of a licensed doctor under the auspices of the competent TCM department of the people's government of the provinces, autonomous regions or municipalities directly under the Central Government. After conducting practice registration according to the examination content, he or she may be engaged in TCM medical activities in the form of individual business operation or working in medical institution within the registered scope of practice. The competent TCM department of the State Council shall draft the measures for the categorized examination of the personnel described in this paragraph according to the safety risks of TCM techniques, and report the measures to the health administration department of the State Council for review and issuance.

【Article 16】 A TCM institution shall be mainly equipped with TCM professionals and technicians, mainly providing TCM services. TCM practitioners who have obtained physician qualification upon examination may, in accordance with relevant provisions of China, adopt modern scientific and technological methods related to their professions in their medical practice after obtaining training and passing the examination. The modern scientific and technological methods applied in the medical activities shall be conductive to preserving and giving full play of TCM features and advantages.

The community health service centers, township health centers, community health service stations and qualified village clinics shall reasonably assign TCM professional technicians, and apply and promote appropriate TCM techniques.

【Article 17】 TCM service shall be carried out by taking TCM theories as the guidance and applying TCM techniques and comply with basic requirements for TCM service formulated by the competent TCM department under the State Council.

【Article 18】 The people's government at or above the county level shall develop TCM in services of prevention and health care and incorporate them into basic public health service items for overall planning and implementation in accordance with the relevant provisions of China.

The people's government at or above the county level shall allow TCM to fully play its role in emergency response to sudden public health events, and strengthen the reserves of TCM emergency response supplies, equipment, facilities, technologies and talents.

Medical and health institution shall actively apply TCM theories and techniques in disease prevention and control.

【 Article 19 】 A medical institution that plans to release a TCM medical advertisement shall be subject to the revision and approval of the competent TCM department of the people's government of the province, autonomous region or municipality directly under the Central Government; and shall not issue the advertisement without revision and approval. The content of the issued TCM medical advertisement shall be consistent with the content approved upon revision, and comply with the relevant provisions of the *Advertisement Law of the People's Republic of China*.

【 Article 20 】 The competent TCM department under the people's governments at or above the county level shall strengthen the supervision and inspection of TCM services, and make the following items as the focus of the supervision and inspection:

(1) Whether the TCM medical institutions or practitioners conducts medical activities beyond the registered scope;

(2) Whether the TCM service complies with the basic requirements for TCM services formulated by the competent TCM department under the State Council;

(3) Whether the release of medical advertisements related to TCM complies with the provisions of this law.

The competent TCM department shall carry out supervision and inspection according to the laws, and the relevant units and individuals shall cooperate with it and shall not refuse or obstruct it.

## Chapter III   Protection and Development of TCM

【 Article 21 】 The state shall formulate the technical specifications and standards for the cultivation, collection, storage and initial processing of Chinese materia medica and strengthen the quality supervision and management during the whole process of production and circulation to guarantee the quality safety of Chinese materia medica.

【 Article 22 】 The state shall encourage the development of standardized cultivation of Chinese materia medica, strictly control the use of pesticides, fertilizers and other agricultural inputs, prohibit the use of highly poisonous or toxic pesticides during the cultivation of Chinese materia medica, and support the breeding of fine varieties of Chinese materia medica to improve the quality.

【 Article 23 】 The state shall establish the evaluation system of genuine regional materia medica, support the variety breeding of genuine regional materia medica, support the launch of production base of genuine regional materia medica, strengthen the ecological environment protection of the production base of genuine regional materia medica, and encourage the protection of genuine regional materia medica by geographical indication and other measures.

The genuine regional materia medica in the proceeding Article refer to those selected by long-term clinical application of TCM, produced in certain areas with better quality and efficacy compared with the same species produced in other regions, and thereby with stable quality and high popularity.

〖 Article 24 〗 The department of the pharmaceutical supervision and administration under the State Council shall organize and strengthen the quality monitoring of Chinese materia medica and regularly publish the results. The relevant departments under the State Council shall cooperate in the accomplishment of the quality monitoring of Chinese materia medica.

The collection and storage of Chinese materia medica and their initial processing shall conform to the relevant technical specification, standard and administrative regulation of China.

The state shall encourage the development of modern distribution system of Chinese materia medica, improve the technological standards for packaging and warehousing of Chinese materia medica and establish the circulation traceability system for Chinese materia medica. The pharmaceutical manufacturers shall establish a system of inspection and record for the purchase of Chinese materia medica.

The proprietors of Chinese medicinal shall establish an inspection system for the purchase of goods and registration system for the buying and selling and indicate the geographical origin of the Chinese materia medica.

〖 Article 25 〗 The state shall protect the medicinal wildlife resources, carry out dynamic monitoring and regular general-survey on the medicinal wildlife resources, establish a germplasm gene bank for the medicinal wildlife resources, encourage the development of artificial cultivation and breeding, and support the development of the protection, breeding and relevant research of precious and endangered medicinal wildlife according to the law.

〖 Article 26 〗 TCM practitioners from village medical institutions and countryside doctors with Chinese materia medica knowledge and identification skills may plant and collect Chinese materia medica for the application in the clinical activities in accordance with relevant provisions of the state.

〖 Article 27 〗 China protects the traditional processing techniques for decoction pieces of Chinese crude drugs, supports the application of traditional processing techniques in processing decoction pieces of Chinese crude drugs.

〖 Article 28 〗 For the decoction pieces of Chinese crude drugs which are not supplied on the market, a medical institution may process and use them within the medical institution based on corresponding formulas prescribe by physician of this institution. Medical institutions shall abide by relevant provisions on the processing of decoction pieces and take charge of drug quality to ensure safety. The processing of decoction pieces of Chinese crude drugs by medical institutions should be reported to the department of pharmaceutical supervision and administration under the local municipal people's government for the record.

According to the needs of clinical medication, a medical institution may reprocess decoction pieces of Chinese crude drugs based on the formulas prescribed by physicians of the institution.

【Article 29】 China encourages and supports the development and production of new Chinese materia medica.

The state shall protect traditional processing techniques and procedures of Chinese materia medica, support the production of traditional dosage form of Chinese patent medicine, and encourage the application of modern science and technology to study and develop traditional Chinese patent medicine.

【Article 30】 For the production of compound preparation of Chinese materia medica derived from ancient classical formulas meeting the national prescribed condition, it may only provide non-clinical safety research materials when applying for the drug approval number. Specific regulations shall be developed by the department of pharmaceutical supervision and administration under the State Council in conjunction with the competent TCM department.

The ancient classical formulas in the proceeding Article refer to prescriptions that are still widely used, with definite efficacy and outstanding characteristics and advantages recorded in the ancient classics of TCM. The specific catalogue shall be formulated by the competent TCM department under the State Council in conjunction with the department of pharmaceutical supervision and administration.

【Article 31】 The state shall encourage medical institutions to prepare and use Chinese medical preparation according to their clinical needs, and support the application of traditional techniques in preparing Chinese medicinal preparation and the development of new TCM drugs on the basis of Chinese medicinal preparation.

Medical institutions shall obtain the *Pharmaceutical Preparation Certificate for Medical Institution* in accordance with the *Pharmaceutical Administration Law of the People's Republic of China,* or entrust a pharmaceutical manufacturing enterprise that has obtained *Drug Manufacturing Certificate* or other medical institutions that have obtained the *Pharmaceutical Preparation Certificate for Medical Institution* to prepare Chinese medicinal preparation. The documents of Chinese medicinal preparation should be submitted to the department of pharmaceutical supervision and administration under the people's government of the province, autonomous region of municipality directly under the Central Government where the entrusting party files on record.

Medical institutions shall be responsible for the quality of self-made Chinese medicinal preparation. For the entrustment of preparation, the entrusting party and entrusted party shall respectively bear the corresponding responsibilities for the quality of Chinese medicinal preparation.

【Article 32】 Medical institutions shall obtain the preparation approval number according to the law for the self-made Chinese medicinal preparation products. However, the approval number is not required for the Chinese medicinal preparation products prepared simply with traditional techniques, and they shall be reported to pharmaceutical supervision and administration department under the local people's government of the province, autonomous region or municipality directly under the Central Government for record.

Medical institutions shall strengthen monitoring on adverse reactions caused by registered Chinese medicinal preparation products and report the cases in accordance with the relevant provisions of China. The pharmaceutical supervision and administration department shall strengthen the supervision and inspection on the preparation and use of the self-made Chinese medicinal preparation products on record.

## Chapter IV  Education and Training of Traditional Chinese Medicine

【Article 33】 The TCM education should follow the development rules of TCM talents, with TCM as the main content, and shall reflect the cultural features of TCM and emphasize TCM classical theories and clinical practice, as well as the combination of modern and traditional education methods.

【Article 34】 The state shall improve the education system for TCM universities and vocational schools, and support the development of higher education institutions, secondary vocational schools and other educational institutions that specialized in the implementation of TCM education.

【Article 35】 The state shall develop TCM master-disciple education and support TCM physicians and technical TCM personnel with rich clinical experience and technical expertise to impart theories and technical methods to disciples in practice and medical activities to train professional TCM technician personnel.

【Article 36】 The state shall strengthen the education and training for TCM physicians and professional TCM technical personnel at the community level in urban and rural areas.

The state shall develop education for integrated Chinese and Western medicine to cultivate high-level talents integrating TCM and Western medicine.

【Article 37】 The competent TCM department under the local government at or above the county level shall organize and develop TCM continuing education plans and strengthen basic TCM knowledge and skills training towards medical personnel, especially those TCM technicians at the community level in urban and rural areas.

Professional TCM technical personnel shall participate in further education in accordance with the provisions, and local institutions shall create favorable conditions to support them.

## Chapter V    Scientific Research of TCM

【Article 38】 The state shall encourage scientific research institutions, higher education schools, medical institutions and pharmaceutical manufacturers to carry out scientific research on TCM by applying both modern scientific and technological research methods and TCM research techniques, strengthen the study on integration of Chinese and Western medicine, so as to promote the inheritance and innovation of TCM theories and technical methods.

【Article 39】 The state shall take measures to support the collation, study and use of the ancient TCM literature, academic thoughts and diagnostics and treatment experience of famous TCM experts, and folk TCM technical techniques.

The state shall encourage organizations and individuals to donate TCM literature, secret or proved formulas, and diagnostic and treatment methods and techniques with great value in scientific research and clinical application.

【Article 40】 The state shall establish and improve the scientific and technological innovation system, evaluation system and administrative system that conform to TCM features so as to promote TCM scientific and technological progress and innovation.

【Article 41】 The state shall take measures to strengthen the scientific research of basic TCM theories and treatment according to syndrome differentiation methods, prevention and treatment for common diseases, frequently occurring diseases, chronic diseases, major difficult diseases and major infectious diseases by means of TCM, and research projects, playing significant roles in the promotion of theoretical and practical TCM development.

## Chapter VI    Inheritance and Cultural Communication of TCM

【Article 42】 The competent TCM departments under the people's governments at or above the provincial level should organize the selection of academic heritage projects and successors of TCM within their respective administrative regions to carry forward TCM theories and technical methods with significant academic values and create favorable conditions for the inheritance. The inheritors shall carry out heritage activities to cultivate successors, and collect, collate and properly preserve relevant academic materials. The inheritance activities for representative projects of intangible cultural heritage shall be carried out in accordance with the relevant provisions of the *Law of the People's Republic of China on the Protection of Intangible Cultural Heritage.*

【Article 43】 The state shall establish the database, list and system for the protection of traditional knowledge of TCM.

Practitioners possessing TCM knowledge shall have the right to inherit and use their own knowledge. They shall have informed consent and shared interest for their TCM knowledge to be obtained and applied by other.

The state shall implement special protection for the composition and manufacturing process of China secret prescriptions of traditional TCM identified according to the law.

【Article 44】 The state shall encourage the development of TCM health care and health preservation services and support non-government investment to launch standardized TCM health care institutions. The standards and criteria of TCM health care services shall be formulated by the competent TCM department under the State Council.

【Article 45】 The people's governments at or above the county level should strengthen the public education of TCM knowledge and culture, and encourage organizations and individuals to create TCM cultural and popular works.

【Article 46】 The activities for publicity and popularization TCM culture and knowledge should be carried out in compliance with the relevant provisions of the state. No organization or individual shall make any false or exaggerated TCM publicity, nor shall they make fraudulent use of TCM to seek illegitimate interests.

The radio, television, newspaper, internet and other media shall employ professional TCM technical personnel when promoting TCM knowledge.

## Chapter VII    Safeguard Measures

【Article 47】 The people's governments at or above the county level should provide policy and material support for the TCM development, and incorporate the funds for the TCM development in the financial budgets of the governments at corresponding levels.

The people's governments at or above the county level and relevant government authorities should invite the competent TCM department in drafting and developing policies for basic medical insurance payment, drug administration and other medical and health issues, so as to fully exploit TCM advantages to encourage practice and application of TCM services.

【Article 48】 The people's governments at or above the county level and their relevant departments shall rationally set the charge items and standards of TCM services according to the statutory authority for price management, and reflect the cost of services and professional and technical values of TCM services.

【Article 49】 In accordance with the provisions of the state, the relevant departments of the people's government at or above the county level shall incorporate qualified TCM institutions into the medical institutions designated for basic medical insurance with the inclusion of qualified TCM diagnostic and treatment projects, TCM decoction pieces, Chinese patent medicine and self-made TCM preparation into the scope of basic medical insurance payment.

【Article 50】 The state shall strengthen the construction of TCM standard system, develop standards for the technical requirements that need to be unified according to the TCM features and revise them in time.

The national and industrial TCM standards shall be formulated or revised by the relevant departments under the State Council in accordance with their responsibilities and be published on their websites for free-access to the public.

The state shall promote the establishment of the TCM international standard system.

【Article 51】 The evaluation, assessment and appraisal of TCM required by the law and administrative regulations shall be carried out with the launch of special organizations or the participation of TCM experts.

【Article 52】 The state shall take measures to strengthen support towards ethnic minority medicine in inheritance and innovation, application-oriented development and talent cultivation and enhance the launch of medical institutions and establishment of physician team, so as to promote and standardize the development of ethnic minority medicine.

## Chapter VIII  Legal Liability

【Article 53】 The competent TCM department of the people's government at or above the county level and other relevant departments that fails to perform their duties as required by this Law shall be instructed for rectification by the people's government at the same level or the relevant departments of the people's government at the next higher levels. If the circumstances are serious, the person directly in charge and other persons directly responsible shall be penalized according to law.

【Article 54】 Any TCM clinic, in violation of the provisions of this Law, that carries out medical activities beyond the registered practice scope shall be instructed to rectify by the competent TCM department under the local people's government at the county level, and the illegal gains shall be confiscated and imposed with a fine of not less than 10,000 *yuan* but not more than 30,000 *yuan*. If the circumstances are serious, it shall be instructed to cease the practice.

For any TCM clinic instructed to cease the practice, the person directly in charge shall be barred from being engaged in the management of medical institutions within five years from the issuance date of the penalty decision. For any medical institution that hires the above-mentioned persons to engage in the management work, the medical practice license shall be revoked by the former license issuance department or the institution shall be instructed to cease the practice by the former registration department.

【Article 55】 Any TCM physician obtained qualification of a licensed doctor after passing the examination who is engaged in medical activities beyond the registered practice scope, in violation of the provisions of this Law, shall be instructed to suspend the practice for no less than six months but not more than one year by the competent TCM departments under the people's governments at or above the county level and imposed a fine of no less than 10,000 *yuan* but not more than 30,000 *yuan*. If the circumstances are serious, his/her medical practice license shall be revoked.

【Article 56】 In case of failure in record keeping of filling with false materials in launching TCM clinic, processing decoction pieces or entrusting others to prepare Chinese medicinal preparation in violation of the provision of this Law, offenders shall be instructed to rectify by the competent TCM department and pharmaceutical supervision and administrative department according to their respective responsibilities. The illegal gains shall be confiscated and a fine of no more than 30,000 *yuan* shall be imposed and the relevant information should be publicized. If offenders refuse to rectify, they shall be instructed to cease the practice or the processing of TCM decoction pieces and the entrusted TCM preparation, and the person directly responsible shall be barred from being engaged in any TCM activities within five years from the date of the issuance of the penalty decision.

Any TCM institution fails to record on files when applying traditional process to prepare Chinese medicinal preparation in violation of the provisions of this Law, or fails to make Chinese medicinal preparation in accordance with the requirements stated clearly in the record files shall be penalized as producing counterfeit.

【Article 57】 In case of releasing a TCM advertisement not in conformity with the reviewed and approved edition, in violation of the provisions of this Law, the regulatory department responsible for the approval will revoke the approval document for the advertisement and dismiss the application for advertising review submitted by this medical institution with one year.

In violation of the provision of this Law, other illegal actions when releasing TCM advertisement, offenders shall be penalized in accordance with the provisions of the *Advertising Law of the People's Republic of China*.

【Article 58】 In case of using high-toxic pesticides in the process of planting Chinese materia medica, in violation of the provisions of this Law, offenders shall be penalized in accordance with the relevant laws and administrative regulations; If the circumstances are serious, the person directly in charge or other persons directly responsible may be detained by the public security organ for no less than five days but not more than 15 days.

【Article 59】 In the case of causing personal or property damage in violation of the relevant provisions of this Law, the offender shall bear civil liability in accordance with the Law. In case of violations of this Law involving criminal offenses, the offenders shall be prosecuted in accordance with the law.

## Chapter IX   Supplementary Provisions

【Article 60】 The administration of TCM that is not specified by this Law shall apply to the provisions of the relevant laws and administrative regulations such as the *Law of the People's Republic of China on Medical Practitioners and the Drug Administration Law of the People Republic of China*.

The administration of TCM in the armed forces shall be organized and implemented by the military health authorities in accordance with this Law and the relevant provisions of the armed forces.

【Article 61】 Autonomous Regions of ethnic minorities may formulate measures to promote and standardize the development of local ethnic minority medicine based on their practical situations, in accordance with the *Law of the People's Republic of China on Regional National Autonomy* and the relevant provisions of this Law.

【Article 62】 If the blind obtain qualification for braille medical massage personnel in accordance with the relevant provisions of China, medical massage services could be provided in the form of an individual business or within a medical institution.

【Article 63】 The Law shall come into force as of July 1st, 2017.

**Notice of the CPC Central Committee and the State Council on Issuing the *Outline of the Healthy China 2030 Plan***

(No. 23 [2016] of the CPC Central Committee)

The Party committees and people's governments of all provinces, autonomous regions and municipalities directly under the Central Government, all departments of the Central Committee of the CPC, all ministries and commissions under the State Council, all headquarters of the Chinese People's Liberation Army, all large entities, and all people's organizations, the *Outline of the Healthy China 2030 Plan* is hereby printed and distributed to you, please earnestly implement them in light of your actual situation.

The CPC Central Committee and the State Council

October 17th, 2016

## 9. *Outline of the Healthy China 2030 Plan*

### Foreword

Health is a must for human development and a basis for socio-economic development. Health and longevity are an important token of national wealth and prosperity, representing the common wishes of people of all ethnic groups in the country.

The Communist Party of China (CPC) and the government have always attached great importance to the health of the population. Since the establishment of New China, especially with the reform and opening up, the health sector has seen successful reforms and development, with a better urban and rural environment, intensified health promotion campaigns, an improved medical care system, and continuously enhanced health and wellbeing among the population. In 2015, the average life expectancy reached 76.34 years; infant mortality, under-five mortality and the maternal mortality rate were reduced to 8.1‰, 10.7‰ and 20.1 per 100,000 respectively. With main health indicators outperforming the averages seen in upper middle-income countries, the Chinese health system has laid a solid foundation for building an all-round moderately prosperous society. Meanwhile, industrialization, urbanization, aging population, a changing disease spectrum, ecosystem and lifestyles complicate the situation and pose new challenges to maintaining and promoting health. There are prominent conflicts between health needs and health supply, and health development and socio-economic development are still lacking coordination. Long-term strategic solutions for key and profound issues are needed.

A healthy China is fundamental for the country to achieve an all-round moderately prosperous society and the modernization of socialist society. "Healthy China 2030" is a national strategy for improving the health of the population and coordinating health and socio-economic development, and a major means for the country to participate in global health governance and meet targets set in the *2030 Agenda for Sustainable Development*. The next 15 years will be a key period for improving the population's health. Economic growth at medium to high speed provides a solid foundation for health improvement. Upgrading of consumption may mean more opportunities for development of the healthcare market. With more mature and fixed institutional arrangements and great momentum in science and technology innovation, sustainable development of the healthcare system will be guaranteed.

To build a healthy China and raise the health status of the people, we have developed the outline of a plan based on the decisions made at the Fifth Plenary Session of the 18th CPC Central Committee. This outline of the plan will be a blueprint and action plan for facilitating the development of Healthy China. The entire society will take responsibility and make commitments to achieving the goal, and contribute to the rejuvenation of the nation and advancement of human civilization.

## Part I  Overall Strategy

## Chapter I  Principles

To build a healthy China, we need to hold high the great banner of socialism with Chinese characteristics. We need to implement the guiding principles of the 18th National Congress of the CPC and the third, fourth and fifth plenary sessions of the 18th CPC Central Committee. We must follow the guidance of Marxism-Leninism, Mao Zedong Thought, Deng Xiaoping Theory, the Theory of Three Represents, and the Scientific Outlook on Development. The guiding principles from General Secretary Xi Jinping's major policy addresses must be put into practice. Work must be carried out in accordance with the plan for promoting all-round economic, political, cultural, social and ecological progress, and the Four-Pronged Comprehensive Strategy. Decisions made by the CPC Central Committee and the State Council must be carried out. The people-centered and new vision of development must be followed, and the right health policies must be stuck to. With people's health at the center, we need to reform and innovate institutional arrangements, and make healthy living, healthcare services, health security, healthy environment, and the healthcare market as our five priorities. We should incorporate health into all policies, and transform the development modes of the healthcare sector, and ensure people's health at all stages of life by improving their health and health equity. Ultimately, this will lay a solid health foundation for the great rejuvenation of the Chinese nation and realization of the "two centenary goals".

The following principles need to be adhered to:

**Health as a top priority.** Health should be at the top of the development agenda. Based on national conditions, health promotion should be a part of the public policymaking process. Healthy lifestyles, the ecosystem, and socio-economic development models should be put into place to pursue the coordination of health and economic and social development.

**Reform for innovation.** With the market playing its due role, government-led reforms in key fields will free people's minds and thoughts, break vested interests and eliminate institutional barriers. Sci-tech innovation and information technology application should have a steering and supportive role in forming an institution that contributes to improving people's health, with Chinese characteristics.

**Scientific development.** We need to identify rules for health development, and adhere to "prevention first, combining prevention with control, and supporting both traditional Chinese and Western medicine." Healthcare delivery systems should become integrated, moving from an extensive development mode based on scale to an intensive one focusing on quality and efficiency. Efforts should be made in the complementary development of both traditional Chinese medicine (TCM) and Western medicine, as well as overall enhancement of healthcare delivery.

**Equity and fairness.** Rural and primary health will be prioritized. We will aim to achieve equity of public health services, ensuring that access and the non-profit nature of basic medical care and health services to reduce urban-rural, regional and sub-group health inequalities. Universal coverage and social equity in health care services will be realized.

## Chapter II   Strategic Themes

To "contribute and share to build a healthy nation" is the theme for the Healthy China strategy. Centered around population health, with momentum in terms of reform and innovation, the strategy takes the principle: "health in all, health by all, health for all". It will prioritize primary health care, focus on prevention, give equal stress to the development of Chinese and Western medicine, incorporate health care into all policies, and encourage people to contribute and share. Targeting risk factors of health related to lifestyles, working and living environments, and healthcare services, the strategy will be led by the government and actively implemented by society. All interventions and programs will be participated in and contributed to by all, and results shared by all. Prevention measures will be emphasized alongside healthy lifestyles to prevent diseases and ensure early diagnosis, treatment and rehabilitative care, and to improve the population's health.

"Contribute and share" is the basic method to build a healthy China. Supply-side and demand-side reforms integrating individual, institutional and social factors will provide momentum to maintain and protect people's health. There will be an emphasis on encouraging social participation. Cross-sector cooperation will be strengthened, and military and civilian healthcare delivery integrated. Motivating the initiative and creativity of social forces, we will protect the environment, ensure food and drug safety, prevent and reduce harm, control health risks and environmental hazards, and form a social co-regulation system encompassing multiple levels and multiple stakeholders. To drive supply-side reforms, sectors such as health, family planning and sports will deepen institutional reform in optimizing health resource allocation and service delivery, developing underdeveloped areas, upgrading the healthcare industry, and meeting increasing healthcare needs. Individuals will be held accountable for their own health. Health literacy will be improved. Self-motivated and self-disciplined living habits need to be explored by citizens based on their own needs, so as to control factors affecting health, and create a social environment nurturing, pursuing and supporting good health.

The fundamental goal of building Healthy China is to maintain a healthy population. Focusing on the lifelong needs of all people, we need to provide equitable, accessible, comprehensive and continuous care to achieve better health. To ensure universal benefits, we need to innovate institutional arrangements, expand coverage, improve healthcare quality, ensure access to quality and affordable preventive, curative, rehabilitative health care, while focusing on priority groups such as women, children, the elderly, the disabled and low-income groups. To cover lifelong health needs, we need to deal with key health issues, identify priorities, and step up interventions, to provide "cradle-to-grave" care and protection.

## Chapter III    Strategic Targets

By 2020, a universal primary healthcare system with Chinese characteristics will cover both urban and rural citizens; enhance health literacy; deliver greatly improved health care; ensure universally accessible primary medical and healthcare services and sports facilities; develop a healthcare industry with sound structure and rich content; maintain health indicators ranked top in upper middle-income countries.

By 2030, we will further improve institutional arrangements supporting implementation of the Healthy China strategy; develop a more coordinated healthcare sector; promote more healthy living styles; enhance healthcare service quality and health protection levels; revitalize the healthcare industry; achieve health equity; maintain health indicators equal high-income countries. By 2050, we will build a healthy China complemented with a modernized socialist country.

The following targets will be met by 2030:

Continuously improved health of the people. Physical fitness of the population will be significantly improved, with average life expectancy increased to 79 years.

Key health risk factors under effective control. Health literacy of the population will be greatly increased and healthy lifestyles widely advocated. Living and working environment favoring health improvement will be formed, with effective food and drug safety. A batch of major diseases will be eliminated.

Increased healthcare service delivery capacity. Effective and integrated medical and healthcare service delivery systems will be built. Public sports and fitness services covering all citizens will be developed. Health security systems will be improved. World-leading health sci-tech innovation capacity will be fostered. Healthcare service quality will be enhanced.

Significantly expanded healthcare industry. A healthcare industry with complete and optimal structure will be established. Large businesses with a track record of strong innovation and a global competitive edge will become a mainstay of the national economy.

A well-developed health promotion system. Policy and legislation will be strengthened and modernized. A health governance system will be built up.

**Main indicators for the healthy China strategy**

| Domain | Indicators | 2015 | 2020 | 2030 |
|---|---|---|---|---|
| Health status | Life expectancy (year) | 76.34 | 77.3 | 79.0 |
| | Infant mortality (‰) | 8.1 | 7.5 | 5.0 |
| | Under-five mortality (‰) | 10.7 | 9.5 | 6.0 |
| | Maternal mortality (1/100,000) | 20.1 | 18.0 | 12.0 |
| | People meeting the fitness standards defined in the National Physical Fitness Standards (%) | 89.6 (2014) | 90.6 | 92.2 |
| Healthy living | Health literacy (%) | 10 | 20 | 30 |
| | Frequent physical exercises (100 million) | 3.6 (2014) | 4.35 | 5.3 |
| Health service and protection | Premature death rate from major chronic diseases (%) | 19.1 (2013) | 10% lower than 2015 | 30% lower than 2015 |
| | Practicing or assistant physicians per 1,000 | 2.2 | 2.5 | 3.0 |
| | Out-of-pocket payment as a share of total health expenditures (%) | 29.3 | Around 28 | Around 25 |
| Healthy environment | Percentage of days with good air quality in cities at prefecture or above level (%) | 76.7 | >80 | Continuous improvement |
| | Percentage of surface waters at or above level III | 66 | >70 | Continuous improvement |
| Healthcare industry | Total size of healthcare industry (trillion Yuan) | — | >8 | 16 |

## Part II    Healthy Living for All

## Chapter IV    Strengthening Health Education

### Section One    Improving Health Literacy

An emphasis will be placed on healthy living among urban and rural residents by providing health mentoring and interventions to households and high-risk groups, and by launching programs on weight control, as well as dental and bone health. By 2030, all county-level areas nationwide will be covered by such programs. Appropriate techniques and products for healthy living will be developed and promoted. Effective publicity for core information and health knowledge will be developed. The monitoring of health literacy and healthy living will cover all the country. Health education will be increased and strengthened, and health knowledge will be made available for all, with special focus on children and teenagers. Stressing spiritual awareness, health culture will be nurtured, obsolete habits and customs discarded, and good living habits cultivated. Media institutions at different levels will advocate good health knowledge; health-related broadcasting or TV programs will be actively developed and standardized, and health education expanded via new media.

### Section Two    Promoting School Health Education

Health education will be part of the national curriculum and relevant classes made available for students at all levels as essentials for quality education. Making primary and middle school education a priority, school-based health education will be explored. Subject-based education will be combined with theme-based in-class and outdoor education. This will be advocated at regular and centralized levels. Health education faculties need to be trained, and health education will be conducted in the whole process of vocational training of sports teachers.

## Chapter V    Encouraging Healthy Habits in Individuals

### Section One    Developing Well-balanced Diet

A national nutritional plan will be developed and implemented. Research and nutritional assessments of food (both at farm and table) will be carried out. Nutritional knowledge will be widely disseminated; dietary guidance of population sub-groups publicized; citizens coached to develop healthy dietary habits; and healthy culinary culture promoted. Nutrition monitoring will be established to monitor progress, with nutritional interventions in key areas and population groups, specifically focusing on micronutrient deficiency and excessive intake of high-calorie foods, such as fat, to improve problematic diets. Clinical nutritional interventions will be carried out. Meanwhile, guidance to schools, kindergartens, and nursing homes will be strengthened. Demonstration health canteens and restaurants will be nominated. By 2030, nutritional knowledge and literacy rates will be significantly improved, incidence of nutrition deficiency greatly reduced, average daily salt intake reduced by 20%, and increase in the overweight and obese population slowed down.

### Section Two  Tightening Tobacco and Alcohol Control

The World Health Organization Framework Convention on Tobacco Control will be implemented fully, with tobacco prices tightly controlled through pricing, taxation and other legal means. Advocacy and education on tobacco control will be launched, smoke-free environments actively built, and supervision and law enforcement of smoking bans in public places enhanced. The smoking ban in public places will be fully enforced, and the indoor smoking ban will gradually cover all public venues. Officials will take the lead in implementing the smoking ban in public places, and Party and government buildings will become smoke-free areas. Smoking cessation services will be strengthened. By 2030, the population of smokers aged 15 or above will be reduced to 20%. Education on alcohol control will be intensified to control excessive alcohol intake and reduce alcohol abuse. Monitoring of harmful alcohol use will be stepped up.

### Section Three  Protecting Mental Health

Mental health services will be further developed and orderly managed. Mental health advocacy will be strengthened to increase understanding of mental health. Common mental disorders, psychological or behavioral problems, such as depression and anxiety, will be targeted and intervened with, and more emphasis placed on early detection and intervention for mental disorders in priority groups. The national registry will be improved, and rescue and medical aid given to patients with severe mental illnesses. Community-based rehabilitation for patients with mental illnesses will be fully encouraged. Overall ability to implement interventions in emergency cases of psychological crisis will be enhanced. By 2030, competence in identifying and intervening in common mental disorders will be greatly enhanced.

### Section Four  Reducing Unsafe Sexual Behaviors and Drug Abuse

Comprehensive harnessing of social security will be strengthened. Education and intervention on sexual morality, sexual health and safe sex (focusing on teenagers, young women and migrants) will help high-risk groups reduce unplanned pregnancy and curb sexually transmitted diseases. Drug related harm will be actively addressed, with knowledge and treatment options improved. Nationwide drug-use services will be strengthened to provide drug addicts with access to early detection services and treatment. Drug maintenance therapy for detoxification will be linked with community-based drug rehabilitation as well as compulsory rehabilitation services. A comprehensive rehabilitation mode will be established, offering a variety of services including abstinence, psychological rehabilitation, employment support and return to the community, to minimize social harm caused by drugs.

## Chapter VI    Improving Physical Fitness for All

### Section One    Improving Physical Fitness Services

Public facilities and infrastructure for physical fitness services will be uniformly planned and developed. More walking paths, bike lanes, public fitness centers, sports parks and community sports grounds will be built. By 2030, networks of public sports facilities at village, township and county levels will be established, with sports ground of no less than 2.3 $m^2$ per capita. In urban areas, sports facilities will be within 15 minutes' walking distance. Public sports facilities will be free or at less charge, and all public sports facilities and those of non-government institutions, which meet criteria for opening, should be made available for public use. Networks of public fitness clubs will be set up, and support and guidance provided to support the development of community-based sports organizations.

### Section Two    Launching a Nationwide Fitness Campaign

A nationwide plan for public physical exercise will be continuously made, knowledge of physical exercises and body fitness publicized, and public fitness exercises made routine. Mentoring of social sports activities will be organized to provide guidance in public fitness exercises. National criteria on physical exercise will be introduced. Common fitness and leisure exercises will be developed to enrich and improve public fitness. Exercises favored by communities will be adopted and developed. Sports events suitable for specific population groups or geographic areas will be encouraged, and traditional, cultural and historic sports exercises such as Tai Chi or Qigong will be supported and encouraged.

### Section Three　Integrating Sports Exercises with Medical Care and Strengthening Non-medical Health Interventions

Guidelines on sports and fitness exercises will be published, with a database of prescriptions for different population groups, different contexts, and different physical statuses established to develop an innovative mode of disease management and healthcare services by combining sports exercise with medical care. In this way, public fitness exercises can play an active role in improved health as well as the prevention and rehabilitation of chronic diseases. Platforms or centers for fitness technology innovations and supporting fitness services will be created. Physical fitness assessments will be carried out; monitoring systems for fitness and health will be improved; big data on national physical fitness monitoring will be developed and applied; and risk assessment of sports exercises carried out.

### Section Four　Promoting Physical Exercise among Priority Groups

Tailored intervention plans will be made on fitness and health of priority groups, such as teenagers, women, elderly, occupational groups and the disabled. Plans on promoting sports among teenagers will be implemented to cultivate teenagers' interests in sports. Teenagers will master at least one sports skill, and students will spend no less than one hour doing sports exercises on campus every day. By 2030, 100% of sports facilities and devices at schools will meet national standards; young students will attend moderate-intensity physical exercises at least three times a week; and at least 25% of students will maintain excellent health status and physical fitness according to national standards. With enhanced mentoring, women, elderly and occupational groups will be mobilized to participate in public fitness exercises. Working interval fitness programs will be adopted; newly built working infrastructures will have proper space designated for fitness exercises. Rehabilitative sports and fitness exercises for the disabled will be widely promoted.

## Part III　Optimizing Healthcare Services

## Chapter VII　Promoting Universal Access to Public Health Services

### Section One　Preventing and Controlling Major Illnesses

A comprehensive strategy for prevention and control of chronic diseases will be implemented. National demonstration sites for such diseases will be further developed. Early screening and diagnosis for chronic diseases will be strengthened.

For areas with high cancer prevalence, early diagnosis and treatment programs for major cancers will be launched. Opportunistic screening for cancers, stroke and coronary heart disease will be encouraged. Management and intervention programs for hypertension and diabetes will cover all target demographics. Appropriate technologies for early diagnosis and treatment for major chronic diseases such as cancer and strokes will be included in diagnosis and treatment routines. Control and prevention of common illnesses among students, such as short-sightedness and obesity, will be intensified. By 2030, chronic disease care and management will cover lifelong needs of all people. The overall five-year survival rate of cancer patients will increase by 15%. Dental health will be improved, with the prevalence of cavities among the under 12-years kept within 25%.

Control and prevention of major infectious diseases will be strengthened. Early warning systems for infectious diseases will be improved. The Expanded Program on Immunization will be continuously implemented. Inoculation rate of vaccines included in the national immunization program for eligible children will be maintained at a relatively high level. Compensation and insurance systems will be developed for vaccination anomalies. HIV/AIDs detection, antiviral therapy and follow-up management will be further improved. Nucleic acid testing will be performed fully on blood for clinical use and efforts will be made to prevent mother-to-child transmission of HIV. HIV prevalence will be kept at a low level. A comprehensive service model for tuberculosis prevention and control will be established. Screening and monitoring of multi-drug resistant tuberculosis will be enhanced. Diagnosis and treatment of tuberculosis will be standardized. Prevalence of tuberculosis will continue to decrease. Epidemics caused by influenza, foot-and-mouth disease, dengue fever and measles will be effectively dealt with. A control and prevention strategy of schistosomiasis will be continuously adopted with a focus on control of the source of infection. All counties suffering from epidemics will meet standards for eliminating schistosomiasis. Achievements made in eliminating malaria will be consolidated. All counties suffering from epidemics will control prevalence of major parasitic diseases such as hydatidosis. Major endemic diseases will be contained or eliminated, so that such diseases can no longer pose major threats to people's health. Control and prevention of sudden outbreaks of acute infectious diseases will be stepped up. Active measures will be introduced for controlling imported acute infectious diseases. Control and prevention of fulminating infectious diseases such as plague will be strengthened. Infection source of major animal-borne diseases will be tightly controlled.

### Section Two    Improving Management of Family Planning Services

Policymaking processes and systems on population and development will be improved, and policies beneficial for more balanced demographics formulated. Management of family planning services will be reformed to deliver household-based services and build family development policies for reproductive care, child raising, youth development, elderly care, and disability care. The public should be guided to make planned and responsible birth decisions. There will be more well-developed policies concerning technological services for family planning and more investment in techniques supporting second births. Policies on making informed choices will be fully implemented with contraceptive and reproductive health knowledge widely publicized. Allowance, support and special aid programs for families practicing family planning policies will be improved, and dynamic adjustment of the allowances made. Targeted management will be upheld and improved. Long-term systems will be developed to advocate and publicize family planning policy, and to better manage, regulate, serve and promote related work. A monitoring system for newborns will be developed. Continuous efforts will be made to bring the gender ratio at birth under control. By 2030, a natural balance of gender ratio at birth will be achieved.

### Section Three   Equity of Primary Public Healthcare Services

An essential public healthcare service package and major public health service package will be implemented and improved continuously. Studies on the economic burden of diseases will be conducted to make appropriate adjustments to the funding of healthcare packages. Efforts will be made to enrich and expand healthcare services, improve service quality, provide equal access to primary public healthcare services for urban and rural residents, and ensure migrants equal access to both primary public healthcare and family planning services.

## Chapter VIII   Delivery of High Quality and Efficient Medical Care

### Section One   Improving Medical Care Delivery Systems

Integrated medical care delivery systems with complete structures, clear and complementary functions, close coordination, and high performance will be put into place. Primary medical care resources at county and city levels will be planned and distributed based on population and distance to care facilities to ensure universal access to primary medical care services. At provincial regions or above, resources will be allocated on a regional basis, and regional resource pooling and sharing will be encouraged. Balanced allocation of quality medical and health resources will be achieved, with equal access to high quality acute, emergency and specialist care. Based on current health facilities, a group of national centers of clinical excellence with global influence will be developed. A group of regional medical centers and clinical specialties networks will be established to enhance regional medical delivery capacity and competence, and to promote coordinated medical development in areas such as the Beijing-Tianjin-Hebei region and the Yangtze River economic zone. Post-acute medical care facilities, such as rehabilitation, elderly care, long-term care, chronic disease management and hospice palliative care facilities will also be developed. Medical programs for poverty reduction will be implemented, with more medical infrastructure projects needing to be launched in central and western poverty-stricken regions, to increase medical service capacity and protect the poor's health. By 2030, all communities will be within 15 minutes distance of primary medical care facilities, and registered nurses per 1,000 permanent residents will reach 4.7.

### Section Two    Innovating Medical Care Supply Modes

A "3-in-1" control and prevention mechanism for major diseases will be established. It will incorporate professional public health facilities, general and specialty hospitals, and primary medical care facilities, which will share information and coordinate control, prevention and day-to-day management of chronic diseases to achieve integration in prevention and clinical care. Various medical care facilities with different ownership at different levels will collaborate and coordinate with clear targets and defined roles and functions. Care networks, operational mechanisms and incentives will be constantly explored. Primary medical care providers will acquire gate-keeping function for residents. Contract-based care provision by family doctors will be further implemented and improved. Mature mechanisms of coordinated care will be explored, including the gate-keeping functions of primary care providers, two-way referrals, vertical coordination, and the separation of acute and chronic care. Integrated curative, rehabilitative and long-term care will be soundly developed. Bigger public hospitals at Grade 3 will be encouraged to reduce outpatient encounters and focus on acute and emergency care, as well as complex and specialist care. Medical complex or hospital groups will be encouraged to explore coordination between care facilities and to improve system-wide performance. The integration of military and civil medical care delivery will be accelerated; military hospitals need to play a bigger role in serving the people.

### Section Three    Improving Medical Care Quality and Competence

A world-class quality management and control system for medical care will be developed with Chinese characteristics. A three-tier quality control network covering most specialties will be established at city, provincial and national levels, with a batch of international standards and norms. Information platforms will be set up for quality control and management, with precise and real-time management and control, covering all aspects of all hospitals to improve medical care quality and safety. Efforts will be made to increase homogeneity of hospital care quality, and reduce readmission rates, and antibiotics used to catch up with advanced world levels. Clinical pathway management will be implemented to reduce clinical variations, optimize care process and improve patients' experiences. Programs on rational drug use, clinical blood safety and mutual recognition of test results will be further implemented. Medical ethics needs to be encouraged to build good doctor-patient relationships. Crimes, especially violence against doctors, will be cracked down on, with legal backup, to protect the personal safety of medical professionals.

## Chapter IX    Letting Traditional Chinese Medicine Play Its Unique Role

### Section One    Improving the Capacity of Traditional Chinese Medicine

Projects bolstering TCM with clinical advantages will be launched to enhance research on the superior effects of TCM in treating specific conditions. TCM will be better combined with Western medicine to enhance treatment of major, complex and critical conditions as well as acute diseases. Non-medicine therapies will be developed to play a role in preventing and treating common and chronic illnesses. Rehabilitation with TCM will be encouraged. Primary medical care with TCM will be developed to cover both urban and rural communities. General care departments providing TCM will be set up in all township and community health centers. Appropriate technologies will be promoted, and all primary health facilities will be able to deliver TCM. Ethnic medicines will also be encouraged. By 2030, TCM will play a key role in preventing illnesses, treating major illnesses and in rehabilitation.

### Section Two    Developing Preventive and Health Maintenance Services Based on Traditional Chinese Medicine

Projects on TCM-based preventive care will be implemented to explore the strength of TCM in health management. TCM-based health maintenance models will be explored, incorporating health culture, health management and health insurance. Social enterprises will be encouraged to open TCM-based healthcare centers providing standard services to develop healthcare service quickly. The service scope of TCM hospitals will be expanded to offer TCM-based preventive interventions, such as health counseling, assessment, recuperation, and follow-up care. TCM hospitals and doctors are encouraged to provide expertise support, such as health consultancy and recuperation care, for such TCM-based healthcare centers. National programs on TCM promotion will be launched to advocate TCM knowledge and easy-to-understand healthcare techniques and methods. Efforts will be made to protect and carry on the intangible cultural heritage of TCM, as well as to innovate and develop TCM-based health care.

### Section Three    Promoting Preservation and Innovation of Traditional Chinese Medicine

Projects promoting TCM need to be launched to draw special attention to the studies of classic TCM books and reuse of historical theories, trends, approaches and methods. Academic thinking and clinical experiences of well-known and senior TCM experts will be carried forward to extract indigenous clinical techniques and prescriptions, and to preserve and promote TCM. Intellectual property will be established to protect TCM. A list of protected TCM patents will be set up. TCM prescriptions will be studied with the assistance of modern technologies. TCM technologies and new therapeutics for major, complex acute and chronic diseases will be strengthened. TCM theories and clinical practices will be further developed. The TCM market will be expanded, and world-known Chinese brands and multinational companies covering the whole production chain will be created to introduce TCM to the world. Major TCM resources and biodiversity will be preserved. Surveys and dynamic monitoring of TCM resources will be implemented. Plantation bases for large quantities, genuine, or endangered TCM seedlings will be built. Monitoring data of TCM markets will be provided in real time. TCM plantation will be encouraged to pursue green policies.

## Chapter X    Improving Healthcare Services for Priority Groups

### Section One    Improving Maternal and Child Health

Plans to ensure mother and baby safety will be implemented, and healthy births and rearing encouraged. Public subsidies will be made available for hospital deliveries, and free primary care services will be provided for pregnant women for all their pregnancy. Birth defects will be controlled and prevented, and a prevention and control system will be built to cover pre-pregnancy, pregnancy, and post-natal care for both the urban and rural population. A healthy childhood plan will be initiated to support early childhood development, develop pediatrics, strengthen prevention of major children's diseases, expand disease detection services for neonates, and continue to support nutrition projects in priority areas. More women will be screened for common gynecological diseases to ensure early diagnosis and treatment. Projects for protecting maternal and child health, and family planning services will be launched to enhance rescue, acute and emergency care competence.

### Section Two  Promoting Healthy Aging

The development of medical and health care systems for the elderly will expand to communities and households. Coordination between medical facilities and nursing homes will be sought, and nursing facilities will support medical services. Coordinated development of TCM and elderly care will be encouraged, to provide integrated care for the elderly, covering hospital care, rehabilitative care, home care and palliative care. Chronic disease management will link with home care, community care and nursing care. The private sector is also encouraged to open facilities providing both medical and nursing care. Common geriatric illnesses or major chronic diseases will be closely supervised alongside intervention where necessary to develop a holistic health management system for the elderly. Mental health care will be encouraged, and effective interventions for diseases such as dementia will be introduced. Long-term home-based care for the elderly will be developed. Policies for subsidizing the elderly at an advanced age or for disabled elderly with financial difficulties will be fully established. Long-term nursing care insurance programs with multiple-layer designs will be established. More policies will be introduced to make essential drugs more readily accessible for the elderly.

### Section Three  Maintaining Health of the Disabled

Regulations on prevention of disability and the rehabilitation for disabled people will be issued. Medical financial aid for low-income disabled people will also be increased, and eligible medical rehabilitation services for the disabled will be covered by basic medical insurance schemes. A medical assistance system will be established for disabled children. Local governments will be encouraged to subsidize equipment to assist the disabled. Rehabilitation for the disabled will be included in the basic public service package. Tailored rehabilitation will be given to those who need it, and poor or severely disabled people will be provided with primary rehabilitation services. Barrier-free facilities will be developed in medical institutions, and medical services for the disabled will be improved. Rehabilitation systems will be further developed. More rehabilitation and nursing home facilities for the disabled will be built. Two-way referrals will be made possible between medical facilities and rehabilitation centers. Primary medical care providers will give priority to contract-based services for disabled people, providing them with primary medical care and public health management. A national action plan for the prevention of disabilities will be introduced, and public awareness of disability prevention will be raised.

Disability prevention measures targeting the life cycle of all the population will be carried out to effectively control incidences and the development of disabilities. Diseases or risk factors that may cause disabilities will be better controlled. National pilot programs on disability control and prevention will be introduced. Prevention and treatment for the deaf and blind will be continued.

## Part IV    Improving Health Security

## Chapter XI    Strengthening the Medical Insurance System

### Section One    Developing Universal Health Coverage

Multi-level health insurance systems will be developed and improved, and be dominated by basic health insurance, and supplemented by commercial and other forms of insurance. Urban and rural basic health insurance schemes and management systems will be integrated. Sustainable financing and benefit adjustment mechanisms of basic health insurance schemes will be improved to achieve medium to long-term actuarial balance. The premium collection mechanism will be improved to keep organizational and personal contributions at appropriate levels, and rationally determine the share from public funds and private contributions. Individual accounts of the basic medical insurance for urban employees will be reformed to cover outpatient care. Insurance policies for major and catastrophic illness will be further reformed, and the link between basic health insurance schemes, insurance for major illnesses for urban and rural residents, commercial health insurance and medical financial assistance strengthened. A mature form of universal health coverage will be developed by 2030.

### Section Two    Improving Health Insurance Management

Budget management of health insurance schemes will be strictly implemented. Payment reforms will be launched on the active promotion of case payment and capitation, and on the exploration of diagnosis related groups (DRGs) as well as pay for performance methods, to launch multiple payment methods under global budget management. Negotiation and risk sharing arrangements between health insurance organizations and medical organizations need to be improved. Policies on medical billing and making-claims at localities other than home counties, cities or provinces will be quickly implemented. On site billing and claims by retired inpatients in their non-home province, and direct billing claims for inpatients meeting referral requirements will be made possible. Intelligent monitoring of health insurance schemes will be implemented, and supervision of designated health services will be expanded to individual medical professionals. Commercial insurance companies will be encouraged to engage in management of basic health insurance schemes. Basic standards and specifications for basic health insurance schemes will be developed and applied. Management of universal health coverage will be well developed and achieve high performance by 2030.

### Section Three    Promoting Commercial Health Insurance

Favorable policies including taxation will be introduced to encourage enterprises and individuals to join commercial health insurance and other supplementary insurance schemes. More health insurance products will be provided, and insurance policies related to health management services developed. Cooperation between commercial insurance companies and health facilities, as well as examination centers and nursing facilities, will be facilitated. New forms of health organizations such as health maintenance organizations will be developed. By 2030, a modern commercial health insurance industry will be developed, with an increased share of commercial claims in total health expenditure.

## Chapter XII    Improving the Drug Supply Security System

### Section One    Deepening Reforms on Drug and Medical Device Circulation Systems

Upstream and downstream drug and medical device services in the supply chain will be expanded to develop a modern system. Medical e-commerce will be standardized, with drug circulation channels and development models enriched. Modern logistic techniques will be promoted. Modern TCM distribution networks and tracing systems will be improved. Health facilities will play a pivotal role in drug procurement, with joint procurement encouraged. The national drug price negotiation system will be improved, and a tracing system for pricing set up. Availability guarantees and warning of drugs shortages will be developed, and drug reserve and emergency supply chains established. Urban and rural modern drug circulation networks will be built to improve drug security at community level and remote areas.

### Section Two    Meliorating National Drug Policy

The national essential drug system will be consolidated and developed to ensure special groups' access to essential drugs. Drug policy on free treatment will be improved, and free drug supply for prevention and treatment of special diseases such as HIV will be increased. Children's drug supply will be guaranteed. Drug supply for rare diseases will be ensured. A comprehensive clinical evaluation system will be built with a focus on essential drugs. Drug pricing systems will be improved under regulation of the central government and with support of the market. Linkage of pricing, health insurance, and purchasing policies will be strengthened. Category-based management of drugs will be adhered to. Price regulation for expensive medical consumables and drugs with insufficient market competition will be strengthened, and a public drug price monitoring and information disclosure system will be set up. Standards for drug payments by health insurance schemes will be formulated.

## Part V    Building a Healthy Environment

## Chapter XIII    Deepening Patriotic Public Health Campaigns

### Section One    Comprehensively Improving Urban and Rural Environment and Sanitary Conditions

Urban and rural environment and sanitation will continued to be enhanced, with better infrastructure and long-term mechanisms to solve environmental and sanitary problems. Residential environment will be managed well in rural areas with improved garbage disposal and proper domestic sewage treatment. Clean energy will be promoted. By 2030, more rural areas will have beautiful homes suitable for growing old with improved sanitary conditions in residential environments. Rural residents and nature will be developed in a harmonious manner. Projects to ensure the safety of drinking water in rural areas will be implemented, and efforts made to expand urban water supply to rural areas. Centralized water supply in rural areas will be increased, as will access to tap water, better water quality, and adequate water supply. A comprehensive rural water safety system will be built from source to tap. The building of safe public toilets will be accelerated to ensure they can be accessed by all rural residents by 2030. Prevention and control strategy for diseases, with a focus on environmental management will be implemented. By 2030, the share of national sanitary cities will reach 50%, and provinces (autonomous regions, municipalities directly under the Central Government) with favorable conditions will have 100% coverage.

### Section Two    Building Healthy Cities, Towns and Villages

"Building healthy cities, towns and villages" is an important project for healthy China. Land supply for public health infrastructure will be secured, and health-related infrastructure, planning and standards improved. Health will be included in urban and rural planning, construction and management process, and urban development and residents' health will be improved in a coordinated manner. Based on local health needs, plans for healthy cities, towns and villages will be developed and implemented. Healthy communities, healthy enterprises and healthy households will be launched to increase social participation. Also, the building of healthy schools will be emphasized, with the enhancement of student health risk factor monitoring and evaluation, alongside school food-safety management, infectious disease control and other related policies. By 2030, a group of healthy cities, towns and villages will be built for nationwide demonstration.

## Chapter XIV   Strengthening Management of Environmental Problems Affecting Health

### Section One   Strengthening Prevention and Management of Air, Water and Land Pollution

Joint control and prevention, and co-governance of water sources will be strengthened, with a focus on improving the environment. Targets for environmental quality control and strict environmental protection regulations will be implemented to solve outstanding environmental issues that affect people's health. Environmental impact assessment of the development of new industrial parks, districts and cities will be reinforced, with strict control of approval of construction projects and intensive use of preventive measures. Regional measures on air pollution control and prevention will be promoted with regular regional cooperation. A joint warning mechanism will be enhanced to handle heavily polluted air and other conditions. Goals for city air quality will be fully monitored, and city air quality improved significantly. Water source safety management will be developed. Groundwater management and protection will be strengthened, and management and pollution control in excessively pumped areas of ground water will be enhanced. A national land quality monitoring network will be built, with a soil quality assessment system for construction land established, and soil pollution control and repair implemented. With the focus on arable land, categorical management of farmland will be implemented. Full measures for pollution control and prevention will be taken to effectively protect ecosystems and genetic diversity. Noise control and prevention will be strengthened.

## Section Two   Implementing Comprehensive Plan on Discharge Control of Industrial Pollution Sources

A licensing policy for industrial pollution sources will be fully implemented. Self-monitoring and information disclosure of enterprises will be promoted, with disposal accounts established to ensure licensed discharge. Highly pollutant and risky techniques, products and devices will be eliminated quickly. Special pollution control projects for industrial agglomeration areas will be carried out. Renovation projects for discharge control of industries will be accelerated, with a focus on steel, cement and petrochemical industries.

## Section Three   Building Comprehensive Environment and Health Monitoring, Survey and Risk Assessment System

A comprehensive environment and health management system will be gradually established, with health surveys conducted in key areas, fields and industries. A comprehensive monitoring network and risk assessment system will be established to cover pollution sources, environmental quality, and health outcomes. Environment and health risk management will be implemented. Areas of high health risk will be identified, the health impact of environmental pollution on the population studied, and policy on health impact evaluation for major projects in high risk areas will be developed. Environmental health risk communication mechanisms will be set up. A unified platform for publicizing environmental information will be established, and mandatory information disclosure fully launched. Air quality of counties and higher levels will be monitored, and information publicized.

# Chapter XV   Ensuring Food and Drug Safety

## Section One   Strengthening Food Safety Regulation

Food safety standards will be improved to comply with international standards. Food safety risk monitoring and assessment will be strengthened. Nationwide reporting on food safety-risk monitoring and food-borne diseases will be fully established by 2030. Standardized and hygienic agricultural production will be encouraged. Risk assessment of the quality and safety of agricultural products will be carried out, comprehensive management of pesticide residue and heavy metal pollution conducted, and actions taken on animal antibiotics control. Supervision and regulation of the geographical origin of food will be stepped up, and market access control of agriculture products established. An edible agricultural product tracing mechanism will be developed, as will uniform and authoritative food safety regulation armed with a professional inspection taskforce. Regular testing capacity will be improved, and coverage of sample-based checking will be expanded. Regulation of online food businesses will be reinforced. Management of the entrance of imported food will be strengthened, and inspection of safety testing for food with foreign origin conducted. Construction projects of designated ports for imported food will be orderly launched. Local governments will be encouraged to develop demonstration zones on safety and quality control of foods and agricultural products for export. And a food safety credit system will be developed, and policy on food safety information disclosure implemented. A whole-process regulation system will be established, covering activities from production to consumption. Every procedure from farm to table will be closely controlled to provide safe and quality food for consumers.

### Section Two   Strengthening Drug Safety Regulation

Policies on drug (medical device) assessment and regulation will be further reformed, a clinical-effectiveness oriented regulatory system established, and drug (medical device) regulatory standards upgraded. The assessment and approval process for innovative and urgently-demanded clinical drugs (and medical devices) will be accelerated, and bioavailability and bioequivalence study of generics encouraged. The national drug standard system will be improved, medical device standards raised, and global standards of TCM developed. Drug regulation will be enhanced, and regulatory chains on the whole process and all products formed. Medical devices and cosmetics will be closely regulated.

## Chapter XVI   Improving Public Safety Systems

### Section One   Improving Production Safety and Occupational Health

Production safety will be enhanced, and double defense of risk level control and hidden hazard screening established to effectively reduce the frequency and harm of major accidents. Industries will strengthen their ability to regulate and supervise themselves, while enterprises will take the main responsibility; source control of occupational diseases will be strengthened. Production safety supervision and management of mines, dangerous chemicals and other key industries will be enhanced. A census on occupational diseases will be carried out, and tailored health interventions developed. Occupational safety and health standard systems will be further improved, and network on monitoring, reporting and managing of major occupational diseases and risk factors established to control high incidence of pneumoconiosis and occupational poisoning. Tiered and targeted regulation will be established, with special attention given to enterprises with high risk of occupational disease hazards. Ear-marked actions on occupational disease hazards of key industries will be launched. Policies on occupational disease reporting will be strengthened, and employers encouraged to promote occupational health education to control and prevent work-related injuries and occupational diseases. National per capita radiation dose control will be implemented, with radiation harm in radiotherapy controlled and prevented.

### Section Two    Enhancing Road Traffic Safety

Design, planning and construction of road traffic safety facilities will be supported. Highway safety and life protection projects will be launched to control hidden traffic dangers on highways. Road transport safety management will be strictly implemented together with the enhancement of self-discipline in enterprises. Transportation enterprises will be held accountable for safe production. Supervision of safe operations and support of safe production will be enhanced. Regulation for road traffic safety will be further strengthened, standards for vehicle safety techniques raised, and comprehensive quality of automobile drivers, passengers and pedestrians improved. By 2030, deaths caused by road traffic accidents per 10,000 vehicles will decrease by 30%.

### Section Three    Preventing and Reducing Injuries

A comprehensive monitoring system for injuries will be established, and technical guidelines and standards for the interventions of major injuries established. Prevention and intervention of children and elderly injuries will be strengthened; cases of traffic injury, drowning of children and accidental falls among the elderly reduced; and safety standards for children's toys and supplies raised. Suicide and accidental poisoning will be prevented and related cases reduced. Mandatory reporting on consumer goods quality and safety accidents will be enforced, and a product injury monitoring system established. Extra efforts will be taken to strengthen quality and safety supervision in key areas to reduce injuries from consumer goods.

### Section Four    Improving Emergency Management Capacity

Safety awareness education will be conducted among all people. A mechanism for the responsibility in construction and maintenance for urban and rural public firefighting facilities will be clarified and improved, and coverage of urban and rural firefighting facilities reach will 100% by 2030. Disaster prevention capacity and emergency response will be improved. Health emergency response systems will be improved, and capacity of early prevention, timely detection, quick response and effective action enhanced. Emergency medical rescue systems with land, sea and air tactics covering all health facilities including military ones will be established to improve emergency medical rescue capability. By 2030, a more comprehensive emergency medical rescue network will be established, with improved response and rescue capacity equal to that of developed countries. Emergency medical rescue systems and their performance will be further improved. By 2030, road traffic injuries and deaths will be reduced to the levels of moderately developed countries.

### Section Five  Improving Public Health System at Ports

Control and prevention system of infectious diseases at ports will be established, with intelligent monitoring and early warning of global epidemics and accurate quarantine measures, in addition to a prevention and control system handling hazardous nuclear, biological and chemical factors in modern ports. Border public health emergency response systems will be established, based on source control and domestic-foreign joint control and prevention mechanisms. Monitoring and control mechanism of major infectious diseases and port pathogens will be implemented to actively prevent, control and respond to foreign public health emergencies. Core capabilities will be continually consolidated to create world-class healthy airports and ports. An international travel and health information network will be improved to provide timely and effective international travel health guidance; to build a world-class international travel health service system; and to protect the health and safety of cross-border travelers.

Control and prevention capability of plant and animal epidemics will be improved. Risk assessment and access control of quarantine inspection on inbound animals and plants will be implemented. Efforts should be made for detention, detection and identification, elimination, monitoring and control of imported diseases, epidemics and hazardous life. An accountability system will be enhanced to investigate individual or institutional buyers and carriers of plants and animals to prevent and control international plant and animal-borne epidemics and cross-border transmission. Biological safety inspection mechanisms in gateways will be enhanced to effectively prevent the loss of species and invasion of foreign species.

## Part VI  Developing Healthcare Industry

### Chapter XVII  Optimizing Pluralistic Structure of Medical Care Services

Policies will be further optimized to support the development of non-profit private health services, and treatment for profit private hospitals and public hospitals will be equal. Physicians are encouraged to use their free time to practice in primary health institutions or to open clinics, as are retired physicians. The establishment of private clinics will not be bound by regional health planning. Unreasonable restrictions and invisible barriers for private health services will be eliminated. Scope for health services with foreign investment will be expanded gradually. Public procurement of services will be increased. The insurance sectors will be supported in investing in and opening health services and non-public hospitals will be encouraged to develop to a higher level and achieve economies of scale. Development of professional hospital management groups will be encouraged. Government regulation, industry self-discipline and social supervision will be enhanced to support the development of non-public health services.

## Chapter XVIII   Developing New Types of Health Services

Nursing care, tourism, the Internet, fitness and leisure, and food sectors will be integrated with the health sector to develop new health industries, businesses and care models. Development of Internet-based health services, physical checkups and consultations will be promoted to foster a personalized health management service industry. Wearable devices, intelligent electronic products and mobile health will be explored and developed. Maternal and childcare services will be standardized. Health culture and sports rehabilitation industry will be cultivated. The healthcare tourism industry will be standardized, and medical tourism destinations with global competitiveness developed. TCM health tourism will be promoted. Efforts will be made to nurture the positive development of leading brands of healthcare businesses and to support the development of micro, small and medium-sized enterprises.

Development of professional medical centers including medical laboratories, health imaging centers, pathological diagnosis and blood dialysis centers will be guided and supported. Development of third party healthcare evaluation, health management services, as well as health market research and consultation services will be supported. The private sector is encouraged to provide food and drug testing services. Science and technology intermediary systems will be developed, and professional and market-oriented transformation of medical knowledge greatly promoted.

## Chapter XIX   Promoting Fitness, Leisure and Sports Industry

The market environment will be improved and pluralistic ownership supported.

The private sector will be encouraged to construct and operate fitness and leisure facilities. Reforms in sports associations and separation of management rights from sport organization ownership will be launched. Sports resources will be made available to the public, with innovative fitness leisure sports popularized. Policy and mechanisms in favor of public procurement of sports services will be developed, to create a comprehensive fitness and leisure service system. The development of various forms of fitness clubs will be encouraged, amateur sports enriched, and consumption-based sports including ice and snow, mountain, water, automobile, aviation, extreme, equestrian, and other fashionable leisure sports developed. Fitness and leisure industry demonstration zones and industrial belts with regional characteristics will be created.

## Chapter XX    Promoting Development of Medical Industry

### Section One    Strengthening Medical Technology Innovation

A system of innovation will be developed to promote innovation and transformation, with coordination between government, industry, universities, research institutions and users. Innovation capacity of patent drugs, new TCM, new type of formulations, and advanced medical equipment will be built. Development of generics for expired patent drugs of major diseases will be promoted. Biological medicine, new types of chemical drugs, quality TCM, medical devices with high performance, new packaging materials and drug manufacturing devices will be developed. Major drugs will be industrialized, medical devices transformed and upgraded quickly, and international competitiveness of medical diagnostics and supplies with independent intellectual property rights will be developed. Business of rehabilitation assistive devices will be developed speedily, and independent innovation capability increased. Quality standard systems and quality control technology will be improved by launching projects on green and intelligent transformation and upgrading. By 2030, quality standards of drug and medical equipment will fully meet international standards.

### Section Two    Enhancing Development of Healthcare Industry

Development of professional medical industrial parks, and formation of business alliances or consortiums will be supported to build innovation-driven, green and low-carbon, intelligent, efficient and advanced manufacturing systems; increase industrial concentration; and enhance the supply capacity of high-end products. Trade in healthcare services will be strongly promoted to help pharmaceutical enterprises go abroad to intensify international collaboration, and to improve their international competitiveness. By 2030, global market share of new drugs and medical devices with independent intellectual property rights will be substantially increased, and the localized production of high-end medical devices greatly promoted. The medical industry will develop at a medium-to-high speed and march toward medium and high-end markets, so that China will become a country with a strong pharmaceutical industry. The pharmaceutical distribution industry will be transformed and upgraded to reduce intermediate links in distribution, improve market concentration, and form a batch of large multinational pharmaceutical distribution enterprises.

## Part VII   Improving Supportive and Guarantee Mechanisms

## Chapter XXI   Deepening Reforms in Institutional Arrangements

### Section One   Putting Health in All Policies

Cross-ministerial and industrial communication and cooperation will be strengthened to form a joint health promotion force. Evaluation system for conducting health impact assessment will be established to systemically assess the health impact of economic and social development plans and policies, as well as major projects. Associated supervision mechanisms will be developed. Channels of public participation will be opened, and social supervision strengthened.

### Section Two   Deepening Healthcare System Reforms

The establishment of a more mature primary healthcare system will be facilitated, effectively maintaining the welfare of government-sponsored healthcare services; containing unreasonable growth of medical cost; and continuing to improve people's access to essential healthcare services. Administration will be kept away from health institutions, while management and operation of government-owned hospitals will be separated to ensure proper relationships between publicly-owned health institutions and the government, and to establish modern management systems in public hospitals. Health administration powers between central and local governments and governments at all levels will be clearly distributed to set up a territory-based and sector-wide health management structure. Military hospitals will be covered by urban public hospital reform initiatives and national reform programs for developing tiered healthcare delivery systems. A sector-wide supervision system will be built covering all aspects of health and family planning.

### Section Three   Improving Health Financing Mechanisms

Public input in health will be increased and relevant mechanisms improved. Budgetary structures of public finance will be adjusted and optimized. Total public health spending increased, the share of financing responsibilities between the central and local governments clarified, and public financing for primary healthcare services ensured. Economically underdeveloped areas will be favored in the transfer payment plans of the central government, and effectiveness of funding use improved. Result-based health financing will be established and monitoring and evaluation of health input performance launched. Social organizations and enterprises will be fully mobilized to form a diversified health financing pattern. Financial institutions will innovate products and services and improve supportive measures. The development of charity, including social and personal donations as well as mutual assistance, will be encouraged.

### Section Four   Speeding up Transformation of Government Functions

Decentralization and reduction of administrative interference, power delegation and regulation, and optimization of public services will be further promoted. Approval policy of drugs and health institutions will be reformed, and opening of health facilities orderly supervised. Health authorities and agencies will abide by the law, and disclose public affairs and information. Regulatory innovation in health care, family planning, sports, food and drug and other health-related fields will be accelerated, with the establishment of pre and post regulatory systems. The "randomized sampling of subjects and inspectors by industrial and commercial agencies and market regulation and publicity of inspection results" will be fully implemented. Comprehensive supervision and inspection systems will be established, and self-discipline and credit systems will be developed. Development of industry associations will be encouraged so that social forces will play a role in supervision. Fair competition will be promoted and health-related industries developed. Public service processes will be simplified, administrative services optimized, and productivity of public services improved.

## Chapter XXII   Developing Human Resources for Health Care

### Section One   Strengthening Health Personnel Training

Health and education policies will be better coordinated, and the supply and demand balance of medical personnel training achieved. Medical education systems will be reformed to speed up the construction of the health education system integrating college education, post-graduate education and continuous education, reflecting features in the health sector. Quality assurance systems in medical education will be improved, with the establishment of health professionals licensing systems equivalent to internationally-recognized health education programs. With a focus on general practitioners, primary healthcare human resources will be cultivated. Training programs of resident and specialist doctors will be improved, and programs for high-level professionals with training in both public health and clinical medicine. Continuous medical education will be strengthened for all medical professionals. More supports will be given to primary healthcare staff and those working in remote areas. Education and training of those specialties in great shortage, such as general medicine, pediatrics, obstetrics, psychiatry, pathology, nursing, midwifery, rehabilitation, and mental health, will be strengthened. Capacity building for interdisciplinary talents including pharmacists and TCM care providers, health emergency staff, and health information specialists will be increased. Training of high-level international academic leaders will be strengthened, and leading experts with global recognition will be cultivated. Professionalism and specialization in health management staff will be enhanced. The range of medical specialties in health education will be adjusted and optimized to meet human resource demands of the healthcare industry. More healthcare talents including nurses, physiotherapists and psychiatrists will be trained. Health education cloud platforms will be established based on national open universities of health and medical care and supported by the Chinese open online courses on health and medical care to provide lifelong training support for health staff. A taskforce of social sports mentors will be built, and a target of 2.3 instructors per 1000 achieved by 2030.

### Section Two    Incentives for Innovative Talents

Health facilities will be given more autonomy in personnel management, and a contract-based employment system implemented, so that flexible employment measures encouraging inward and outward flow of staff can be applied. Policies on the remuneration of primary healthcare staff will be firmly implemented. Medical personnel employment, mobility and practice models will be reformed, with efforts to actively explore self-employed practice, and practice based on contract with health institutions or medical groups organized by physicians. Medical personnel and remuneration-systems characteristic of the health sector will be established. Assessment of nurses, midwives, medical auxiliary staff, health technicians and other professionals will be further improved based on common international practices. Assessment of talented staff will be reformed, with less attention on academic publications, foreign languages and scientific professional titles. Assessment of talented general practitioners will be reformed to meet specialty requirements.

## Chapter XXIII   Promoting Science and Technology Innovation in Health Care

### Section One   Building National Medical Innovation Systems

National clinical research centers and collaborative innovation networks will be developed with significant efforts, and more laboratories, engineering centers and other research bases built. TCM clinical research bases and institutions will be developed from existing facilities, and capacity increased. Distribution and layout of health research and scientific research bases will be optimized. Resource integration and data interchange will be enhanced, with comprehensive integration of national resource platforms, including biomedical big data, biological samples, and laboratory animal resources, etc. Clinical data demonstration centers will be established for cardio-cerebrovascular diseases, cancer, and geriatric diseases, etc. The national project on health and medical for the Chinese Academy of Medical Sciences will be implemented. Construction of biomedical and health industrial bases will be accelerated, high-tech healthcare enterprises fostered, and several medical research and health innovation centers established. Integration among healthcare delivery, health research and development, and the health industry will be enhanced. Effective cooperation among health facilities, research institutes, universities and enterprises will be encouraged. A platform for transformation and promotion of medical research and development results will be developed to facilitate transformation and promotion of innovations. Better incentives for medical innovation and application-oriented assessment measures will be designed. Scientific research bases, bio-safety, technology assessment, medical research standard, ethics and scientific integrity, and intellectual property rights will all be improved. Integration of science and health policies will be strengthened; civilian and military health research coordinated; central and provincial cooperation also strengthened. Capacity for fundamental frontier research, key common research, public welfare research and strategic high-tech research will be increased.

### Section Two   Promoting Medical Science and Technology Progress

Major scientific and technological projects and programs in areas including brain science, brain-like intelligence technology, and health protection, etc. will be initiated. Ear-marked major national science and technology projects will be promoted, as will ear-marked R&D programs and other major science plans. Advanced medical technologies such as omics technology, stem cell technology and regenerative medicine, new vaccines, and biotherapy will be developed. Breakthroughs in key technologies, such as control and prevention of chronic diseases, precision medicine, and e-Health will be promoted. New drug R&D, domestic production of medical equipment, and modernization of TCM will be carefully planned. Science and technology will play a major supportive role in prevention and treatment of major diseases and development of the healthcare industry. By 2030, the impact of scientific and technological papers and the total number of triadic patents will reach top international rankings. Scientific and technological innovation will contribute more to the growth of the pharmaceutical industry, and innovation transformation will increase.

## Chapter XXIV  Developing Digital Health Information Services

### Section One  Improving Population Health Information Service

Common, authoritative and well-connected information platforms on the population's health will be established. "Internet + healthcare" services will be standardized and promoted, and Internet-based healthcare services innovated. National health information services will be continuously developed in a bid to cover the whole life cycle of prevention, treatment, rehabilitation and self-health management. Cloud service plans for Healthy China will be implemented, a comprehensive telemedicine system established, and digital health services with better accessibility developed. Standards and security for public health information will be established. Soldiers' electronic health records will be shared continuously before and after military service. By 2030, a standard health information platform for the population's health connecting county, city, provincial and national levels will be established. Standard digital health records will be available for all, and health cards with complete functions also available for all. Telemedicine will cover all health facilities at township, county, city and provincial levels. All population health information will be managed and used in a standard format. Information needs of personalized and precision medicine will be met.

### Section Two  Promoting Use of Big Data in Health

Use of big data in health will be promoted. Open sharing, deep mining and wide application of big data in health will be promoted based on regional population health information platforms. Barriers to data sharing will be eliminated. Coordination and unification of cross-departmental and cross-sector data sharing will be established in a bid to realize data extraction, sharing and integration of public health, family planning, health services, health protection, drug supply and comprehensive management. A national health data resources directory system will be established and improved. Health data utilization will be used in supporting health governance, clinical and scientific research, public health, education and training. New business models of big data use in health will be developed. Regulations and standards of big data in health will be established. Capacity of national and regional population health information technology will be improved. Policies and regulations on data classification, domain classification and application will be developed. Credited information systems will be built. Network system, content, data and technology security will be strengthened to ensure health data security and patient privacy protection. Internet-based health services supervision will be enhanced.

## Chapter XXV    Strengthening Health Legislation

Basic health law and TCM law will be developed and issued, and the Drug Administration Law amended. Legislation and revision will be enhanced in key areas. Departmental and local health regulations will be improved, and all health-related standards and guidelines developed. Government's regulatory responsibilities in health, food, medicine, environment, sports and other health-related areas will be strengthened. Supervision and management systems combining government regulation, industry self-regulation and social supervision will be established. Supervision on health law enforcement systems and relevant capacity building will be enhanced.

## Chapter XXVI    Intensifying International Exchanges and Cooperation

China's global health strategy will be implemented, and all-round international cooperation in population health promoted. Based on bilateral partnership, the mode of cooperation will be innovated and cultural exchanges strengthened, to promote China's Belt and Road Initiative in international health cooperation. "South-South cooperation" will be intensified, and China-Africa cooperation in public health implemented. Health professional teams will be dispatched to developing countries, medical assistance in areas such as maternal and child health emphasized, and major support given to development of disease control and prevention systems. International exchanges and cooperation in TCM will be encouraged. By establishing high-level strategic dialogues between countries, China will encourage putting health on the diplomatic agenda of major countries. China will actively participate in global health governance, play a key role in research, negotiation and establishment of standards, regulations, guidelines, and gain international influence and a strong voice in building institutional health.

**Part VIII    Strengthening Organization and Implementation**

## Chapter XXVII    Strengthening Organization and Leadership

Implementation and coordination mechanisms for Healthy China will be established to promote the overall strategic agenda. Deliberations on key programs, important policies, large-scale infrastructure development plans, major issues and arrangements will be initiated. Strategic planning will be emphasized to provide guidance to ministries, agencies and local governments.

Local governments, ministries and agencies will put Healthy China on top of the policy agenda, and improve leadership and working mechanisms. Healthy China will be incorporated into local economic and social development plans, and key health indicators used for merit assessment of all Party committees and government departments. Assessment and accountability will be improved to ensure actual implementation of relevant tasks and missions. Trade unions, communist youth leagues, women's federations, federations of the disabled, and representatives of other social organizations, non-communist parties and persons without party affiliation will be supported to play their roles. Social consensus will be reached and joint taskforces formed as much as possible.

## Chapter XXVIII    Creating Favorable Social Conditions

Major strategic thinking of the Party and the government's policies on maintaining and improving population health will be strongly advocated. The significance of building Healthy China, its overall strategy, objectives and tasks and major initiatives, will be publicized. Positive publicity, public opinion supervision, scientific guidance and reports on typical cases will be encouraged to help create social awareness of building Healthy China, and create favorable conditions to support its implementation.

## Chapter XXIX    Conducting Implementation Monitoring

The Five-Year Plan for Health and Family Planning and other policy documents will be formulated and implemented. Details of policies and measures stated in the outline of the plan will be constructed, and major infrastructure development programs, key projects and policies in all stages defined. Regular and standardized supervision and assessment mechanisms will be identified to strengthen incentives and accountability. Monitoring and evaluation mechanisms will be established and improved, detailed task distribution among main departments or agencies and monitoring and evaluation strategies developed, and annual evaluation of progress and outcomes of implementation conducted. Necessary adjustments will be made to the objectives and tasks in an appropriate and timely manner. Initiatives and innovations by the people will be respected. Good local practices and effective experiences will be summarized in timely fashion, and actively scaled up during implementation.

**Notice Forwarded by the General Office of the CPC Central Committee and the General Office of the State Council Concerning *Several Opinions of the Leading Group for Deepening the Reform of the Medical and Healthcare System under the State Council on Further Publicizing the Experience in Deepening the Reform of the Medical and Healthcare System***

(No. 36 [2016] of the General Office of the CPC Central Committee and the General Office of the State Council)

The CPC committees and the people's governments of all provinces, autonomous regions and municipalities directly under the Central Government, all ministries and commissions of the Central and State organs, all major units of the People's Liberation Army, all departments of the Central Military Commission, and all people's organizations,

The *Several Opinions of the Leading Group for Deepening the Reform of the Medical and Healthcare System under the State Council on Further Publicizing the Experience in Deepening the Reform of the Medical and Healthcare System*, with the consent of the leaders of the CPC Central Committee, is hereby forwarded to you for your conscientious implementation in combination with the reality.

The General Office of the CPC Central Committee
The General Office of the State Council
October 23rd, 2016

**10. *Several Opinions of the Leading Group for Deepening the Reform of the Medical and Healthcare System under the State Council on Further Publicizing the Experience in Deepening the Reform of the Medical and Healthcare System***

Deepening the reform of the medical and healthcare system is a major policy decision made by the CPC Central Committee and the State Council. It is also an important task for comprehensively deepening the reform and building a moderately well-off society in an all-round way. To further consolidate and expand the achievements of healthcare reform, the following opinions on publicizing the experience in deepening the reform of medical and healthcare system are hereby put forward.

### I. Achieving major progress and significant results in deepening the healthcare reform

Since the start of a new round of healthcare reform, especially since the 18th CPC National Congress, all relevant departments in all regions have conscientiously implemented the decisions and arrangements of the CPC Central Committee and the State Council. What's more, they have adhered to the core concept of providing the people with basic medical and healthcare system as public goods, and to the basic principle of ensuring basic medical services, bolstering support at the community level and building sound institutions. Sticking to the basic path of making overall arrangements, highlighting priorities and advancing step by step, the departments have overcome obstacles and made solid progress in all aspects of the reform. As a consequence, major progress and significant results have been achieved in deepening healthcare reform, which are as follows. A universal healthcare system has been basically established, with the rate of signing up for the basic healthcare insurance remaining 95% or above and coverage of over 1.3 billion people. The year 2016 witnessed a fiscal subsidy of 420 *yuan* per capita for urban-rural residents' healthcare insurance. And the insurance for urban-rural residents' critical illnesses has been fully promoted to reach a high level of security. With the comprehensive reform of public hospitals extending and deepening continuously, the comprehensive reform of public hospitals at the county level has been pushed forward in an all-round way in 1,977 counties (county-level cities) across the country; there have been 200 pilot cities for the comprehensive reform of public hospitals. And the scientific management system and operation mechanism are taking shape. Due to the continuous improvement of primary-level healthcare service system, there have been health centers in nearly all townships and clinics in nearly all villages, and the service capabilities have been significantly improved. With a substantial increase in the level of equal access to basic public health services, 45 items of national basic public health services projects in 12 categories have been implemented, covering the whole process of residents' lives and benefiting millions of people. What's more, the guarantee system of drug supply has been further improved, with the implementation of the national basic drug system, and the promotion of open, transparent and centralized online procurement at the provincial level for drugs of public healthcare institutions. Consequently a market-oriented mechanism for drug pricing has been gradually established. With the construction of hierarchical diagnosis system accelerated, the trials for initial visits at primary-level healthcare institutions have been conducted at more than half of the counties (county-level cities) nationwide; as a result there has been 80% or above of the initial visits within the counties. The proportion of personal health expenditure in total health expenditure has continued to decline, from 40.4% in 2008 to less than 30%. The accessibility to basic medical care and healthcare services has improved significantly, with 80% of residents reaching medical facilities in 15 minutes. The people's health has significantly improved, with the average life expectancy reaching 76.34 years, an increase of 1.51 years over 2010. In general, the people's health is better than the average level of middle- and high-income countries. And higher health performance has been achieved with less investment. Practice has proved that deepening the reform of medical and healthcare system is in the right direction, with the clear path and effective measures. Reform efforts have widely benefited the people and played an important role in solving the problems of seeking medical treatment, improving the people's health quality, safeguarding social fairness and justice, and promoting socioeconomic development.

Under the strong leadership of the CPC Central Committee and the State Council, deepening healthcare reform has gradually shifted from laying a good foundation to improving quality, from forming a framework to system building, and from single breakthroughs to system integration and comprehensive promotion. Furthermore, top-level design has continued to improve, local initiative and creativity have been strengthened and key and difficult problems have been gradually dealt with. Some typical areas that dare to fight hard, explore and innovate have emerged, forming a number of practical, replicable and propagable experience and practices.

At present, the deepening of healthcare reform has entered the deep water zone and tough period, with the interest adjustment more complicated and the contradictions among systems and mechanisms highlighted. In the critical period of tough reform, summarizing and publicizing the good practices and matured experience in the early stage of deepening healthcare reform, as well as giving full play to the role of typical experience in demonstration, breakthrough and leading for global reform, are conducive to further unifying our thinking, strengthening our conviction, and conquering obstacles. Moreover they are helpful to innovations in systems and mechanisms, and breaking through barriers of interest. What's more, they are beneficial to accelerating the improvement of the basic medical and healthcare system, and achieving the goal of universal access to basic medical and healthcare services. In brief, they lay a solid foundation for building a healthy China and building a moderately well-off society in an all-round way.

### II. Utilizing typical experience to push healthcare reform further

**(1) Establish a powerful leadership system and a working mechanism for the linkage of medical care, medical insurance and medicine to provide organizational guarantee for deepening healthcare reform.**

1) Efforts shall be made to strengthen the leadership of the Party committee and the government over healthcare reform. Top officials of local Party committees and governments at all levels shall be responsible for deepening healthcare reform. Responsible officials or one responsible official of the Party committee and the government shall serve as group leader(s) of the leading group for healthcare reform. Efforts shall be made to give full play to the overall coordination role of the leading group for healthcare reform and effectively fulfill the government's responsibilities of leadership, security, management and supervision for healthcare reform.

2) Efforts shall be made to establish and improve a mechanism for advancing our work. Attention shall be focused on the mechanism for division of responsibilities to establish and reform the task accounting system, and put the responsibilities in place. Attention shall be paid to the mechanism for the implementation of supervision and inspection to conduct special supervision and inspection for the key reform tasks as an important basis for annual assessment. Importance shall be attached to the mechanism for assessment and accountability to include the completion of healthcare reform tasks in the performance appraisal for the comprehensive deepening of the reform and the performance appraisal for government target management. Furthermore, regions and individuals that have failed to advance the reform shall be subject to serious accountability, while regions and individuals shall be commended or given awards for their positive innovations and remarkable achievements.

**(2) Abolish the compensation system for the medical cost through drug-selling profits to establish and improve a new mechanism for running public hospitals.**

3) Efforts shall be made to gradually straightening out the price of healthcare services in accordance with the basic path of making room, adjusting the structure and ensuring the connection. The reform of medical service prices should be promoted positively yet prudently. Under the premise of ensuring the healthy operation of public hospitals, affordable medical insurance fund, and no overall increase in the people's burden, efforts should be made to give classification guidance to and straighten out the price comparison between different levels of medical institutions and medical service items, as requested by the total amount control, structural adjustment, ups and downs, and being gradually in place. Cancelling drug

price additions, all public hospitals shall take into full account the compensation policies made by local governments, accurately calculate the price adjustment level, and adjust the medical service price simultaneously. The medical service price shall be dynamically adjusted through standardizing diagnosis and treatment practices, and reducing the cost of medicines and consumables. Price adjustment shall focus on raising the prices of medical treatment items, such as diagnosis, surgery, nursing, rehabilitation and traditional Chinese medicine (TCM) that embody the value of medical workers' technical work. In addition, the prices of examination, treatment and testing with large-size medical equipment should be lowered; meanwhile a good job should be done in conjunction with policies such as healthcare insurance payment, hierarchical diagnosis and treatment, and cost control. Through comprehensive measures, we shall gradually increase the proportion of medical service revenue (excluding the revenue from drugs, consumables, inspection and testing) in total hospital revenue for establishing a new mechanism for the operation of public hospitals.

4) Efforts shall be made to implement classified procurement of pharmaceuticals in public hospitals. Different situations with pharmaceuticals shall be distinguished for reasonable procurement pricing by means of bidding, negotiation, direct interconnection, and designated production. Adhering to the principle of centralized procurement with a certain quantity, provincial-level pharmaceutical procurement agencies should seek bidding and purchasing for basic drugs and non-patented drugs manufactured by a large number of pharmaceutical enterprises with large clinical dosage, high purchase costs. In the pilot cities for the comprehensive reform of public hospitals, pharmaceuticals can be purchased on the provincial-level centralized procurement platform for pharmaceuticals with the city as the unit. Cross-regional joint procurement and joint procurement of specialist hospitals shall be encouraged. Medical consumables shall be purchased in an open, transparent and scientific way, while the centralized procurement for high-value medical consumables, testing reagents and large-sized medical equipment shall be conducted. And an open, transparent and multi-party price negotiation mechanism shall be established for some patented drugs and exclusively manufactured drugs. The results of the negotiations shall be announced on the national comprehensive management information platform for the supply and guarantee of drugs, and hospitals shall purchase them according to the results of the negotiations. Efforts shall be made to make a good connection with the medical insurance payment policy, and include eligible negotiating drugs into the scope of medical insurance compliance expenses in accordance with the regulations.

5) Efforts shall be made to implement step by step the "two-invoice system" in the procurement of pharmaceuticals in public hospitals. Local governments

should gradually implement the "two-invoice system" for the procurement of pharmaceuticals in public healthcare institutions according to local actual conditions (An invoice shall be paid from the manufacturing enterprise to the circulation enterprise, and in turn an invoice shall go from the circulation enterprise to the medical institution.) Other medical institutions shall be encouraged to implement the "two-invoice system" to reduce the intermediate links of drug circulation, improve the concentration of circulation enterprises, crack down on "money laundering", lower the high drug price, and purify the circulation environment. By integrating the resources of storage and transportation of trading pharmaceutical enterprises, we shall accelerate the development of modern pharmaceutical logistics, and encourage the urban-rural integration of regional pharmaceutical distribution to provide basic conditions for promoting the "two-invoice system." We shall also establish a blacklist system for commercial bribery enterprises, and disqualify the drug production and distribution enterprises that engage in commercial briberies such as kickbacks.

6) Efforts shall be made to standardize the behavior of diagnosis and treatment. All the medical behaviors and expenses of outpatient and inpatient in medical institutions shall be monitored and assessed by means of intelligent audit, which can be used for pre-warning, in-case control and post-event audit. Comments should be made on prescriptions to strengthen information disclosure and social supervision. With the monitoring of rational use of drugs and adverse reactions strengthened, a catalogue for the key monitoring for drugs with high prices, large dosage, and non-therapeutic assistance shall be established to carry out tracking and monitoring and extraordinary early warning. Key drugs may be purchased on record, and procurement quantity and doctors making prescriptions shall be specified to register with the drug purchasing department upon the approval of the person in charge of the medical institution. And the overgrowth of public hospitals shall be strictly controlled.

7) Efforts shall be made to implement the input responsibility of the government. The government's policy of investment in public hospitals shall be fully implemented. In accordance with relevant regulations, the long-term liabilities of public hospitals that conform to the regulations shall be gradually repaid and resolved.

**(3) Give full play to the fundamental role of healthcare insurance to strengthen the external constraints on medical services.**

8) Efforts shall be made to strengthen the management function of medical insurance. The basic healthcare insurance system for urban and rural residents shall be integrated to achieve the unification of coverage, financing policies, guaranteed treatment, medical insurance catalogs, designated management and fund management. The management system shall be straightened out to unify the

management of basic healthcare insurance. It is possible to carry out trials for the establishment of a healthcare insurance fund management center to assume the functions of fund payment and management, drug procurement and cost settlement, negotiation of medical insurance payment standards, and the agreement management and settlement of designated institutions. We shall give full play to the role of healthcare insurance in supervising and restricting the production and distribution of drugs in enterprises, hospitals and doctors to provide effective measures for the linkage reform. The unified healthcare insurance agency should intensify the reform of the mode of medical insurance payment, and further exert the control of healthcare insurance on the unreasonable increase of medical expenses.

9) Efforts shall be made to comprehensively promote the reform of the payment method. Payment by the item shall be gradually reduced to improve the control over the total amount of medical insurance payment. The compound payment methods of capitation, per-diem payment by bed and scale payment shall be promoted with Diagnosis Related Group System (DRGs) as the focus. The implementation of DRGs method shall be encouraged to gradually extend the reform of medical insurance payment method to all medical institutions and medical services. Where conditions permit, point system shall be combined with budget management and DRGs to promote orderly competition among healthcare institutions and rational allocation of resources. An incentive and restraint mechanism for the retention of balances and reasonable over-expenditure sharing shall be established to stimulate the endogenous power of standard behavior and cost control of medical institutions.

10) Efforts shall be made to create a new model for handling basic healthcare insurance. The professionalization of healthcare insurance agencies shall be promoted in accordance with the principle of separation of administration and management. On the premise of ensuring the safety and effective regulation of the fund, qualified commercial insurance institutions and other social forces entrusted by means of government purchasing service shall participate in the services provided by the basic healthcare insurance agency. In addition, they shall undertake critical illness medical insurance for urban and rural residents, and introduce a competition mechanism to improve the efficiency and quality of management services of healthcare insurance. And the development of commercial health insurance shall also be encouraged.

**(4) Promote the separation of government affairs and administration to establish a modern hospital management system.**

11) Efforts shall be made to straighten out the system of state-owned hospitals. All local authorities should explore effective forms of organization and coordinate the implementation of the government's responsibilities in handling medical affairs in light of local conditions.

12) Efforts shall be made to exercise autonomy in the operation and management of public hospitals. To transform government functions, administrative authorities at all levels shall change from direct management of public hospitals to industry management, and shall strengthen the formulation, supervision and guidance of policies and regulations, industry planning and standards. With the corporate governance structure of public hospitals improved, autonomy shall be exercised in internal personnel management, institutional setup, income distribution, deputy position recommendation, appointment and removal of middle-rank officials, and annual budget implementation. Efforts shall be made to improve the internal decision-making and restriction mechanisms of public hospitals, make their affairs more open, give full play to the functions of staff congress, and strengthen democratic management.

13) Efforts shall be made to implement the performance assessment of public hospitals. A public welfare oriented assessment and evaluation system shall be established to highlight functional orientation, performance of duties, social satisfaction, cost control, operational performance, financial management, and other indicators. The performance assessment of public hospitals and the performance of annual and term target liabilities of the dean shall be organized on a regular basis. The assessment results shall be linked to the hospital's financial subsidy, medical insurance payment, total performance salary, dean's salary, appointment and dismissal, rewards and punishment, etc., and thus an incentive and restraint mechanism shall be established.

14) Efforts shall be made to strengthen the sophisticated management of public hospitals. The medical quality and safety management system as well as the quality monitoring and evaluation system shall be improved. And the clinical pathway management and continuous improvement of medical quality shall be promoted. Through comprehensive budget management and cost accounting, a comprehensive analysis shall be conducted of revenue and expenditure, budget implementation, cost efficiency and debt solvency, which can be an important basis for hospital operation and management decisions. What's more, a third party accounting audit supervision system shall be implemented to strengthen the regulation over the state-owned assets and economic operations of hospitals.

**(5) Establish a personnel remuneration system in line with the characteristics of the industry to arouse the enthusiasm of medical staff.**

15) Efforts shall be made to establish a flexible employment system. With the way of staffing management of public hospitals innovated and the measures of staffing management improved, the pilot reform of staffing management of public hospitals shall be actively explored and carried out. Within the existing total local

staffing, the total public hospital staffing shall be determined to implement a filling system step by step. And the reform of staffing management in some Grade III A public hospitals in large and medium-sized cities shall be carried out for the trial of total staffing management. Personnel management systems such as employment system, post management system and open recruitment system shall be implemented. In simplifying the recruitment process for professional and technical personnel, professional and technical personnel or high-level talents that are in short supply in hospitals shall be recruited on an inspection basis as required by hospitals. The proportion of senior and middle posts in primary-level healthcare institutions shall be increased to expand the space for medical workers to develop professionally.

16) Efforts shall be made to promote the reform of compensation system. Local governments shall, in light of the actual situation, reasonably determine the remuneration level of public hospitals in accordance with relevant regulations, and gradually increase the proportion of personnel expenditure in business expenditure. Public healthcare institutions that have more work beyond the working hours, converging of high-level medical talents, and heavy target tasks of public welfare, and that develop family doctor's contracted service shall be tilted when verifying the total amount of merit pay. With long-term incentives for medical workers strengthened, a performance appraisal mechanism that is oriented towards public welfare shall be established. And on the basis of maintaining the current level, a moderate increase in compensation shall be achieved. Public healthcare institutions shall autonomously allocate merit pay based on the assessment results within the approved total amount of merit pay. The verification of the total compensation and the allocation of individual merit pay shall not be linked to the business income of healthcare institutions such as pharmaceuticals, consumables and large-scale medical examinations. Since the compensation allocation reflects technical content, risks and contribution of the post, it shall be strictly prohibited to set income- generating targets for medical workers. Primary-level healthcare institutions shall, in accordance with financial regulations and provisions, draw out welfare funds and incentive funds for staff and workers from the verified balance of income and expenditure.

**(6) Accelerate the establishment of a hierarchical diagnosis and treatment system with the family doctor's contracted service and medical complex as the important starting point.**

17) Efforts shall be made to promote the family doctor's contracted service. A contracted service team with family doctors as the core and specialists providing technical support shall be established to provide residents with long-term and continuous basic medical care, public health and health management services. Efforts shall be made to optimize the connotation of contracted services, and implement

differentiated policies for contracted residents in terms of medical treatment, referral, medication, and healthcare insurance to promote initial visit at primary-level medical institutions. Efforts shall also be made to improve the performance appraisal system based on standardized workload. Residents or families can be guided to choose a secondary hospital and a tertiary hospital voluntarily while signing a contract with the family doctor team. Furthermore a combined contracted service model of "1+1+1" shall be established, in which residents can choose whatever a medical institution they want for treatment within the combined contracted service. In the case of treatment beyond the combined contracted service, the family doctor shall refer the patient to the other doctor, so that residents can be guided to change their habits in seeking medical advice and form a reasonable order for medical treatment.

18) Efforts shall be made to establish a medical complex. In accordance with the principle of government-led model, voluntary combination, regional coordination, and convenience for the people, and with the goal of resource sharing and talent serving for primary-level healthcare institutions, a longitudinal complex of medical resources shall be established to improve the community-level service capacity. Within the medical complex, the responsibilities, rights and interests of urban tertiary hospitals, secondary hospitals, and primary-level healthcare institutions shall be defined, two-way referral agreements be signed, and related management, operation, and assessment mechanisms be improved. Efforts shall be made to promote the availability of community-level healthcare workers in townships and villages, and establish flexible mechanisms for the flow of talents to take turns serving community-level healthcare institutions. Efforts shall be redoubled to assist counterparts, give accurate assistance to the construction of specialized programs and talent training at community-level healthcare institutions, and promote the balanced allocation of medical resources between urban and rural areas. With the channel of counterpart support to integrate medical resources, the support for the medical and health care in the old revolutionary base areas, ethnic minority areas, border areas and poverty-stricken areas shall be intensified. And further efforts shall be made to provide group-type assistance of medical talents for medical and healthcare in Tibet and Xinjiang.

19) Efforts shall be made to give full play to the advantages of the service of Traditional Chinese Medicine (TCM). The construction of TCM clinics at community-level healthcare institutions shall be strengthened to promote the comprehensive service model of TCM, widely promote and employ appropriate TCM techniques, and give full play to the role of TCM in the prevention and control of common diseases, frequently-occurring diseases and chronic diseases. On the basis of raising the price of medical service of TCM to reflect the value of technical service of TCM, the payment standard of TCM by type of disease shall be reasonably set. In areas where the service

system of TCM at the community level is not perfect and the capacity is relatively weak, the outpatient TCM diagnosis and treatment service of TCM hospitals shall be included in the range of initial visit, so as to meet the people's demand for the initial visit at TCM hospitals. And there shall be innovative model of TCM.

20) Efforts shall be made to improve the supporting policies for hierarchical diagnosis and treatment. The responsibilities of medical treatment in healthcare institutions at all levels shall be reasonably divided and implemented. The procedures and standards for referral shall be clarified, and the responsibility system for initial visit and the accountability system for referral approval shall be implemented. Efforts shall be made to give full play to the role of medical insurance in adjusting and link the implementation of medical institutions' medical responsibilities and referral status to performance assessment and the allocation of medical insurance funds. Explorations shall be made in how to pay for the total amount of medical insurance in the division of collaboration such as medical complex in vertical cooperation, in order to give guidance to two-way referral. Differentiated payment policies of medical insurance of medical institutions at different levels shall be improved to promote initial visit at primary-level medical institutions. Medicare reimbursement policy for patients referred as required shall be made favorably.

**(7) Make full use of Internet technology to improve the people's experience in seeking medical advice.**

21) Efforts shall be made to strengthen the infrastructure of health information. A platform of population health information at the national, provincial, municipal and county level for people to share information and work together shall be constructed. The basic database with residents' electronic health records, electronic medical records and electronic prescriptions as the core shall be improved. Channels for sharing data resources among various medical and health institutions shall be opened up to improve the hierarchical medical information system based on the Internet and big data technology, which shall provide technical support for achieving continuous, collaborative and integrated medical and healthcare services.

22) Efforts shall be made to promote the service for the convenience and benefit of the people. Efforts shall also be made to optimize the diagnosis and treatment process, improve the medical environment, make overall arrangements for appointments, inspections, diagnosis and treatment, referrals, payment and settlement, etc., and promote applications such as online appointment triage, mobile payment, clinic settlement, and results query. The mechanism for mutual recognition of inspection and testing results shall be improved while the radiation effect of high-quality resources shall be amplified to make it convenient for people to visit doctors nearby. Technologies such as mobile clients and the Internet of Things shall be utilized

to establish a communication platform for both doctors and patients, which shall facilitate health consultation, patient feedback, and health management. Efforts shall be made to make full use of information technology to provide telemedicine service, and give priority to the opening of telemedicine systems in 834 poverty-stricken counties. Promoting residents' health card, social security card application integration, such as activating residents electronic health records applications, strengthen information publishes, connectivity, to promote prevention, treatment, rehabilitation and health management of electronic health services

The integration of applications of residents' health cards and social security cards shall be promoted to activate the application of electronic health records of residents. The military and local information convergence and interconnection shall be strengthened, whereas the integration of e-health services in prevention, treatment, rehabilitation and health management shall be promoted. Medical resources shall be reasonably allocated to make scientific arrangements for the number of physicians for each specialty, ensure adequate time for diagnosis and inspection, and improve the quality of medical services.

**(8) Develop and standardize nongovernmental hospitals to meet the needs of diversified medical services.**

23) Efforts shall be made to enhance the development of nongovernmental hospitals. Regional health planning and medical institution setup planning shall provide sufficient space for nongovernmental hospitals to give priority to non-profit medical institutions. The development environment for nongovernmental hospitals shall be optimized to promote the same treatment for public medical institutions and nonpublic medical institutions in terms of market access, designated hospitals of social insurance, key specialty construction, job title assessment, academic exchanges, rating review, and technical access. Efforts shall be made to support the chain operation, the establishment of brands and group development of nongovernmental hospitals to provide high-end services as well as services in shortage such as rehabilitation and elderly care. Nongovernmental organizations shall be encouraged to establish independent institutions, in accordance with relevant regulations, of laboratory medicine, medical imaging diagnosis, disinfection supplies and blood purification.

24) Efforts shall be made to enhance standardized management. Territorial management shall be promoted to strengthen the oversight of the whole industry. Unified plan, unified access and unified regulation for all medical institutions shall be implemented to regulate the practice of nongovernmental medical institutions in accordance with the law. Efforts shall be made to crack down on illegal medical practice. In accordance with the relevant requirements of the reform of "simplification of administration, integration of simplification of administration and fair regulation,

and optimization of services, we shall streamline and optimize the procedures for review and approval to strengthen regulation during the event and post-event regulation. Efforts shall be made to strengthen the regulation of the ownership of property rights, financial operations and the use of fund balances of non-profit private medical institutions to promote the healthy development of nongovernmental hospitals.

### III. Intensifying our efforts to promote and enhance the initiative and creativity for deepening healthcare reform

(1) Attach great importance to the work of promotion. Fully understanding the importance of promoting the experience in deepening healthcare reform, Party committees and governments at all levels shall seriously organize and learn from healthcare reform experience, and thoroughly study the reform ideas, steps, and approaches. They shall also include the promotion of relevant reform measures as the priority in the region to enhance the concentration on the reform and intensify the reform. Efforts shall be made to shape the employment orientation of reformers and non-reformers to push forward the reform in a down-to-earth manner, and to ensure that the experience of the reform takes root and produce practical results.

(2) Explore and innovate in light of local conditions. All local authorities shall closely integrate their own realities, respect primary-level initiative, take institutional innovation as the core task, and further emancipate their minds and make bold innovation around key links and key areas. In addition, they shall explore effective ways to implement the reform and clarify the internal logic and policy mix of the reform to implement detailed management of the reform, and to encourage regional linkage. We shall be highly responsible in our efforts to achieve our goals, achieve them accurately, explore and innovate, track their effectiveness and ensure their mechanisms, in order to gain more reform experience that can be replicated and popularized.

(3) Strengthen the supervision and guidance to the promotion. All relevant departments shall implement the relevant requirements on streamlining administration, strengthen the guidance according to their responsibilities, and provide policy support. The State Council's Office of the Leading Group for Deepening the Reform of the Medical and Healthcare System, together with relevant departments, shall intensify the supervision and inspection, analyze and resolve emerging problems in time, and prevent the arbitrariness and uncertainty in the promotion of the experience. Efforts shall be made to further summarize the mature experience accumulated in various regions to escalate it to policies in a timely manner,

so as to further summarize, consolidate and develop the results of the reform.

(4) Push the publicity work forward. Efforts shall be made to continue to strengthen the search and publicity of typical experience in medical reform, reflect the fresh practice and progress of medical reform, and strengthen confidence in the reform and build consensus on reform. We shall adhere to the correct orientation of public opinion, respond to social concerns in a timely manner, reasonably guide social expectations, and create a favorable public opinion environment for deepening healthcare reform.

**(Shan Yongxiang)**

## Order of the State Council of the People's Republic of China

(No. 668)

The Decision of the State Council on Amending the *Regulation on the Administration of Circulation and Vaccination of Vaccines*, approved at the 129th session of the State Council on April 23<sup>th</sup>, 2016, is now issued and will be effective from the date of issuance.

Premier Li Keqiang
April 13<sup>th</sup>, 2016

## 11. The Decision of the State Council on Amending the *Regulation on the Administration of Circulation and Vaccination of Vaccines*

According to the decision of the State Council, the *Regulation on the Administration of Circulation and Vaccination of Vaccines* is amended as the following:

I. Article 10 is amended as: "Vaccines shall be purchased through provincial public resource trading platforms."

II. Article 15 is amended as: "Provincial disease prevention and control institutions shall organize the centralized procurement of Class II vaccines through provincial public resource trading platforms, and county disease prevention and control institutions shall, after purchasing vaccines from vaccine production enterprises, supply them to inoculation entities within their respective administrative regions."

"Vaccine production enterprises shall directly distribute Class II vaccines to county disease prevention and control institutions or authorize enterprises with cold chain storage and transport conditions to distribute them. The enterprises that distribute Class II vaccines upon authorization shall not authorize distribution. "

"County disease prevention and control institutions that supply Class II vaccines to inoculation entities may charge vaccine fees and storage and transport fees.

Vaccine fees shall be charged at the purchase price, and storage and transport fees shall be charged according to the provisions of provinces, autonomous regions, and municipalities directly under the Central Government. The charging information shall be disclosed to the public."

III. Article 16 is amended as: "Disease prevention and control institutions, inoculation entities, vaccine production enterprises, and enterprises that distribute vaccines upon authorization shall abide by the rules on the administration of vaccine storage and transport, and guarantee the quality of vaccines. Vaccines shall be stored and transported in the environment with the prescribed temperature during the entire process, shall not be isolated from the cold chain, and temperature shall be monitored and recorded at regular time. Provincial disease prevention and control institutions shall require the attachment of temperature control labels to the vaccines that are transported in cold chain for a long time and need to be distributed to remote regions."

"The rules on the administration of storage and transport of vaccines shall be developed by the competent health department and drug administrative department of the State Council."

IV. Item One of Article 17 is amended as: "A vaccine production enterprise shall, when selling vaccines, provide a photocopy of the inspection conformity or examination and approval certificate lawfully issued by the drug inspection institution for each batch of biological products, and affix its enterprise seal. If the enterprise sells imported vaccines, it shall also provide a photocopy of the customs clearance list of imported drugs, and affix its enterprise seal."

V. Article 18 is amended as: "A vaccine production enterprise shall, in accordance with the *Pharmaceutical Administration Law* and the provisions of the drug administrative department of the State Council, set up true and complete sales records, and retain them until two years after the expiration of validity term of the vaccines for future reference."

"A disease prevention and control institution shall, in accordance with the provisions of the competent health department of the State Council, set up true and complete records on purchase, storage, distribution and supply, ensure consistency among bills, account books, goods and payments, and retain them until two years after the expiration of validity term of the vaccines for future reference. The disease prevention and control institution shall, when receiving or purchasing vaccines, request the temperature monitoring records during the entire process of vaccine storage and transport; and if the records on temperature monitoring during the entire process cannot be provided or temperature control fails to satisfy the relevant requirements, the disease prevention and control institution shall not receive or purchase the vaccines, and shall immediately report it to the drug administrative department and competent health department."

VI. Item One of Article 23 is amended as: "An inoculation entity that receives Class-I vaccines or purchases Class-II vaccines shall request records on temperature monitoring during the entire process of vaccine storage and transport, set up and retain true and complete receipt and procurement records, and ensure consistency among bills, account books, goods and payments. If the records on temperature monitoring during the entire process cannot be provided or temperature control fails to satisfy the relevant requirements, the inoculation entity shall not receive or purchase the vaccines, and shall immediately report it to the drug administrative department and competent health department of the county people's government at the place where it is located."

VII. Item Two of Article 25 is amended as: "Medical and health staff members shall inoculate the persons complying with inoculation conditions, and according to the provisions of the competent health department of the State Council, record the categories and production enterprises of vaccines, the information on the identification of minimum packing units, term of validity, inoculation time, medical and health staff members that perform inoculations, and inoculated persons, among others. Inoculation records shall be retained for not less than five years."

VIII. Item Two of Article 46 is amended as: "Where a vaccinated person needs to be compensated due to the abnormal action to a Class-I vaccine, the compensation shall be covered with the working expenses by the financial department of a province (autonomous region or municipality directly under the central government). Where a vaccinated person needs to be compensated due to the abnormal action to a Class-II vaccine, the compensation shall be shouldered by the vaccine manufacturer. The state shall encourage the establishment of the mechanism of compensation with commercial insurance and other channels for persons with abnormal reaction to vaccination. "

IX. Article 52 is amended as: "The competent health department and drug administrative department shall make timely report to each other and share the information when discovering the issues like quality problems of vaccines and abnormal reaction to vaccination."

X. One article is added as Article 54: "The state shall establish the whole-course tracing system of vaccines. The competent health department of the State Council shall joint with the drug administrative department of the State Council to formulate the uniformed technical standards for the vaccine tracing system."

"Vaccine production enterprises, disease prevention and control institutions and inoculation entities shall, in accordance with the *Pharmaceutical Administration Law*, the *Regulation on the Administration of Circulation and Vaccination of Vaccines* and the provisions of the competent health department and drug administrative department of the State Council, set up the vaccine tracing system, make authentic records of the distribution and usage of the vaccines and realize the whole-course traceability of the vaccines in the smallest unit of package during the production, storage, transportation and usage."

"The competent health department of the State Council shall joint with the drug administrative department of the State Council to establish the collaboration mechanism for the whole-course trace of vaccines."

XI. One article is added as Article 55:"Disease prevention and control institutions and inoculation entities shall make authentic record of the vaccines that are with unrecognizable packages, expired, isolated from the cold chain, unqualified upon inspection and of unidentified source and make report to the drug administrative department of the local county government, which shall joint with the competent health department at the same level to supervise the destruction of the vaccines. Disease prevention and control institutions and inoculation entities shall make authentic record of the destruction and the record shall be kept for at least 5 years."

XII. Article 54 is changed into Article 56 and amended as: "The competent health department and drug administrative department above the county level, in violation of the provisions in this *Regulation* with one of the following conditions shall be instructed to rectify and be given a criticism by circulating a notice; the person directly in charge and other persons directly responsible shall be punished by law if serious consequences occur, like physical harm to the vaccinated persons or transmission and prevalence of infectious diseases; if the consequence is particularly serious, the main responsible person shall also resign to assume responsibility; and in case of criminal offenses, the offenders shall be prosecuted in accordance with the law."

(1) It fails to carry out supervision and inspection or fails to carry out timely investigation and punishment upon finding out illegal activities;

(2) It fails to timely verify and deal with the report on the negligence of duty in supervision and administration by the subordinate competent health department and drug administrative department;

(3) It fails to organize immediate investigation and handling of the relevant report on discovering cases and suspected cases of abnormal reaction to vaccination;

(4) It carries out unauthorized group vaccination;

(5) Other relevant acts of malpractice or dereliction of duty.

XIII. Article 55 is changed into Article 57 and amended as: "The people's government above the county level that fails to provide guarantee for inoculation and vaccination in accordance with the provisions of this Regulation shall be instructed to rectify and given a criticism by circulating a notice by the people's government at the higher level; where physical harm to the vaccinated persons, transmission and prevalence of infectious diseases or other serious consequence occurs, the person directly in charge and other persons directly responsible shall be punished by law; where a particularly serious quality and safety issue of vaccine occurs or a successive series of such issues occur, the person chiefly in charge of the local people's government shall resign; and in case of criminal offenses, the offenders shall be prosecuted in accordance with the law."

XIV. Article 56 is changed into Article 58 and Item One is amended as: " Where a disease prevention and control institution has one of the following conditions, it shall be instructed to rectify, criticized with a circular notice and given a warning by the competent health department of the people's government above the county level; and in case of refusing to rectify, the person chiefly in charge, the executives directly responsible and other persons directly responsible shall get punishment ranging from warning to demotion in accordance with the law."

(1) It fails to distribute Class I vaccines to the subordinate disease prevention and control institutions, inoculation entities and township medical and health institutions;

(2) It fails to set up and keep the records on the procurement, storage, distribution and supply of vaccines;

(3) It fails to request the temperature monitoring record, accepts and purchases unqualified vaccines or fails to make reports in accordance with the regulation."

XV. Article 57 is changed into Article 59 and amended as: "Where the inoculation entity has one of the following conditions, it shall be instructed to rectify and given a warning by the competent health department of the local people's government at the county level; in case of refusing to rectify, the person chiefly in charge and the executives directly responsible shall get punishment ranging from warning to demotion in accordance with the law and the responsible medical and health personnel shall be instructed to suspend the practice for a period of more than 3 months and less than 6 months."

(1) "It fails to request the temperature monitoring record, accepts and purchases unqualified vaccines or fails to make reports in accordance with the regulation;"

(2) " It fails to set up and retain true and complete receipt and procurement records;"

(3) "It fails to display the types and inoculation methods of Class I vaccines at an eye-catching place in the inoculation facilities;"

(4) "The medical and health personnel fail to inform and inquire the inoculated person or his/her guardian the related information;"

(5) "Medical and health staff members that perform inoculations fail to fill in and retain the inoculation record;"

(6) "It fails to record and make report of the vaccine inoculation in accordance with the regulations."

XVI. Article 58 is changed into Article 60 and amended as: "Where a disease prevention and control institution and an inoculation entity has one of the following conditions, it shall be instructed to rectify and given a warning by the people's government at or above the county level; the illegal gains shall be confiscated if they are obtained; in case of refusing to rectify, the person chiefly in charge, the executives directly responsible and other persons directly responsible shall get punishment ranging from warning to removal from the office in accordance with the law; where physical harm to the vaccinated persons and other serious circumstances occur, the person chiefly in charge and the executives directly responsible shall be discharged and the medical practicing licenses of the medical staff who are responsible shall be revoked by the former license issuance department; In case of criminal offenses, the offenders shall be prosecuted in accordance with the law."

(1) "It violates the provisions of this *Regulation* and fails to purchase vaccines at the provincial public resources trading platform;"

(2)"It violates the provisions of this *Regulation* and purchases Class II vaccines from an entity or an individual other than a vaccine production enterprise or a disease prevention and control department at the county level;"

(3) "It fails to observe the working norms of inoculation, the vaccination procedures, the guiding principles for application of vaccines and the vaccine plans;"

(4) "It fails to make timely response or report upon discovering cases or suspected cases of abnormal reaction to vaccination; "

(5) "It carries out unauthorized group vaccination;"

(6) "It fails to make records and reports on vaccines that are with unrecognizable package, expired, isolated from the cold chain, unqualified upon inspection and of unknown source or fails to make records on the destruction of these vaccines."

XVII. Article 61 is changed into Article 63 and amended as: "Where the vaccine production enterprises fail to set up and retain records on the storage and sales of vaccines, they shall be punished in accordance with the provisions in Article 78 of the *Pharmaceutical Administration Law of the People's Republic of China*."

XVIII. Article 63 is changed into Article 65 and amended as: "Where vaccine production enterprises sell Class II vaccines to entities or individuals other than disease prevention and control department at the county level, the vaccines sold illegally shall be confiscated by the drug administrative department and a fine two times higher and 5 times less than the value of the vaccines shall be imposed; the illegal gains shall be confiscated if they are obtained; in case of serious circumstances, the production qualifications shall be revoked or the import permission certificates shall be withdrawn in accordance with the law, and the executives directly responsible and other persons directly responsible shall be forbidden to carry out pharmaceutical production and sales within 10 years; and in case of criminal offenses, the offender shall be prosecuted in accordance with the law."

XIX. Article 64 is changed into Article 66 and amended as: "Where disease prevention and control department, inoculation entities, vaccine production enterprises and enterprises that distribute vaccines upon authorization fail to store and transport the vaccines in cold chain conditions in accordance with the regulations, they shall be instructed to rectify and given a warning by pharmaceutical administrative department and the vaccines that are stored or transported by them shall be destroyed; the person chiefly in charge, the executives directly responsible and other persons directly responsible shall get punishment ranging from warning to removal from office by competent health department, and in case of serious circumstances, they shall be discharged and the inoculation qualifications of the inoculation entity shall be revoked in accordance with the law; the vaccine production enterprises and the vaccine production enterprises and enterprises that distribute vaccines upon authorization shall be instructed to stop production and distribution to rectify by the pharmaceutical administrative department, a fine two times more and five times less than the value of the vaccines that are stored and transported shall be imposed and in case of serious consequences, in case of serious circumstances, the production qualifications shall be revoked or the import permission certificates shall be withdrawn in accordance with the law, and the executives directly responsible and other persons directly responsible shall be forbidden to carry out pharmaceutical production and sales within 10 years; and in case of criminal offenses, the offender shall be prosecuted in accordance with the law."

XX. Article 68 is changed into Article 70 and amended as: "Where an entity or an individual other than the vaccine production enterprises or disease prevention and control department at the county level, in violation of the provisions of this Regulation, carries out sales of vaccines, the entity or the person shall be punished in accordance with the provisions of Article 72 of the *Pharmaceutical Administration Law*."

XXI. Article 72 is changed into Article 74 and one item is added as Item 5: "Vaccine production enterprises refer to both the domestic vaccine production enterprises and the agency of overseas vaccine manufacturers within the border of China."

XXII. One article is added as Article 75: "The *Measures for the Management of Vaccination of Entry and Exit* shall be separately formulated by the state entry-exit inspection and quarantine department."

XXIII. "Vaccine wholesale businesses" in Article 12, Article 13 and Item Two of Article 17, Article 33, Article 49 and Article 62 shall be deleted.

XXIV. Article 60 is changed into Article 62 and the content "Article 87" in it is amended as "Article 86". Besides, the orders of the items and some words are revised accordingly. This *Decision* shall come into force from the date of issuance.

The *Regulation on the Administration of Circulation and Vaccination of Vaccines* shall be amended in accordance with this *Decision* and reissued.

## 12. *Regulation on the Administration of Circulation and Vaccination of Vaccines*

Promulgated on March 24$^{th}$, 2005 as the Decree [No. 434] of the State Council and amended on the April 23$^{rd}$, 2016

## Chapter I    General Provisions

【 Article 1 】  The *Regulation* is formulated in accordance with the *Pharmaceutical Administration Law of the People's Republic of China* (hereinafter referred to as the *Pharmaceutical Administration Law*) and the *Law of the People's Republic of China on Prevention and Treatment of Infectious Diseases* (hereinafter referred to as the *Law on Prevention and Treatment of Infectious Diseases*) so as to strengthen the administration of circulation and vaccination of vaccines, prevent and control the occurrence and spread of infectious diseases, and guarantee human health and public sanitation.

【 Article 2 】  Vaccines mentioned in this *Regulation* shall mean the preventive biotic products of the vaccine type, which are used for human vaccination for the sake of preventing and controlling the occurrence and spread of infectious diseases.

Vaccines are divided into two classes. Vaccines of Class I shall mean the vaccines provided by the government to citizens free of charge, which shall be vaccinated to citizens in accordance with the government provisions. Vaccine of this class include the vaccines determined in the State's immunity planning, the vaccines added by the people's government of provinces, autonomous region, and municipalities directly under the Central Government in the implementation of the State's immunity planning, and the vaccines used in the emergent inoculation or mass vaccination organized by people's government at the country level or above or their respective competent health departments. Vaccines of Class II shall mean other vaccines with which the citizens are voluntarily inoculated at their own expenses.

【 Article 3 】  The expenses for inoculation with vaccines of Class I shall be borne by the government, while the expenses for inoculation with vaccines of Class II shall be borne by the inoculated persons or their respective guardians.

【 Article 4 】  The circulation and vaccination of vaccines and the supervision and administration thereof shall be governed by this *Regulation*.

【Article 5】 The competent department of health under the State Council shall, in light of such factors as the spread of infectious diseases within China, the crowd's immunity condition, etc., formulate the State's immunity planning; and shall, jointly with the department of public finance under the State Council, draft vaccine varieties which are included into the State's immunity planning, and promulgate them upon approval of the State Council.

The people's government of the province, autonomous region, or municipality directly under the Central Government may, when implementing the State's immunity planning increase the vaccines varieties supplied to citizens free of charge in light of such factors as the spread of infectious diseases, the crowd's immunity conditions, etc. within its own administrative region, and report to the competent department of health under the State Council for archival purposes.

【Article 6】 The State applies a planned vaccination system, carries out and enlarges the immunity planning.

Those who need to be inoculated with vaccines of Class I shall be inoculated in accordance with this *Regulation*. If the inoculated person is a minor, his guardian shall cooperate with the relevant disease prevention and control institution, medical institution, or other medical and health institution, so as to guarantee the said minor to be inoculated in time.

【Article 7】 The responsibility to supervise and administer the vaccination throughout the country shall remain with the competent department of health under the State Council. The competent health department of the local people's government at the country level or above shall be responsible for supervising and administering the vaccination within its own administrative region.

The responsibility to supervise and administer the quality and circulation of vaccines throughout the country shall remain with the drug administration department under the State Council. The drug administration department of the people's government of the province, autonomous region, or municipality directly under the Central Government shall be responsible for supervising and administering the quality and circulation of vaccines within its own administrative region.

【Article 8】 The medical and health institution designated by the competent health department of a people's government at the county level in accordance with this *Regulation* (hereinafter referred to as the inoculation entity) shall undertake the vaccination work. The competent health department of the people's government at the country level shall, when designating an inoculation entity, clarify the area of its responsibilities.

The people's government at the country level or above shall reward the inoculation entities and their personnel who undertake vaccination work and have made prominent achievement and contributions.

【Article 9】 The State supports and encourages entities and individuals to participate in vaccination. The people's government at each level shall improve relevant systems so as to facilitate the entities and individuals to take part in the activities of vaccination work including publicity, education and donation, etc.

Residents' committees and villages' committees shall cooperate with relevant department in carrying out the propaganda and education relating to vaccination, and assist in organizing residents and villagers to be invocation with vaccine of Class I.

## Chapter II Circulation of Vaccines

【Article 10】 Vaccines shall be purchased through provincial public resource trading platforms.

【Article 11】 The disease prevention and control institution at the provincial level shall, in light of the State's immunity planning and needs in preventing and controlling the occurrence and spread of infectious diseases in the local area, make the plan on use of vaccines of Class I in the local area (hereinafter referred to as use plan), and report it to the department responsible for procuring vaccines of Class I in accordance with the relevant provisions of the State, and meanwhile report it to the competent health department of the people's government at the same level for archival purposes.

The use plan shall include such contents as the varieties and quantity of the vaccines, the channel and method of supply, etc.

【Article 12】 The department responsible for procuring vaccines of Class I in accordance with the relevant provisions of the State shall conclude a government procurement contract with a vaccine production enterprise in accordance with law, stipulating the varieties, quantity and prices, etc. of the vaccines.

【Article 13】 A vaccine production enterprise shall, according to the stipulation in the government procurement contract, supply vaccines of Class I to the disease prevention and control institutions at the provincial level or other disease prevention and control institution designated by the aforementioned institutions, and shall not supply vaccines of Class I to any other entities or individuals.

The vaccine production enterprise shall mark the words of "Free of Charge" and the special mark of "Immunity Planning" set forth by the competent department of health under the State Council at an eye-catching position of the smallest exterior packing of the vaccines included into the State's immunity planning which it supplies. The specific administrative measures shall be formulated by the drug administration department under the State Council jointly with the competent department of health under the State Council.

【Article 14】 A disease prevention and control institution at the provincial level shall do a good job in organizing the distribution of vaccines of Class I, and shall organize the distribution of vaccines of Class I to the disease prevention and control institution at the prefecture level or at the country level according to the use plan. Each disease prevention and control institution at the county level shall distribute the vaccines of Class I to the inoculation entities and the medical and health institution at the township level according to the use plan. Each medical and health institution at the township level shall distribute the vaccine of Class I to the village medical and health institution undertaking the vaccination work. No medical and health institution shall distribute vaccines of Class I to any other entity or individual. An institution that distributes vaccines of Class I may not charge any fee.

When an infectious disease breaks out or spreads, the local people's government at the county level or above or its competent health department needs to take emergent inoculation measures, the disease prevention and control institution at the prefecture level or above may distribute vaccines of Class I directly to the inoculation entities.

【Article 15】 Provincial disease prevention and control institutions shall organize the centralized procurement of Class II vaccines through provincial public resource trading platforms, and county disease prevention and control institutions shall, after purchasing vaccines from vaccine production enterprises, supply them to inoculation entities within their respective administrative regions.

Vaccine production enterprises shall directly distribute Class II vaccines to county disease prevention and control institutions or authorize enterprises with cold chain storage and transport conditions to distribute them. The enterprises that distribute Class II vaccines upon authorization shall not authorize distribution.

County disease prevention and control institutions that supply Class II vaccines to inoculation entities may charge vaccine fees and storage and transport fees. Vaccine fees shall be charged at the purchase price, and storage and transport fees shall be charged according to the provisions of provinces, autonomous regions, and municipalities directly under the Central Government. The charging information shall be disclosed to the public.

【Article 16】 Disease prevention and control institutions, inoculation entities, vaccine production enterprises, and enterprises that distribute vaccines upon authorization shall abide by the rules on the administration of vaccine storage and transport, and guarantee the quality of vaccines. Vaccines shall be stored and transported in the environment with the prescribed temperature during the entire process, shall not be isolated from the cold chain, and temperature shall be monitored and recorded at regular time. Provincial disease prevention and control institutions shall require the attachment of temperature control labels to the vaccines that are transported in cold chain for a long time and need to be distributed to remote regions.

The rules on the administration of storage and transport of vaccines shall be developed by the competent health department and drug administrative department of the State Council.

【Article 17】 A vaccine production enterprise shall, when selling vaccines, provide a photocopy of the inspection conformity or examination and approval certificate lawfully issued by the drug inspection institution for each batch of biological products, and affix its enterprise seal. If the enterprise sells imported vaccines, it shall also provide a photocopy of the customs clearance list of imported drugs, and affix its enterprise seal.

Disease prevention and control institution or an inoculation entity shall, when receiving or purchasing vaccines, ask for the testimonials prescribed in the preceding paragraph from the vaccine production enterprise, and reserve them for checking until 2 years after expiry of duration of validity of the vaccines.

【Article 18】 A vaccine production enterprise shall, in accordance with the *Pharmaceutical Administration Law* and the provisions of the drug administrative department of the State Council, set up true and complete sales records, and retain them until two years after the expiration of validity term of the vaccines for future reference.

A disease prevention and control institution shall, in accordance with the provisions of the competent health department of the State Council, set up true and complete records on purchase, storage, distribution and supply, ensure consistency among bills, account books, products and payments, and retain them until two years after the expiration of validity term of the vaccines for future reference. The disease prevention and control institution shall, when receiving or purchasing vaccines, request the temperature monitoring records during the entire process of vaccine storage and transport; and if the records on temperature monitoring during the entire process cannot be provided or temperature control fails to satisfy the relevant requirements, the disease prevention and control institution shall not receive or purchase the vaccines, and shall immediately report it to the drug administrative department and the competent health department.

## Chapter III    Inoculation with Vaccines

【Article 19】 The competent department of health under the State Council shall formulate and promulgate the rules on vaccination work, and shall, according to the national standards of vaccines, and the information on the surveys on epidemiology of infectious disease, formulate and promulgate the immunity procedure for the vaccine included into the State's immunity planning, and the immunity procedures or guiding principles for use of other vaccines.

The competent health department of the people's government of a province, autonomous region, or municipality directly under the Central Government shall, according to the immunity procedures and the guiding principles for use of the vaccine formulated by the competent department of health under the State Council and in light of the situation on spread of infectious diseases within its administrative region, formulate the inoculation program for its region, and report it to the competent department of health under the State Council for archival purposes.

【Article 20】 The disease prevention and control institution at all level shall, upon their respective duties, and according to the State's immunity planning or inoculation program, carry out propagandas, trainings, technical guidance, monitoring, appraisals, epidemiological surveys and emergent treatment, etc. related to vaccination, and make records thereof in accordance with provisions of the competent department of health under the State Council.

【Article 21】 An inoculation entity shall meet the following conditions;

(1) Having a medical institution practicing permit;

(2) Having practicing doctors, assistant practicing doctors, nurses or village doctors who have accepted the professional vaccination trainings organized by the competent health department of a people's government at the county level and who are assessed to be qualified; and

(3) Having the refrigerating facilities or equipment and refrigerating custody systems which conform to the administrative rules on storage and transport of vaccines.

An urban medical and health institution undertaking vaccination work shall set up an outpatient ward for vaccination.

【Article 22】 An inoculation entity shall undertake the vaccination work within its own responsible area, and accept the technical guidance provided by the local disease prevention and control institution at the country level.

【Article 23】 An inoculation entity that receives Class I vaccines or purchases Class II vaccines shall request records on temperature monitoring during the entire process of vaccine storage and transport, set up and retain true and complete receipt and procurement records, and ensure consistency among bills, account books, products and payments. If the records on temperature monitoring during the entire process cannot be provided or temperature control fails to satisfy the relevant requirements, the inoculation entity shall not receive or purchase the vaccines, and shall immediately report it to the drug administrative department and competent health department of the county people's government at the place where it is located.

An inoculation entity shall, in light of needs in vaccination, formulate the plans on the demands for vaccines of Class I and on the purchase of vaccines of Class II, and shall report them to the competent health department of the people's government at the country level and disease prevention and control institution at the country level.

【 Article 24 】 An inoculation entity shall, when inoculating vaccines, abide by the rules on vaccination work, the immunity procedures, the guiding principles for use of the vaccines and the inoculation program, and shall announce the varieties and inoculation methods of the vaccines of Class I at an eye-catching position of its inoculation place.

【 Article 25 】 A medical and health staff member shall, before carrying out the inoculation, inform the inoculated person or his guardian of the variety, function, contraindication and ill response of the inoculated vaccine and the points for attention, inquire about the inoculated person's health and his information on whether he has contraindication to the inoculation, etc., and shall truthfully record the informed and inquired particulars. The inoculated person or his guardian shall know about the relevant knowledge on vaccination, and shall truthfully provide the information on the inoculated person's health and his contraindication to the inoculation, etc.

Medical and health staff members shall inoculate the persons complying with inoculation conditions, and according to the provisions of the competent health department of the State Council, record the categories and production enterprises of vaccines, the information on the identification of minimum packing units, term of validity, inoculation time, medical and health staff members that perform inoculations, and inoculated persons, among others. Inoculation records shall be retained for no less than five years.

For a person who cannot be inoculated due to his contraindication to the inoculation, the medical and health staff shall propose medical suggestions to this person or his guardian.

【 Article 26 】 The State applies a vaccination certificate system to children. Within 1 month after a child is born, his guardian shall go to the inoculation entity undertaking vaccination work at the child's residential locality to obtain the vaccination certificate for the child. The inoculation entity shall check the child's vaccination certificate when carrying out the inoculation, and shall make records.

During the period when the child is not in his original residential locality, the responsibility to carry out the inoculation shall remain with the inoculation entity undertaking vaccination work at the child's present residential locality.

The format of the vaccination certificate shall be set forth by the competent health department of the people's government of the province, autonomous region, or municipality directly under the Central Government.

【 Article 27 】 When a child enters a nursery, kindergarten or school, the nursery, kindergarten or school shall check his vaccination certificate. If it finds that the child is not inoculated according to the State's immunity planning, it shall report to the local disease prevention and control institution at the county level or the inoculation entity undertaking vaccination work at the child's residential locality, and shall cooperate with the disease prevention and control institution or the inoculation entity in urging his guardian to have his child inoculated in time at the inoculation entity after the child enters the nursery, kindergarten or school.

【 Article 28 】 An inoculation entity shall, according to the State's immunity planning, inoculate those who live in its responsible area and need inoculation with vaccines of Class I, and shall reach the invocation rate as required by the State's immunity planning.

The disease prevention and control institution shall distribute vaccines of Class I in time to the inoculation entities.

Where the inoculated person or his guardian requests inoculation with the same variety of vaccine as that in vaccines of Class I at his own expenses, the inoculation entity providing the service shall inform him of the expenses, the method of compensating abnormal reaction, and the relevant contents prescribed in Article 25 of this *Regulation*.

【 Article 29 】 An inoculation entity shall, in accordance with the provisions of the competent department of health under the State Council, register the information on inoculation, and report to the competent health department of the local people's government at the country level and the local disease prevention and control institution at the county level. The inoculation entity shall, after completing the State's immunity planning, report the remaining vaccines of Class I, if any, to the original vaccine distribution entity, and state the reasons thereof.

【 Article 30 】 An inoculation entity shall not charge any fee for inoculation of vaccines of Class I.

An inoculation entity may charge service fees and inoculation consumption fee for inoculation of vaccines of Class II. The specific fee rates shall be ratified by the competent price department of the local people's government of the province, autonomous region, or municipality directly under the Central Government.

【 Article 31 】 Where the competent health department of a local people's government at the country level or above needs to carry out mass vaccination in some areas within its region on the basis of the information on monitoring and forewarning infectious disease in order to prevent and control the break-out and spread of infectious disease, it shall report to the people's government at the same level for decision, and report to the competent health department of the people's government of the province, autonomous region, or municipality directly under the Central Government for archival purposes. If it needs to carry out mass vaccination within the whole region of the province, autonomous region, or municipality directly under the Central Government, the competent health department the people's government of the province, autonomous region, or municipality directly under the Central Government shall report to the people's government at the same level for decision, and report to the competent department of health under the State Council for archival purposes. If it needs to carry out mass vaccination throughout the whole country or in a large area covering different provinces, autonomous regions, or municipalities directly under the Central Government, the decision shall be made by the competent department of health under the State Council. If a decision on approval is made, the people's government or the competent department of health under the State Council shall organize relevant departments to make staff trainings, propaganda, education, transfer of goods and materials, and so on.

No entity or individual shall carry out unauthorized mass vaccination.

【 Article 32 】 When an infectious disease breaks out or spreads, the local people's government at the county level or above or its competent health department shall, if necessary, take emergent inoculation measures in accordance with the *Law on Prevention and Treatment of Infectious Diseases* and the *Regulation on Urgent Response to Public Health Emergencies*.

【 Article 33 】 The competent department of health under the State Council or the competent health department of a people's government of the province, autonomous region, or municipality directly under the Council Government may, on the basis of the information on monitoring and forewarning infectious diseases, promulgate the information on suggesting inoculation of vaccines of Class II, while no other entity or individual may promulgate such information.

The information on suggesting inoculation of vaccines of Class II shall include such contents as the knowledge on prevention and control of the targeted infectious disease, the relevant inoculation program, etc. provided that it shall not involve any specific vaccine production enterprise.

## Chapter IV   Safeguarding Measures

【 Article 34 】 The people's government at the county level or above shall include the vaccination work related to the State immunity planning into the plans on national economy and social development for its own region, guarantee the expenses necessary for vaccination work, warrant the inoculating rate as required by the State's immunity planning, and ensure the implementation of the State's immunity planning.

【 Article 35 】 The people's government of a province, autonomous region, or municipality directly under the Central Government shall, in light of the spreading trend of the infectious diseases within its region, determine the projects related to vaccination within its region within the scope of infectious disease prevention and control projects determined by the competent department of health under the State Council, and ensure the implementation of such projects.

【 Article 36 】 The people's government of a province, autonomous region, or municipality directly under the Central Government shall guarantee the expenses needed in purchasing and transporting vaccines of Class I, and ensure the construction and operation of the cold chain systems of the disease prevention and control institution and the inoculation entities within its region.

The State may, if necessary, provide adequate supports to the vaccination work in the poverty-stricken areas.

【 Article 37 】 The people's government at the county level shall ensure the necessary expenses for carrying out vaccination with the State's, immunity planning, and shall, in accordance with the relevant provisions of the State, provide adequate subsidies to the village doctors engaging in vaccination and to other community-level prevention and healthcare personnel as well.

The people's government of a province, autonomous region, or municipality directly under the Central Government and the people's governments at the prefecture level shall provide necessary subsidies to the people's governments at the country level in the poverty-stricken areas for carrying out the work related to vaccination.

【 Article 38 】 The responsibility to reserve vaccines and other relevant products and materials for the sake of transfer shall remain with the people's governments at the county level or above.

【 Article 39 】 The expenses arranged by the public finance departments at all levels for vaccination shall be used for this particular purpose, and may not be misappropriated or occupied by any entity or individual. The expenses used by relevant entities and individuals for vaccination shall be lawfully subject to the auditing organ's audit and supervision.

## Chapter V  Dealing with Abnormal Reactions to Vaccination

【 Article 40 】 Abnormal reactions to vaccination shall mean the ill response of medicine which causes damage to the inoculated person's tissues, organs or functions in the process of or after regularized inoculation of a qualified vaccine, and for which no relevant part has any fault.

【Article 41】 The following circumstances do not belong to abnormal reactions to vaccination:

(1) Common reactions of post inoculation caused by the vaccine's features;

(2) Damage to the inoculated person due to disqualification of the vaccine's quality;

(3) Damage to the inoculated person due to the inoculation entity's violation of the rules on vaccination work, immunity procedures, guiding principles for use of the vaccines, or inoculation program;

(4) The inoculated person was in the delitescence or prodromal phase of a certain disease at the time of inoculation, and is attacked by the disease by coincidence after inoculation;

(5) The inoculated person has the contraindication to the inoculation as stated in the vaccine directions, but the said inoculated person or his guardian fails to truthfully provide the information on the inoculated person's health and contraindication to the inoculation, etc. prior to the inoculation, and the inoculated person's original disease recrudesces urgently or becomes worse after the inoculation; and

(6) Individual or mass psychogenic responses due to psychological factors.

【Article 42】 Where a diseases prevention and control institution or an inoculation entity or any of its medical and health staff finds any abnormal reaction to vaccination, suspected abnormal reaction to vaccination or receives any relevant report, it/he shall deal with the matter in time in accordance with the rules on vaccination work, and immediately report to the competent health department and the drug administration department of the local people's government at the county level. The competent health department and the drug administration department that receive the report shall immediately organize an investigation into the matter.

【Article 43】 The competent health department and the drug administration department of a local people's government at the county level or above shall report the information on the abnormal reactions to vaccination which occur within their own region and the information on dealing with the responses separately and level by level to the competent department of health under the State Council.

【Article 44】 After a dispute over abnormal reaction to vaccination arises, the inoculation entity or the inoculated person may ask the competent health department of the people's government at the county level at the inoculation entity's locality for settlement.

Where, due to vaccination, an inoculated person die or becomes heavily disabled, or any suspected group of people suffer from abnormal reaction to vaccination, and the inoculation entity or the inoculated person asks the competent health department of the people's government at the county level for settlement, the competent health department receiving such request shall take necessary emergent measures to deal with the matter, to the competent health department of the people's government at the next higher level for settlement.

【Article 45】 The authentication of abnormal reactions to vaccination shall be conducted by referring to the *Regulation on Handling Medical Malpractices*, and specific measures shall be formulated by the competent department of health under the State Council jointly with the drug administration department under the State Council.

【Article 46】 Where, due to abnormal reaction to vaccination, an inoculated person die or becomes heavily disabled, or any of his organs or tissues is damaged, he shall be paid a lump-sum of compensation.

Where an inoculated person needs to be compensated due to the abnormal action to a Class I vaccine, the compensation shall be covered with the working expenses by the financial department of a province (autonomous region or municipality directly under the Central Government). Where an inoculated person needs to be compensated due to the abnormal action to a Class II vaccine, the compensation shall be covered by the vaccine manufacturer. The state shall encourage the establishment of the mechanism of compensation with commercial insurance and other channels for persons with abnormal reaction to vaccination.

The specific measures for compensation for abnormal reactions to vaccination shall be formulated by the people's government of each province, autonomous region, on municipality directly under the Central Government.

【Article 47】 Where an inoculated person is harmed due to disqualification of a vaccine's quality, the matter shall be dealt with in accordance with the relevant provision of the *Pharmaceutical Administration Law*. If he is harmed due to the inoculation entity's violation of the rules on vaccination work, the immunity procedures, the guiding principles for use of the vaccines, or the inoculation program, the matter shall be dealt with in accordance with the relevant provisions of the *Regulation on Handling Medical Malpractices*.

## Chapter VI   Supervision and Administration

【Article 48】 The drug administration department shall, in accordance with the relevant provisions of the *Pharmaceutical Administration Law* and the *Regulation for the Implementation*, supervise and inspect the quality of vaccines in the process of storage, transport, supply, sale, distribution and use, etc., and circularize the result of inspection in time to the competent health department at the same level. If the drug administration department samples and inspects a vaccine upon the needs in supervision and inspection, the entity or individual concerned shall cooperate, and shall not refuse the sampling and inspection.

【Article 49】 A drug administration department may, in its supervision and inspection, seal up or distain the vaccine which is proved by any evidence as likely to harm human health and the relevant materials thereof, and shall make a handling decision within 7 days. If the vaccine needs to be inspected, the drug administration department shall make a handling decision within 15 days as of the day when the inspection report is sent out.

Where a diseases prevention and control institution, an inoculation entity, a vaccine production enterprise finds any fake, inferior vaccine or any vaccine whose quality is suspicious, it shall immediately cease the inoculation, distribution, supply or sale, and immediately report to the competent health department and the drug administration department of the local people's government at the county level, and may not deal with the matter by itself. The competent health department that receives the report shall immediately organize the disease prevention and control institution and the inoculation entity to take necessary emergent measures, and meanwhile report to the competent health department at the higher level. The drug administration department that receives the report shall lawfully take such measures as sealing up or distaining the fake, inferior vaccine or the vaccine whose quality is suspicious.

【Article 50】 The competent health department of the people's government at the county level or above shall perform the following supervision and inspection duties within the scope of its own duties:

(1) Supervising and inspecting the information on implementation of the State's immunity planning by the medical and health institution;

(2) Supervising and inspecting the publicity, trainings and technical guidance related to vaccination, which are carried out by the disease prevention and control institution; and

(3) Supervising and inspecting the information on the distribution and purchase of vaccines by medical and health institutions

A competent health department shall perform its supervision and administration duties mainly through inspecting the records made by medical and health institution in accordance with this *Regulation* on distribution, storage, transport and inoculation, etc. of vaccines. When necessary, it may conduct on-site supervision and inspections.

The competent health department shall record the information on supervision and inspection, and shall, when finding any illegal act, order the relevant entity to make a correction immediately.

【Article 51】 There shall be no less than 2 persons when the personnel of a competent health department or drug administration department perform their supervision and inspection duties in accordance with law. They shall show their testimonials, and keep confidential the commercial secrets of the inspected part.

【Article 52】 The competent health department and drug administrative department shall make timely report to each other and share the information when discovering the issues like quality problems of vaccines and abnormal reaction to vaccination.

【Article 53】 Any entity or individual shall have the right to expose to the competent health department or the drug administration department the act violating this *Regulation*, and to expose to the people's government at the same level or the relevant department of the people's government at the higher level the competent health department's or the drug administration department's failure to lawfully perform its supervision and administration duties. The people's government, the competent health department or the drug administration department that receives the exposure shall verify the information and deal with the matter in time.

## Chapter VII   Legal Liabilities

【Article 54】 The state shall establish the whole-course tracing system of vaccines. The competent health department of the State Council shall joint with the drug administrative department of the State Council to formulate the uniformed technical standards for the vaccine tracing system.

Vaccine production enterprises, disease prevention and control institutions and inoculation entities shall, in accordance with the *Pharmaceutical Administration Law*, the *Regulation on the Administration of Circulation and Vaccination of Vaccines* and the provisions of the competent health department and drug administrative department of the State Council, set up the vaccine tracing system, make authentic records of the distribution and usage of the vaccines and realize the whole-course traceability of the vaccines in the smallest unit of package during the production, storage, transportation and usage.

The competent health department of the State Council shall joint with the drug administrative department of the State Council to establish the collaboration mechanism for the whole-course trace of vaccines.

【Article 55】 Disease prevention and control institutions and inoculation entities shall make authentic record of the vaccines that are with unrecognizable packages, expired, isolated from the cold chain, unqualified upon inspection and of unidentified source and make report to the drug administrative department of the local county government, which shall joint with the competent health department at the same level to supervise the destruction of the vaccines. Disease prevention and control institutions and inoculation entities shall make authentic record of the destruction and the record shall be kept for at least 5 years.

【Article 56】 The competent health department and drug administrative department above the county level, in violation of the provisions in this *Regulation* with one of the following conditions shall be instructed to rectify and be given a criticism by circulating a notice; the person directly in charge and other persons directly responsible shall be punished by law if serious consequences occur, like physical harm to the inoculated persons or transmission and prevalence of infectious diseases; if the consequence is particularly serious, the main responsible person shall also resign to assume responsibility; and in case of criminal offenses, the offenders shall be prosecuted in accordance with the law.

(1) It fails to carry out supervision and inspection or fails to carry out timely investigation and punishment upon finding out illegal activities;

(2) It fails to timely verify and deal with the report on the negligence of duty in supervision and administration by the subordinate competent health department and drug administrative department;

(3) It fails to organize immediate investigation and handling of the relevant report on discovering cases or suspected cases of abnormal reaction to vaccination;

(4) It carries out unauthorized group vaccination;

(5) Other relevant acts of malpractice or dereliction of duty.

【Article 57】 The people's government above the county level that fails to provide guarantee for inoculation and vaccination in accordance with the provisions of this *Regulation* shall be instructed to rectify and given a criticism by circulating a notice by the people's government at the higher level; where physical harm to the inoculated persons, transmission and prevalence of infectious diseases or other serious consequence occurs, the person directly in charge and other persons directly responsible shall be punished by law; where a particularly serious quality and safety issue of vaccines occurs or a successive series of such issues occur, the person chiefly in charge of the local people's government shall resign; and in case of criminal offenses, the offenders shall be prosecuted in accordance with the law.

【Article 58】 Where a disease prevention and control institution has one of the following conditions, it shall be instructed to rectify, criticized with a circular notice and given a warning by the competent health department of the people's government above the county level; and in case of it refusing to rectify, the person chiefly in charge, the executives directly responsible and other persons directly responsible shall get punishment ranging from warning to demotion in accordance with the law.

(1) It fails to distribute Class I vaccines to the subordinate disease prevention and control institutions, inoculation entities and township medical and health institutions;

(2) It fails to set up and keep the records on the procurement, storage, distribution and supply of vaccines;

(3) It fails to request the temperature monitoring record, accepts and purchases unqualified vaccines or fails to make reports in accordance with the regulation.

【 Article 59 】 Where the inoculation entity has one of the following conditions, it shall be instructed to rectify and given a warning by the competent health department of the local people's government at the county level; in case of it refusing to rectify, the person chiefly in charge and the executives directly responsible shall get punishment ranging from warning to demotion in accordance with the law and the responsible medical and health personnel shall be instructed to suspend practice for a period of more than 3 months and less than 6 months.

(1) It fails to request the temperature monitoring record, accepts and purchases unqualified vaccines or fails to make reports in accordance with the regulation;

(2) It fails to set up and retain true and complete receipt and procurement records;

(3) It fails to display the varieties and inoculation methods of Class I vaccines at an eye-catching place in the inoculation facilities;

(4) The medical and health personnel fail to inform and inquire the inoculated person or his/her guardian the related information;

(5) Medical and health staff members that perform inoculations fail to fill in and retain the inoculation record;

(6) It fails to record and make report of the vaccine inoculation in accordance with the regulations.

【 Article 60 】 Where a disease prevention and control institution and an inoculation entity has one of the following conditions, it shall be instructed to rectify and given a warning by the people's government at or above the county level; the illegal gains shall be confiscated if they are obtained; in case of it refusing to rectify, the person chiefly in charge, the executives directly responsible and other persons directly responsible shall get punishment ranging from warning to removal from the office in accordance with the law; where physical harm to the inoculated persons and other serious circumstances occur, the person chiefly in charge and the executives directly responsible shall be discharged and the medical practicing licenses of the medical staff who are responsible shall be revoked by the former license issuance department; and in case of criminal offenses, the offenders shall be prosecuted in accordance with the law.

(1) It violates the provisions of this *Regulation* and fails to purchase vaccines at the provincial public resources trading platform;

(2) It violates the provisions of this *Regulation* and purchases Class II vaccines

from an entity or an individual other than a vaccine production enterprise or a disease prevention and control department at the county level;

(3) It fails to observe the working norms of inoculation, the vaccination procedures, the guiding principles for application of vaccines and the vaccine plans;

(4) It fails to make timely response or report upon discovering cases or suspected cases of abnormal reaction to vaccination;

(5) It carries out unauthorized group vaccination;

(6) It fails to make records and reports on vaccines that are with unrecognizable package, expired, isolated from the cold chain, unqualified upon inspection and of unknown source or fails to make records on the destruction of these vaccines.

【 Article 61 】 Where a disease prevention and control institution or an inoculation entity violates this *Regulation* to charge fees in the process of distributing or supplying vaccines or in the process of inoculation, it shall, under supervision of the competent health department of the local people's government at the county level, refund the illegally charged fees to the original entity or individual that paid the fees, and shall be penalized by the price competent department the people's government at the county level or above in accordance with law.

【 Article 62 】 Where a pharmaceutical inspection institution issues a false vaccine inspection report, it shall be penalized in accordance with Article 86 of the *Pharmaceutical Administration Law of the People's Republic China.*

【 Article 63 】 Where the vaccine production enterprises fail to set up and retain records on the storage and sales of vaccines, they shall be punished in accordance with the provisions in Article 78 of the *Pharmaceutical Administration Law of the People's Republic of China.*

【 Article 64 】 Where a vaccine production enterprise fails to comply with the provisions to mark the words of "Free of Charge" and the special mark of "Immunity Planning" on the smallest exterior packing of the vaccines included into the State's immunity planning, it shall be ordered to make a correction and be warned by the drug administration department. Where it refuses to make a correction, it shall be fined 5,000 *yuan* up to 20,000 *yuan*, and its vaccines involved shall be sealed up and preserved.

【 Article 65 】 Where vaccine production enterprises sell Class II vaccines to entities or individuals other than disease prevention and control department at the county level, the vaccines sold illegally shall be confiscated by the drug administrative department and a fine two times higher and 5 times less than the value of the vaccines shall be imposed; the illegal gains shall be confiscated if they are obtained; in case of serious circumstances, the production qualifications shall be revoked or the import permission certificates shall be withdrawn in accordance with the law, and the executives directly responsible and other persons directly responsible shall be forbidden to carry out pharmaceutical production and sales within 10 years; and in case of criminal offenses, the offender shall be prosecuted in accordance with the law.

【 Article 66 】 Where disease prevention and control department, inoculation entities, vaccine production enterprises and enterprises that distribute vaccines upon authorization fail to store and transport the vaccines in cold chain conditions in accordance with the regulations, they shall be instructed to rectify and given a warning by pharmaceutical administrative department and the vaccines that are stored or transported by them shall be destroyed; the person chiefly in charge, the executives directly responsible and other persons directly responsible shall get punishment ranging from warning to removal from office by competent health department, and in case of serious circumstances, they shall be discharged and the inoculation qualifications of the inoculation entity shall be revoked in accordance with the law; the vaccine production enterprises and the vaccine production enterprises and enterprises that distribute vaccines upon authorization shall be instructed to stop production and distribution to rectify by the pharmaceutical administrative department; a fine two times more and five times less than the value of the vaccines that are stored and transported shall be imposed and in case of serious circumstances, the production qualifications shall be revoked or the import permission certificates shall be withdrawn in accordance with the law; the executives directly responsible and other persons directly responsible shall be forbidden to carry out pharmaceutical production and sales within 10 years; and in case of criminal offenses, the offender shall be prosecuted in accordance with the law.

【 Article 67 】 Whichever entity violates this *Regulation* by promulgating the suggested information on inoculation of vaccines of Class II shall be ordered to eliminate the effect via a mass media and be warned by the competent health department of the people's government at the county level at its locality or at the locality of occurrence; its illegal gains, if any, shall be confiscated, and this entity shall be fined one time to 3 times of the amount of the illegal gains. If a crime is constituted, it shall be subject to criminal liabilities in accordance with law.

【 Article 68 】 Whichever entity discretionarily engages in inoculation without being lawfully designated by the competent health department shall be ordered to make a correction and be warned by the competent health department of the people's government at the county level at its locality or at the locality of occurrence; the illegally held vaccines or the illegal gains, if any, shall be confiscated. If it refuses to make a correction, its principal responsible persons, directly responsible person in charge, and other persons directly held liable shall be warned or degraded in accordance with law.

【Article 69】 When a child enters a nursery, kindergarten or school, the nursery, kindergarten or school fails to check his vaccination certificate in accordance with the provisions, or fails to report to the disease prevention and control institution or the inoculation entity after finding any child who is not inoculated in accordance with the provision, it shall be ordered to make a correction and be warned by the educational administration department of the local people's government at the county level or above. If it refuses to make a correction, its principal responsible person, directly responsible person in charge, and other persons directly held liable shall be imposed upon sanctions in accordance with law.

【Article 70】 Where an entity or an individual other than the vaccine production enterprises or disease prevention and control department at the county level, in violation of the provisions of this *Regulation*, carries out sales of vaccines, the entity or the person shall be punished in accordance with the provisions of Article 72 of the *Pharmaceutical Administration Law* of *the People' Republic of China*.

【Article 71】 Where a competent health department, a disease prevention and control institution, an entity or individual other than inoculation entities violates this *Regulation* to conduct group vaccination, it shall be ordered by the competent health department of the people's government at the county level or above to make a correction immediately, its illegally held vaccines shall be confiscated, and this entity shall be fine twice to 5 times of the amount of the value of the illegally held vaccines; and its illegal gains, if any, shall also be confiscated.

【Article 72】 An entity or individual shall bear civil liabilities in accordance with law when violating this *Regulation* and causing any personal or property damage to an inoculated person.

【Article 73】 Whoever provokes a quarrel and makes trouble, and disturbs the inoculation entity's normal medical treatment order or authentication of any abnormal reaction to vaccination on the pretext of abnormal reaction to vaccination shall be imposed upon penalties of public security administration in accordance with law.

If a crime is constituted, he shall be subject to criminal liabilities in accordance with law.

## Chapter VIII   Supplementary Provisions

【Article 74】 The following terms in this *Regulation* shall have their meanings as follows:

The State's immunity planning shall mean the planned vaccination carried out among the population according to the vaccine varieties, immunity procedures or inoculation programs determined by the State or the government of the province, autonomous region, or municipality directly under the Central Government, so as to prevent and control the occurrence and spread of certain infectious diseases.

Cold chain shall mean the refrigerating facilities and equipment for storage and transport which are installed in order to guarantee the quality of vaccines in the process from the vaccine production enterprise to the inoculation entity.

Common reaction shall mean the reaction occurring after the immunity inoculation and caused from the vaccine's own intrinsic features, which will only result in transient impediment in physiological functions to the body. Common reactions mainly include becoming feverish or partially red and swollen, which may possibly be accompanied with such comprehensive symptoms as discomfort from head to foot, tiredness, poor appetite, short of strength, etc.

Vaccine production enterprises refer to both the domestic vaccine production enterprises and the agency of overseas vaccine manufacturers within the border of China.

【 Article 75 】 The *Measures for the Management of Vaccination of Entry and Exit* shall be separately formulated by the state entry-exit inspection and quarantine department.

【 Article 76 】 This *Regulation* shall come into force on June 1st, 2005.

(Qu Yang)

## 13. *Opinions of the State Council on Integrating Basic Medical Insurance System for Urban and Rural Residents*

(No. 3 [2016] of the General Office of the State Council, January 3rd, 2016)

The people's governments of all provinces, autonomous regions, and municipalities directly under the Central Government; all ministries and commissions of the State Council; and all institutions directly under the State Council,

Integrating the basic medical insurance for urban residents (hereinafter referred to as urban residents' medical insurance) and the new rural cooperative medical care (hereinafter referred to as the new rural cooperative medical system), and establishing a unified system of the basic medical insurance for urban and rural residents (hereinafter referred to as urban and rural residents' medical insurance) are important measures for promoting the reform of the medical and health system, having fair accessibility to basic medical insurance rights and interests for urban and rural residents, promoting social fairness and justice, and promoting people's well-being. It is of much significance for promoting the coordinated development of urban and rural economy and society, and building a moderately prosperous society in all respects. On the basis of accumulating the experience of medical insurance for urban residents and the operation of the new rural cooperative medical system, and the experience of exploration and practice in local areas, the following opinions are proposed on integrating and establishing the medical insurance system for urban and rural residents.

## I. General requirements and basic principles

### (1) General requirements

Guided by the important thoughts of Deng Xiaoping Theory and "Three Represents", and scientific development concept, the spirit of the important speeches of the Party's 18th National People's Congress, the 2nd, 3rd, 4th and 5th Plenary Sessions of 18th CPC Central Committee, and General Secretary Xi Jinping should be conscientiously implemented. The requirements of the CPC Central Committee and the State Council on deepening medical and health care system reform should be implemented. In accordance with full coverage, guarantee of the basic, multi-level, and sustainable policies, overall coordination and top-level design should be strengthened. The principle of prioritizing the work from the easy to the difficult should be followed. It is necessary to start from improving policies to promote the institutional integration of urban residents' medical insurance and new rural cooperative medical care, gradually establish a unified urban and rural residents' medical insurance system nationwide, promote fairer security, more standardized management services, and more effective use of medical resources, and promote the sustainable and healthy development of the national health insurance system.

### (2) Basic principles

1) Overall plan and coordinated development. It is necessary to integrate the medical insurance system of urban and rural residents into the development of the national medical insurance system and deepening of the overall medical reform, make overall arrangements and rational planning, highlight the linkage of medical insurance, medical care and medicine, strengthen basic medical insurance, major illness insurance, medical assistance, disease emergency assistance, and commercial health insurance, etc. and strengthen the system to make it systemic, holistic and synergistic.

2) Being based on the basic and guaranteeing fairness

It is necessary to ensure accurate location and scientific design, be based on the level of economic and social development, the burden of urban and rural residents and the capability of the funds, fully consider and gradually narrow the gap between urban and rural areas and the gap between different regions, ensure that urban and rural residents have fair access to basic medical insurance and achieve the sustainable development of medical insurance system for urban and rural residents.

3) Advancing in accordance with local conditions and priorities

It is necessary to be practical, comprehensively analyze and judge the actual situation, comprehensively formulate implementation plans, strengthen the link before and after integration, ensure smooth and orderly transition of work, ensure that the basic medical insurance benefits of the people are not affected, and ensure the safety of the medical insurance funds and the stable operation of the system.

4) Innovating mechanisms and improving efficiency. It is necessary to adhere to the separation of management and administration, implement government responsibilities, improve management and operation mechanisms, further promote the reform of payment methods, and improve the efficiency of medical insurance funds and the effectiveness of management services. The role of market mechanism should be given full play to. Social forces should be mobilized to participate in basic medical insurance services.

**II. Integration of basic institutional policies**

**(1) Unifying coverage**

Medical insurance system for urban and rural residents covers all those who have current urban residents' medical insurance and all those who should have new rural cooperative medical insurance (cooperative), that is, all urban and rural residents are covered except those who should have employees' basic medical insurance. Migrant workers and flexible employees participate in basic medical insurance for employees in accordance with the law. If they have difficulties, they can participate in medical insurance for urban and rural residents in accordance with local regulations. All localities should improve the way they have insurance, promote the full coverage of insurance, and avoid repeated insurance.

**(2) Unifying fundraising policies**

It is necessary to adhere to multi-channel fundraising, continue to implement the combination of personal payment and government subsidies, and encourage collective organizations, entities or other social and economic organizations to provide support or funding. All localities must take into account the needs of urban and rural residents' medical insurance and major illness insurance, and rationally determine the unified fundraising standards for urban and rural areas in accordance with the principle of balance of funds. In areas where the gap between the urban residents' medical insurance and the new rural cooperative medical insurance standard is relatively large, a differential payment method can be adopted to make a gradual transition in 2-3 years. The actual per capita fundraising and individual contributions after integration should not be lower than those at the current level.

The dynamic adjustment mechanism of fundraising should be improved. On the basis of actuarial balance, a stable fundraising mechanism will be gradually established that is compatible with the level of economic and social development and the capability of all parties. A mechanism for linking individual payment standards with per capita disposable income of urban and rural residents should be gradually established. It is necessary to make reasonable division of government and individual fundraising responsibilities, and appropriately increase the proportion of individual contributions while enhancing government subsidy standards.

### (3) Unifying security treatment

It is necessary to follow the principle of appropriate security and balance of payments, balance urban and rural security treatment, and gradually unify the security scope and payment standards to provide fair basic medical security for the insured. It is necessary to handle the special security policies before integration and make a good transition and connection.

The urban and rural residents' medical insurance funds are mainly used to pay for the insured's inpatient and outpatient medical expenses. The security level of hospitalization should be stabilized, and the proportion of hospitalization expenses paid within the policy range should remain at around 75%. The outpatient overall plans should be further improved. The level of outpatient security should be gradually improved. It is necessary to gradually narrow the gap between the proportion of payments within the policy and the actual proportion of payments.

### (4) Unifying medical insurance catalogue

It is necessary to unify the drug catalogue and the catalogue of medical service items for urban and rural residents' medical insurance, and clarify the scope of payment for drugs and medical services. All provinces (autonomous regions and municipalities directly under the Central Government) shall follow the relevant provisions of the national basic medical insurance drug administration and the essential medicine system, and follow the principles of clinical necessity, safety and effectiveness, reasonable price, appropriate technology, and affordable funds. Based on the current urban residents' medical insurance and the new rural cooperative medical catalogue, due consideration should be given to the changes in the needs of the insured , which are subject to increase or decrease, control and expansion, and the types are basically complete and the structure is reasonable as a whole. The management of medical insurance catalogues should be improved. It is necessary to implement graded management and dynamic adjustment.

### (5) Unifying designated area management

The methods for managing designated institutions of urban and rural residents' medical insurance should be unified. The management of designated service agreements should be strengthened. A sound assessment and evaluation mechanism and a dynamic access and exit mechanism should be established and improved. The same designated area management policy should be applied to non-public medical institutions and public medical institutions. In principle, the overall planning regional management institutions should be responsible for the access, exit and supervision of the designated agencies. The provincial management institutions should be responsible for formulating the access principles and management methods for the designated institutions, and focusing on strengthening the guidance and supervision of provincial and municipal designated medical institutions outside the overall planning region.

### (6) Unifying fund management

The medical insurance for urban and rural residents should implement the national unified funds and financial system, accounting system, and fund budget and final account management system. The urban and rural residents' medical insurance funds should be included into the financial special accounts, and the "two lines of revenue and expenditure" management should be implemented. The funds' independent accounting and special account management should be implemented. The funds should not be used by any entity or individual.

Combined with the fund budget management, the total payment control should be comprehensively promoted. The use of the funds should follow the principle of expenditures based on revenues, the balance of revenues and expenditures, and a slight balance to ensure that the expenses are payable on time and in full, and the funds' current balance ratio and accumulated balance ratio are reasonably controlled. The warning mechanism for fund operation risks should be established and improved. Fund risks should be prevented. The usage efficiency should be improved.

The internal audit and external supervision of the funds should be strengthened. It is necessary to adhere to the information disclosure of the funds' revenue and expenditure, publicize the information system for settlement of medical expenses, and strengthen social supervision, democratic supervision and public opinion supervision.

### III. Rationalizing the management system

### (1) Integrating the operation agency

Qualified regions should be encouraged to rationalize medical management system and unify the basic medical insurance administrative functions. It is necessary to make full use of current urban residents' medical insurance and new rural cooperative medical resources, integrate urban and rural residents' medical insurance operation agencies, personnel and information systems, standardize the operation procedures, and provide unified operation services. The internal and external supervision and control mechanisms of the operation agencies should be improved, and training and performance appraisal should be strengthened.

**(2) Innovating operation and management**

Management and operation mechanism should be improved. Service means and management methods should be improved. Operation process should be optimized. Management efficiency and service level should be improved. Qualified regions should be encouraged to innovate operation service models. The separation of management and operation should be promoted. Competition mechanism should be introduced. Qualified commercial insurance institutions and other social forces should be entrusted by means of government's buying services to participate in the basic medical insurance operation services, and stimulate the vitality of the operation, while ensuring the safety and effective supervision of the funds.

### IV. Improving service efficiency

#### (1) Improving the level of overall planning

In principle, the medical insurance system for urban and rural residents should implement and steadily promote overall planning at the municipal (prefecture) level around the key points of unified treatment policies, fund management, information system, settlement of medical expenses, etc. It is necessary to do well in the transfer of medical insurance relations and settlement of medical expenses in places away from home. According to the economic development and medical service level of all counties (county-level cities, ds) in the coordination regions, the graded management of the funds should be strengthened. It is necessary to fully mobilize the enthusiasm and initiative of the fund management of the county-level governments and the operation management institutions. Qualified regions should be encouraged to implement provincial-level coordination.

#### (2) Improving information systems

It is necessary to integrate current information systems to support the operation and function expansion of urban and rural residents' medical insurance system. It is necessary to promote the business collaboration and information sharing between the urban and rural residents' medical insurance information system and the designated institution information system, and the medical assistance information system, and do well in necessary information exchange and data sharing for the urban and rural residents' medical insurance information system and the information system of the commercial insurance institutions participating in the services. Information security and the privacy protection of patient information should be strengthened.

**(3) Improving payment methods**

The system promotes the reform of the composite payment methods based on the combination of capitation, case-based payment, payment based on time of inpatient treatment, total prepayment, etc. The negotiation and consultation mechanism and risk sharing mechanism of medical insurance operation agencies, medical institutions and drug suppliers should be established and improved. Reasonable medical insurance payment standards should be promoted and formed. It is necessary to guide the designated medical institutions to standardize service behaviors and control the unreasonable growth of medical expenses.

It is necessary to promote the construction of hierarchical diagnosis and treatment system, and gradually form new order of medical treatment such as primary diagnosis, two-way referral, division of acute and chronic treatment, and up and down linkage by taking measures such as supporting insured residents to carry out contracting services with primary medical institutions and general practitioners, and formulating differentiated payment policies.

**(4) Strengthening the supervision of medical services**

The supervision methods for medical insurance services for urban and rural residents should be improved. It is necessary to fully utilize the management of agreements and strengthen the monitoring role of medical services. Medical insurance agencies at all levels should use information technology to promote medical insurance smart audits and real-time monitoring, and promote rational diagnosis and medication. The health and family planning administrative departments should strengthen the supervision of medical services and regulate the behavior of medical services.

**V. Carefully organizing implementation to ensure smooth integration**

**(1) Strengthening organizational leadership**

Integrating the medical insurance system for urban and rural residents is one of the key tasks of deepening medical reform, has a bearing on the vital interests of urban and rural residents, and involves a wide range of interests and strict policies. All departments in various localities involved should fully understand the significance of the work in accordance with the strategic layout requirements for comprehensive deepening reforms, strengthen leadership, and meticulously organize relevant parties to ensure smooth and orderly integration. The provincial medical reform leading groups should strengthen overall coordination and do timely research on and solve problems in the integration process.

**(2) Clarifying work progress and division of responsibilities**

All provinces (autonomous regions and municipalities directly under the Central Government) should make plans and deployment, clear timetables and roadmaps for the integration of urban and rural residents' medical insurance work, improve work progress mechanism, and assessment and evaluation mechanism, strictly implement the responsibility system, and ensure that all policies and measures should have been enforced by the end of June 2016. Each integrated region should have had a specific implementation plan by the end of December 2016.

The pilot provinces for comprehensive medical reform should consider integrating the medical insurance for urban and rural residents as the key reform content, strengthen the overall coordination with other medical reforms, and accelerate the promotion of social security of human resources at all localities. Health and family planning departments should improve relevant policies and measures, and strengthen the link of urban and rural residents' medical insurance systems before and after integration; the financial departments should improve the fund's financial accounting system, and work with relevant departments to do fund supervision; the insurance supervision departments should strengthen qualification review of the operation institutions and supervision of service quality and market behavior of commercial insurance institutions; the development and reform departments should include the integration of the urban and rural residents' medical insurance system into the national economic and social development plans; the compilation management departments should play a functional role in the integration of the operation resources and management system; the medical reform offices should coordinate relevant departments to do well in tracking evaluation, experience accumulation and promotion.

**(3) Doing well in publicity**

It is necessary to strengthen positive publicity and public opinion guidance, and timely and accurate interpretation of policies, publicize local experience, properly respond to public concerns, reasonably guide social expectations, and strive to create a good environment for the integration of urban and rural residents' medical insurance systems.

**(Wang Guimin)**

**Notice of the State Council on Issuing the *Outline for the Planning of the Development Strategy of Traditional Chinese Medicine (2016-2030)***

(No.15 [2016] of the State Council)

The people's governments of all provinces, autonomous regions and municipalities directly under the Central Government, all ministries and commissions of the State Council, and all institutions directly under the State Council,

The *Outline for the Planning of the Development Strategy of Traditional Chinese Medicine* is hereby issued to you for your conscientious implementation.

The State Council

February 22<sup>nd</sup>, 2016

### 14. *Outline for the Planning of the Development Strategy of Traditional Chinese Medicine (2016-2030)*

Traditional Chinese medicine, a unique resource in terms of healthcare, an economic resource with great potential, a scientific and technological resource with originality advantages, an outstanding cultural resource and an ecological resource of great importance, has come to play an increasingly significant role in the social and economic development. With development in industrialization, information, urbanization and modern agriculture and acceleration of aging population, healthcare services develop prosperously and people have growing demands for the services of traditional Chinese medicine, so it is imperative that every effort be made to inherit, develop and make good use of traditional Chinese medicine, fully play its role in deepening the reform of the medical care and health system and serve people's health. The *Outline for the Planning of the Development Strategy of Traditional Chinese Medicine* is hereby formulated to define the development direction and key tasks in the forthcoming 15 years and promote a sound development of the services of traditional Chinese medicine.

### I. Current situations

Since the establishment of new China, particularly since the reform and opening up, the Party Central Committee and the State Council have always attached great importance to traditional Chinese medicine, formulated a series of policies and measures on promoting the development of the services of traditional Chinese medicine and remarkable achievements have been made. The scope of traditional Chinese medicine has kept expanding and development level and service capacity have been improving gradually so that a new development structure has been formed initially, integrating TCM clinical practice, healthcare, research and development, education, industry and culture, and traditional Chinese medicine has done greater contributions to the social and economic development. Statistics collected at the end of 2014 show that there were 3,732 hospitals of traditional Chinese medicine across the country, (including hospitals of ethnic minority medicine and hospitals of integrated Chinese and Western medicine) and 755,000 beds in such hospitals; there were 398,000 practicing or assistant physicians of traditional Chinese medicine (including practicing or assistant physicians of ethnic minority medicine and integrated Chinese and Western medicine) and 531 million visits to TCM medical and healthcare service institutions across the country that year. The role of traditional Chinese medicine in the prevention and treatment of common diseases, frequently occurring diseases, difficult and complicated diseases, chronic diseases and major infectious diseases has been better played and traditional Chinese medicine is more accepted by the rest of the world. In 2014, there were 3,813 TCM pharmaceutical enterprises and the total output value of the TCM pharmaceutical industry was 730.2 billion *yuan*. Traditional Chinese medicine has spread to 183 countries and regions around the world.

However, there are some problems for the development of traditional Chinese medicine. Lack of available resources of traditional Chinese medicine, decreasing service areas and weak service capacity at community-level medical and healthcare institutions lead to insufficient development in TCM service coverage and capacity, which fails to satisfy people's health need. There is a shortage of high-level talented professionals and attention shall be attached to inheritance and innovation. Low concentration ration of TCM pharmaceutical industry, severe destruction of the resources of wild Chinese medicinal plants and decreased quality of some Chinese medicinal materials have negative impacts on the sustainable development of traditional Chinese medicine. Legal and policy systems conforming to the development laws of traditional Chinese medicine are to be perfected; restrictions and barriers to introduction of traditional Chinese medicine to the rest of the world shall be eliminated and global competitiveness of traditional Chinese medicine shall improve further. TCM governance system and capacity and modernization need further improvement and it is a urgent need to strengthen "top-down" design and overall planning.

Currently, it is a crucial time for our country's building of a moderately prosperous society in all respects. For satisfaction of people's need for simple, convenient and low-cost services of traditional Chinese medicine, it is urgently needed to energetically develop TCM health services and expand its service areas; for deepening the reform of the medical care and health system and accelerating the construction of healthy China, it is imperative to play the unique role of traditional Chinese medicine in building the basic medical system with Chinese characteristics; for adaptation to the development trend of transforming from disease-treatment-oriented medicine to health-care-oriented medicine and from bio-medical model to bio-psycho-social model, it is high time to inherit and develop the green health outlook, the holistic view on the unity of the heaven and humanity, the treatment on the basis of syndrome differentiation and harmony in the functions of the various body organs, the naturalistic prevention and treatment, and the whole life-cycle health care services. For promoting economic transformation and upgrading and fostering the new economic growth functions, more support is urgently required to further motivate the originality advantages of traditional Chinese medicine and improve the quality and effectiveness of the industry of traditional Chinese medicine. For carrying on and spreading excellent Chinese traditional culture, efforts shall be made to further popularize and spread the knowledge on traditional Chinese medicine. Promotion of innovation and development of traditional Chinese medicine worldwide is also a pressing demand for carrying out the "go global" strategy and the Belt and Road Initiative. All regions and departments concerned shall correctly understand current situations and seize the opportunities to earnestly promote the sustained and healthy development of traditional Chinese medicine.

## II. Guidelines, basic principles and development goals

### (1) Guidelines

Efforts shall be made to implement the guiding principles of the 18th National Congress of the CPC and the third, fourth and fifth plenary sessions of the 18th CPC Central Committee, put into practice the guiding principles from General Secretary Xi Jinping's major addresses, carry out work in accordance with the Four-Pronged Comprehensive Strategy (this refers to making comprehensive moves to finish building a moderately prosperous society in all respects, deepen reform, advance the law-based governance of China, and strengthen Party self-governance) and the decisions made by the CPC Central Committee and the State Council, follow the new vision of development of innovation, coordination, green, opening-up and sharing, pay equal attention to traditional Chinese medicine and Western medicine, and accord to traditional Chinese medicine and Western medicine equal status in terms of ideological understanding, legal status, academic development and practical application. Laws for the development of traditional Chinese medicine shall be adhered to, and with promoting inheritance and innovation as the theme, promotion of the development of traditional Chinese medicine as the center, perfection of management systems and policy mechanisms in accordance with TCM characteristics as the key task, and improvement and safeguard of people's health as the goal, efforts shall also be made to expand TCM service scope, promote combination of traditional Chinese medicine and Western medicine, play the unique role of traditional Chinese medicine in the development of health, economy, science and technology, culture, and ecological civilization, push forward the overall revitalization and development of the services of traditional Chinese medicine, and do contributions for deepening the reform of the medical care and health system, promoting the construction of healthy China and an all-round moderately prosperous society, and realizing the "two centenary goals".

**(2) Basic principles**

The basic principles are: putting people first, and making traditional Chinese medicine serve people. Satisfaction of people's demands for healthcare is both the starting point and the ultimate objective. Traditional Chinese medicine shall serve the people and the achievements in the development of traditional Chinese medicine shall be accessible to everyone to enhance the wellbeing of the people and ensure that the people can get access to safe, efficient and convenient services of traditional Chinese medicine.

Sticking to inheritance and innovation and highlighting the characteristics of traditional Chinese medicine. Inheritance and innovation shall run through all the work of traditional Chinese medicine and efforts shall be made to ensure appropriate relationship between inheritance and innovation, carry on and fully play the TCM characteristic advantages and original thought, make full use of modern scientific technologies and methods to promote TCM theories and practices to develop unceasingly, advance modernization of traditional Chinese medicine, form new characteristics and advantages in innovation, and let traditional Chinese medicine pass on from generation to generation.

Deepening reform and maximizing vitality. Efforts shall be made to reform and optimize the systems and mechanisms for the development of traditional Chinese medicine, let the market play a full and decisive role in allocating resources, stimulate investment and consumption, promote adjustment of industrial structure, bring the government's role into full play in the formulation of plans and policies, the introduction of funds, and the regulation of market, and strive to create a market environment characterized by equal participation and fair play so as to maximize the potential and vitality of traditional Chinese medicine.

Making overall planning for coordinated development of traditional Chinese medicine. Efforts shall be made to make traditional Chinese medicine and Western medicine complementary to each other, let each play to its strengths, promote integration of traditional Chinese medicine and Western medicine, and develop traditional Chinese medicine in opening up. All the fields and links of traditional Chinese medicine shall be taken into overall consideration and attention shall be attached to the coordination of the development in urban and rural areas and in different regions, and the development home and abroad so as to push forward the overall development in TCM clinical practice, healthcare, research and development, education, industry and culture and the coordinated development of traditional Chinese medicine, and accelerate the overall and systematic development of traditional Chinese medicine.

**(3) Development goals**

By 2020, universal primary services of traditional Chinese medicine shall be accessible to everyone; TCM clinical practice, healthcare, research and development, education, industry and culture shall develop comprehensively and coordinately, and constant improvement shall be made in TCM standardization, information, industrialization and modernization. TCM healthcare service capacity shall improve obviously and with further broadened service coverage, the medical care network of traditional Chinese medicine shall be more perfect. With ward beds per 1000 residents in TCM hospitals reaching 0.55, more people shall get access to the services of traditional Chinese medicine, which shall effectively alleviate the burden of medical care on the people and further augment the benefits of reform for the people. Great progress shall be made in the research on the basic theories of traditional Chinese medicine, and the prevention and treatment of major diseases and the capacity for disease prevention and treatment with traditional Chinese medicine shall improve remarkably. A training system for the professionals of traditional Chinese medicine shall be built initially; a majority of TCM talents having advanced professional knowledge and excellent medical skills and ethics shall come to the fore, and TCM practicing or assistant physicians per 1,000 residents shall reach 0.4. Significant improvement shall be made in the modernization of the industry of traditional Chinese medicine, and with the total output value of the TCM pharmaceutical industry accounting for above 30 percent of the total generated by the country's pharmaceutical industry, TCM industry shall become a new source of growth in China's economy. International exchange and cooperation in traditional Chinese medicine shall be more extensive; systems of law, standard, supervision and policy shall be basically established in accordance with the TCM development laws and systems for management of traditional Chinese medicine shall be more perfect.

By 2030, modernization of the governance systems and capacity of traditional Chinese medicine shall be significantly improved, and with cover-all TCM service scope and improved service competence, TCM leading role in preventive healthcare, the collaborative role in the treatment of major diseases and the key role in rehabilitation shall be brought into full play. Science and technology of traditional Chinese medicine shall be remarkably improved. A TCM taskforce composed of about a hundred of country-level TCM masters, tens of thousands of well-known TCM experts, millions of TCM physicians and tens of millions of TCM workers shall be basically set up. People's health literacy shall greatly improve. New achievements shall be gained in the industry intelligence of traditional Chinese medicine and more contributions shall be made to the economic and social development. China's leading position in the development of traditional medicine in the world shall be more consolidated and the goal of developing traditional Chinese medicine with inheritance and innovation, overall coordination, ecological green, openness and inclusiveness and people's universal access to the services of traditional Chinese medicine shall be realized, which shall lay a solid foundation for building healthy China.

### III. Key tasks

#### (1) Improving the service capacity of traditional Chinese medicine earnestly

1) Perfecting the TCM medical care network covering both urban and rural areas. A TCM medical care network covering both urban and rural areas shall be established throughout the country, with hospitals of traditional Chinese medicine as the main body, TCM clinical departments of general hospitals and other hospitals as the backbone, community-level medical and healthcare institutions as the basis, and TCM service centers and clinics as the complement. Local people's governments at or above the county level shall rationally allocate resources of traditional Chinese medicine in local health plans; in principle, there shall be one TCM hospital in each city and county and there shall be TCM-related departments in general hospitals, maternal and child health centers, and other non-TCM medical institutions. Departments offering comprehensive services of traditional Chinese medicine shall be established in township clinics and community health centers, and allocation of equipment and assignment of professionals of traditional Chinese medicine shall be enhanced. Construction of rehabilitation department in hospitals of traditional Chinese medicine shall be strengthened; support shall be rendered to the establishment of TCM departments in rehabilitation hospitals and staffing for TCM rehabilitation shall be improved.

2) Improving the capacity for disease prevention and treatment with traditional Chinese medicine. Projects on fostering clinical advantages of traditional Chinese medicine shall be implemented and construction of provincial and municipal TCM hospitals that play a leading role and have outstanding capacity for scientific research shall be strengthened. A network shall be established for traditional Chinese medicine to participate in public emergency response, so shall a coordinated mechanism for emergency medical rescue, and the capability for medical rescue and the prevention and control of serious infectious diseases with traditional Chinese medicine shall be improved tremendously. Continuous efforts shall be made to improve the service

capacity of traditional Chinese medicine at the community level so as to heighten the TCM superior effects in treating specific diseases and the integrated service competence of county-level TCM hospitals and community-level medical and healthcare institutions. TCM monitoring systems and information management systems for chronic diseases shall be established and establishment of the community health management mode with involvement of traditional Chinese medicine shall be promoted. Health interventions among high-risk groups with traditional Chinese medicine shall develop and TCM health management at the community level shall improve. Non-pharmacological alternative approaches in traditional Chinese medicine shall develop energetically and the unique role of these approaches in the prevention and treatment of common diseases, frequently occurring diseases and chronic diseases shall be brought into full play. The network and mechanisms for TCM hospitals' coordinated work with the community-level medical and healthcare institutions and the disease prevention and control institutions in the prevention and treatment of chronic diseases shall be established to accelerate the separation of acute and chronic care.

3) Promoting traditional Chinese medicine to combine with Western medicine. Efforts shall be made to integrate the resources of traditional Chinese medicine and Western medicine, fully play each strength, and make collaborative innovation. Construction of the platforms for the collaboration and innovation of integrated traditional Chinese medicine and Western medicine shall be intensified and efforts shall be made to improve the collaboration on clinical practices and the joint research on the treatment of major difficult and complicated diseases and work out therapies with unique characteristics of integrated traditional Chinese medicine and Western medicine to improve clinical effectiveness in the treatment of major difficult and complicated diseases, and acute and severe diseases. Exploration shall be conducted to establish and perfect the mechanisms and the modes for the collaboration of traditional Chinese medicine and Western medicine in the treatment of major difficult and complicated diseases so as to improve the service capacity. Efforts shall be made to create conditions for constructing hospitals of integrated Chinese and Western medicine, optimize the policies and measures on cultivation of the doctors who have a good knowledge on both traditional Chinese medicine and Western medicine, formulate better systems for encouraging doctors of Western medicine to learn traditional Chinese medicine, create opportunities for doctors of Western medicine to have full-time learning from their TCM counterparts, and enhance the cultivation of high-level talents specializing in both traditional Chinese medicine and Western medicine.

4) Improving the development of ethnic minority medicine. The development of

ethnic minority medicine shall be included in the economic and social development plans of the regions with concentrations of ethnic minorities and the ethnic minority autonomous areas and construction of the institutions of ethnic minority medicine shall be strengthened. Encouragement shall be rendered to the ethnic minority regions with favorable conditions to run hospitals of ethnic minority medicine, to medical and healthcare institutions in ethnic minority regions to establish departments of ethnic minority medicine and pharmacology, and to private investors to establish hospitals and clinics of ethnic minority medicine. Efforts shall be made to strengthen the inheritance and protection and the theoretical research of ethnic minority medicine and pharmacology, and the rescue and collation of the literature. Standardization of ethnic minority medicine shall be promoted and quality of ethnic drugs shall be improved to accelerate the growth of ethnic drugs and promote the development of ethnic pharmaceutical industry.

5) Expanding the service access of traditional Chinese medicine. Reform shall be conducted in TCM practitioners' qualification admittance, practice scope and practice management system and exploration shall be carried out on classified management on the basis of professional skills. Archive-filing management shall be applied to the practitioners of traditional Chinese medicine running clinics of traditional Chinese medicine. Admittance systems for traditional master-apprenticeship and qualification of the practitioners with special professional skills shall be reformed and licensed village TCM doctors with special professional skills shall be allowed to open TCM clinics in towns and villages. Private investors shall be encouraged to establish TCM chain medical institutions and the programs on the establishment of medical institutions and the local plans for health development shall not impose any restriction on the layout of the clinics that are run by private investors and offering the services of traditional Chinese medicine exclusively. Qualified professionals of traditional Chinese medicine, well-known TCM experts in particular, shall be encouraged to open clinics of traditional Chinese medicine and drug trading enterprises shall also be encouraged to establish the clinics with TCM practitioners working in. Medical institutions of traditional Chinese medicine run by nongovernmental sectors and the government shall be entitled to equal right in access and in medical practice.

6) Promoting "Internet + TCM medical care". Endeavors shall be made to develop new TCM service modes, including long-distance medical care, mobile medical care and WIT120 (Wise Information Technology of 120). Information sharing systems, integrating medical images, test reports and health records together, shall be constructed and standards for cross-hospital sharing and exchange of TCM medical data shall be established gradually. Efforts shall be made to explore the ways of taking the advantage of the Internet to provide medical services of traditional Chinese

medicine, such as delivering doctor's order and description, and more information technologies shall be used to render convenient medical services, including online appointment making, appointment reminding, drugs pricing and paying, report inquiring and drug delivering.

### (2) Energetically developing TCM-based health maintenance services

7) Accelerating the construction of the service system of health maintenance based on traditional Chinese medicine. Policies and measures on promoting health maintenance based on traditional Chinese medicine shall be formulated and private investors shall be encouraged to open TCM-based health maintenance centers and develop into corporate groups or chains. The health promotion project featuring preventive treatment of diseases shall be implemented and construction of the departments for preventive treatment of diseases in hospitals of traditional Chinese medicine shall be enhanced to provide TCM-based preventive interventions, such as health counseling and assessment, recuperation care and follow-up care. TCM-based health maintenance models shall be explored, incorporating health culture, health management and health insurance. Hospitals and physicians of traditional Chinese medicine shall be encouraged to offer health counseling and expertise guidance on recuperation care, medicated food, etc. to TCM-based health maintenance centers.

8) Improving the capacity for TCM-based health maintenance services. TCM medical institutions and TCM-based health maintenance centers shall be encouraged to go to government buildings, schools, factories, communities, villages and families to advocate and popularize TCM knowledge on health maintenance and easy-to-understand healthcare techniques and methods, such as physiotherapy and medical massage. Institutions of traditional Chinese medicine shall be encouraged to make full use of modern scientific technologies in biology, bionics and intelligence to develop healthcare foods, healthcare products and healthcare instruments. Systems of the technology and the industry for TCM-based preventive treatment of diseases shall be constructed and healthy styles of work and life based on TCM disease prevention shall be advocated.

9) Developing TCM-based healthy elderly care. Coordinated development of traditional Chinese medicine and elderly care shall be pushed forward and medical resources of traditional Chinese medicine shall be made good use of in nursing homes, communities and residents' homes. Cooperation of the nursing homes and the medical institutions of traditional Chinese medicine shall be encouraged; emergency green channels shall be established and medical institutions of traditional Chinese medicine shall be encouraged to provide home medical service, physical examination and healthcare counseling for the elderly. Physicians of traditional Chinese medicine shall be encouraged to offer healthcare counseling and recuperation care in nursing

homes. Efforts shall be made to encourage private investors to establish TCM healthcare-based nursing homes and rehabilitation centers for the elderly, explore the ways to establish the institutions with the characteristic of TCM integrated treatment and convalescence, and build a batch of such demonstration bases.

10) Developing TCM-based health tourism. Endeavors shall be made to promote an organic linkup between health services and health tourism based on traditional Chinese medicine and develop TCM-based health tourism, with spreading and experiencing the culture of traditional Chinese medicine as the main theme, incorporating TCM convalescence, rehabilitation, health maintenance, culture transmission, exhibition, survey on Chinese medicinal materials and tourism. TCM-based health tourist products and routes with regional features shall be developed, and so shall the TCM-based tourist demonstration bases and the TCM-based health tourist complex. Tourist goods featuring TCM culture shall be developed and produced and standards for TCM-based health tourism shall be set to promote the standardized and specialized services of TCM-based health tourism. The activity of "China's TCM-based Health Tourism Year" shall be launched and support shall be rendered to mounting international exhibitions, conferences and forums on TCM-based health tourism.

**(3) Promoting the inheritance of traditional Chinese medicine**

11) Strengthening the inheritance of the theories, approaches and methods of traditional Chinese medicine. Projects shall be launched to reuse historical theories, trends, approaches and methods and efforts shall be made to carry forward well-known veteran TCM experts' academic thinking and clinical experience comprehensively and systematically, and summarize the superior effects of traditional Chinese medicine in treating specific diseases. Collation of classic books on traditional Chinese medicine shall be incorporated into the national projects on the collation of Chinese classics, and efforts shall be made to carry out surveys on the resources of TCM ancient books and literature, rescue endangered rare and precious ancient books, promote digitalization of TCM ancient books, compile and publish the *Collection of Classics of Chinese Medicine* and promote TCM books in foreign countries to be photographed and come back to China.

12) Enhancing the protection of the traditional knowledge on traditional Chinese medicine and the rediscovery of its techniques. Database, a list of protected patents, and intellectual property shall be established to protect the traditional knowledge on traditional Chinese medicine. Screening of appropriate techniques for clinical practice, health maintenance and rehabilitation shall be promoted and the catalog of TCM medical techniques and the specification for operating the medical techniques shall be optimized. The inheritance and application of the techniques for traditional ways of

preparation, evaluation, and processing of Chinese medicinal materials and that of the skilled pharmaceutical workers' experience shall be enhanced. Efforts shall be made to survey, rediscover, categorize, research, evaluate, spread and apply TCM folk medical techniques featuring unique characteristics and protect the time-honored brands of traditional Chinese medicine.

13) Improving the master-apprenticeship training of traditional Chinese medicine. A system for master-apprenticeship training shall be established and master-apprenticeship training shall run through college, post-graduate and continuing education. Medical institutions of traditional Chinese medicine shall be encouraged to develop the master-apprenticeship training, which shall be a normal system in cultivating professionals of traditional Chinese medicine. Systems for management of the physicians of traditional Chinese medicine shall be established; studios shall be set up for carrying forward the prominent veteran TCM masters' expertise and encouragement shall be offered to the prominent veteran TCM masters and the TCM experts working at the community level permanently to cultivate multi-level talents of traditional Chinese medicine.

**(4) Pushing forward the innovation of traditional Chinese medicine**

14) Perfecting the collaborative innovation system for traditional Chinese medicine. A multidisciplinary and cross-departmental TCM collaborative innovation system shall be improved to optimize the layout of scientific research on traditional Chinese medicine, with national and provincial TCM scientific research institutions as the core, colleges and universities, medical institutions and enterprises as the main body and TCM scientific research bases and platforms as the support. Overall plans shall be made for the programs, the projects and the funds related to the scientific research on traditional Chinese medicine and efforts shall be made to support TCM scientific and technologic innovation, improve innovation capacity, accelerate development of independent intellectual property rights, and promote commercialization and industrialization of technological innovation achievements.

15) Enhancing the scientific research on traditional Chinese medicine. Approaches and methods of both modern science and technology and traditional Chinese medicine shall be used to enhance the research on the TCM fundamental theories, the theory and methods for syndrome differentiation treatment, the specificities of acupoints, the TCM pharmaceutical theory, the theory of the compatibility of medicinal ingredients, and the material foundation and the effectiveness mechanisms of Chinese medicine compounds and a theoretical framework with explicit concepts and a reasonable structure shall be established. Interdisciplinary efforts shall be made to jointly research the treatment and control of the major difficult and complicated diseases and the major infectious diseases as well as the prevention and treatment

of common diseases, frequently occurring diseases, and chronic diseases with traditional Chinese medicine and achieve major curative products and technological achievements in the prevention and treatment of major diseases and in the preventive treatment of diseases. Endeavors shall be made in the application of modern science and technology to research and develop a batch of new medical devices and equipment on the basis of the theories of traditional Chinese medicine. Exploration shall be carried out on the new modes of developing drugs in accordance with the characteristics of traditional Chinese medicine to push forward the development of major TCM drugs. Encouragement shall be given to the research and development of the new TCM drugs based on the classic prescriptions of traditional Chinese medicine and the Chinese medicine preparations of TCM medical institutions. For new drug targets, efforts shall be made to find out new candidate drugs from Chinese medicinal materials.

16) Perfecting the evaluation systems for the scientific research on traditional Chinese medicine. Standards and systems for evaluation of the scientific research of traditional Chinese medicine shall be built and optimized in accordance with the characteristics of traditional Chinese medicine and incentive policies beneficial to innovation shall be perfected. Management efficiency and research capacity shall be improved by the peer review and the third-party evaluation. Transformation of research achievements shall be accelerated constantly; efforts shall be made to evaluate clinical effectiveness of the research achievements, conduct research on transformation and application, and establish the evaluation systems suited to the characteristics of traditional Chinese medicine.

**(5) Improving the overall development of TCM pharmaceutical industry**

17) Strengthening the protection and application of Chinese medicinal resources. Efforts shall be made to carry out projects on the protection of wild Chinese medicinal resources, perfect the systems for classified protection of Chinese medicinal resources and wild Chinese medicinal species, build the reserves for endangered wild medicinal animals and plants, the bases for cultivation of wild Chinese medicinal resources and the bases for breeding and planting rare and endangered Chinese medicinal resources, and strengthen research on the protection and breeding of rare and endangered wild Chinese medicinal animals and plants. National Chinese medicinal animal and plant germplasm banks and systems integrating surveys and dynamic monitoring of Chinese medicinal resources shall be established. Chinese crude drugs and decoction pieces shall be further improved in the national drug reserve and private investors shall be encouraged to build such bases as parks, exhibitions and gardens of Chinese medicinal plants and animals for protection and breeding of Chinese medicinal plants and animals. Exploration shall be conducted on the construction of eco-economic

demonstration zones for planting Chinese medicinal plants on desertification soil.

18) Pushing forward standardized seeding and planting of Chinese medicinal materials. Plans shall be worked out for major planting regions; the national catalog for genuine Chinese medicinal materials shall be formulated and construction of the bases for seed-breeding and standardized breeding and planting of Chinese medicinal materials shall be enhanced. Efforts shall be made to promote the green development of Chinese medicinal materials, establish technique standards for planting, breeding, collecting and storing of Chinese medicinal plants and animals, intensify guidance on scientific planting and breeding of Chinese medicinal materials, develop professional cooperation, and promote large-scaled standardized planting and breeding of Chinese medicinal materials. Support shall be rendered to the development of including production of Chinese medicinal materials in insurance provisions, and the system of marking the geographic origin of Chinese medicinal materials shall be established and perfected. Campaigns on promoting the development of the industry of Chinese medicinal materials shall be launched in poverty-stricken areas to lead low-income families to participate in the production and promote targeted poverty relief.

19) Promoting the transformation and upgrading of pharmaceutical industry of traditional Chinese medicine. Endeavors shall be made to promote digital, networked and intelligent development in the TCM pharmaceutical industry, improve technological integration and innovation, advance equipment manufacturing level, accelerate standardization and modernization of TCM drug manufacturing technique and process, and increase the application of the intellectual property in TCM pharmaceutical industry to gradually develop TCM pharmaceutical enterprises into large-scaled corporate groups and industry clusters. On the basis of modern science and technology industrial bases, the campaign of technology entrepreneurship shall be launched in the TCM all-round health industry and the integrated development of primary, secondary and tertiary TCM pharmaceutical industries shall be promoted. Chinese patent medicines shall be reevaluated after marketing and greater efforts shall be made to redevelop Chinese patent medicines, carry out large-scaled standardized clinical tests, and develop a batch of outstanding TCM drugs with international competitiveness. TCM drug manufacturing machines and equipment shall also be developed to improve the techniques and the scale merit of TCM pharmaceutical industry. Plans on the standardization of TCM drugs shall be carried out and high-quality standard systems for all links of TCM pharmaceutical industry shall be built. Efforts shall be made to implement the project on green manufacturing TCM drugs, establish various newly-emerging green industrial systems, decrease gradually the amount of heavy metals and chemical compounds applied, and adhere strictly to the *Standards for Discharge of Water Pollutants by TCM Pharmaceutical Manufacturers*

*(GB21906-2008)* to build a green TCM pharmaceutical manufacturing system.

20) Constructing a modern circulating system for Chinese medicinal materials. Endeavors shall be made to formulate plans on construction of the circulating systems for Chinese medicinal materials and build a number of standardized, intensive, large-scaled and traceable centers for pre-processing, storing and circulating genuine Chinese medicinal materials that are closely connected with the TCM drug manufacturers' and suppliers' management systems and the TCM drug quality tracing systems. E-commerce for Chinese medicinal materials shall be promoted and big data shall be used to gather the information on producing Chinese medicinal materials, dynamically monitoring and analyzing drug prices, forecasting and early warning. Projects on guarantee of the quality of Chinese medicinal materials shall be conducted; quality management systems and quality tracing systems shall be established throughout the whole process of circulation, and the third-party testing platforms shall be constructed.

**(6) Energetically advocating the culture of traditional Chinese medicine**

21) Thriving and developing the culture of traditional Chinese medicine. The concept of "mastership of medicine lying in proficient medical skills and lofty medical ethics" shall be advocated and construction of professional ethics shall be intensified in a bid to establish a high standard of professional conducts. Projects on promotion of TCM health and culture literacy shall be launched to enhance the protection TCM relics and facilities and the inheritance of the intangible cultural heritage of traditional Chinese medicine. Endeavors shall be made to promote more TCM-based non-pharmacological therapies to be included in the *Representative List of the Intangible Cultural Heritage of Humanity* by UNESCO and the *Representative List of National Intangible Cultural Heritage* and more ancient books on traditional Chinese medicine to be listed in the Memory of the World Register. Spread of TCM culture to the rest of the world shall be promoted to demonstrate the unique charm of Chinese culture and improve China's cultural soft power.

22) Developing the cultural industry of traditional Chinese medicine. Integrated development of traditional Chinese medicine and its cultural industry shall be promoted and exploration shall be conducted to include the culture of traditional Chinese medicine in the programs for the development of cultural industry. Efforts shall be made to produce creative products and cultural masterpieces embodying the culture of traditional Chinese medicine, and promote effective integration of traditional Chinese medicine with radio, film & television, press & publication, digital publishing, animation & game, tourism & catering, and sports & entertainment to develop new-type cultural products and services. Well-known brands and enterprises shall be built and integrated development of traditional Chinese medicine and its

cultural industry shall be promoted.

**(7) Actively promoting the globalization of traditional Chinese medicine**

23) Promoting international exchange and cooperation in traditional Chinese medicine. Efforts shall be made to promote the exchange and cooperation with foreign governments, the World Health Organization (WHO) and the International Organization for Standardization (ISO), actively participate in the formulation of international regulations and standards and create an environment beneficial to the global development of traditional Chinese medicine. Projects on boosting the global development of traditional Chinese medicine shall be launched to promote TCM techniques, drugs, standards and services to develop overseas and make them accepted by the rest of the world. With non-governmental sectors' as the main force and supported by the government, exploration shall be conducted to establish TCM centers overseas to serve local people and create a win-win situation. Institutions of traditional Chinese medicine shall be encouraged to participate in international cooperation and competition in all fields of traditional Chinese medicine and the role of non-governmental TCM organizations shall be brought into full play. More services of traditional Chinese medicine shall be provided in foreign medical aid. Multi-level educational exchange and cooperation in traditional Chinese medicine with foreign countries shall be promoted to attract more foreign students to China for academic education, non-academic education, short-term training and clinical practice, and traditional Chinese medicine shall be a key component in people-to-people communication between China and the rest of the world.

24) Expanding international trade in traditional Chinese medicine. TCM international trade shall be included in the national overall strategy for foreign trade and development and efforts shall be made to construct supporting policies, eliminate legislation, policy and technology barriers to the overseas development of traditional Chinese medicine, strengthen the protection of TCM intellectual property in foreign countries, and expand international market access for TCM service trade. Institutions of traditional Chinese medicine shall be encouraged to participate in the Belt and Road Initiative and expand foreign investment and trade of traditional Chinese medicine, and overall public resource guarantee shall be provided for the development of TCM service trade. Institutions of traditional Chinese medicine shall be encouraged to set up TCM hospitals, chain clinics, and TCM-based health maintenance centers in foreign countries. Support shall be rendered to the overseas exploitation of Chinese medicinal materials and the quality management of the production and circulation of Chinese medicinal materials in foreign countries shall be strengthened. Enterprises of traditional Chinese medicine shall be encouraged to go abroad to accelerate the building of the multinational companies offering whole-industry-chain services

and world-famous brands. Efforts shall be made to attract foreigners to the health tourism of traditional Chinese medicine, outsource TCM medical services, and improve integral publicity and promotion to foreign countries for the service trade in traditional Chinese medicine.

### IV. Supporting Measures

**(1) Improving the legal systems for traditional Chinese medicine.** Efforts shall be made to promote the promulgation and implementation of the *Law of the People's Republic of China on Traditional Chinese Medicine*, discuss and formulate supporting polices, laws and departmental rules, promote the amendment of the *Law on Practicing Doctors of the People's Republic of China*, the *Pharmaceutical Administrative Law of the People's Republic of China*, the *Regulation on the Administration of Medical Institutions*, the *Regulation on the Protection of Traditional Chinese Medicines*, and other laws and regulations, further improve the laws and regulations concerning the classification and administration of TCM practitioners and medical institutions, the approval and administration of TCM drugs, and the protection of traditional knowledge on traditional Chinese medicine, construct the legal and regulatory systems suited to the development of traditional Chinese medicine, and lead local governments to strengthen the formulation of local laws and regulations on traditional Chinese medicine.

**(2) Perfecting the standard systems for traditional Chinese medicine.** For guarantee of the quality and the safety of the services of traditional Chinese medicine, TCM standardization projects shall be launched to formulate, popularize and apply the clinical practice guidelines, the technique operating norms, and the standards for assessment of therapeutic effectiveness in traditional Chinese medicine. Standards for TCM preventive treatment of diseases, medicated food, and health products shall be discussed and formulated systematically. Standard systems for TCM drugs shall be improved and perfected and safety management for Chinese medicinal materials shall be strengthened, with a special attention attached to setting the standards for processing and evaluation of Chinese medicinal materials and the standards for Chinese materia medica preparations, TCM formula granules and genuine Chinese medicinal materials. Construction of digital standards for Chinese medicinal materials and the specimens of Chinese medicinal plants shall be accelerated, and so shall the transformation of domestic standards to international standards. Construction of the supervisory systems for traditional Chinese medicine shall be strengthened and supervisory information data platforms shall be built. TCM certification administration shall be promoted and supervisory role of nongovernmental sectors shall be brought into play.

**(3) Providing more policy support to traditional Chinese medicine.** The government's investment policy shall be implemented. Efforts shall be made to reform TCM drug pricing systems, rationally determine the items and prices of the services of traditional Chinese medicine, lower extortionate prices on Chinese patent drugs, and abolish the system of charging more for medicines to make up for low prices for medical services. The markup policy for decoction pieces of Chinese medicinal materials shall be implemented continually. The number of Chinese patent drugs shall increase further in the national essential drug list and the quality of the Chinese patent drugs in the list shall be improved unceasingly. Local governments at all levels shall plan for the development of traditional Chinese medicine comprehensively in the general plan for utilization of land and in the urban and rural planning and expand land supply for the clinical practice of traditional Chinese medicine, the TCM-based health maintenance, the TCM health services for the elderly, etc.

**(4) Strengthening the construction of talented professionals of traditional Chinese medicine.** A training system for the professionals of traditional Chinese medicine that features an organic linkup between college, post-graduate and continuing education, with master-apprenticeship training running through, shall be established and optimized, with a focus on the cultivation of leading talents in the TCM key disciplines and specialties and the TCM clinical scientific research. Cultivation of the talented TCM general practitioners, the community-level TCM talents and the skilled professionals for ethnic minority medicine and integrated Chinese and Western medicine shall be strengthened and the training in TCM knowledge and skills for clinical physicians and village doctors shall be conducted. Manning quota shall be set for the technical professionals of traditional Chinese medicine and posts shall be reasonably established for TCM healthcare services. Efforts shall be made to reform the education of traditional Chinese medicine, establish the certification system for TCM-related majors, explore cultivation modes suited to the classified management of TCM physicians' licensed practice, enhance the building of a batch of key disciplines of traditional Chinese medicine, encourage the ethnic minority regions and the colleges and universities with favorable conditions to establish the majors of ethnic minority medicine for college and postgraduate education, and build a number of world-famous TCM universities and disciplines. The system for election and commendation of the national TCM masters shall be improved and evaluation systems for the talents of traditional Chinese medicine shall be perfected. Guarantee and long-term incentive mechanisms for attracting and stabilizing the professionals of traditional Chinese medicine at the community level shall be established.

**(5) Promoting the information construction of traditional Chinese medicine.** In accordance with the plan for use of big data in health, efforts shall be made to strengthen the use of big data of traditional Chinese medicine in the cloud service program for building healthy China. Building of TCM hospital information infrastructure shall be strengthened and information systems of hospitals of traditional Chinese medicine shall be perfected. Online systems for verification of the authenticity and effectiveness of patients' descriptions shall be established and information on people's health shall be shared throughout the country. Building of the system for TCM information statistics shall be optimized and the national systems for online direct report of comprehensive statistics of traditional Chinese medicine shall be established.

### V. Organization and implementation

**(1) Strengthening organization and implementation of the *Outline for the Planning of the Development Strategy of Traditional Chinese Medicine.*** The system for joint inter-ministerial meeting of the State Council for traditional Chinese medicine shall be further perfected and leaders of the State Council shall be the organizers of the meetings. The office of the joint inter-ministerial meeting of the State Council for traditional Chinese medicine shall strengthen overall planning and coordinating, work out detailed policies and measures for the development of traditional Chinese medicine, solve major problems coordinately, and intensify the leadership, supervision and inspection in the implementation of the *Outline for the Planning of the Development Strategy of Traditional Chinese Medicine*. Departments concerned shall discuss and formulate plans for implementing this *Outline for the Planning of the Development Strategy of Traditional Chinese Medicine* and make plans for constructing a number of national pilot areas for the comprehensive reform of traditional Chinese medicine to ensure implementation of all the measures. Local governments at all levels shall incorporate the work of traditional Chinese medicine into local economic and social development plans, strengthen organization and leadership, optimize coordinated mechanisms and working systems for the development of traditional Chinese medicine, work out plans for implementation of this *Outline for the Planning of the Development Strategy of Traditional Chinese Medicine* according local conditions, and improve systems for evaluation and supervision.

**(2) Improving the management system for traditional Chinese medicine.** In line with the requirements for modernization of the governance systems and capacity for traditional Chinese medicine, efforts shall be made to innovate management patterns, establish and perfect national, provincial, municipal and township management systems for traditional Chinese medicine, optimize leading mechanisms further, and enhance the management of traditional Chinese medicine earnestly. All departments concerned shall strengthen communication and coordination within the scope of the respective functions and duties and make concerted efforts to promote the development of traditional Chinese medicine.

**(3) Creating a sound social environment for the development of traditional Chinese medicine.** Efforts shall be made to make use of traditional media, such as broadcast, television, newspaper and new carriers, including digital intelligent terminal, mobile terminal, etc. to energetically disseminate the culture and the knowledge of traditional Chinese medicine as well as the significant role of traditional Chinese medicine in the economic and social development. Traditional Chinese medicine shall be promoted to spread in schools, communities, villages and families and the fundamental knowledge of traditional Chinese medicine shall be taken as a part of the course of traditional culture and health in primary school and middle school. Meanwhile, endeavors shall be made to fully play social organizations' role and build a sound social environment in which everyone believes in traditional Chinese medicine, love traditional Chinese medicine, and treat diseases with traditional Chinese medicine, and a favorable landscape that joint efforts shall be made to develop traditional Chinese medicine.

(Zhao Yinghong)

## Notice of the State Council on Issuing the *Health and Wellness Plan for the 13th Five-Year Plan Period*

(No. 77 [2016] of the State Council)

The people's governments of all provinces, autonomous regions and municipalities directly under the Central Government, and all ministries and commissions and institutions directly under the State Council,

The *Health and Wellness Plan for the 13th Five-Year Plan Period* is hereby issued to you for your serious implementation.

The State Council
December 27th, 2016

## 15. *Health and Wellness Plan for the 13th Five-Year Plan Period*

In order to promote the building of a healthy China, this *Plan* is formulated based on the *Outline of the 13th Five-Year Plan for National Economic and Social Development of the People's Republic of China* and the *Outline of the Healthy China 2030 Plan*.

### I. Plan background

(1) Achievements in the 12th Five-Year Plan period. During the 12th Five-Year Plan period, the reform of the medical and health systems was deepened and implemented at an accelerated pace, considerable progress was made in the health undertakings and the people's health continued to improve. The year 2015 witnessed life expectancy at 76.34 years, 1.51 years over 2010; infant mortality rate dropped from 13.1‰ to 8.1‰; mortality rate of children under five, from 16.4‰ to10.7‰; and maternal mortality rate, from 30/100,000 to 20.1/100,000. In general, the main health indicators of residents were better than the average level of middle- and high-income countries, with the annual natural growth rate of population being 4.97‰ on the average. Consequently the main targets and tasks identified in the 12th Five-Year Plan for health undertakings have been completed on schedule.

As the reform of the medical and health system was further advanced, significant progress and remarkable achievements were made. With the universal healthcare insurance system speeded up, the participation rate of basic healthcare insurance remained above 95%, and critical illness insurance, medical aid for major diseases and emergency medical assistance of urban-rural residents were fully promoted. With steady progress made in the reform of public hospitals, the comprehensive reform of county-level public hospitals was fully implemented, the pilots for the comprehensive reform of urban public hospitals continued to expand and deepen, and positive progress was achieved in the pilots for the comprehensive healthcare reform at the provincial-level. The national basic drug system was consolidated and improved, and the comprehensive reform of community-level healthcare institutions was continuously deepened. The development of nongovernmental hospitals was accelerated. The proportion of personal health expenditure in total health expenditures decreased from 35.29% to 29.27%. The medical and health service system was unceasingly improved and the service capacity was greatly enhanced. In 2015, the number of beds in medical and health institutions per thousand people increased to 5.11, the number of practicing (assistant) physicians increased to 2.22, and the number of registered nurses increased to 2.37. The infrastructure of medical and health institutions continued to improve. A standardized training system for resident physicians was initially established, and the construction of the team of community-level medical and health talents focusing on general practitioners was accelerated. And as a result, there were 1.38 general practitioners per 10,000 people in 2015. The construction of a hierarchical diagnosis and treatment system in an orderly manner was promoted. Activities such as the "action plan for further improvement of the medical service" were widely carried out. A long-term mechanism for preventing and resolving medical disputes was preliminarily established. And the construction of population health information was comprehensively strengthened.

The childbearing policy was gradually adjusted and improved, and the reform of service management of family planning was carried out as a whole. The universal two-child policy was steadily implemented. By the end of 2015, nearly two million couples (either of them was the only child born to his /her parents) applied to have another child. Efforts were made to study and start up the universal two-child policy. The reform of maternal and child healthcare and family planning institutions was carried out in an orderly manner, and solid progress was made in the reform of service management for family planning. The gender ratio at birth dropped for seven consecutive years. The national free pre-pregnancy health inspection program was extended to all counties (county-level cities and districts) across the country, and comprehensive prevention and control of birth defects had been advancing. The coverage of free family planning service for floating population reached 89.2%.

The equalization of basic public health services was steadily raised, and the prevention and control efforts of major diseases were very effective. The per capita subsidy standard for basic public health services was raised to 40 *yuan*, and the service content was increased to 45 items in 12 categories. HIV/AIDS was controlled in low prevalence, the reported incidence of tuberculosis dropped to 63.4/100,000, and all counties where schistosomiasis was prevalent met the transmission control standards. As a result, the hazards of key pandemic diseases was basically eliminated or controlled. A system for the prevention and control of chronic diseases was preliminarily established, and the network for the prevention and control of severe mental disorders was constantly improved. The patriotic health campaign was launched in a deep-going manner. Residents' health literacy was steadily enhanced. Efforts were made to promote blood screening for nucleic acid testing, and thus blood safety level was further raised. The working mechanism of joint prevention and joint control was constantly improved, and acute infectious diseases and public health emergencies such as human infection with avian flu were successfully prevented and handled. The comprehensive supervision and law enforcement of health and family planning were further strengthened. The evaluation of the standards and surveillance of food safety was solidly promoted.

The service capacity of traditional Chinese medicine (TCM) was continuously improved, and the cause of TCM developed rapidly. A multi-tiered and widely-covered TCM service network was basically established. With the community-level TCM service capacity improved significantly, more than 95% of the national community health service centers, 90% of the township health centers, 80% of the community health service stations, and 60% of the village clinics could provide service of TCM. Efforts were made to promote the technological advances in TCM and continue to expand the new business model of TCM health services. TCM has taken important steps toward "going global".

Since the differences between urban and rural residents' health were further narrowed, the accessibility of medical and health services, the quality of services, the efficiency of services and the satisfaction of the public have been significantly improved. And the international influence of the health and health industry has been highlighted. All of the above have made important contributions to maintaining steady growth, promoting the reform, adjusting the structure and benefiting the people's livelihood, and laid a solid foundation for building a moderately well-off society in an all-round way and achieving basic medical and health services for all.

(2) Opportunities and challenges in the 13th Five-Year Plan period. Attaching great importance to the development of the health and health undertakings, the CPC Central Committee and the State Council have proposed to promote the construction of a healthy China, and placed the development of health and health undertakings in an important position in the overall economic and social development. The people's pursuit of a better life in a moderately well-off society in an all-round way has stimulated the multi-tiered and diversified health needs, which creates a broader space for the development of health services. Further progress shall be made in comprehensively governing the country in accordance with the law, which provides a solid legal guarantee for the improvement of the modern level in health management system and management capacity. The development of health is facing a rare historical opportunity.

Meanwhile, the development of health is facing new challenges. The problem of population structure is becoming more and more serious, and the quality of birth population remains to be improved. With the universal two-child policy implemented, the aging process will be accelerated, and the urbanization rate is increasing; thus the contradiction between supply and demand of medical and health resources in some areas will become more prominent. In the process of economic and social transformation, rapid changes will take place in the residents' living environment and lifestyle, and chronic diseases will become the main health problem. Threats of major infectious diseases and key parasitic diseases will persist. More and more frequent exchanges at home and abroad will increase the risk of infectious diseases and vector biological importation. Atmospheric and other environmental pollution and food safety problems will seriously affect the people's health. With economic development entering a new normal, the rapid development of emerging information technologies like the Internet requires that there should be faster transformation of development modes and innovation of service modes and management modes in health field.

In addition, the internal structural problems that constrain the reform and development of health and health undertakings remain. Firstly, the insufficient amount of resources and the unreasonable distribution structure remain fundamentally unchanged, and the quality medical resources are especially lacking. Secondly, the community-level service capacity is still an outstanding weak link, the technical level of medical staff at the community-level needs to be improved urgently, and the service facilities and conditions remain to be continuously improved. Thirdly, deepening the reform requires that we shall further resolve the deep-seated system and mechanism contradictions. Fourthly, the idea and method of family planning work need to be changed urgently.

## II. Guiding ideology and development goals

(1) Guiding ideology. Efforts shall be made to hold high the great banner of socialism with Chinese characteristics. We need to implement the guiding principles of the 18th National Congress of the CPC and the Third, Fourth, Fifth and Sixth Plenary Sessions of the 18th CPC Central Committee. With Marxism-Leninism, Mao Zedong Thought, Deng Xiaoping Theory, the Important Thought of Three Represents, and the Scientific Outlook on Development as the guidance, we shall thoroughly implement the guiding principles of General Secretary Xi Jinping's series of important speeches. Work must be carried out in accordance with the plan for promoting all-round economic, political, cultural, social and ecological progress, and the Four-Pronged Comprehensive Strategy. Decisions and arrangements of the CPC Central Committee and the State Council must be implemented to firmly establish and implement the development concept of innovation, coordination, greenness, openness and sharing. Efforts shall be made to adhere to the people-oriented development philosophy, the correct guidelines for health work, and the basic state policy on family planning. And health should be at the top of the development agenda. With the people's health at the center, and driven by reform and innovation, we will focus on promoting health, shifting the model, bolstering support at the community level, and stressing the safeguard. More attention should be paid to prevention first and health promotion; more attention should be paid to the decentralization of work and resources transfer to the lower level; and more attention should be paid to improving the service quality and level. We will shift the development model from treating diseases as the center to health care as the center, significantly improve the people's health, and work hard to build a healthy China.

(2) Development goals. By 2020, the basic medical and health care system covering both urban and rural residents will have been basically established, and everyone will

have had access to basic medical and health services, with the average life expectancy increased by one year on the basis of 2015.

—*The system will have become more mature and established.* With the legal system for health and family planning further improved, the modernization of the governance system and governance capacity will have been continuously enhanced, and positive progress will have been made in integrating health into all policies.

—The health service system will have continued to improve. The medical and healthcare capacity will have been significantly enhanced to better satisfy the people's needs for basic medical and healthcare, as well as diversified and multi-level needs for health.

—*Marked effects will have been produced in disease prevention and control.* In line with an emphasis on prevention, efforts shall be made to popularize a healthy lifestyle, improve health literacy of residents, effectively control health risk factors, and eliminate a number of major diseases.

—*The health service model will have been transformed.* The division of labor and collaboration among institutions will have been closer. There will have been full coverage of contracted service system for family doctors, and a hierarchical medical system will have been basically established in line with the national conditions.

—*A moderate childbearing level will have been maintained.* With the universal two-child policy implemented smoothly, the family planning service management system will have been relatively perfect.

### Main Development Indicators

| Domain | Main Indicators | Units | 2020 | 2015 | Indicator Properties |
|---|---|---|---|---|---|
| health status | life expectancy | years | >77.3 | 76.34 | anticipated |
| | maternal mortality | /100,000 | <18 | 20.1 | anticipated |
| | Infant mortality | ‰ | <7.5 | 8.1 | anticipated |
| health status | mortality in children under 5 | ‰ | <9.5 | 10.7 | anticipated |
| disease prevention and control | status of residents' health literacy | % | >20 | 10 | anticipated |
| | vaccination rates for immunization program for children of appropriate age in townships (towns, sub-districts) | % | >90 | >90 | obligatory |
| | incidence of TB | /100,000 | <58 | 63.4 | anticipated |
| | premature mortality from cardi-ovascular and cerebrovascular diseases, cancer, chronic respir-atory diseases and diabetes | % | 10% lower than 2015 | 18.5 | anticipated |

*Continued*

| Domain | Main Indicators | Units | 2020 | 2015 | Indicator Properties |
|---|---|---|---|---|---|
| women's and children's health | rates of maternal system management | % | >90 | >90 | obligatory |
| | rates of system management for children under 3 | % | >90 | >90 | obligatory |
| | coverage of pre-pregnancy eugenic health check for target population | % | >80 | >80 | anticipated |
| medical services | average length of hospital stay in Grade III hospitals | days | <8 | 10.2 | anticipated |
| | nosocomial infection rates | % | <3.2 | 3.5 | anticipated |
| | 30-day re-hospitalization rate | % | <2.4 | 2.65 | anticipated |
| | use rates of antibiotics on outpatient prescriptions | % | <10 | <11 | anticipated |
| family planning | total population | 100 million | about 1.42 billion | 13.7 billion | anticipated |
| | total childbearing rates | | about 1.8 | 1.5-1.6 | anticipated |
| | sex ratios at birth | | <112 | 113.5 | obligatory |
| healthcare service system | beds at healthcare institutions per 1,000 | beds | <6 | 5.11 | anticipated |
| | practicing (assistant) physicians per 1,000 | physicians | >2.5 | 2.22 | anticipated |
| | registered nurses per 1,000 | nurses | >3.14 | 2.37 | anticipated |
| | general practitioners per 1,000 | practitioners | >2 | 1.38 | obligatory |
| | proportion of beds at nongovernmental hospitals in total hospital beds | % | >30 | 19.4 | anticipated |
| healthcare security policy | proportion of hospitalization expenses covered by basic healthcare insurance | % | 75% or so | 75% or so | anticipated |
| | proportion of personal health expenditures in total health expenditures | % | 28% or so | 29.27% | obligatory |

## III. Main tasks

### (1) Strengthen the prevention and control of major diseases.

Efforts shall be made to promote the combination of prevention and control. A "three-in-one" major disease prevention and control mechanism for professional public health institutions, general hospitals and specialty hospitals, and community-level healthcare institutions shall be established for information sharing and interconnection to promote the integrated development of prevention, treatment and management of chronic and mental diseases. Efforts shall also be made to implement the compensation policy for healthcare institutions to assume public health tasks and improve the government's mechanism for purchasing public health services. (The National Health and Family Planning Commission and the Ministry of Finance shall be in charge of the above task.)

Efforts shall be made to implement the comprehensive prevention and control of chronic diseases. A government-led coordination mechanism for comprehensive prevention and control of chronic diseases shall be improved to optimize the prevention and control strategy. And the construction of national demonstration zone of comprehensive prevention and control shall be strengthened to cover more than 15% of the counties (county-level cities, districts) nationwide. With the strengthening of screening and early detection of chronic diseases, such as stroke, early diagnosis and early treatment of key cancer types in high incidence areas shall be carried out to reach the early diagnosis rate of 55%, and improve the 5-year survival rate. There shall be full implementation of blood pressure measurement at initial diagnosis for people aged over 35 years of age. And the disease risk assessment and intervention guidance for high-risk groups of chronic diseases, such as elevated blood pressure and blood glucose levels, dyslipidemia, overweight and obesity, will be conducted step by step. In addition, oral examinations and lung function testing shall be included in routine physical examinations. The number of people with hypertension and diabetes under health management shall reach100 million and 35 million respectively. We shall improve the system for the monitoring of causes of death, the registration reports of tumors, and the monitoring of chronic diseases and nutrition. Injury prevention and intervention shall be strengthened. (The National Health and Family Planning Commission shall be in charge of the above task.)

Efforts shall be made to strengthen the prevention and control of major infectious diseases. With the capacity building for monitoring and early warning, and prevention and control of infectious diseases strengthened, the reported rate of statutory infectious diseases shall reach 95% or above for timely investigation and handling of the epidemic situation. Besides the infection rate of hepatitis B virus in the whole population shall be reduced. HIV/AIDS testing, intervention and follow-up shall be strengthened to spot infected people and patients to the greatest extent, so as to provide all eligible HIV-infected individuals and patients who are willing to receive treatment with antiviral treatment to control the epidemic to a low prevalence level. Efforts shall be made to launch a pilot program for the services of comprehensive prevention and treatment of tuberculosis, and intensify tuberculosis discovery among average patients. Furthermore, active screening among key populations shall be reinforced, whereas the screening and monitoring for multi-drug resistant tuberculosis shall be strengthened, in order to standardize the management of the entire course of treatment. There shall be effective response to the outbreaks of priority infectious diseases, such as cholera, influenza, hand-foot-mouth disease and measles. A comprehensive treatment strategy for human and animal diseases such as rabies, brucellosis, avian influenza and so on shall be implemented, with emphasis on infection source control. And the hazards of leprosy shall be eliminated. A reserve mechanism for the prevention and control of serious infectious diseases shall be established. (The National Health and Family Planning Commission shall take the lead, with the participation of the Ministry of Agriculture and other departments.) The construction of the capacity for port sanitation and quarantine inspections shall be strengthened, while the monitoring, early warning and emergency handling of infectious diseases from abroad shall be enhanced. Free testing of suspected infectious diseases for passengers at ports shall be promoted to prevent the introduction of foreign major infectious diseases. (The General Administration of Quality Supervision, Inspection and Quarantine shall be in charge of the above task.)

Efforts shall be made to intensify the prevention and control of mental diseases. Report registration, service management and rescue assistance for patients with severe mental disorders shall be strengthened, with over 80% of the management rate of those in the register with serious mental disorders. A community rehabilitation service system for those with mental disorders shall be established and improved step by step. Trials for early screening and intervention for common mental disorders, such as anxiety and depression, shall be carried out, with the treatment rate of depression significantly raised. Efforts shall be made to strengthen mental health service. (The National Health and Family Planning Commission shall take the lead, with the participation of the Ministry of Public Security, the Ministry of Civil Affairs, China Disabled Persons' Federation and some other relevant departments.)

Efforts shall be made to implement the Expanded Program on Immunization (EPI). With the routine immunization strengthened, a good job shall be done in supplementary immunization and checking for missed immunization, so as to promote the standardized construction of vaccination clinics, and improve the quality of vaccination management. Nationwide implementation of alternative inactivated poliovirus vaccines (IPV) shall be provided to continue to maintain polio-free status. As required by the disease prevention work, the vaccine types of the national immunization program shall be adjusted in a timely manner to gradually incorporate safe, effective and financially affordable vaccines into the national immunization program. The surveillance of vaccine-preventable infectious diseases shall be enhanced. The establishment of a compensatory insurance mechanism for abnormal vaccination response shall be explored. Efforts shall be made to reform and improve the centralized procurement mechanism for type ii vaccines to strengthen the management of the cold chain of vaccines, and promote the establishment of a whole-process traceability system for vaccines. (The National Health and Family Planning Commission shall take the lead, with the participation of the Ministry of Finance, China Food and Drug Administration, the General Administration of Quality Supervision, Inspection and Quarantine, and some other relevant departments.)

Efforts shall be made in the prevention and control of key parasitic diseases and endemic diseases. The comprehensive prevention and control strategy of schistosomiasis mainly based on infection source control shall be adhered to. The control of mosquito-borne infectious diseases such as dengue fever and malaria shall be enhanced to achieve the goal of eliminating malaria across the country. The comprehensive prevention and control strategy shall be implemented to basically bring the prevalence of echinococcosis under control. There shall be continuous elimination of iodine deficiency hazards to keep the iodine nutrition in population in general at an appropriate level. Efforts shall be made to maintain the basic elimination of Kaschin-Beck disease, Keshan disease, and fluorine and arsenic poisoning hazards induced by coal-burning pollution to effectively control the hazards of endemic fluorine and arsenic poisoning induced by drinking water and endemic fluorosis induced by drinking tea. (The National Health and Family Planning Commission shall take the lead, with the participation of the Ministry of Water Resources, the Ministry of Agriculture, and some other relevant departments.)

Efforts shall be made to promote the prevention and control of occupational diseases. The general survey and prevention and control of occupational diseases shall be conducted to strengthen the monitoring of key occupational diseases such as pneumoconiosis and occupational health risk assessment. And the level of medical radiation protection monitoring and hazard control shall be improved. Efforts shall also be made to improve the capacity of medical and health institutions to report occupational diseases, conduct occupational health checks and diagnose, identify and treat occupational diseases. With the health education of the working population strengthened, the main responsibility for occupational disease prevention and control of employers shall be promoted, and a pilot program for promoting occupational health in employers shall be launched. (The National Health and Family Planning Commission and the State Administration of Work Safety shall be in charge of the above task.)

Efforts shall be made to enhance public health emergencies. The capacity building for comprehensive monitoring, rapid detection, risk assessment and timely early warning of public health emergencies, especially acute infectious diseases, shall be strengthened. The level of early warning, response capacity and commanding effectiveness of health emergency monitoring for emergencies shall be enhanced, with the response rate of early warning information of public health emergencies reaching more than 95%. The building of health emergency response teams shall be strengthened to improve the capacity of medical and health institutions at all levels to prepare for and handle health emergencies. On-site standardized disposal rate of acute infectious diseases such as plague and human avian influenza shall reach 95% or above. The military and civilian joint prevention and control mechanism for medical assistance for major natural disasters and public health emergencies shall be improved. The national coordination mechanism for bio-safety shall be established and improved to advocate social participation in health emergencies. (The National Health and Family Planning Commission and the Health Bureau of Logistics Department under the Central Military Commission shall be in charge of the above task.)

**Column I   Programs for Prevention and Control of Major Diseases**

The comprehensive prevention and control of chronic diseases: demonstration area for comprehensive prevention and control of chronic diseases; surveillance and comprehensive intervention for chronic diseases and nutrition; early diagnosis and early treatment of cancer; screening and intervention for stroke, cardiovascular disease and chronic respiratory disease; health intervention for people at high risks of hypertension and diabetes; and comprehensive intervention in key populations with oral disease.(The National Health and Family Planning Commission shall be in charge of the above task.)

The prevention and control of major infectious diseases: prevention and control of AIV/AIDS; prevention and control of tuberculosis; monitoring of flu and unexplained pneumonia; monitoring and early intervention for hand-foot-mouth disease, rabies, brucellosis, dengue fever, leprosy and other infectious diseases; and prevention and control of emergent acute infectious diseases. (The National Health and Family Planning Commission shall be in charge of the above task.)

The prevention and control of mental illnesses: management and treatment of patients with severe mental disorders; mental health service; and pilot program of comprehensive management of mental health. (The National Health and Family Planning Commission shall be in charge of the above task.)

The Expanded Program on Immunization (EPI): Expanded Program on Immunization (EPI); and monitoring of acute flaccid paralysis cases and key vaccine-preventable diseases such as measles and hepatitis B. (The National Health and Family Planning Commission shall be in charge of the above task.)

The prevention and control of key parasitic diseases and endemic diseases: prevention and control of schistosomiasis; prevention and treatment of malaria, echinococcosis and other key parasitic diseases; and prevention and control of key endemic diseases. (The National Health and Family Planning Commission shall be in charge of the above task.)

The prevention and treatment of occupational diseases: monitoring of key occupational diseases and occupational health risk assessment; occupational radiation disease surveillance and occupational health risk assessment; and medical radiation protection monitoring at healthcare institutions. (The National Health and Family Planning Commission shall be in charge of the above task.)

Items for basic public health service: residents' health records, health education, vaccination, children's health management, maternal health management, health management of the elderly, health management of patients with chronic illnesses (hypertension, type II diabetes), health management of patients with severe mental disorders, health management of TB patients; health management of traditional Chinese medicine (TCM), regulation and assistance for health and family planning, and report and handling of infectious diseases and public health emergencies. (The National Health and Family Planning Commission, the State Administration of Traditional Chinese Medicine and the Ministry of Finance shall be in charge of the above task.)

**(2) Promote patriotic health campaign and health.**

Efforts shall be made to improve the urban and rural environmental hygiene. With intensified efforts to promote the establishment of health towns, the proportion of national health cities shall be raised to 40%, and the proportion of national health counties (townships), 5%. Campaigns shall be launched to clean up the environment in urban and rural areas, with an emphasis on the weak areas of urban environmental sanitation, and rural waste water treatment and toilet system renovation. Moreover the infrastructure and long-term management mechanism for the urban and rural environmental sanitation shall be improved to accelerate the rural domestic sewage treatment and the building of innocuous sanitation toilet system. As a result, the penetration rate of rural sanitation toilets shall reach more than 85%, and a special campaign for the treatment of rural household garbage shall be launched. The implementation of a project to strengthen and improve rural drinking water safety shall be accelerated to extend urban water supply facilities to rural areas. And centralized rural water supply safety inspection shall cover over 90% of towns and townships. There shall be scientific prevention and control of vector organisms. The comprehensive prevention and control of multi-pollutants and environmental management shall be promoted. The comprehensive control of air pollution shall be enhanced to improve the quality of the atmosphere. The prevention and control of water pollution in key river basins and the treatment and restoration of soil contamination shall be promoted. The comprehensive surveillance and risk evaluation for environment and health shall be strengthened. (The National Health and Family Planning Commission, the Ministry of Ecology and Environment, the Ministry of Housing and Urban-Rural Development and the Ministry of Water Resources shall be in charge of the above task.)

Efforts shall be made to comprehensively promote the construction of healthy cities and healthy towns & villages. The comprehensive demonstration construction of healthy cities shall be carried out to form a model for building healthy cities that can be popularized. Efforts shall also be made to extensively build healthy communities, health organizations, healthy schools and healthy families, and innovate ways of social mobilization and public participation in our work. Social organizations shall be encouraged to carry out activities, such as voluntary services, self-management groups of health and community health workshops. The effect evaluation of healthy city construction shall be conducted to achieve scientific and dynamic management. The building of healthy villages & townships shall be promoted to improve rural residents' health quality and health level. With the working system of healthy cities and healthy villages and townships basically improved, and the working model of health management established, a number of demonstration cities for healthy city construction, and a number of demonstration villages &towns shall be built. (The National Health and Family Planning Commission shall be in charge of the above task.)

Efforts shall be made to launch campaigns for universal health education and health promotion. Efforts shall also be made to extensively carry out activities to promote universal health literacy and promote health in China. Knowledge on proper nutrition, rational drug use, scientific medical treatment and self-rescue and mutual aid in disasters shall be popularized to improve universal health literacy. The standardized management of health science popularization shall be strengthened to establish a sound system for releasing core information of health knowledge and skills. Efforts shall be made to advocate a healthy and civilized lifestyle, implement national nutrition programs, and guide the public to strengthen self-health management. An action for a healthy lifestyle for all shall be promoted, with the focus on reducing salt, oil, sugar, oral health, healthy body weight and healthy bones. Efforts shall be made to extensively disseminate knowledge on health popularization, such as reasonable diet, moderate exercise, smoking cessation, alcohol restriction and psychological balance, and provide strengthened guidance and intervention on family's and high-risk individuals' healthy lifestyle. The capacity building for health education shall be enhanced to promote health education and health promotion in medical institutions. Efforts shall be made to comprehensively promote the implementation of tobacco control contracts, speed up legislation on tobacco control, vigorously develop a smoke-free environment, comprehensively promote smoking bans in public places, strengthen smoking cessation services, and prevent and control passive smoking. The monitoring system for health literacy and tobacco prevalence shall be improved, with the prevalence rate of tobacco use in people over the age of 15 kept under 25% or below. (The National Health and Family Planning Commission shall take the lead, with the participation of the Propaganda Department under the CPC Central Committee, the Ministry of Industry and Information Technology, the General Administration of Sport, the Legal Affairs Office of the State Council, and some other relevant departments.)

Efforts shall be made to improve the people's health. The construction of the basic public sports service system shall be pushed forward, while the integrated construction of the national fitness facilities shall be under way. Furthermore the network of facilities and 15-minute fitness circle in urban community shall be built, with sports area reaching 1.8 square meters per capita. Efforts shall be made to open public sports facilities to the public free of charge or at low cost, and gradually open sports and fitness centers, such as school stadiums and gymnasiums, to the public. Nationwide fitness campaigns shall be extensively organized and carried out to vigorously develop the people's fitness and leisure programs. The implementation of the workroom fitness regulations shall be encouraged, whereas it shall be ensured that primary and secondary school students shall have one-hour campus sports activities every day. The building of universal fitness organizations and talent training shall be strengthened. National physical fitness monitoring and surveys on the situations of universal fitness shall be conducted to provide individualized scientific fitness guidance services for the public. And 435 million people shall regularly take part in physical exercise. (The General Administration of Sport and the Ministry of Education shall be in charge of the above task.)

### Column II　Programs for Patriotic Health and Health Promotion

Healthy cities and health townships & villages: comprehensive pilot projects for healthy cities and health townships & villages; rural latrine improvement; monitoring of vector organisms; and construction of urban-rural demonstration villages for environmental sanitation improvement (The National Health and Family Planning Commission shall be in charge of the above task.)

Surveillance of hazard factors for environmental health: hygienic monitoring of urban-rural drinking water; monitoring of rural environmental sanitation; monitoring of health risk factors in public places; monitoring of influence of air pollution on population health; and bio-monitoring of human body(The National Health and Family Planning Commission shall be in charge of the above task.)

Healthy lifestyle for all: action to reduce tobacco hazards; and special action to promote the reduction of salt, oil, and sugar, oral health, healthy body weight and healthy bones (The National Health and Family Planning Commission shall be in charge of the above task.)

Health education: action to promote health literacy; action to promote health in China; and healthy families (The National Health and Family Planning Commission shall be in charge of the above task.)

Universal fitness program: construction of facilities for universal fitness; special action for fitness promoting health; and promotion plan for juvenile physical exercise (The General Administration of Sport shall be in charge of the above task.)

**(3) Strengthen maternal and child healthcare and reproductive health service.**

Efforts shall be made to safeguard maternal and child health. The basic healthcare service throughout the whole process of childbirth shall be provided for pregnant women to further enhance the capacity for treating maternal and neonatal critical illnesses, and effectively reduce maternal and infant mortality. The special management of programs for high-risk pregnant women shall be strengthened to prevent mother-to-child transmission of HIV/AIDS, syphilis and hepatitis B, and ensure both maternal and infant safety. Efforts shall be made to vigorously promote pre-marital check-up, continue to implement free pre-pregnancy check-up for eugenics, and implement three-level preventive measures for birth defects. A service system covering birth defect prevention and treatment at all stages of pre-pregnancy, pregnancy and new-born babies in both urban and rural areas shall be established to effectively reduce the incidence of birth defects. Efforts shall be intensified to prevent and control common diseases among women, with the rate of regular screening for common diseases among women reaching over 80% or above. The coverage of screening programs for women's two cancers (cervical cancer and breast cancer) shall be gradually expanded to raise the rates of early diagnosis and early treatment of cervical cancer and breast cancer. The prevention and treatment of children's diseases and accidental injuries shall be strengthened. Efforts shall be made to vigorously promote breastfeeding, and provide guidance over infant nutrition and feeding, growth and development, and psychological behavior. In addition, the coverage of programs for improving children's nutrition and screening for newborn diseases in poverty-stricken areas shall be extended, with the growth retardation rate for children under 5 kept below 7%, and the rate of low weight reduced to less than 5%. The technical service for family planning shall be enhanced to implement the basic projects for free technical services for family planning as prescribed by the state. Efforts shall be made to comprehensively promote informed choice, popularize contraceptive birth control, eugenics and reproductive health knowledge, improve the accessibility and convenience of drugs and devices, provide guidance over technical service for reproduction, and raise the level of reproductive health. (The National Health and Family Planning Commission and the Ministry of Finance shall be in charge of the above task.)

Efforts shall be made to care for adolescent health. School health shall be strengthened with the focus on primary and secondary schools. The surveillance and evaluation for schoolchildren's health hazards shall be conducted to strengthen the prevention and control of common diseases such as myopia, dental caries and obesity. Efforts shall be intensified to promote school health education and health promotion, and integrate healthy education into the national education system. Based on the summary of the national pilot experience, the nutrition improvement plan for schoolchildren under rural compulsory education shall be implemented. The system for the monitoring and evaluation of schoolchildren's nutrition and health shall be established to intensify the regulation and guidance over the food safety and nutritional quality of collective meal at school. The prevention and control of infectious diseases such as tuberculosis and HIV/AIDS and mental health service in schools shall be enhanced. Efforts shall be made to care for teenagers' reproductive health to reduce unwanted pregnancies. The healthcare work of child-care institutions shall be strengthened to achieve full coverage of their healthcare guidance. (The National Health and Family Planning Commission, the Ministry of Education and China Food and Drug Administration shall be in charge of the above task.)

**(4) Develop health services for the elderly.**

Efforts shall be made to improve the health literacy of the elderly. Health guidance and comprehensive intervention for common diseases and chronic diseases in the elderly shall be carried out to disseminate appropriate technologies, with the focus on chronic disease management, traditional Chinese medicine (TCM) and nutritional and exercise intervention for the elderly. And the health management rate among the elderly above 65 shall reach 70% or above. The nutritional and health status of the elderly shall be effectively improved to reduce the risk of disability. Efforts shall be made to carry out trials for long-term care insurance to explore ways to establish a long-term care insurance system. Mental health and mental care services for the aged shall be carried out for the prevention and treatment of Alzheimer's disease. (The

National Health and Family Planning Commission, the Ministry of Human Resources and Social Security, and China Insurance Regulatory Commission shall be in charge of the above task.)

Efforts shall be made to improve the health service system for the elderly. Priority shall be given to the development of community-based health and old-age care services to improve the capacity of community-based healthcare institutions to provide home-based services for the elderly. All healthcare institutions shall open green channels for providing convenient services such as registration and medical treatment for the aged. Efforts shall be made to strengthen the construction of the departments of geriatrics of general hospitals. The proportion of beds for rehabilitation and nursing in community-based healthcare institutions shall be raised to encourage them to add beds for old-age care and palliative care based on the service needs. The chain of treatment-rehabilitation-long-term care shall be improved to develop and strengthen continuing healthcare institutions for rehabilitation, senile diseases, long-term care, chronic disease management and palliative care. (The National Health and Family Planning Commission shall be in charge of the above task.)

Efforts shall be made to promote the integrated development of healthcare and old-age care. The resources of healthcare and old-age care services shall be coordinated to create the model of health and old-age care services, and establish and improve the business cooperation mechanism between healthcare institutions and old-age care institutions. General hospitals at or above the secondary level shall be encouraged to give counterpart assistance and collaborate with old-age care institutions. Efforts shall be made to promote referrals and collaboration between general hospitals at or above the secondary level and nursing homes for the aged, rehabilitation institutions, and healthcare institutions established within old-age care institutions. Old-age care institutions shall be supported to establish healthcare institutions in accordance with regulations. And services such as senile diseases, rehabilitation, nursing, traditional Chinese medicine (TCM) and palliative care shall be provided. The combination of TCM and old-age care shall be promoted to give full play to the advantages of TCM in healthcare and disease rehabilitation.(The National Health and Family Planning Commission and the Ministry of Civil Affairs shall take the lead, with the participation of the State Administration of Traditional Chinese Medicine.)

**(5) Promote the health of key populations such as impoverished people.**

Efforts shall be made to implement the project of health poverty alleviation. Efforts shall also be made to ensure that impoverished people shall have access to basic healthcare services and strive to prevent poverty from illness and returning to poverty due to illness. According to the regulations, the individual payment of basic healthcare insurance for urban and rural residents of impoverished people who are eligible shall be subsidized by the government. The New Rural Cooperative Medical System (NCMS) and major disease insurance system shall have a preferential policy for the impoverished population—outpatient coordination shall be the first to cover all poverty-stricken areas. The impoverished population shall be brought into medical assistance for major and severe diseases as prescribed. The rural impoverished people who suffer from major diseases and chronic diseases shall be classified for treatment. And health cards for impoverished population shall be filed. Medical service capacity in poverty-stricken areas shall be significantly improved. Efforts shall be made for Grade III military and local hospitals to steadily and continuously provide one-to-one assistance for county-level hospitals in closely grouped poverty-stricken areas and counties and key counties for national poverty alleviation and development work. Efforts shall be made to further promote healthcare institutions at or above the second level to give partner assistance to township health centers in poverty-stricken counties. In addition, the extension of telemedicine services to poverty-stricken areas shall be positively promoted. (The National Health and Family Planning Commission shall take the lead, with the participation of the State Council Leading Group Office of Poverty Alleviation and Development, the Ministry of Civil Affairs, the Ministry of Human Resources and Social Security, the Ministry of Finance, the Health Bureau of Logistics Department under the Central Military Commission, China Insurance Regulatory Commission, the State Administration of Traditional Chinese Medicine and some other relevant departments.)

Efforts shall be made to maintain the health of shifting population. According to the allocation of resources for resident population (or service population), shifting population shall be included in the health and family planning service system at inflow areas. Equal access to basic public health and family planning services for shifting population shall be comprehensively promoted, with the coverage of basic public health and family planning services for target population among shifting population reaching 90%. Efforts shall be made to improve measures for the transfer and continuation of basic healthcare insurance formalities to raise the level of medical safeguard for shifting population. Greater efforts shall be made to respond to public health emergencies in settlements of shifting population. Health promotion activities for shifting population shall be extensively carried out to improve their health literacy. The development of the national "situation as a whole" mechanism for shifting population shall be deepened. Efforts shall be made to take care of and care for left-behind people, especially left-behind children. The health education program for left-behind children in 40 counties shall be launched to promote social integration. (The National Health and Family Planning Commission, the Ministry of Human Resources and Social Security and the Ministry of Civil Affairs shall be in charge of the above task.)

Efforts shall be made to ensure access to health services for the disabled. The disabled in urban and rural areas generally shall have access to basic healthcare insurance. Medical assistance for eligible low-income disabled people shall be intensified to gradually include medical rehabilitation programs for eligible disabled people in the coverage of basic healthcare insurance payments as prescribed. Accessibility facilities for healthcare institutions shall be improved. With targeted rehabilitation services implemented, and with disabled children and disabled people with certificates as the focus, there shall be 80% of disabled people with rehabilitation needs receiving basic rehabilitation service. And the health management and community rehabilitation for the disabled shall be strengthened. (China Disabled Persons' Federation, the National Health and Family Planning Commission, the Ministry of Human Resources and Social Security, the Ministry of Civil Affairs and some other relevant departments shall be in charge of the above task.)

### Column III   Programs for Health Improvement of Key Populations

Healthy aging: health management of the elderly; mental health and psychological care for the elderly; pilot demonstration for combination of medical treatment and old-age care; and pilot of long-term care insurance (The National Health and Family Planning Commission, the Ministry of Human Resources and Social Security and the Ministry of Civil Affairs shall be in charge of the above task.)

Maternal and child health: examination of two cancers (cervical cancer and breast cancer) for rural women; basic items for technical services for family planning and contraceptives; technical services for reproduction; and prevention of mother-to-child transmission of HIV/AIDS, syphilis and hepatitis B (The National Health and Family Planning Commission and the Ministry of Finance shall be in charge of the above task.)

Comprehensive prevention and treatment of birth defects: free pre-pregnancy check-up for rural couples; supplement of folic acid to prevent neural tube defects; prenatal screening and prenatal diagnosis of Down's syndrome during pregnancy; neonatal screening; prevention and control of thalassemia; and prevention and treatment of congenital heart disease (The National Health and Family Planning Commission and the Ministry of Finance shall be in charge of the above task.)

Adolescent health: monitoring and prevention of health hazards and common diseases in schoolchildren; and mental health education (The National Health and Family Planning Commission and the Ministry of Education shall be in charge of the above task.)

Health poverty alleviation: medical assistance for eligible people in poverty due to illness; building of provincial mobile medical teams; partner assistance of Grade III hospitals for hospitals in key poverty-stricken counties; and partner assistance of healthcare institutions of Grade II or above for health centers in poverty-stricken counties (The National Health and Family Planning Commission, the State Council Leading Group Office of Poverty Alleviation and Development and the Ministry of Civil Affairs shall be in charge of the above task.)

Health maintenance of shifting population: equal access to basic public health and family planning services for shifting population; health promotion action for shifting population; and dynamic monitoring of health and family planning for shifting population (The National Health and Family Planning Commission shall be in charge of the above task.)

### (6) Improve family planning policy.

Efforts shall be made to implement the universal two-child policy. Resources such as maternal and child healthcare, child care, pre-school, elementary and secondary education, and social security shall be rationally allocated to meet new public service needs. Classified guidance shall be strengthened to encourage childbearing by policy. The family planning policy and relevant socioeconomic policies should be linked up well before and after the policy adjustment, so as to safeguard the legitimate rights and interests of the people. Policy interpretation and advocacy shall be strengthened to investigate and punish multiple births beyond the policy in accordance with law and regulations, and maintain a sound childbearing order. The information management of the population at birth shall be improved to strengthen the monitoring and early warning of the population at birth, and grasp the dynamics of the population at birth in time. (The National Health and Family Planning Commission shall take the lead, with the participation of the National Development and Reform Commission, the Ministry of Education, the Ministry of Human Resources and Social Security and some other relevant departments.)

Efforts shall be made to reform and improve the management of family planning service. The childbearing policy, the service management system, the support system for family development and the comprehensive reform of governance mechanism shall be coordinated as a whole. Population and family planning work shall be promoted to simultaneously shift mainly from controlling the population quantity to controlling the total amount, improving quality and optimizing the structure, from the management to giving priority to stressing serving families, and from mainly relying on government forces to co-governing of the government, the society and citizens. In addition, more attention shall be paid to publicity and advocacy, service and care, policy guidance, and law-based administration. Efforts shall be made to deepen the establishment of exemplary organizations providing quality family planning services. The capacity building for family planning services and management shall be strengthened to stabilize the working networks and teams at the primary level. A birth registration system shall be implemented. An online service and commitment system shall be comprehensively promoted. Efforts shall be made to give full play to the role of mass organizations such as family planning associations and other social organizations, and deepen family planning in good faith and autonomous activities of the people at the primary level. (The National Health and Family Planning Commission shall be in charge of the above task.)

Efforts shall be made to enhance the development capability of planned-parenthood families. The award and assistance system of planned-parenthood families shall be improved to intensify the support for planned-parenthood families, and strengthen the support and care for special planned-parenthood families. Efforts shall be made to continue to implement a reward and assistance system for some rural planned-parenthood families and a special assistance system for planned-parenthood families. And dynamic adjustment for assistance standard shall be implemented. In western China, where there is a high fertility rate, fragile ecological environment and the arduous task of poverty alleviation, efforts should be made to reward and assist planned-parenthood families. Efforts shall be made to stick to gender equality to severely crack down on gender identification of fetuses and artificial termination of pregnancy by gender selection for non-medical needs, and comprehensively address the problem of high gender ratio among the population at birth. Campaigns to care for girls shall be launched to provide assistance for eligible girls in planned-parenthood families and girls' families, and enhance their family development capabilities. (The National Health and Family Planning Commission and the Ministry of Finance shall be in charge of the above task.)

Efforts shall be made to adhere to and improve the target management responsibility system for family planning. Effort shall also be made to adhere to the practices of the head of the Party and government personally in charge of family planning work and assuming overall responsibility. And the system of part-time family planning commission members and leading groups shall be adhered to. What's more, the work pattern under the joint management of all local departments in all localities shall be enhanced. Efforts shall be made to establish and improve a scientific, reasonable, convenient and efficient appraisal system and an operational mechanism for the target management responsibility system for family planning, which shall be in line with the situation and tasks of the new era, and implement the "one-vote veto" system. (The National Health and Family Planning Commission shall be in charge of the above task.)

**Column IV Programs for Family Planning Service Management**

Family planning service management: adjustment and improvement of childbearing policy surveillance; capacity building of community-based family planning service management; balanced promotion of gender structure of population at birth; promotion of social gender equality; award and assistance for some rural planned-parenthood families; special assistance for planned-parenthood families; follow-up study on family development; and creation of happy families (The National and Family Planning Commission and the Ministry of Finance shall be in charge of the above task.)

### (7) Improve medical care service.

Efforts shall be made to implement hierarchical diagnosis and treatment. With the focus on improving the capacity of community-based medical care service, and with the hierarchical diagnosis and treatment of common diseases, frequently-occurring diseases and chronic diseases as a breakthrough, a scientific and rational medical order shall take shape, basically achieving initial diagnosis at community-based healthcare institutions, two-way referral, joint efforts and separation of acute diseases and chronic diseases. With the functional orientation of diagnosis and treatment services of various healthcare institutions at all levels defined, the scale of general outpatient services in tertiary hospitals shall be controlled to support and guide patients to visit primary-level healthcare institutions first. Primary-level healthcare institutions shall gradually undertake the services of general outpatient, stable and recovery rehabilitation, and chronic disease care of public hospitals. Hospitals above the secondary level shall be encouraged to establish departments of general medicine. The enhanced competence of general practitioners (family doctors) and electronic health records shall be promoted to play the role of "gatekeeper" for residents' health of general practitioners (family doctors). In addition, the implementation of signing the family doctor service system shall be given priority to covering the elderly, pregnant women, children, the disabled, as well as patients with chronic diseases such as hypertension, diabetes, tuberculosis and severe mental disorders, etc. Doctors' multi-sited practice shall be promoted and standardized. Policies on differentiated medical insurance payments and prices for healthcare institutions at different levels shall be improved to promote the establishment of the mechanism for division of labor and coordination among healthcare institutions at all levels. And military healthcare institutions shall be integrated into the system of hierarchical diagnosis and treatment. (The National

Health and Family Planning Commission shall take the lead, with the participation of the National Development and Reform Commission, the Ministry of Human Resources and Social Security, the Health Bureau of the Logistics Department under the Central Military Commission and some other relevant departments.)

Efforts shall be made to improve medical quality and safety. The clinical pathway shall be comprehensively implemented to strengthen the standardized management of diagnosis and treatment of major diseases, and ensure medical safety. The team building of pharmacists shall be strengthened to implement the national action plan to curb bacterial resistance. Moreover rational drug use with emphasis on antimicrobial drugs shall be promoted to strengthen prescription supervision, and improve the safety and effectiveness of clinical drug use. Medical quality regulation shall be strengthened to improve the clinical application management system of medical technology. Efforts shall be made to strengthen the regulation over medical quality and improve the management system for the clinical application of medical technology. The national, provincial and prefecture-level network for medical quality control shall be gradually improved. A scientific medical performance evaluation mechanism and a dynamic monitoring and feedback mechanism for medical quality control shall be established to improve the medical security system, and achieve continuous improvement of medical quality and medical security. Nursing technique shall be continuously improved to play the positive role of nursing in enhancing medical quality. Efforts shall be made to strengthen the management of medical practitioners and improve the system for regular physician assessment. Efforts shall also be made to improve the registration of healthcare institutions and the registration system for physicians, and adopt electronic information such as electronic certificates to realize the dynamics of medical practice activities and the whole process of management. An internal audit system focusing on controlling unreasonable expenses shall be established to standardize medical and health services for medical staff. (The National Health and Family Planning Commission and the Health Bureau of the Logistics Department under the Central Military Commission shall be in charge of the above task.)

Efforts shall be made to strengthen the capacity building of clinical service. The planning, guidance and support for the development of clinical specialty construction shall be strengthened to improve the overall service capacity and level of clinical specialty. With the construction of key clinical specialties strengthened, a number of high-level clinical specialties shall be established with the aim of developing high-quality medical resources. Priority shall be given to improving the capacity of key specialties in the diagnosis and treatment of tumor, cardiovascular and cerebrovascular diseases, pediatrics, mental health, infection, maternity and other weak areas. Efforts shall be made to give full play to its role as a model, leader, driver and radiation to promote the coordinated development of the medical service system. The construction of weak specialties shall be strengthened, based on the present situation and development needs of provincial specialties. And the total quantity of high-quality medical resources shall be increased to improve the comprehensive service capacity of specialties, and reduce the rate of out-of province medical treatment. Effort shall be made to strengthen the construction of related specialties in common diseases and frequently occurring diseases, as well as the clinical specialties in infectious diseases, mental illness and emergency rescue, critical medicine, hemodialysis, gynecology and obstetrics, pediatrics, and traditional Chinese medicine (TCM) in the county. Thus the comprehensive capacity of county-level public hospitals shall be enhanced in an all-round way, to raise the rate of hospital visits in the county to approximately 90%, and basically prevent major diseases from leaving the county. The building of the service capacity of community-level healthcare institutions shall be strengthened to improve their services capacity to diagnose, treat and rehabilitate common, frequently occurring and chronic diseases. The functions of the central township health centers shall be expanded to improve their medical service capacities in emergency rescue, routine operations below the secondary level, normal childbirth, high-risk maternal screening, and pediatrics. Efforts shall be made to continue to prevent and treat blindness and deafness. (The National Health and Family Planning Commission and the Ministry of Science and Technology shall be in charge of the above task.)

Efforts shall be made to improve medical care service. The layout of facilities in the clinic waiting area shall be optimized to create a warm and inviting environment for medical treatment. The appointment diagnosis and treatment service shall be promoted to effectively divert patients. Resources for diagnosis and treatment shall be rationally allocated to promote day surgery, strengthen emergency work, and make emergency green access unimpeded. Efforts shall be made to give full play to the advantages of information technology to promote electronic medical records, provide services such as diagnosis and treatment information, fee settlement and information inquiry, improve the service procedures for hospitalization, discharge and transfers, and improve patients' medical experience. In addition, quality care service shall be implemented comprehensively. Efforts shall be made to vigorously promote the mutual recognition of inspection and testing results in the healthcare institutions of medical complex, and the mutual recognition of inspection and testing results of healthcare institutions at the same level in the same city. And patients' safety management shall be intensified. Projects to improve community health services and activities to build public health centers in townships shall be promoted. Efforts shall be made to stick to the high-pressured situation for the illegal and criminal behavior related to medical practice. The system of organic combination for court mediation, the people's mediation, judicial mediation, and medical risk sharing mechanism shall be improved to properly resolve medical disputes, and build a harmonious doctor-patient relationship. (The National Health and Family Planning Commission, the Ministry of Public Security and China Insurance Regulatory Commission shall be in charge of the above task.)

Efforts shall be made to improve the mechanism for ensuring blood supply. Efforts shall also be made to continue to raise the rate of blood donation among the population, so that the number of unpaid blood donors and the quantity of blood donation shall be commensurate with the growing demand for local medical services. Blood safety risk monitoring shall be carried out to consolidate the full coverage of blood nucleic acid testing, improve the system of blood quality control and improvement, and promote rational use of blood in the clinic. (The National Health and Family Planning Commission shall be in charge of the above task.)

**Column V   Programs for Medical Service Improvement**

Community-based healthcare service: electronic health records (EHR); and health cards (The National Health and Family Planning Commission shall be in charge of the above task.)

Hierarchical diagnosis and treatment: pilot project for integrated diagnosis and treatment services for chronic diseases; and family doctors' contracted service (The National Health and Family Planning Commission shall be in charge of the above task.)

Medical service capacity: capacity building of clinical specialties (The National Health and Family Planning Commission and the Ministry of Finance shall be in charge of the above task.)

Management of medical quality safety: construction of medical quality management and control system; monitoring of hospital infection management and continuous improvement of quality; and blood safety (The National Health and Family Planning Commission shall be in charge of the above task.)

**(8) Promote the inheritance and innovation of traditional Chinese medicine (TCM).**

Efforts shall be made to strengthen the inheritance and innovation of TCM. The development of TCM medical services shall be accelerated to improve the system of TCM medical services covering both urban and rural areas. What's more, the construction of key specialties in TCM shall be strengthened to establish the service model of TCM hospitals. Efforts shall be made to make full use of TCM technology and modern science and technology, improve the capacity of TCM diagnosis and treatment service for critical and severe diseases and refractory diseases, and improve TCM outpatient service for dominant TCM diseases. Efforts shall be made to vigorously develop TCM healthcare services, disseminate TCM healthcare technique and methods, and promote the standardized development of TCM healthcare institutions. The construction of clinical research bases and research institutions for TCM shall be strengthened to intensify theoretical and basic research on TCM, and promote the standardization and modernization of TCM. With the protection of TCM knowledge strengthened, *Chinese Medical Collection* shall be compiled and published and a database for the protection of TCM knowledge shall be set up. Efforts shall be made to improve the system for training TCM talents, accelerate the training of TCM talents at all levels and of various types, improve the system for selecting and honoring TCM masters, and improve the evaluation mechanism for TCM talents. The inheritance and development of TCM culture shall be promoted to carry forward the essence of TCM culture, and implement the project for improving health and cultural literacy of TCM. Efforts shall be made to carry out a census of TCM resources to strengthen the protection of TCM resources. The standardized planting and breeding of TCM materials shall be promoted to strengthen the construction of the system for ensuring the efficacy and quality of TCM. The mechanism for tracing the circulation of TCM shall be improved to promote the sustainable development of TCM resources, and raise the development level of TCM industry. In addition, ethnic minority medicine shall be positively developed. And appropriate TCM technology shall be disseminated. (The State Administration of Traditional Chinese Medicine, the National Health and Family Planning Commission, the National Development and Reform Commission, the Ministry of Industry and Information Technology, the Ministry of Education, the Ministry of Science and Technology, the Ministry of Commerce and the Ministry of Agriculture shall be in charge of the above task.)

Efforts shall be made to promote the coordinated development of TCM and western medicine. The health service system for TCM, which is supplementary to modern medicine and benefits the public, shall be improved. The integration of TCM and western medicine shall be strengthened to promote the organic combination of original thinking of TCM and modern and rapidly developed new technologies and methods. Efforts shall be made to find innovative ways and means to prevent and cure diseases, and promote the coordinated development of TCM and western medicine. The collaboration between TCM and western medicine in clinical practice shall be strengthened to improve the clinical efficacy of major, refractory and critical diseases. Efforts shall be made to strengthen the training of high-level talents in the integration of TCM and western medicine, and encourage western medicine doctors to learn

TCM comprehensively and systematically. Based upon clinical needs, TCM doctors shall use modern medical methods and technologies related to their own specialties and attend the training course for special access to medical technology related to their own specialties. Support shall be provided for non-traditional Chinese medicine practitioners to learn theoretical knowledge and skills of TCM and apply them in clinical practice. Efforts shall be made to carry out the project to upgrade the service capacity of community-based TCM institutions, and improve the comprehensive service capacity of community-based western medicine and TCM. Efforts shall be made to strive to equip all community health service institutions, township health centers and 70% of village clinics with TCM service capacities that are appropriate to their functions. (The State Administration of Traditional Chinese Medicine, the National Health and Family Planning Commission and the National Development and Reform Commission shall be in charge of the above task.)

**Column VI    Programs for Inheritance and Innovation of TCM**

> Inheritance and innovation of TCM: comprehensive improvement of facilities of TCM hospitals; support for the establishment of TCM museum. Improvement of the scientific research capacity of provincial TCM institutions. Support for the development of key disciplines and key specialties (special diseases) of TCM. Strengthening of TCM talent training. A census of TCM resources. Implementation of the project of inheriting TCM, the project of developing clinical advantages of TCM, and the project of improving the service capacity of community-based TCM (The State Administration of Traditional Chinese Medicine, the National Health and Family Planning Commission, the National Development and Reform Commission and the Ministry of Education shall be in charge of the above task.)

**(9) Intensify comprehensive supervision and law enforcement and regulation of food and drug safety.**

Efforts shall be made to strengthen the construction of supervision and law enforcement system. Comprehensive supervision of administrative law enforcement of health and family planning shall be reformed and improved to integrate resources for health and family planning law enforcement. The health and family planning supervision and law enforcement system shall be improved to push the focus of law enforcement down to lower levels. The regulatory mechanism shall be improved to strengthen the oversight after and during incidents, implement the "double-random" spot inspection mechanism, and strengthen the regulation of the entire industry. A network of the national key oversight and spot checks shall be established and improved. Administration in accordance with the law shall be intensified to strictly enforce administrative law, and improve the administrative law enforcement capacity and level of health and family planning. Efforts shall be made to supervise and inspect the implementation of important health and family planning laws and regulations. The system of administrative law enforcement shall be improved to vigorously carry out special rectification, the key supervision and inspection and regular inspection, and crack down on illegal activities, with the focus on the prominent problems, which arouse great social concern and affect the vital interests of the people. The liability system and accountability system for oversight and law enforcement shall be established and improved. The building of a comprehensive supervision and administrative law enforcement team for health and family planning shall be strengthened. With the construction of oversight and law enforcement capacity intensified, the regulatory information system shall be improved to promote information disclosure, and improve the efficiency of oversight and law enforcement. Efforts shall be made to establish and improve the industry integrity system and the joint disciplinary mechanism for breach of trust, and establish a "blacklist" system for medical and healthcare industries. (The National Health and Family Planning Commission shall be in charge of the above task.)

Efforts shall be made to intensify the regulation of food and drug safety. The food safety strategy shall be implemented to improve the food safety laws and regulations. The national food safety standard system shall be improved to perfect the standard management system. Efforts shall be made to accelerate the formulation of key food safety standards for heavy metals, pesticide residues and veterinary drug residues, with the completion of the formulation and revision of no less than 300 standards. The network of food safety risk monitoring and evaluation shall be improved to promote food safety risk monitoring, food consumption survey and total dietary study, with the systemic completion of risk assessment for 25 items of food chemistry pollutants. Efforts shall be made to establish and improve the epidemiological investigation mechanism for food safety accidents, and the network for monitoring and reporting food-borne diseases shall cover counties, townships and villages. The national action plan for improving drug standards shall be implemented to conduct consistency evaluation for the quality and efficacy of generic drugs. Efforts shall be made to improve the technical support system for the regulation of pharmaceuticals and medical devices, improve its inspection and testing capacities, and improve their monitoring and evaluation of adverse events and risk early warning. The establishment of institutions of clinical trial on drugs shall be strengthened. The strict, highly efficient and community-based management system for food and drug safety shall be improved. Efforts shall be intensified to improve the safety management of food and drug products in rural areas, and improve the oversight of online sales of food and drug products. The regulation of the imported foods and drugs shall be strengthened. (The National Health and Family Planning Commission, China Food and Drug Administration, the Ministry of Agriculture, the General Administration of Quality Supervision, Inspection and Quarantine and the Health Bureau of the Logistics Department under the Central Military Commission shall be in charge of the above task.)

**Column VII Programs for Comprehensive Supervision and Food Safety**

The construction of the network for national key supervision and spot check: national key supervision and spot check; supervision and spot check of healthcare and prevention and control of infectious diseases in healthcare institutions; supervision and sampling inspection for public places, schools and water supply units; supervision and spot check of the implementation of laws and regulations; and supervision and spot check of technical service institutions of family planning, blood collection and donation institutions, service institutions of radiation health; and disinfection manufacturing enterprises, and manufacturing enterprises of water-related products (The National Health and Family Planning Commission shall be in charge of the above task.)

Food safety standards and monitoring assessment: construction of food safety standard system; construction of the network of food safety risk evaluation surveillance and reporting network of food-borne disease surveillance with the integration of existing resources; and capacity building for food-borne disease management and epidemiological investigation of food safety accidents (The National Health and Family Planning Commission shall be in charge of the above task.)

**(10) Speed up the development of healthcare industry.**

Non-governmental healthcare institutions shall be vigorously developed. Nongovernmental sectors shall be encouraged to set up healthcare service. With no less than 1.5 beds per 1,000 permanent residents, planned space shall be reserved for nongovernmental sectors to run medical services, with simultaneous reservation of allocation space for medical services and large medical equipment. And private clinics shall not be restricted by the planning layout. Priority shall be given to supporting the establishment of non-profit healthcare institutions to promote equal treatment for non-profit privately-owned hospitals and public hospitals. The service requirements of nongovernmental sectors in establishing healthcare institutions shall be eased to support their participation in healthcare services in various forms. Efforts shall be made to develop professional hospital management groups and promote the development of nongovernmental sectors in healthcare institutions at a higher level.

Nongovernmental sectors shall be encouraged to develop services for scarce resources and services to meet diverse needs in pediatrics, psychiatry, senile diseases, long-term care, oral care, rehabilitation and palliative care. Multi-site practice of physicians shall be vigorously promoted to encourage them to practice in community-level healthcare institutions. Efforts shall be made to vigorously develop third-party services and guide the development of professional medical inspection centers and imaging centers. In regions with abundant resources of public hospitals, nongovernmental sectors shall participate in the restructuring and reorganizing of some public hospitals in various ways, such as the healthcare institutions run by state-owned enterprises. Public hospitals and nongovernmental sectors shall be encouraged to jointly establish new non-profit healthcare institutions to meet the needs of the public for multi-tiered medical services. Efforts shall be made to strengthen industry regulation and self-discipline, standardize market order, and ensure medical quality and safety. (The National Health and Family Planning Commission, the National Development and Reform Commission, the Ministry of Commerce and the State-owned Assets Supervision and Administration Commission of the State Council shall be in charge of the above task.)

Efforts shall be made to positively develop new forms of healthcare services. Health management and promotion services shall be improved. The development of curative tourism shall be promoted to develop featured TCM tourism products, and enhance the internationalization of medical services. New business models of big data application of healthcare shall be developed. Standardized management of physical examination shall be strengthened. And TCM health service shall be developed. Efforts shall be made to establish a group of well-known brands and a virtuous circle of healthcare service industry groups, and form certain international competitiveness to explore and develop international travel health services. (The National Health and Family Planning Commission, the General Administration of Quality Supervision, Inspection and Quarantine, the National Tourism Administration and the State Administration of Traditional Chinese Medicine shall be in charge of the above task.)

Efforts shall be made to accelerate the development of commercial healthcare insurance. Enterprises and individuals shall be encouraged to address the needs beyond basic healthcare by participating in commercial insurance and in various forms of supplementary insurance. Commercial insurance agencies shall be encouraged to actively develop health insurance products related to health management services, and strengthen health risk assessment and intervention. Efforts shall be made to accelerate the development of medical liability insurance and medical accident insurance, and explore various forms of medical practice insurance. (China Insurance Regulatory Commission shall be in charge of the above task.)

Efforts shall be made to innovatively develop industries such as pharmaceuticals and medical devices. The introduction of innovative drugs and clinically needed varieties shall be encouraged. On the basis of strengthening the industry standards, the development of new technologies such as gene detection and cell therapy shall be promoted. Enterprises shall be guided to improve the quality of innovation and cultivate major products. Efforts shall be made to support the merger and reorganization and partnerships of enterprises, foster large enterprises with international competitiveness, and improve industrial concentration. Intelligent medical equipments shall be vigorously developed. Efforts shall be made to support the improvement of the industrialization capacity and quality of medical equipments to promote its development and application. Efforts shall be made to develop wearable physiological information monitoring equipment, portable diagnostic equipment and other mobile medical products, telemedicine system that shall achieve remote monitoring, diagnosis and treatment guidance. (The Ministry of Industry and Information Technology, the National Health and Family Planning Commission, China Food and Drug Administration, the Ministry of Science and Technology and the National Development and Reform Commission shall be in charge of the above task.)

**Column VIII    Programs for Healthcare Industry Development**

Development of healthcare service industry: demonstration institutions for nongovernmental hospitals; demonstration institutions for health management and promotion services; and construction of demonstration bases for curative tourism (The National Health and Family Planning Commission, the National Development and Reform Commission, the Ministry of Finance and the National Tourism Administration shall be in charge of the above task.)

**(11) Strengthen the construction of the service system for health and family planning.**

Efforts shall be made to optimize the service system for medical and healthcare. For overall plans for regional health resources, military hospitals shall be integrated into the relevant planning of the resident areas in accordance with the strategy of integrating military and civilian development. The distribution of healthcare institutions shall be optimized to promote the coordinated development of medical and health services in Beijing-Tianjin -Hebei Region. Medical resources shall be promoted to favor the central and western regions, the communities and rural areas, so as to narrow the gap in basic medical and health services between regions. With the support at the community level bolstered and weak links improved, medical service capacity in maternal and child health, public health, tumor, psychiatry, obstetrics, pediatrics, rehabilitation, nursing and other areas with urgent needs shall be improved. The integrated medical and healthcare service system shall be established to improve the efficiency of resource utilization and avoid repeated construction. (The National Health and Family Planning Commission and the Health Bureau of the Logistics Department under the Central Military Commission shall be in charge of the above task.)

Efforts shall be made to promote the scientific development of public hospitals. For newly-built urban areas, suburban areas, satellite towns and other weak areas, the government shall establish public medical and health institutions in a planned and step-by-step way to meet the basic medical and health needs of the people. Rapid expansion of public hospitals shall be controlled. Based on the existing resources, national medical centers and regional medical centers at the national and provincial levels shall be reasonably planned and established. Efforts shall be made to continue to strengthen the construction of county-level public hospitals, improve their operational housing and equipment, and improve their service capacities. The allocation planning and access management of large medical equipments shall be strengthened to strictly control abnormal equipments in public hospitals, and gradually establish a mechanism for sharing and co-manage large equipments. (The National Health and Family Planning Commission and the National Development and Reform Commission shall be in charge of the above task.)

Efforts shall be made to strengthen the construction of health emergency response system. Based on the existing institutions, a national emergency medical rescue base and a regional emergency medical rescue center shall be laid out and established. An emergency medical rescue network of the land, the sea and the air shall be constructed, while the emergency medical rescue network for nuclear radiation and poisoning shall be improved, in order to raise the emergency medical rescue level for major emergencies. The capacity to treat acute infectious diseases shall be improved. Efforts shall be made to strengthen the construction of county-township first-aid system. (The National Health and Family Planning Commission, the National Development and Reform Commission and the Health Bureau of the Logistics Department under the Central Military Commission shall be in charge of the above task.)

Efforts shall be made to strengthen the construction of the service capacity of community-based healthcare institutions. With focus on poverty-stricken areas, the standardized construction of township health centers and community healthcare service institutions shall be strengthened to raise the service capacity and level of community-level healthcare. The integrated management of township health centers and village clinics shall be promoted. With the number of beds in community-based healthcare institutions reaching 1.2 per 1,000 permanent residents, priority shall be given to strengthening the provision of nursing and rehabilitation beds. (The National Health and Family Planning Commission shall be in charge of the above task.)

Efforts shall be made to strengthen the construction of the capacity of the professional public health institutions. With the establishment of disease prevention and control institutions strengthened, there shall be one laboratory within each provincial disease prevention and control institution that shall reach level 3 of bio-safety. In addition, there shall be one laboratory at level 2 of bio-safety within the prefectural and county-level disease prevention and control institutions where there shall be need. Laboratories at level 3 of bio-safety of the testing and quarantine system shall be established and improved. The capacity of psychiatric service shall be improved. The infrastructures of maternal and child health and family planning service institutions shall be comprehensively improved. The technical and service capacities of maternal and child health service institutions in maternal healthcare, birth defect prevention and treatment, child health care, women's healthcare and family planning shall be enhanced. The constructions of occupational disease prevention and control capacity, comprehensive supervision and law enforcement capacity for health and family planning, and technical support system for food safety shall be strengthened. Efforts shall be made to accelerate the improvement of operational housing of blood banks. (The National Health and Family Planning Commission, the National Development and Reform Commission and the General Administration of Quality Supervision, Inspection and Quarantine shall be in charge of the above task.)

**Column IX   Programs for Construction of Health and Family Planning Service System**

Construction of community-based service capacities in poverty-stricken areas: support for operational housing construction of county-level hospitals (including TCM hospitals) with focus on poverty-stricken areas; promotion of township health centers construction; the standardization rate of the community-based healthcare institutions reaching 95% or above; and a 30-minute circle of community-based healthcare service established (The National Health and Family Planning Commission and the National Development and Reform Commission shall be in charge of the above task.)

Construction of maternal and child health and family planning service capacities: strengthening the construction of the capacity to treat critical and severe diseases of pregnant women and newborn babies; support for the building of service capacity of maternal and child health service institutions at the provincial, prefectural and county levels; and comprehensive improvement of maternal and child health service with an addition of 89,000 obstetric tables (The National Health and Family Planning Commission and the National Development and Reform Commission shall be in charge of the above task.)

Capacity building for public health services: enhancing our emergency response capacity; establishing a national mobile emergency response platform and a provincial-level medical treatment base for nuclear radiation based on the existing institutions; strengthening the operational housing construction of disease prevention and control institutions at the provincial, prefectural and municipal and county levels; strengthening the infrastructure construction of provincial-level prevention and control institutions for occupational diseases, infectious disease, endemic diseases and tuberculosis; and supporting the building of operational houses for provincial and municipal blood centers (The National Health and Family Planning Commission and the National Development and Reform Commission shall be in charge of the above task.)

Capacity building for the diagnosis and treatment of refractory diseases:

Giving support for the establishment of provincial-level or ministerial-level general or specialized hospitals in weak areas such as cancer, cardiovascular and cerebrovascular diseases and respiratory diseases (The National Health and Family Planning Commission and the National Development and Reform Commission shall be in charge of the above task.)

**(12) Strengthen the construction of talent team.**

Efforts shall be made to optimize the size and structure of talent team. The ratio of doctors to nurses shall reach 1:1.25, while the ratio of beds to nurses in hospitals at the municipal level or above shall not be less than 1:0.6. And the number of public health personnel per thousand permanent residents shall reach 0.83. The size of talent team shall be in line with the people's health service needs of our country. The distribution of medical and health talents in urban and rural areas and regions shall become more reasonable, and all types of talents shall be coordinated and developed. (The National Health and Family Planning Commission shall be in charge of the above task.)

Efforts shall be made to improve the system for talent training. With the medical and educational collaboration strengthened, a supply and demand balance mechanism between medical talent training and the needs of health and family planning professionals shall be established. Efforts shall be made to strengthen the macro-control of medical universities and colleges establishments, regional layout, medical discipline structure, academic level and enrollment scale, and increase the supply of graduates for provinces with shortage of talents. Qualified universities and colleges shall be supported to establish undergraduate programs in pediatrics and psychiatry, and universities and colleges shall be supported to reasonably determine the enrollment scale of undergraduate programs in pediatrics and psychiatry according to the needs of the industry. Efforts shall be intensified to support medical institutions of higher learning in the central and western regions and narrow the gap in training levels between regions, institutions and disciplines. The medical education system after graduation shall be improved. Efforts shall be made to fully implement a standardized training system for resident physicians, expand the size of enrollment, and give priority to majors in urgent need, such as general family medicine, pediatrics and psychiatrics. By 2020, all new clinicians entering the medical position shall have received standardized training for resident physicians. A standardized training system for specialized physicians shall be established step by step. The construction of training bases and teaching staff shall be strengthened. Efforts shall be made to consolidate and improve the continuing medical education system, establish a number of education bases for continuing medical science, and comprehensively improve the comprehensive professional quality and professional service capacities of all kinds of health and family planning personnel at all levels. A standardized training system for clinical medical talents that connects the three stages of university education, post-graduation education and continuing education in an organic way shall be basically established. Education quality of colleges and universities shall be significantly improved, post-graduation shall be popularized, and continuing education shall be fully covered. (The National Health and Family Planning Commission, the Ministry of Education, the Ministry of Finance, the Ministry of Human Resources and Social Security and the State Administration of Traditional Chinese Medicine shall be in charge of the above task.)

Efforts shall be made to intensify talent training. The building of a community-based medical and health team with the focus on general practitioners shall be promoted. Preferential policies shall be formulated to train medical students free of charge for rural order and orientation. The implementation of training for assistant general practitioners shall be started. Efforts shall be made to continue to implement the plan for establishing special posts for general practitioners in community-based healthcare institutions, and give priority to arranging for them to work in township health centers in linked poverty-stricken areas. Efforts shall be made to strengthen the training of shortage talents in obstetrics, pediatrics, psychiatry, geriatrics, pharmacy, nursing, first aid and rehabilitation, as well as skilled health service talents such as reproductive health consultants and nursing assistants. The building of the ranks of high-level talents and public health professionals shall be strengthened. Vocational training for hospital deans shall be strengthened. Efforts shall be made to strengthen the ranks of village doctors. (The National Health and Family Planning Commission, the Ministry of Education, the Ministry of Finance, the Ministry of Human Resources and Social Security and the State Administration of Traditional Chinese Medicine shall be in charge of the above task.)

Efforts shall be made to innovate the mechanism of employment, management and evaluation of talents. The employment mechanism of public institutions focusing on the employment system and post management system shall be improved. Efforts shall be made to establish a personnel compensation system that is in line with the characteristics of the medical industry, try hard to reflect the value of technical services of medical workers, and optimize the career development environment for medical workers. With the incentive and restraint mechanisms for people at the community level and in short supply improved, the internal distribution of community-based healthcare institutions to the staff of key positions, business backbone and who has made outstanding achievements, in order to narrow the actual income gap among healthcare institutions at different levels. Efforts shall be made to implement the policy of professional titles assessment for community-level health professionals to establish a talent evaluation mechanism that shall conform to the reality of community-level medical and health work. Through the integration of human resources service and flexible introduction, the talent management and service mode of improving the linkage between urban and rural areas shall be established. With innovations in the management of organization structure of public hospitals made, the measures for the management of staffing of public hospitals shall be improved to actively explore and carry out pilot reform of staffing management of public hospitals, and give them the right to choose their own employees. With the economic and social development, the treatment of rural doctors shall be improved little by little, and the pension policy of village doctors shall be improved to stabilize and optimize the ranks of village doctors. (The National Health and Family Planning Commission, the Ministry of Human Resources and Social Security, the State Commission Office of Public Sectors Reform and the Ministry of Finance shall be in charge of the above task.)

**Column X   Programs for Talent Development**

Capacity building for community-based healthcare and family planning talents with the focus on general practitioners: training for general practitioners through standardized training for resident doctors with general practice specialty, training for assistant general practitioners, job-transfer training for general practitioners, and training for medical students free of charge for rural order and orientation medical students; training for teaching staff in general practice medicine; and strengthening the training for key talents in community-based urban and rural healthcare institutions (The National Health and Family Planning Commission, the Ministry of Education, the Ministry of Human Resources and Social Security and the State Administration of Traditional Chinese Medicine shall be in charge of the above task.)

Standardized training for physicians: standardized training for 500,000 resident doctors; strengthening the construction of standardized training bases; launching a pilot program to standardize training for specialized physicians; and training resident doctors for qualification (The National Health and Family Planning Commission, the Ministry of Human Resources and Social Security and the State Administration of Traditional Chinese Medicine shall be in charge of the above task.)

Training for key physicians at county-level hospitals: training key clinicians at county-level hospitals with the focus on pediatrics, obstetrics, psychiatry, pathology, rehabilitation, geriatrics and pre-hospital care; comprehensively improving the service capacity and level of county-level hospitals (The National Health and Family Planning Commission shall be in charge of the above task.)

Improving the safeguard of service talents for birth policy: intensifying the training for professionals in the area of maternal and child health; extensive post training and job-transfer training for medical workers in obstetrics and pediatrics; striving to increase the number of obstetricians and midwives by 140,000 in various forms (The National Health and Family Planning Commission shall be in charge of the above task.)

Construction of medical and health innovation talent team: attracting, selecting and cultivating a number of medical leaders with internationally leading levels; cultivating a new generation of outstanding academic leaders of young and middle age; attracting, stabilizing and training a number of outstanding young professionals who shall be interested in medical and health care; and supporting the discipline development with national priority and the outstanding innovation teams in frontier areas of international science and technology (The National Health and Family Planning Commission shall be in charge of the above task.)

**(13) Strengthen information technology for population health.**

Efforts shall be made to promote the sharing of information on population health. Based on the platform of information on regional population health, the continuous records of electronic health records and electronic medical records as well as the information sharing among different levels and types of healthcare institutions shall be achieved. Data fusion, dynamic interaction and sharing shall be realized in the three databases of population information, electronic health records and electronic medical records, which shall basically cover the entire population and achieve dynamic update of information. Efforts shall be made to build population health information platforms for unity, authority and interconnectivity at the national, provincial, prefectural and municipal, and county levels. Resource sharing and business collaboration among six business application systems shall be available, including public health, family planning, medical service, medical security, drug supply and comprehensive management. With the residents' health cards popularized and applied, the application integration of residents' health cards, social security cards and other public service cards shall be positively promoted to realize one-card application of residents' health management and medical services. Based on the national e-government network and the government data sharing and exchange platform, the interconnection and information sharing between various platforms and various health and family planning institutions at all levels shall be realized. The standard system for population health information shall be established and improved to strengthen the standard construction and application management. Faced with the online medical and health information service, the network security strategy shall be implemented to strengthen the construction of the information security protection system. Efforts shall be made to guide the development and application of independently controllable standardized information products. (The National Health and Family Planning Commission, the National Development and Reform Commission, the Office of the Central Cyberspace Affairs Commission, the Ministry of Industry and Information Technology and the Ministry of Human Resources and Social Security shall be in charge of the above task.)

Efforts shall be made to actively promote the rapid and orderly development of new forms of healthcare information. The "Internet plus" health and medical services for the people shall be fully implemented, whereas smart medical services that integrate telemedicine and online and offline services for the central and western regions and community-based healthcare institutions shall be developed. The in-depth integration of information technologies such as cloud computing, big data, the Internet of things, mobile Internet and virtual reality with health services shall be promoted to enhance the capacity of health information services. The establishment of regional telemedicine business platforms shall be encouraged to promote the vertical flow of high-quality medical resources, and telemedicine services shall cover more than 50% of the counties (districts, county-level cities).

Efforts shall be made to deepen the application of big data in health care. The governance of the healthcare industry, clinical and scientific research and the application of big data on public health shall be promoted to enhance the security of medical data and the protection of patients' privacy. The technology of Internet of things, wearable devices, etc. shall be utilized to explore new models of health services, develop smart health services for the convenience of the people, reinforce the fine service for prevention, treatment and rehabilitation and residents' business collaboration of health information management, and improve the service capacity and management level. Efforts shall be made to actively develop online services such as disease management and residents' health management, and promote online services such as online booking, online payment, online follow-up, health counseling and online query of inspection and test results. Based on residents' electronic health records, residents' health management and medical information resources shall be integrated. Residents' medical and health information services shall be provided to improve residents' self-management abilities. Efforts shall be made to improve the statistical system to strengthen the ability to analyze statistics. (The National Health and Family Planning Commission, the National Development and Reform Commission, the Office of the Central Cyberspace Affairs Commission and the Ministry of Industry and Information Technology shall be in charge of the above task.)

**Column XI   Programs for Population Health Information Construction**

Population Health Information Construction: Improving platforms at the provincial, prefectural and county levels in accordance with the principle of evening up and filling in the gaps; connecting platforms at the provincial level with those at the national level; and making platforms within the province interconnect and work together. Consolidating and improving the report and management of prevention and control of infectious diseases, vaccination, and severe mental disorders, and highlighting dynamic updating of electronic medical records and electronic health records. Launching a pilot project for big data and telemedicine applications. Promoting big data application for healthcare; strengthening the demonstration work of regional clinical medical health data, and pushing forward telemedicine (imaging, pathology, ECG), appointment diagnosis and treatment, two-way referral and other services benefiting the people (The National Health and Family Planning Commission, the National Development and Reform Commission and the Office of the Central Cyberspace Affairs Commission shall be in charge of the above task.)

**(14) Strengthen the construction of the system for medical science and technology innovation.**

Efforts shall be made to fully promote the innovation in health science and technology. Centering on health issues such as malignant tumor, cardiovascular disease and other major diseases and rare diseases as well as the needs for healthcare industry development, efforts shall be made to strengthen the forefront of basic research of medical science, key technology research and development, transfer and transformation of achievements, pharmaceutical product development and appropriate technology dissemination. The major healthcare projects for 2030 shall be launched and implemented. Efforts shall be made to continue to organize and implement the state key scientific research programs of the "development of major new drugs" and the "prevention and control of major infectious diseases such as HIV/AIDS and viral hepatitis". A number of state key research and development plans such as "precision medical research" shall be organized and implemented. The development and industrialization of new technologies of diagnosis and treatment, pharmaceuticals and medical devices shall be accelerated to significantly improve capacity of prevention and control of major diseases and the scientific support for the development of healthcare industry. Efforts shall be made to strengthen the constructions for the state major scientific infrastructure of translational medicine, the national clinical medicine research center and collaborative research network. Efforts shall be made to promote the capacity improvement of the existing number of state key laboratories and other state scientific research bases. Key laboratories at the commission level shall be adjusted and improved, and a platform system for standard, integrated and efficient medical science bases shall be gradually established. The construction of environment for medical science innovation policy shall be strengthened to improve the safeguard mechanism for innovative talent training, new technology evaluation, standards and norms of medical research, medical ethics and research integrity, and intellectual property rights. The rate of transfer and conversion of medical scientific achievements shall be greatly increased. Efforts shall be made to give full play to the role of the national center for clinical medicine research and the collaborative research network, and promote the popularization of appropriate technologies, guidelines for diagnosis and treatment, and technical specifications. (The Ministry of Science and Technology, the National Health and Family Planning Commission and the National Development and Reform Commission shall be in charge of the above task.)

### Column XII   Programs for Health Technology

Major projects and projects in health technology: major health care projects; state key scientific research programs of the "development of major new drugs" and the "prevention and control of major infectious diseases such as HIV/AIDS and viral hepatitis"; state key research and development plans such as "precision medicine research", research on the prevention and control of major, chronic non-infectious diseases, and research on reproductive health and prevention and control of major birth defects; innovation project of medical science and health technology of Chinese Academy of Medical Sciences (The Ministry of Science and Technology and the National Health and Family Planning Commission shall be in charge of the above task.)

Results transformation and appropriate technology promotion: transfer and transformation of health technology achievements; promotion of appropriate technology in community-based medical and health services (The Ministry of Science and Technology and the National Health and Family Planning Commission shall be in charge of the above task.)

### IV. Safeguard measures

(1) Comprehensively deepen the reform of the medical and healthcare system. Efforts shall be made to carry out coordinated reform of medical care, healthcare insurance and drugs, and establish and improve a basic medical and healthcare system that shall cover both urban and rural residents. A universal healthcare insurance system shall be improved. Efforts shall be made to strengthen major illness insurance and medical assistance for major diseases for urban and rural residents, and improve the emergency aid system for diseases. Efforts shall be made to improve the mechanism for sustainable financing and adjusting the proportion of reimbursement for basic healthcare insurance. Efforts shall be made to integrate basic healthcare insurance policy for urban and rural residents and agency management. Efforts shall be made to accelerate the direct settlement of basic healthcare insurance for out-of town medical treatment. The comprehensive reform of public hospitals shall be comprehensively promoted. A modern hospital management system shall be established to improve the corporate governance mechanism and external regulation mechanism of hospitals. The unreasonable growth of medical expenses shall be controlled. The mechanism for ensuring drug supply shall be improved to make perfect the national drug policy system. The basic drug system shall be consolidated and improved to establish a comprehensive clinical evaluation system for drugs. And the basic drug safeguard for children, the elderly and other special groups shall be strengthened. Equal access to basic public health services shall be promoted to improve the national basic public health services, and continue to implement the major national public health services. Efforts shall be made to consolidate and improve the community-based new operating mechanism. (The Office of Medical and Healthcare System Reform under the State Council, the National Health and Family Planning Commission, the National Development and Reform Commission,

the Ministry of Finance, the Ministry of Human Resources and Social Security, China Food and Drug Administration and the Ministry of Civil Affairs shall be in charge of the above task.)

(2) Establish a fair, effective and sustainable financing system. Efforts shall be made to further clarify the government, social and individuals' responsibilities for health and family planning, improve the mechanism for rational sharing, and ease the financial burden of personal medical treatment. The leading role of the government in providing public health and basic healthcare service shall be defined to increase government investment in healthcare, and ensure the people's needs for basic medical and healthcare services. Efforts shall be made to encourage and guide social forces to increase their investment in health and health programs, and establish a medical care system with diversified sources of investment and diversified investment. (The National Health and Family Planning Commission, the Ministry of Finance and the Ministry of Human Resources and Social Security shall be in charge of the above task.)

(3) Improve the legal system for health and family planning. Efforts shall be made to promote legislation on the basic medical and health law. The system of laws and regulations on healthcare and family planning shall be improved to strengthen the formulation and revision of laws and regulations in key areas such as medical care, drugs, healthcare insurance, public health and family planning. There shall be reestablishment, revision, annulment and interpretation for departmental rules and regulations. The legality review of normative documents shall be reinforced to improve the legal decision-making mechanism. Regular clearing of regulatory and normative documents and review of standards shall be carried out to maintain the coordination and consistency of the system of medical and health laws and regulations. The system of health standards shall be improved to promote the implementation of mandatory health standards. The reform of the administrative examination and approval system shall be deepened to further promote streamlining administration and delegating powers to lower-levels, the integration of oversight with management, and optimize the reform of services. Besides, efforts shall be made to bring forth new ideas to the administrative management of health and family planning, and accelerate the transformation of government functions. The standardization of administrative examination and approval shall be promoted to prohibit the continuing and disguised examination and approval of administrative approval items that have been canceled. The capacity building of undertaking institutions shall be reinforced to ensure the implementation of the de-delegated items. Efforts shall be made to make government affairs more open. (The Legislative Affairs Office of the State Council, the National Health and Family Planning Commission, the Ministry of Human Resources and Social Security and China Food

and Drug Administration shall be in charge of the above task.)

(4) Strengthen publicity and guidance. Efforts shall be made to strengthen positive publicity and typical publicity, and enhance the general public awareness of health and family planning. Efforts shall be made to seek strong support from all sides to ensure effective implementation of the plan. With social publicity strengthened, public awareness of health and family planning shall be raised by widely publicizing laws and regulations related to health and family planning and the situation and challenges facing them through television, radio broadcasting, newspaper and network. Efforts shall be made to strengthen publicity on the health and family planning law. The professional spirit of health and family planning shall be vigorously carried forward and practiced to carry out in-depth publicity and promotion of professional spirit. The press release system and the work system for online public opinion shall be improved to respond promptly to online public opinion and social concerns. And the construction of guidance team for online public opinion shall be strengthened to enhance the ability of news publicity and public opinion guidance. Health culture shall be developed to strengthen the cultural construction and culture and ethical progress in health and family planning. Efforts shall be made to establish a base for the publicity on health and family planning culture and a cultural promotion platform. (The Propaganda Department of the CPC Central Committee, the National Health and Family Planning Commission and the Office of the Central Cyberspace Affairs Commission shall be in charge of the above task.)

(5) Carry out international exchanges and cooperation. Efforts shall be made to develop China's global health strategy to implement the multi-level and multi-channel cooperative strategies adapted to the characteristics of different countries, regions and organizations, and enhance China's influence in the global health diplomacy and international voice. Health exchanges and cooperation in the construction of the Belt and the Road shall be promoted. Efforts shall be made to strengthen cooperation in the 2030 agenda for sustainable development, global health, medical and health research, population and development, and introduce the intellectual and technological resources needed for health and family planning reform and development. Our working model shall be innovated to continue to strengthen health assistance to foreign countries. The training and development of global health talents shall be reinforced. Efforts shall be made to deepen medical and health cooperation and exchanges with Hong Kong, Macao and Taiwan. And South-South cooperation shall be promoted. Medical equipment and drugs shall be promoted to go global. Efforts shall be made to vigorously develop international trade in medical and health services, and strengthen international exchanges and cooperation in TCM. (The National Health and Family Planning Commission, the State Administration of

Traditional Chinese Medicine, the National Development and Reform Commission, the Ministry of Commerce and China Food and Drug Administration shall be in charge of the above task.)

(6) Strengthen organization and implementation. Governments at all levels shall further raise their awareness from the height of building a moderately prosperous society in all respects and promoting the building of a healthy China. They shall also strengthen their leadership and put health work on the agenda. All relevant departments shall, according to the division of responsibilities, refine their goals and fulfill the implementation of relevant tasks. An evaluation system for health influence assessment shall be established gradually. With a monitoring and evaluation mechanism set up and improved, the National Health and Family Planning Commission shall be responsible for taking the lead in the formulation of monitoring and evaluation plan. They shall also conduct yearly monitoring and mid-term assessment for the planned implementation progress and effects to supervise the implementation of major projects. The implementation of major projects shall be supervised to find problems in the implementation in time, and study solutions. Local people's government at all levels shall regularly organize the inspection and supervision for the local implementation of the plan, so as to ensure smooth implementation. (The National Health and Family Planning Commission shall take the lead in the above task.)

**(Shan Yongxiang)**

## Circular of the State Council on Printing and Issuing the *Program on Deepening the Reform of the Medical and Health Care System during the 13th Five-Year-Plan Period*

(No. 78 [2016] of the State Council)

The people's governments of all provinces, autonomous regions, and municipalities directly under the Central Government; all ministries and commissions of the State Council; and all institutions directly under the State Council:

The *Program on Deepening the Reform of the Medical and Health Care System during the 13th Five-Year-Plan Period is hereby* printed and distributed to you, please implement it fully.

December 27th, 2016

## 16. *Program on Deepening the Reform of the Medical and Health Care System during the 13th Five-Year-Plan Period*

The *Program* herein is formulated with a view to deepen the reform of the medical and health care system comprehensively in the light of *Outline of the 13th Five-Year*

*Plan for the National Economic and Social Development of the People's Republic of China,* *Opinions of the State Council on Deepening the Reform of Medical and Health Care System* and *the Outline of Healthy China 2030 Plan.*

## I. Background of the *Program*

Under the strong leadership of the CPC Central Committee and the State Council, all the localities and all the relevant departments promoted medical and health care reform with significant progress and remarkable achievements since the 12th Five-Year Plan, especially the 18th National Congress of CPC. The completion of the national medical security system has been accelerated, with the participation rate of basic medical insurance being over 95%, medical insurance schemes for the urban and rural residents gradually integrated, fund raising and guarantee levels further improved, insurance for major illnesses for urban and rural residents, medical assistance for major and catastrophic illness and assistance for medical emergency response carried out, and commercial health insurance developed quickly. The comprehensive reform of county-level public hospitals has been fully carried out, the pilot of comprehensive reform of urban public hospitals has been further expanded and deepened, the reform of medical services and drug prices has been pushed forward in an orderly manner, and the management system and operation mechanism for public hospitals have been continually improved. The construction of tiered medical diagnosis and treatment has picked up pace, the comprehensive reform of the medical and health institutions at the community level has been continuously deepened, the division and coordination of responsibility among medical and heath institutions have been gradually enhanced and the equity of primary public healthcare services has been improved steadily. The national essential drug system has been consolidated and bettered, the reform of drug distribution has been intensified and the system of drug supply and guarantee has been gradually completed. Hospitals and universities have cooperated to deepen the reform of cultivating clinical medical talents, the standardized training system for residential physicians has been preliminarily established, the construction of talent teams with the general physicians as the priority has been continually enhanced and the initiatives of the medical staff has been further mobilized. Medical and health supervision and management has been continually strengthened and the construction of informationalization has been actively pushed forward. The policies and mechanisms for the development of the traditional Chinese medicine (TCM) have been gradually perfected to let it better play its role and better benefit the people. The policies and environment for healthcare service industry have been remarkably improved and the development of hospitals operated by non-governmental agencies has been sped up. The pilot of comprehensive medical and health reform has been implemented with the province as the entity and useful experience has been accumulated. After years of endeavor, the average life expectancy of the residents in 2015 increased 1.51 over the year 2010, the out-of-pocket payment as a share of total health expenditures dropped from 35.29% to 29.27%,over 80% of the residents could get to the nearest medical institution within 15 minutes, the health of the people have been generally better than the average of the middle- and high-income countries, the irrational excessive rapid growth of medical expenses has been preliminarily kept under control and the equity and accessibility of primary healthcare service have been improved remarkably. As has been proved, the direction of deepening medical and health care reform is correct, methods clear, measures effective, and achievements remarkable; more health results have been achieved with less investment; the issues of difficult and expensive access to medical service have been significantly relieved; people's sense of benefits has been intensified and the role of deepening medical and health care reform in the development of national socio-economic development has become increasingly important.

The 13th Five-Year Plan period is the decisive stage in building a moderately prosperous society in all respects and a critical moment for establishing and completing primary healthcare system and promoting the building of Healthy China. At present, people's demands for health keeps rising with the improvement of their living standards; however, there still exist some prominent problems such as the inadequate amount of health resources, irrational structure of health resources, unbalanced distribution of health resources, relatively unitary supply subjects and weak service capability at the community level etc., therefore, the institutional system to maintain and promote people's health needs improving constantly. As the medical and healthcare reform enters the critical stage and deep water zone, the restraint function of institutional contradiction at the deep level is becoming increasingly prominent, the adjustment of interest structure more intricate, the reform more holistic, systematic and coordinated and the tasks more arduous. Meanwhile, China's economic development has entered a new normal state, industrialization, urbanization, the acceleration of the aging process of population, the change of the disease spectrum, the change of the ecological environment and life style, and the innovation of medical technology, all of which have put forward higher requirements for the deepening of medical and healthcare reform. Facing the new situations and challenges, we need to, on the basis of consolidating the achievements of the previous reform and conscientiously summing up the experience, further unify ideas, strengthen convictions, enhance determination, and further strengthen organizational leadership, institutional innovation, and key breakthroughs so as to promote medical and healthcare reform from laying a good foundation to improving quality, from forming a framework to establishing a system, from a single breakthrough to system integration and comprehensive promotion, solve the worldwide difficult problem of medical reform with a Chinese approach, and provide new impetus to safeguard the health of the people and promote economic and social development.

## II. Guiding ideology, basic principles and overall objectives

### (1) Guiding ideology

We need to hold high the great banner of socialism with Chinese characteristics. We need to implement the guiding principles of the 18th National Congress of the CPC and the third, fourth and fifth plenary sessions of the 18th CPC Central Committee. We must follow the guidance of Marxism-Leninism, Mao Zedong Thought, Deng Xiaoping Theory, the Theory of Three Represents, and the Scientific Outlook on Development. The guiding principles from General Secretary Xi Jinping's major policy addresses must be put into practice. Work must be carried out in accordance with the plan for promoting all-round economic, political, cultural, social and ecological progress, and the Four-Pronged Comprehensive Strategy. Decisions made by the CPC Central Committee and the State Council must be carried out. New vision of development must be established and implemented that is innovative, coordinative, green, open and shared. People-centered concept of development must be followed and the right medical and health policies must be stuck to. The vision of comprehensive health must be established. The innovation of theory, institution, management and technology in the medical and health sector must be propelled forcefully to speed up the establishment of the primary medical and health system which suits the national conditions of China. The development modes must be transformed from treatment-centered to health-centered. The modernization of medical and health governance system and governance capability must be pushed forward. Ultimately, this will lay a solid health foundation for promoting Healthy China, building a moderately prosperous society in all aspects, realizing the "two centenary goals" and the great rejuvenation of the Chinese nation.

### (2) Basic principles

We shall adhere to the principle of focusing on people's health. We shall give strategic priority to people's health, aim at equitable and accessible health services and the people benefiting, stick to the bottom line and improve drawbacks, make more effective institutional arrangements, and maintain the welfare of basic medical and healthcare services, so that all the people shall have more sense of benefit from "Contribute and Share".

We shall adhere to the principle of ensuring basic levels of health care, strengthening health services at the community level and building up health care networks. We shall offer basic health care services to all people as a public good. The medical and health service shall focus more on the communities and we shall make more healthcare resources available for the community-level programs. We shall make the occupation of medical and healthcare service at the community-level more appealing and enhance its service capability. We shall promote institutional innovation and make breakthroughs oriented by problem solving.

We shall adhere to the principle of combining the government's dominant role with giving full play to the role of market mechanism. In the sector of basic medical and health care service, we shall stick to the dominance of the government, implement the responsibility of the government and introduce mechanism of moderate competition. While in the sector of non-basic medical and health care service, we shall give full play to the market's vigor, strengthen normative guidance, and try to meet the diverse, differentiated and individualized demands for health.

We shall adhere to driving the supply-side reform. We shall separate the functions of government from those of institutions, the functions of supervision institutions from those of enforcement institutions, the functions of prescribing from those of dispensing, and the functions of profitable institutions from those of non-profitable institutions. We shall optimize the governance capacity and allocation of factors on the supply side and improve service efficiency and quality. We shall provide scientific guidance on the supply side, rationally divide the responsibility of the government, the society and the individuals and promote social co-regulation.

We shall adhere to coordinated reform of medical services, medical insurance and the medicine industry. In accordance with the requirements of vacating space, adjusting structures and ensuring connection, we shall propel the construction of management system, price system, payment system and salary system etc. in a coordinated manner and improve the capacities of policy connection and system integration. We shall implement the responsibility of the departments, emancipate our mind, take initiative actions, and propel reform in the spirit of self-revolution to form powerful joint force.

We shall adhere to highlighting the key points, pilot demonstration and gradually advancing. We shall straighten out the inner logic of reform, highlight the important fields and key links, summarize and spread the experience from the localities in time and give full play to the breakthrough action of key reform and the driving effect of pilot programs. We shall keep the intensity and pace of reform under control, make overall plan and advance reform vigorously and steadily.

**(3) Overall objectives**

By 2017, a systematic policy framework for the basic medical and health system shall have been established. The policy system of tiered medical diagnosis and treatment shall have been gradually improved, the construction of modern hospital management system and comprehensive supervision system shall have been sped up, the basic medical security system more effective and the policies regarding the production, and the distribution and use of drugs more completed. By 2020, the following systems and mechanism shall have been established, including a comparatively complete public health service system and medical service system, a comparatively complete medical security system, a comparatively standard security system and a comprehensive supervision system for drug supply and a comparatively scientific management system and operation mechanism for medical and health institutions. With continual efforts, the primary medical and healthcare service system covering both the rural and urban residents shall have been established, universally accessible primary medical and healthcare services achieved, and people's multi-layer demands for medical services primarily met, with average life expectancy increased by one year over the year 2015, maternal mortality dropped to 18 per 100,000 persons, infant mortality declined to 7.5 per 1,000, and under-five mortality dropped to 9.5 per 1,000. The main health indicators of the Chinese shall rank top in upper middle-income countries and the out-of-pocket payment as a share of total health expenditures shall drop to around 28 percent.

### III. Key tasks

In the 13th Five-Year-Plan period, new breakthroughs shall be made in the construction of five systems, i.e. the systems of tiered diagnosis and treatment, modern hospital management, public medical insurance, drug supply security and comprehensive supervision etc. and reform in relevant fields shall be pushed forward.

**(1) Establishing scientific tiered diagnosis and treatment system.** We shall adhere to the willingness of the residents, first diagnosis at the community level, guidance by policies and innovation of mechanisms. Family doctors and contract services shall be used as the major means and various modes of tiered diagnosis and treatment shall be encouraged to practice in different localities in combination with their respective situations to propel the formation of new orders of seeking medical services featuring first diagnosis at the community level, two-way referral treatment, different treatments for acute and chronic diseases and interconnection between different levels. By 2017, policies for tiered diagnosis and treatment shall have been gradually improved with over 85 percent of cities launching the pilot. By 2020, the mode of tiered diagnosis and treatment shall have gradually formed and a system of tiered diagnosis and treatment in accordance with our national conditions shall have primarily been established.

1) Improving medical and healthcare service system. The layout of medical and healthcare resources shall be optimized, the functions of medical and healthcare institutions at various levels clearly defined, collaboration enhanced and the integration of functions and sharing of resources promoted. The number and size of public comprehensive hospitals shall be kept under rational control. The construction of telemedicine system shall be forcefully pushed forward which will serve the communities, remote and underdeveloped areas. We shall encourage the second level and third level hospitals to provide distant service for medical and healthcare institutions at community level, improve the capability of telemedicine, promote the vertical mobility of medical resources with information methods and improve the accessibility of quality medical resources and the overall efficiency of medical services.

We shall promote the sharing of resources and collaboration of business between big hospitals and medical and healthcare institutions at the community level and between general physicians and specialist physicians, and complete the information system of tiered diagnosis and treatment that is based on the Internet and big data technology. We shall encourage non-government organizations to run medical examination institutions, pathological diagnosis institutions, medical image inspection institutions, disinfection supply institutions and blood purification institutions as well as encourage public hospitals to provide relevant services to the whole regions to achieve the sharing of resources within the regions. We shall enhance quality control of medical service, and promote the mutual recognition of testing and examination results between medical institutions at the same level as well as between medical institutions and independent medical examination institutions.

We shall launch the projects of traditional Chinese medicine (TCM) preservation and innovation, promote the dynamic integration of the service resources and clinical research of traditional Chinese medicine, enhance the application of appropriate health technology of traditional Chinese medicine and let traditional Chinese medicine play its key role in preventing illnesses, treating major illnesses and in rehabilitation. In areas where the service system of traditional Chinese medicine at the community level is imperfect and capacities are weak, the outpatient diagnosis of traditional Chinese medicine at the TCM hospitals shall be included in first diagnosis. In light of the development strategy of integrating military and civilian resources, the military medical institutions shall be fully integrated into the tiered diagnosis and treatment system. A medical first-aid network for emergent, acute and infectious diseases shall be established and perfected and a three-dimensional emergency medical rescue network covering the land, the sea and the air shall be constructed.

2) Improving the medical and healthcare service capabilities at the community

level. Focusing on the diagnosis and differential diagnosis of common diseases, we shall enhance the capability construction of basic medical service at township hospitals and health service centers at community level. We shall improve the medical service capabilities of township hospitals of emergency rescue, routine surgeries under grade two, normal delivery, primary screening of high-risk pregnant and lying-in women, pediatric department, mental diseases, geriatric diseases, traditional Chinese medicines, and rehabilitation etc. We shall enhance the construction of comprehensive capability and disciplines at county-level public hospitals, focusing on the construction of departments of common diseases within the counties and the construction of clinic specialty departments in great demands of to further reduce the outpatient rate outside the counties. We shall regulate the management of community health service and launch projects to promote the health service at the communities. We shall spread appropriate technologies to benefit all the people. We shall establish a security system for drug supply which is compatible with the tiered diagnosis and treatment and able to fulfill the practical demands of medical institutions at community level so as to achieve the cross-level coordination and mutual interconnection of drug use. We shall spread the technology of big hospitals to the communities by encouraging physicians to go to the communities and retired doctors to run clinics as well as enhancing counter-part medical assistance, offering telemedicine and promoting the construction of healthcare consortiums. We shall implement the action plan for projects of improving capacity of traditional Chinese medicine at the community level during the 13th Five-Year-Plan period. We shall endeavor to equip all the healthcare service institutions at community level, township hospitals and over 70 percent of village infirmaries with the capacity of traditional Chinese medicine as well as the corresponding capacity of medical rehabilitation.

We shall improve the management and operating mechanism at the at community level. We shall strengthen the legal person's status of medical institutions at the community level, granting them autonomy in personnel, operation and income distribution etc. We shall further improve the performance-based salary system for medical institutions at the community level and the surplus part of income and expenditure may be withdrawn as welfare funds and incentive funds for the stuff in accordance with regulations. We shall consolidate and improve the mechanism of multi-channel compensation, implement the financial management methods of medical institutions at the community level such as checking and ratifying tasks, checking and ratifying income and expenditure and subsidizing for performance evaluation; strengthening performance evaluation shall not only mobilize the medical institutions and medical stuff at the community level but also prevent new form of profit-seeking behaviors. We shall establish the performance evaluation mechanism for the basic medical and health institutions and the responsible person, implement the tenure goal responsibility system for the responsible person of the institutions, and for other stuff members, we shall attach more attention to the workload, service quality, code of conduct, technical difficulty, risk level and satisfaction of service objects etc. We shall encourage localities with suitable conditions to implement an integrated management in the township and village health institutions.

3) Guiding public hospitals to participate in tiered diagnosis and treatment. We shall further improve and implement payment by medical insurance and price policies for medical services, mobilize the enthusiasm and initiative of third-level public hospitals to participate in tiered diagnosis and treatment, guide third-level public hospitals to admit and treat patients with complicated and critical diseases and gradually guide patients of common diseases and patients at stable or convalescent stages to the lower-level hospitals. We shall encourage the breaking of regional administrative restrictions, the building of medical consortium, and the integration of medical insurance and telemedicine, so as to achieve a suitable combination and integration of medical resources. Taking sharing resources and guiding talents downwards to the community medical institutions as guidance, we shall build medical consortium into community of shared interest, community of shared responsibility and community of shared development so as to form a regional collaborative service model which clearly divides responsibility, power and benefit. We shall guide the smooth transferring mechanism within the medical consortium by allowing doctors to practice in multiple places, enhancing the drug equipping at the community medical institutions and practicing global payment by medical insurance for the mode of division and collaboration adopted by the medical consortium with cross-level cooperation.

4) Promoting and establishing the continual service mode of medical treatment, rehabilitation and long-term care. We shall clarify the service procedure of different treatments for acute and chronic diseases at the medical institutions, establish and improve the mechanism of division and collaboration, keep the referral channel open between hospitals, community-level medical institutions, and medical institutions for chronic diseases such as rehabilitation hospitals and nursing homes, and form a rational pattern of seeking medical service, i.e. treating minor diseases at the community, major diseases at the hospitals and rehabilitating back at the community. Big hospitals in cities shall mainly offer diagnosis and treatment to the acute serious diseases and difficult and complicated diseases and chronic patients whose diagnosis are clear and conditions are stable and patients at convalescent stage shall be transferred to medical institutions at a lower level or chronic medical institutions such as rehabilitating hospitals or nursing homes. Community-level medical institutions

and chronic medical institutions shall provide treating, rehabilitating and nursing care services to chronic patients with clear diagnosis and stable conditions, patients at convalescent stage, patients with senile diseases, patients with advanced tumors, and the disabled. Medical institutions for chronic diseases shall be provided with much more medical resources such as rehabilitation and long-term nursing care services. We shall improve relevant policies and measures to gradually promote day surgery. We shall explore establishing the insurance system for long-term nursing care. We shall strengthen the construction of specialized rehabilitation institutions for the disabled and establish a working mechanism with close cooperation and interaction between medical institutions and specialized rehabilitation institutions for the disabled.

5) Guiding people's demands for medical service scientifically and rationally. We shall establish and improve the system of contract-based family doctor and encourage rural and urban residents to sign contracts with community doctors or family doctor teams by means of improving service capacity at the community level, payment by medical insurance, price adjustment and bringing convenience and benefit to the public etc. By 2017, the coverage rate of contract-based family doctors shall be over 30 percent, and the coverage rate of contract-based family doctors among the key groups shall be over 60 percent. By 2020, endeavors shall be made to expand the service of contract-based family doctors to all the groups of people so that the whole coverage of contract-based family doctor system shall be primarily achieved.

Efforts shall be made to follow the laws of medical science, clarify the scopes of medical services by the county-level and township-level medical institutions while combing the definition of their functions, and provide referral service to the patients with diseases beyond the functional positioning and service capacity. We shall improve procedures for two-way referral, establish and improve the guidance list for the referral, focusing on smoothing the channel for the downward referral and gradually achieve the orderly referral between medical institutions of different levels and different types. We shall improve differentiated medical insurance payment policies for medical institutions at different levels and appropriately increase the proportion of medical insurance payments for community medical institutions, and rationally guide people for medical service. The starting line shall be calculated continually for the patients who meet the requirement of referral. We shall reasonably formulate and adjust the price of medical service to form an effective incentive mechanism for medical institutions to implement functional positioning and patients to reasonably choose medical institutions.

(2) **Establishing scientific and effective management system for modern hospitals.** We shall further the comprehensive reform for county-level public hospitals and speed up and propel the comprehensive reform public hospitals in

cities. By 2017, we shall have launched comprehensive reform for all kinds of public hospitals at all levels in all respects and preliminarily established a management system and governance mechanism for decision-making, implementing, supervising mutual coordination, mutual balance and mutual promotion. By 2020, we shall have preliminarily established a management system for modern hospitals with Chinese characteristics which has clear definition of responsibility and right, scientific management, perfect governance, efficient operation and forceful supervision, and established a scientific and rational compensation mechanism and a new operation mechanism which can maintain public benefits, mobilize the enthusiasm and safeguard sustainability.

1) Improving the management system for public hospitals. We shall properly deal with the relationship between hospitals and the government, separate the functions of government from those of institutions, the functions of supervision institutions from those of enforcement institutions, and push forward the transformation of management pattern and operation mode of hospitals. We shall enhance the macro management of the government in orientation, policies, guidance, planning and evaluation etc., intensify supervision of medical behaviors, medical expenditures etc. and dwindle the management in hospitals' personnel establishment, department setting, position appointment and income distribution etc. We shall gradually eliminate the administrative ranking of hospitals. We shall rationally define the supervision responsibility of the government as a contributor and the independent operation and management authority of public hospitals. We shall improve the government-run medical system and actively explore various effective ways to separate the functions of supervision institutions from those of enforcement institutions. We shall take effective measures to coordinate the functions of the government in running hospitals to build up synergy. We shall strengthen industry-wide supervision on public hospitals run by governments, the armed forces, enterprises, institutions and other entities, and clarify the responsibilities, rights and obligations of all parties. We shall implement the independent legal status of public hospitals. We shall improve the corporate governance mechanism of public hospitals, and give them the autonomy to manage internal personnel, set up institutions, distribute income, recommend vice positions, appoint and remove middle-level cadres, and implement annual budgets etc. We shall implement the system of accountability for the president, improve the system for selecting and appointing the president, and implement the system of tenure and the tenure goal responsibility system for the president. Public hospitals shall formulate regulations by law. We shall establish and improve the comprehensive budget management system, cost accounting system, financial reporting system, general accountant system, third-party

auditing system and information disclosure system for public hospitals.

2) Establishing standard and efficient operating mechanism. We shall cancel markups of drug prices (excluding herbal pieces of traditional Chinese medicines), set up a scientific and rational compensation mechanism by adjusting prices for medical services, increasing investment of the government, reforming ways of payment and cutting the operation costs of hospitals etc. We shall gradually establish a dynamic adjustment mechanism for medical service prices on the basis of structure change of cost and income and, in accordance with the principle of "total amount control, structural adjustment, coexistence of increase and decrease and gradually in place," increase prices for items that reflect the value of the medical personnel's technical services such as diagnosis and treatment, operation, rehabilitation, nursing and traditional Chinese medicine services while decreasing the prices of drugs, medical consumables and checks & exams with large medical equipment. We shall strengthen guidance on classification and straighten out the price relations between medical institutions at different levels and different medical services. We shall reduce expenditures on drugs and consumables by regulating diagnosis and treatment behaviors and cost-control of medical insurance and strictly control the unreasonable exam fees to make room for adjusting medical service prices and engage with other measures such as medical cost containment, salary system, payment by medical insurance and tiered diagnosis and treatment etc. We shall authorize the medical institutions to price special medical services and other medical services which are faced with sufficient market competition and strong personalized demands. We shall continue to promote the socialization of logistics services in public hospitals. In the comprehensive reform of public hospitals, we shall establish a new operational mechanism to facilitate the development of the advantages of traditional Chinese medicine while taking into account the characteristics of traditional Chinese medicine comprehensively. We shall encourage military hospitals to participate in the comprehensive reform of local public hospitals. We shall regulate the restructuring of public hospitals, and promote the transfer & separation and restructuring of the pilot of hospitals affiliated to state-owned enterprises. In principle, special hospitals run by the government shall not be restructured, including the infectious hospitals, mental hospitals, occupational disease prevention and control hospitals, maternal and child health care and maternity hospitals, children's hospitals, and hospitals of traditional Chinese medicine (minority ethnic hospitals). We shall strive to reduce the proportion of drug income (excluding herbal pieces of traditional Chinese medicines) in public hospitals to around 30 percent and the income of general healthcare materials to less than 20 *yuan* per hundred medical income (excluding drug income) in pilot cities by 2017.

3) Establishing the system of personnel posts and salary system in line with the characteristics of medical and health sector. We shall innovate the management mode of personnel posts in public hospitals, improve the management methods of personnel posts, and proactively explore the pilot of management reform of personnel posts in public hospitals. We shall determine the total number of personnel posts for public hospitals within the total of present personnel posts for the locality, gradually implement the filing system, and carry out the reform of personnel post management and pilot on the total number management of personnel in the Class A tertiary public hospitals in some large and medium-sized cities. We shall confer public hospitals autonomy in choosing and employing stuff members, and hospitals shall be entitled to openly recruit, by means of inspection, high-level talents in urgent need, professionals in shortage of as well as personnel with senior title of technical posts or doctorates. We shall improve the employment relations between medical institutions and medical personnel.

The localities can, in line with the government's relevant regulations and in combination with the practical situations, reasonably determine the salary level for public hospitals, gradually increase the proportion of personnel expenditure in business expenditure, and establish a dynamic adjustment mechanism. While determining the total amount of performance salary, we shall favor those public medical institutions which make more overwork contribution, employ more high-level medical talents, take up arduous non-profits tasks and offer contract-based family doctor services. While distributing performance salary, we shall especially favor those clinical doctors, core members, those working at key posts, as well as those assisting the community-level institutions and those with prominent contribution so as to achieve the goal of more pay for more work and better pay for better work. In line with relevant regulations, public hospitals may explore target annual salary system and negotiated salary. The government department in charge of public hospitals shall conduct inspection and evaluation for the presidents' annual work before determining the presidents' salary to ensure the reasonable proportion between the presidents' salary and the performance salary of the medical staff.

4) Establishing a quality-centered, public-welfare-oriented evaluation mechanism for hospitals. We shall establish a sound evaluation system for hospitals, ensure that agency inspection shall cover the social efficiency, service, quality, comprehensive management and sustainable development etc., and attach importance to public welfare work such as emergency response, counterpart assistance, the implementation of functional positioning and the practicing of tiered diagnosis and treatment etc. We shall integrate the fulfillment of medical reform into the indicators of evaluation for hospitals to enhance the main responsibility of the hospitals and the presidents. The

evaluation for medical stuff shall focus on job workload, service quality, behavioral norms, technical impediments, level of risks and the satisfaction of the service objects etc., and for the persons in charge, the evaluation shall also include the satisfaction of the stuff. The results of the evaluation shall be related to the investment of the government, the payment of the medical insurance and the career development of the personnel.

5) Keeping the unreasonable increase of medical expenses in public hospitals under control. We shall gradually improve the monitoring and evaluating mechanism for controlling medical expenses in public hospitals. We shall set the national targets for controlling medical expenses, and all the provinces (autonomous regions, municipalities directly under the Central Government) shall determine the control requirements and make dynamic adjustments according to the level and growth range of medical expenses in different regions and the functional positioning of different types of hospitals. The prefecture-level cities shall release to the public information about hospitals within their respective jurisdictions such as prices, medical service efficiency and the average medical cost for each treatment etc., and the cost index of the medical institutions shall be ranked, whose results shall be made public at regular intervals. We shall implement the system of prescription review. Health and family planning departments shall trace and monitor public hospitals on drugs, high-valued medical consumables and the inspection of large medical equipment. By 2017, we shall try to keep the growth range of medical expenses in public hospitals under 10 percent nationwide; and by 2020, the growth range shall be stabilized at the rational level.

**(3) Establishing a highly effective universal health insurance system.** In accordance with the principles of ensuring basic medical service, ensuring there is a cushion in place for those most in need, and being sustainable, we shall intensify reform and establish a highly effective medical insurance system for all centering on the three key links of diversification of capital sources, standardization of security system and socialization of management and service. We shall maintain a balanced actuarial system, improve financing mechanism, and improve the quality and efficiency of universal basic health insurance system by reforming the payment modes of medical insurance. We shall establish a comparatively complete interaction and link between basic health insurance schemes, insurance for major illnesses, commercial health insurance and medical financial assistance.

1) Improving sustainable financing and benefit adjustment mechanisms of basic health insurance schemes. We shall improve the premium collection mechanism, clarify the premium collection responsibilities of the government, employers and individuals, and gradually establish a stable and sustainable multi-level financing

mechanism which corresponds to the economic and social development and the affordability of all parties. While improving the fiscal input and raising the subsidy standards by the government, we shall enhance individuals' insurance awareness and appropriately increase the proportion of individual contributions. We shall gradually establish a dynamic financing mechanism that links the payment standard of individual contributions to urban and rural residents' medical insurance with the income of residents, so that the fund-raising standard, the level of security, and the level of economic and social development are in line with each other. By 2020, the participation rate of basic medical insurance shall be stabilized at over 95%.

We shall improve the mechanism for dynamic adjustment of basic medical insurance benefits which commensurate with the level of financing. The basis and decision-making procedure of policy authority adjustment for the determination and adjustment of medical insurance benefits shall be clarified to avoid the randomness of benefit adjustment. The security boundary of basic medical insurance shall be defined, the standards for the benefits of basic medical insurance determined reasonably, and global payment control pushed forward in all respects in combination with the management of medical insurance budget. Personal accounts shall be improved and outpatient expenses shall be pooled. The improvement of fund pooling level shall be sped up in accordance with the basic ideas of tiered management, shared responsibility, adjustment of the pooling of fund and budget assessment. The pooling of fund at the municipal level shall be consolidated in all aspects and that at the provincial level shall be promoted in provinces with suitable conditions. Policies on medical billing and making-claims at localities other than home counties, cities or provinces shall be quickly implemented, nationwide network of basic medical insurance and direct medical billing and making-claims at localities other than home counties, cities or provinces should be pushed forward, and the collaboration between places where premium is collected and where medical service is provided should be enhanced to facilitate the billing claims for the people by reducing the time and energy they spend and their pre-paid fund. Policies and measures for the referral in different places shall be established and improved to promote the direct billing claims of medical services in different places and guiding medical resources downwards to the community level, promote the construction of medical consortium, and establish a tiered diagnosis and treatment system. By 2017, the direct billing claims at localities other than hometowns shall have been achieved as long as they meet the referral requirements. By 2020, a regulating and balancing mechanism for medical insurance fund shall have been established, pooling of fund at provincial level gradually achieved and the reimbursement rate within the range of basic medical insurance policy stabilized at around 75 percent.

2) Deepening reform of payment methods by medical insurance. The payment mechanism by medical insurance and regulating mechanism of benefits shall be improved. Refined management shall be implemented to motivate the medical institutions to regulate their behaviors, control costs, reasonably receive and transfer patients. Multiple payment methods shall be carried out with case payment as the core, combining other methods such as capitation, per-diem payment, global budget etc. and diagnosis related groups(DRGs)shall be encouraged. Case payment, diagnosis related groups and per-diem payment shall be mainly applied to inpatient medical services; while capitation shall be applied to community medical services, and exploration shall be made to combine capitation with the chronic disease management of hypertension, diabetes and hemodialysis etc. and fee-for-service payment and capitation can be applied to complicated cases and outpatient services. Point method (scoring diseases payment) can be combined with budget management and diagnosis related groups (DRGs)where conditions permit to promote the orderly competition among medical institutions and the rational allocation of resources. Open and equal negotiating and counseling mechanism and risk sharing mechanism shall be improved between various medical insurance agencies and medical institutions. An incentive and constraint mechanism of keeping the surplus and rationally sharing the overspending shall be established. Management norms, technical support and supporting policies related to the payment reform shall be established and improved, industry technical standards such as clinical paths formulated which can meet the basic medical needs, the writing of medical history and the home page of medical record standardized, a solid foundation for information management laid, and the names and connotations of service items, disease classification codes, medical service operation codes of the medical institutions nationwide shall be unified. Policies to support traditional Chinese medicine (TCM) services shall be carried on, the scope of traditional Chinese medicine (TCM) preparations, acupuncture, therapeutic massage and other TCM non-drug treatments techniques shall be gradually expanded in medical institutions whose payments are covered by medical insurance, the payment methods in line with the characteristics of traditional Chinese medicine services shall be explored and the provision and use of appropriate TCM services shall be encouraged. By 2017, the government shall select some localities to carry out pilot on diagnosis related groups (DRGs) and encourage all the localities to proactively improve the multiple payment methods including case payment, capitation and per-diem payment etc. By 2020, the payment reform shall gradually cover all the medical institutions and medical services, multiple and compound payment methods by medical insurance shall be implemented nationwide which can apply to different diseases and reflect the features of different services, and the proportion of fee-for-

service shall drop dramatically.

3) Promoting the integration of basic medical insurances. On the basis of unifying covering ranges, financing policies, security benefits, insurance directories, designated management and fund management of basic medical insurance for urban and rural residents, the integration of management institutions for basic medical insurance shall be sped up. The management system shall be straightened out and the administrative functions of basic medical insurance shall be unified. The management of basic medical insurance agencies shall be unified, and pilot on establishing management centers for insurance fund can be launched to take up the functions of fund payment and management, drug purchase and account settlement, negotiation on payment standards of medical insurance and the agreement management and settlement of designated institutions. Reform and innovation shall be enhanced to let medical insurance play its role in controlling the unreasonable increase of medical expenses. The separation of management of medical insurance from that of enforcement shall be sped up to improve the legalization and specialization of medical insurance agencies. The modes of agency service shall be innovated to propel the pattern of diversified competition.

4) Improving the insurance policies for major and catastrophic illness. On the basis of comprehensively implementing insurances for major illness for urban and rural residents, measures shall be taken such as lowering the starting line, improving the proportion of reimbursement and rationally determining the scope of reasonable medical expenses etc. to target the major illness insurance at the needy more accurately. Supplementary medical insurance policies for the employees shall be improved. Medical assistance for major and catastrophic illness shall be provided comprehensively and, on the basis of providing medical assistance to the low-income people and the destitute, the aged, the underage, the severely disabled and patients of major illnesses in low-income families as well as patients in families impoverished by illness shall be covered by the assistance to let it play the role of basic security. Social charity forces and other parties shall be encouraged to participate. A data sharing mechanism between the medical and health institutions and medical insurance agencies shall be gradually established to promote the effective links between the basic medical insurance, insurance for major illness, medical assistance, emergency aid for illness and commercial health insurance and provide one-stop services in all aspects.

5) Promoting the development of commercial health insurance. Commercial insurance institutions shall give full play to their strengths in actuarial techniques, professional services and risk management etc. and they shall be encouraged and supported to join medical insurance agency service to form a new pattern of

diversified agency and multiple competition. On the ground of securing fund safety and effective supervision, the government shall, by means of purchasing service, entrust qualified commercial insurance institutions and other social institutions to join the agency service of basic medical insurance and undertake the insurance for major and catastrophic illness for urban and rural residents. In line with the relevant provisions on government procurement, commercial insurance institutions and other social institutions shall be selected to join medical insurance agencies. The development of medical liability insurance and medical accident insurance shall be sped up and multiple medical practice insurances shall be explored and developed. More health insurance products shall be provided, health insurance as consumption forcefully developed, the development of various health insurance promoted and the security nature of health insurance enhanced. Insurance companies shall be encouraged to develop various commercial health insurance products, such as TCM health care and health care products, health management services with TCM characteristics provided. Preferential policies on fiscal and taxation shall be formulated and improved to support the accelerated development of commercial health insurance. Enterprises and residents are encouraged to meet health needs beyond basic medical insurance by participating in commercial health insurance.

(4) **Establishing standard and orderly drug supply security system.** Reform of the entire process of drug production, distribution and use shall be launched, benefit driven mechanism adjusted, the practices of hospitals funding their operations with profits from overpriced drugs put an end to, medical institutions at all levels encouraged to fully equip themselves with and give priority to the use of essential drugs, a national drug policy system in line with China's national conditions built, drug prices rationalized, restructuring, transformation and upgrading of the pharmaceutical industry promoted and the safety and effectiveness, rational prices and sufficient supply of drugs secured.

1) Deepening reform of drug supply. By means of market reversed transmission and industrial policy guidance, enterprises shall be promoted to improve their capability of innovating and developing to be better and stronger, increase the concentration of industry, push forward the modernization and standardization of Chinese materia medica production, in order that the quality of drug and medical devices reach or get close to advanced world levels and create Chinese standards and Chinese brands. A more scientific and efficient system for drug review and approval shall be established. Quality consistency evaluations and curative effects of generic drugs shall be accelerated, the creation of new drugs encouraged, and innovation of drugs oriented toward clinical value encouraged. Review, evaluation and approval of innovative drugs shall be sped up for AIDS, malignant cancers, serious infectious

diseases, rare diseases as well as pediatric drugs. Drugs with uncertain curative effects or more risks than benefits shall be eliminated. Innovation on medical devices shall be enhanced and the approval of medical devices tightened. The system of drugs marketing authorization holders shall be established. The development and production of drugs for serious infectious diseases and pediatric drugs shall be accelerated. The consistency evaluation of oral solid dosage forms of chemical generic drugs approved for marketing before October 1st, 2007, in the *National Essential Drug List (2012 Version)* shall be finished by the end of 2018. The supply of low-priced drugs, life-saving drugs, orphan drugs and pediatric drugs shall be resolved. The production of low-priced drugs shall be supported to ensure the supply and stabilize the prices. The monitoring and early warning mechanism and tiered responding mechanism for the drugs in short supply shall be established and improved, the production of drugs in short supply promoted, the construction of centralized production base for minor varieties of drugs supported and pilot on the designated production of drugs with small demands yet in imperative need clinically and in short supply in market carried on. The security mechanism for pediatric drugs and health emergency drugs shall be improved. Market monitoring shall be enhanced on drugs with short supply of bulk pharmaceutical chemicals in market and the improvement of their production capacity encouraged.

2) Deepening reform of drug distribution system. The structural adjustment of drug and consumable distribution industries shall be enhanced to guide the balanced allocation of supply capacity, the construction of a drug distribution market pattern accelerated which is unified, open, orderly competitive nationwide to eliminate regional protectionism and establish a new system of modern distribution. The merger and restructuring of drug distributing enterprises shall be pushed forward, the storage resources and transporting resources of drug operating enterprises integrated, the development of modern logistics for drugs accelerated and the urban-rural integration of regional drug distribution encouraged. The transformation from distribution enterprises to smart medical and pharmaceutical service providers shall be promoted, the integrated system of supply chain built and improved and distribution enterprises shall be supported to provide extended service to the upstream and downstream of the supply chain. Big data on distribution shall be made use of to expand the depth and breadth of value-added services and guide the development of the industry. The development of green medical and pharmaceutical logistics shall be encouraged and the third party logistics and cold-chain logistics developed. Drug retailers and consumable retailers shall be supported to practice diversified and differentiating operation. The management and technology of modern logistics shall be applied, the development of on-line medical and pharmaceutical shops regulated, the modern

distribution network and tracing system for Chinese medicinal materials improved, industry structure adjustment promoted and the transparency and efficiency of the industry improved. Efforts shall be made so that by 2020, the traceability mechanism of ex-factory price information of drugs shall have been primarily established, one super drug distribution enterprise will have come into being with over 500 billion *yuan* annual turnover, and the annual turnover of the top one hundred drug wholesale enterprises will account for over 90 percent that of the wholesale market.

3) Improving the centralized procurement system of drugs and high-valued medical consumables. The online centralized procurement system of drugs shall be improved with province (region, city) as unit, category-based procurement of drugs launched for public hospitals, the principle of centralized volume procurement adhered to; pilot cities for the reform of public hospitals can purchase respectively on the provincial centralized procurement platform of drugs by taking the city as the unit and joint procurement across regions and among specialized hospitals shall be encouraged. The links between drug procurement in community hospitals and public hospitals shall be ensured. The integration of trade platforms for public resources shall be promoted. In principle, no more than three dosage forms should be purchased for each drug, and the corresponding specifications of each dosage form should not exceed two in principle. The reform of "two invoice policy" for drug procurement shall be launched (the first invoice refers to the invoice from the manufacturer to the distributor, and the second invoice refers to the invoice from the distributor to the medical service providers.), direct settlements are encouraged for drug billings between hospitals and drug manufacturers and distribution billings between drug manufacturers and distributing enterprises so that payments can be collected strictly by contracts. Hospitals shall further participate in the procurement of drugs, the dominant role of medical institutions must be carried out in drug and consumable procurement, and medical institutions shall be promoted to take initiative actions to control the prices of drugs and consumables. The negotiation mechanism for drug prices shall be improved and drug negotiation system at the national and provincial levels shall be established, which is unified, integrated and coordinated. Open, transparent price negotiation participated by multiple parties shall be launched for some patented drugs and exclusively produced drugs, the number of drug varieties shall be gradually increased for national negotiation and the links with medical insurance policies shall be improved. The acceleration of drug registration approval procedures, patent application and pharmacoeconomic evaluation will be the important content of drug negotiation. For the key drugs to be purchased on record, the amount of drugs to be purchased and the doctors who prescribe shall be clarified, and the persons in charge of the medical institutions shall

file the records with the drug purchasing departments after granting the approvals. The standardized construction of national comprehensive management information platform for drug supply security and provincial centralized procurement platform of drugs shall be strengthened, the service of drug centralized procurement platform and its supervising capacity improved and the collecting and sharing mechanism of procurement information completed.

Centralized procurement of high-valued medical consumables, examining and testing reagents, and large medical equipment shall be carried out. The centralized procurement of high-valued medical consumables shall be standardized and promoted, code standards of high-valued medical consumables unified, and tenders and procurement, negotiated procurement and direct online procurement of high-value medical consumables will be carried out according to different situations, so as to ensure that all links of high-valued medical consumables procurement will operate in the sunshine.

4) Consolidating and improving the essential drug system. The fruits of implementing the essential drug system at the government-run community-level medical institutions and village clinics shall be consolidated, and the unified policies shall be promoted in essential drugs' catalogs, logos, prices, distribution and the equipping and uses etc. The access to essential drugs for some special groups shall be ensured including children, the aged, patients of chronic diseases, patients of tuberculosis, patients of severe psychonosema and the severely disabled. Exploration shall be made to adopt evidence-based medicine and pharmacoeconomic evaluation methods while selecting and adjusting essential drugs. Equal importance shall be attached to both Chinese and western medicine in essential drug category. The system of prior and rational use of essential drugs shall be improved and the dominating role of essential drugs shall be adhered to. The supply system for essential drugs shall be meliorated.

5) Improving national drug policies. The management system shall be improved and the coordinating mechanism for national drug policies shall be established. Separating drug sales from medical services shall be promoted and comprehensive measures shall be taken to cut the chain of interest between hospitals & medical staff and drugs & consumables. Medical institutions shall prescribe medicines in accordance with the generic name of the drugs, and voluntarily offer the prescription to patients without restricting the outflow of prescriptions. The multi-channel drug purchase models for outpatients in hospitals shall be explored so that patients can purchase drugs from retail pharmacies by prescription. Competition and merger and reorganization among enterprises shall be promoted to make the market highly centralized and achieve large-scale, intensive and modernized operation.

Market pattern shall be adjusted so that retail pharmacies will gradually become the important channel of providing drugs and pharmaceutical services to patients.

Drug pricing mechanism shall be further improved. Linkage of pricing, health insurance, and purchasing policies shall be strengthened. Category-based management of drugs will be adhered to. Different models for price management shall be adopted. A system of drug price management shall be gradually established which is in line with the characteristics of Chinese pharmaceutical market. Standards for drug payments by health insurance schemes shall be established and improved, and, in combination with the quality consistency evaluation and the curative effects of generic drugs, standards for drug payments shall be gradually formulated in accordance with the general names. The national medical and drug storage system shall be improved and, on the basis of emergency security, storage for drugs commonly in short supply shall be improved. Policies of traditional Chinese medicine shall be improved, the management of the quality of traditional Chinese medicinal materials strengthened and the clinical use of herbal pieces of traditional Chinese medicine and ethnic medicine encouraged. Exploration on establishing general pharmacist system in hospitals shall be made, and pharmacist management system for medical institutions and retail pharmacies improved so that, in combination with the reform of medical service prices, the value of pharmaceutical services shall be embodied. Comprehensive clinical evaluation system of drugs and comprehensive clinical evaluation mechanism of children's drugs shall be established to improve rational drug use.

**(5) Establishing strict and standardized comprehensive supervision system.** The legal system for medical and health care sector shall be improved, the transformation of government functions accelerated, supervision models improved which is in line with the development of medical and health undertakings, the efficiency and level of comprehensive supervision improved, the legislation and standardization of supervision promoted and the long-term mechanism of comprehensive supervision established and improved which features clarified responsibility, division of labor and collaboration, standardized operation and scientific effectiveness.

1) Deepening reform to delegate power, streamline administration and optimize government services in the medical and health care sector. The reform of administrative examination and approval system for medical and health care sector shall be promoted in accordance with the requirements of decentralization and reduction of administrative interference, power delegation and regulation, and optimization of public services. As for the administrative examination and approval items that must be retained, a system of detailed list shall be established and announced to the public. Supervision concepts shall be transformed, and

supervision mechanism and supervision models innovated. More attention will be paid to strengthening in- and post-supervision to improve the efficacy of supervision. Government services shall be optimized to improve the level of services. The medical institutions shall be propelled to transform their service modes and improve the service quality.

2) Establishing diversified supervision system. A diversified and comprehensive supervision system shall be improved that is led by the government, widely participated by third parties, self-managed by medical institutions and supplemented by social supervision. Cross-department cooperation shall be strengthened to intensify supervision and effectively prevent and reduce violation of laws and regulations that harm people's health rights and interests. The third party shall be guided to participate in supervision by laws and rules. Self-management system of medical institutions shall be established to strengthen connotation management. Whole-process monitoring and intelligent examination shall be conducted by using information technology on the outpatient and inpatient diagnosis and treatment as well as expenditure in all the medical institutions. The application of intelligent examination technology for medical insurance shall be strengthened to propel all the localities with basic medical insurance to use intelligent monitoring system so that comprehensive, timely and efficient monitoring shall be conducted on outpatient services, inpatient services, drug purchases and other medical services. A national public service platform for drug information shall be improved to disclose information about prices and quality etc. A co-governance mechanism by the whole society shall be established and improved, information disclosure and publicity & education shall be strengthened, and channels shall be broadened for the public to participate in supervision so that the medical institutions will initiatively accept supervision from the public.

3) Strengthening comprehensive supervision on the whole sector. Medical and health laws, regulations and standards shall be improved and efforts shall be made to shift the focus of supervision to that of the whole sector. The promulgation of basic laws shall be sped up, TCM laws shall be established and improved and relevant standards and norms shall be improved. Localized supervision shall be practiced, the standardization construction and capacity construction for community-level supervisory institutions shall be strengthened and a security mechanism for comprehensive supervision shall be established and improved. Pilot on comprehensive supervision shall be launched. The "randomized sampling of subjects and inspectors by industrial and commercial agencies" shall be implemented, violation of laws and regulations investigated and handled by law, and the results of sampling and investigation & handling will be disclosed to the public in time. A blacklist system for violation of laws and regulations shall be established, the

institutions and individuals in the blacklist shall be handled severely by laws and regulations and serious violations shall be exposed. The system of performance evaluation for medical institutions shall be improved to evaluate medical institutions' basic standards, service quality, technique level and management level etc. to ensure that all the functions and tasks of the medical institutions shall meet the requirements for medical institutions' establishment planning. The management of clinical path shall be strengthened to improve the technical specifications and make diagnosis and treatment more transparent. Supervision and management shall be strengthened on the property ownership, finance operation and capital surplus of the non-profit private medical institutions, control on the profitability of profit private medical institutions enhanced, and supervision strengthened on medical and health care programs and medical advertisements to promote the sound development of non-government run medical institutions. By 2020, 100 percent of various medical institutions at all levels shall be supervised and inspected.

Improving supervising system for the funds of basic medical insurance and punishment on insurance frauds and other violations of laws concerning medical insurance shall be more severe. The monitoring mechanism of medical insurance on medical services shall be improved and the objects of monitoring shall be extended from the medical institutions to medical staff. Supervision on drug quality shall be strengthened and the circulation order of drug market shall be further regulated. The whole process supervision shall be strengthened on drug registration application, review & approval and production & sales, the tracing system for drug information shall be improved to form a complete tracing and supervising chain covering all the varieties and all the procedures. The management of drug validity date and packing material shall be strengthened and the disposal of expired drugs and other discarded drugs as well as the packing materials shall be regulated. The purchase and sale channels shall be strictly controlled, the management of invoices tightened, intermediate links in circulation reduced, and circulation environment purified. Cross-department cooperation shall be strengthened to severely crack down on violations of laws such as data fraud in the drug registration application, producing and selling counterfeit and inferior drugs, affiliating operation of business, supplying drugs with others' certificates, commercial bribery and illegal operation etc. Supervision on drug prices shall be strengthened and the surveillance and early warning system for drug price information as well as information release system shall be established and completed to proactively guide the industry organizations and market entities to strengthen the development of credit system and consciously maintain the market price order. Price supervision shall be strengthened on drugs and high-valued medical consumables with insufficient market competition. Special investigations shall be carried out in due course for those with frequent and large price changes and violations of laws such as price monopoly, fraud and collusion shall be investigated and punished according to laws.

Guiding and regulating assessment by the third party and self-discipline of the industry. Relevant policies shall be improved to encourage the qualified third party to initiatively carry out or participate in the consultation of the assessment standards, technical support and examination and assessment and promote the transformation of the examination and assessment of medical institutions from the assessment dominated by government to the assessment by the independent third party. Industry associations, colleges and universities and scientific research institutes shall play active roles to cultivate third-party assessment organizations. Self-discipline of the industry shall be strengthened by encouraging industry organizations to establish and improve industry management norms and standards and regulating behaviors of the members. Efforts shall be made to guide and standardize the establishment of an internal audit system for medical institutions, strengthen self-management and self-examination and correction to improve the quality of medical services and ensure medical safety. Management of the supervision information shall be strengthened for the national health care industry to provide effective monitoring basis for the medical institutions to operate and improve quality of services, efficiency of services and degree of satisfaction.

### (6) Promoting reform in relevant areas comprehensively

Improving personnel training & using mechanism as well as incentive assessment mechanism. Efforts shall be made to mobilize the enthusiasm, initiative and creativity of medical staff by improving their remuneration package, development space, practice environment and social status to let them play the main role in medical reform. The training and cultivating system for medical staff shall be improved so that every medical worker has the opportunity for continuous education and vocational retraining. The mechanism for personnel training shall be innovated to build a standardized and normalized training system for medical personnel which integrates college education, post-graduate education and continuous education. The quality assurance mechanism for medical education shall be improved. By 2020, the first round of the certification of undergraduates of clinical medicine major shall be completed with the establishment of health professionals licensing systems equivalent to internationally-recognized health education programs. Reform of medical education shall be deepened, training program for excellent doctors pushed forward and training for medical professionals strengthened. Tuition-waiver education toward order-oriented medical students from rural areas shall be carried on. Policies for post graduation education shall be improved so that by 2020, all the new clinicians with bachelor's degree or above shall receive standardized residency training, and the system for the standardized training for specialists preliminary established, focusing on training specialist doctors for county-level medical institutions and prefectural and municipal hospitals in remote areas. Training of pharmaceutical personnel shall be promoted at the community level. The construction of general physician system shall be promoted forcefully, primary healthcare taskforces shall be built with a focus on general practitioners, and training for general practitioners shall be strengthened by means of standardized training, training for assistant general practitioners and transfer training etc. By 2020, a dynamic system of general practitioners shall be preliminarily established, and a unified and standardized training mode for general practitioners shall be basically established to ensure that two to three qualified general practitioners should be available for every 10,000 urban and rural residents in China by 2020, and the total number of general practitioners will be over 300,000. Projects to promote traditional Chinese medicine and innovative talents shall be launched to promote the preservation and development of traditional Chinese medicine and establish and improve the master-apprentice tutorials of TCM education.

The mechanism for using health talents shall be innovated, the management system for position setting improved, an open recruitment system implemented as well as a contract-based employment system to achieve the classified management of personnel. The practicing environment and remuneration package shall be improved to encourage the medical resources to flow to the mid and western regions and the community-level and rural areas. On the basis of summary and assessment, the special post program for general practitioners shall be carried on. Medical and health institutions shall be allowed to break the current level of wage control in public institutions, the remnant of medical service income shall be allowed to reward the staff after deduction of cost and withdrawals in accordance with regulations, and the specific measures for linking the connotation of medical service income and the performance-based salary shall be formulated separately. The remuneration of the personnel outside the staffing plan shall be determined rationally to gradually achieve the equal remuneration for the same post to mobilize the medical staff. It shall be strictly prohibited to set profit targets for medical personnel and the remuneration of the medical staff shall never be linked to the income from drugs, consumables, inspection, laboratory tests etc. The internal distribution of performance-based salary in community medical and health institutions shall adopt such methods as establishing general practitioner's allowance, which will favor the clinical personnel undertaking the contract-based services. Policies shall be implemented to subsidize staff in poverty-stricken and remote areas or in townships, and the distribution of performance-based salary shall favor the personnel at the community level. Talent assessment mechanism shall be innovated, a scientific and socialized assessment mechanism characteristic of the health talents shall be reformed and improved which is based on the requirements of post responsibility and oriented by morality, capacity and achievements. The system and methods for the promotion of professional titles shall be improved to increase the proportion of senior posts in medical and health institutions and favor the personnel at the community level and broaden the space of the career development for the medical staff. More importance shall be attached to building the taskforce of village doctors, increasing their remuneration reasonably and establishing the expelling mechanism of country doctors in combination with the practical situations. Multi-site practice of doctors shall be encouraged in medical institutions at the community levels, in remote areas, in areas with scarce medical resources or other medical institutions with the demands.

The honor system shall be established to promote medical staff's spirit of "tenacious, dedicated, saving lives with boundless love", the propaganda on the election of "People's Good Doctor" shall be carried out so that the sense of professional honor for medical personnel shall be enhanced by multiple means. Illegal and criminal acts involving medical staff shall be severely cracked down on by law, especially violent crimes against medical staff, emergent cases involving medical staff shall be investigated and handled severely to safeguard the normal medical order and the safety of the medical staff. The mediating mechanism for medical disputes shall be improved, and an institutional system combining in-hospital mediation, people's mediation, judicial conciliation and the medical risk sharing mechanism shall be completed to establish harmonious doctor-patient relations. By 2020, medical liability insurance shall cover all the public hospitals nationwide and over 80 percent of medical institutions at the community level.

Speeding up the formation of pluralistic structure of medical care services. Mass entrepreneurship and innovation shall be carried on in the field of health care service. Private health services shall be encouraged, the scale of supporting industry related to health care service shall be expanded and the environment for the development of health care service shall be optimized. Classified management system for non-profit and profit medical institutions shall be completed. Policies shall be further optimized to urge all the localities to implement equal policies and measures for all the medical institutions in such aspects as market access, designation of social insurance, construction of key specialties, conferring of professional titles, academic status, hospital accreditation etc. Policies for multi-site practice of doctors shall be improved and the system of registration for licensed doctors reformed. The mode of planning and controlling medical resources shall be improved to speed up the development of non-government run medical institutions. Public hospitals shall be allowed, in line with planning and demands, to cooperate with social forces in running new non-profit medical institutions, and cooperation between non-government run medical institutions and public hospitals shall be strengthened to share talents, technology and brands. The scale of special services in public hospitals shall be controlled to keep the proportion of special services under 10 percent of all the services provided. The comprehensive assessment mechanism shall be explored for the non-profit hospitals run by social forces to encourage the social forces to invest in the service sectors that can satisfy people's diverse demands. Financial institutions shall be encouraged and guided to increase investment in healthy industry, pledge of intangible assets and hypothecate of usufruct explored and the credit of health consumption developed. Eligible enterprises shall be supported to raise funds directly, issue bonds and carry out mergers and acquisitions in the capital market to encourage venture capital investment. We shall give full play to the long-term investment advantage of commercial health insurance funds to guide commercial insurance companies to run medical institutions, nursing homes, physical checkup institutions and other health service institutions in the form of investment. Nursing care shall be integrated with medical and health care sector to develop health & nursing care industry. Medical institutions at the community level shall be supported to provide contract-based medical service for families of the aged, the cooperation mechanism between medical institutions and nursing homes established and improved, nursing homes encouraged to provide rehabilitation, elderly care and hospice palliative care, and the private sector shall also be encouraged to open facilities providing both medical and nursing care. The integration of medical care and tourism shall be promoted and policies on access, operation, assessment, supervision and other relevant supporting policies improved to speed up the development of health tourism. The integration of Internet and health shall be promoted to develop the intelligent heath industry. Internet-based health service shall be developed proactively, and in-depth integration of cloud computing, big data, mobile Internet, Internet of things and other information technologies and health services promoted to implant the "core of intelligence" in the health industry. The TCM market will be expanded and the integrated development of TCM and nursing care, tourism etc. promoted to achieve the creative transformation and innovative development of TCM-based health care. By 2017, over 80 percent of the medical institutions shall provide green channels for registration, medical treatment and other convenient services for the elderly, and over 50 percent of the nursing homes shall provide medical and healthcare services for the elderly living in the nursing homes. By 2020, room for no less than 1.5 beds shall be reserved for per 1,000 permanent residents in non-government run hospitals, and meanwhile room shall be reserved for the setting of diagnosis subjects and for the installment of large medical equipment; system & mechanism and policy & regulation for integrated care for the elderly shall be basically established which are suitable to our national conditions; all the medical institutions shall provide green channels for registration, medical treatment and other convenient services for the elderly and all the nursing homes shall provide various medical and healthcare services for the elderly living in the nursing homes.

Promoting the construction of public healthcare system. Professional public healthcare institutions shall collaborate and coordinate with medical institutions and medical institutions at the community level and a mechanism shall be improved for selecting the essential public healthcare service package and major public health service package. By 2020, the system for equity of primary public healthcare services shall be basically completed. Government procurement of public healthcare services shall be promoted. The distribution of public healthcare service package funds shall be improved as well as the mechanisms for the result assessment and incentive and restraint; public healthcare institutions and medical institutions shall play their roles in instructing and evaluating the implementation of the packages, and the results of evaluation and assessment shall be linked with the service funds granted. An incentive mechanism shall be established and improved for the professionals of public healthcare services, and the personnel and operating expenses shall be covered in full by the government budget in accordance with the size of personnel force, funds standards, the fulfillment of tasks and the results of evaluations. Public health institutions specializing in combining prevention with controlling shall be encouraged to obtain reasonable income by providing preventive healthcare and basic medical services and establish a new operation mechanism conducive to combining prevention with controlling. Reform and restructuring of maternal and child health institutions shall be promoted for the integration of healthcare and clinical service. On the basis of rationally determining tasks and the cost expenditure, efforts shall be made to improve the compensation mechanism for medical institutions that undertake the tasks of public healthcare services. The health management for the disabled shall be promoted forcefully and community-based rehabilitation for the disabled shall be strengthened. More TCM services with reasonable costs and definite effects shall be included in the essential public healthcare service package. Existing drug policies shall be improved to alleviate the burden of drug expenses on patients of AIDS, tuberculosis, severe psychonosema and other major diseases as well as emergent infectious diseases. The integration of residents' health cards and social security cards shall be promoted and the application of residents' digital health records shall be activated to promote the digital health service which integrates prevention, treatment, rehabilitation and health management. The health emergency platform system shall be upgraded and renovated to improve the capacity for early detecting public health emergencies. Patriotic public health campaigns shall be deepened.

### IV. Security measures

**(1) Intensifying organization and leadership.** All the localities shall attach great importance to medical and healthcare reform, and the leading group of the medical and healthcare reform shall be headed by the principal leaders of the Party Committees and the governments or primary persons in charge, who shall take charge of the medical and healthcare reform in person, so that the leading groups of the medical and healthcare reform shall bring into full play of their coordinating roles to promote the coordinated medical service, medical insurance, and pharmaceutical reforms. The Party shall take charge of the overall situation and coordinate all parties, give full play to the core leading role of the Party Committees (Party Groups) at all levels, and include the medical and healthcare reform into comprehensively deepening reform with the uniform deployment, uniform requirements and uniform assessment to ensure the fulfillment of planning tasks. In accordance with this planning, all the localities shall, while combining their practical situations, formulate specific implementation plans, make detailed policies and measures and organize implementation carefully. All the relevant departments shall make detailed supporting measures in time, enhance collaboration and cooperation and instruct and urge all the localities to implement the planning tasks.

**(2) Intensifying the implementation of responsibilities.** The responsibilities of the governments at all levels shall be implemented, including leading responsibilities, security responsibilities, management responsibilities and supervision responsibilities and rigid constraint mechanism for the implementation and evaluation of responsibilities shall be established. The government's investment in health sector shall be increased. By 2020, the government shall fully implement its investment policy for public hospitals in line with regional health plans, establish a new mechanism for public hospitals to be compensated by service charge and government's subsidy, implement the government's preferential policies on investment in traditional Chinese medicine hospitals (ethnic hospitals) and gradually repay and dissolve the long-term debts of eligible public hospitals. The construction of Party organizations shall be strengthened in various medical and health institutions at all levels, the overall functions of community-level Party organizations strengthened to let the community-level Party organizations play their powerful roles and Party members play their model roles in medical and healthcare reform to promote the implementation of reform.

**(3) Intensifying reform and exploration.** Initiatives at the community level shall be respected and promoted, power shall be delegated to encourage the local governments to forge ahead with determination and explore baldly according to the local conditions. As for some reform with many contradictions and problems & difficulties, initiative actions and willingness to solve problems are needed to work creatively. Pilot on comprehensive medical and healthcare reform shall be deepened with the provinces as units to promote reform through cross-region cooperation. A regular survey mechanism shall be established and improved to strengthen guidance for the localities, summarize and popularize experience on reform, and upgrade mature experience into policies in timely manners so that the superior governments shall respond promptly to what the local governments call for.

(4) **Intensifying scientific and technological support.** The construction of national innovative system for medical and healthcare science and technology shall be strengthened, major national science and technology projects and key research and development programs shall be carried on to improve the capacity of scientific and technological innovation. Relying on various key laboratories, national clinical medical research centers and collaborative research networks, we will vigorously promote the research and popularization of clinical guidelines and technical specifications. The transformation and application of scientific and technological achievements shall be sped up to provide more medical and healthcare technologies and products that can meet the health needs of the people.

(5) **Intensifying international cooperation.** China's global health strategy shall be formulated and implemented. In combination with the construction of the Belt and One Road Initiative, we will establish and improve international exchange and cooperation mechanisms shall be established and improved, bilateral and multilateral exchanges and cooperation strengthened to take an in-depth part in global health governance and share useful experience in reform and development. An international platform for public services shall be built, the development of trade in medical and health services vigorously promoted, the pace sped up for medical and healthcare institutions to go global, and the scale of medical and healthcare services for overseas personnel in China expanded. With the service trade of traditional Chinese medicine as the focus and the service trade standards as the lead, the global influence of traditional Chinese medicine will be enhanced.

(6) **Intensifying supervision and evaluation.** The supervision and evaluation system shall be established and improved to give full play to the role of third party evaluation, strengthen the application of results and encourage accountability. The real-time and accuracy of monitoring shall be enhanced and the results of the monitoring shall be applied to the whole process of policy formulation, implementation, inspection and rectification. The medical and healthcare reform office under the State Council

shall, in conjunction with relevant departments, supervise, inspect, evaluate and analyze the overall implementation of the programs, plan as a whole on the important problems in the process of program implementation, and major situations shall be reported to the State Council in timely manners. Advice and suggestions from the non-communist party members on deepening medical and healthcare reform shall be encouraged and democratic supervision shall be launched on the major reform tasks.

(7) **Intensifying publicity and guidance.** Public opinions shall be guided correctively, positive publicity and guidance of public opinions intensified to vigorously publicize the progress of the medical and healthcare reform and typical experience and advanced figures; policy interpretation shall be enhanced, the concerns of the society responded in time, the anticipation of the society guided rationally, public awareness and participation in reform improved and the enthusiasm and initiative of medical personnel in the reform encouraged to create a good atmosphere for the whole society to care, understand and support medical reform. Efforts shall be made to develop health culture, purify communication environment, strengthen the dissemination of health knowledge, guide the public to correctly understand the laws of medical development, establish a correct concept of life and medical treatment and improve the health literacy of the public. The ideological and political work shall be strengthened to further guide the establishment of good medical ethics and promote the professionalism of medical personnel. We shall give full play to the advantages of the united front to pool consensus to the maximum extent and push forward the reform to a deeper level.

**Appendix 1: Main Targets of Deepening Medical and Healthcare Reform by 2017**

| | Index Contents |
|---|---|
| 1 | Initiatively forming a more systematic policy framework for the basic medical and health care system. |
| 2 | More than 85 percent of prefectures and cities launching pilot on tiered diagnosis and treatment, gradually improving policy system. |
| 3 | The coverage rate of contract-based family doctor service reaching over 30%, the coverage rate of contract-based service reaching over 60 % . |
| 4 | Various public hospitals at all levels launching comprehensive reform and initially establishing a management system and governance mechanism for decision-making, implementation, supervision, coordination and mutual checks and balances. |
| 5 | The proportion of drugs income (excluding Chinese herbal pieces) in public hospitals in pilot cities dropping to about 30%, income from health materials consumed in one hundred *yuan* of medical income dropped to 20 *yuan* and below. |
| 6 | Gradually establishing and improving the mechanism for monitoring and assessing medical expenses in public hospitals, and the increase in medical costs in public hospitals nationwide expected to be below 10%. |
| 7 | The costs of hospitalization which is eligible for referral can be settled where incurred. |
| 8 | The government selecting some regions to launch pilot on DRG-based hospital payment, encouraging all the localities to initiatively improve bundle payment, capitation, per-diem payment and other payment. |

Appendix 2: Main Targets of Deepening Medical and Healthcare Reform by 2020

| | Index Contents |
|---|---|
| 1 | Average life expectancy of the residents increasing by one year over 2015, maternal mortality dropping to 18 per 100,000, infant mortality to 7.5 ‰ and Under-five mortality to 9.5 ‰. |
| 2 | The out-of-pocket payment as a share of total health expenditures dropping to about 28%. |
| 3 | The mode of tiered diagnosis and treatment gradually taking shape, basically establishing a system of tiered diagnosis and treatment that can meet China's national conditions. |
| 4 | Trying to equip all community health service institutions, township health centers and 70 percent of village health centers with the ability to provide traditional Chinese medicine services and corresponding medical rehabilitation capabilities. |
| 5 | Trying to expand contract-based service to all the residents, basically covering all the residents with contract-based family doctor service. |
| 6 | Basically establishing a modern hospital management system with Chinese characteristics which has clear rights and responsibilities, scientific management, perfect governance, efficient operation and strong supervision; establishing a new mechanisms to safeguard public welfare, mobilize the initiative, and ensure sustainable operation, as well as a scientific and reasonable compensation mechanism. |
| 7 | Stabilizing the rise of medical costs in public hospitals at a rational level. |
| 8 | Stabilizing the participation rate of basic medical insurance at over 95%. |
| 9 | Establishing a mechanism for adjusting and balancing medical insurance funds, gradually achieving provincial pooling of medical insurance, stabilizing the reimbursement rate within the scope of the basic medical insurance policy at about 75%. |
| 10 | Reform on medical payment gradually covering all the medical institutions and medical services, adopting diversified compound medical insurance payments nationwide suitable for different diseases and different features of services, the proportion of fee-for-service payment remarkably declining. |
| 11 | Preliminarily establishing the traceability mechanism of ex-factory price information of drugs. |
| 12 | Cultivating a super drug distribution enterprise with annual sales of more than 500 billion yuan, the annual sales of top 100 pharmaceutical wholesalers accounting for more than 90% of the total wholesale market |
| 13 | 100% supervision and inspection on various medical and health institutions at all levels |
| 14 | Completing the first round of the certification of undergraduates of clinical medicine major, establishing health professionals' licensing systems with Chinese characteristics equivalent to internationally-recognized health education programs |
| 15 | All the new clinicians with bachelor's degree or above receiving standardized residency training, and preliminary establishing the system for the standardized training for specialists |
| 16 | Two to three qualified general practitioners available for every 10,000 urban and rural residents, a total of over 300,000 general practitioners. |
| 17 | Medical liability insurance covering all the public hospitals and over 80% of medical institutions at the community level nationwide. |
| 18 | Preliminarily improving the mechanism for the gradual equity of primary public healthcare service. |
| 19 | Fully implementing the government's investment policy for public hospitals in line with regional health programs, establishing a new mechanism for public hospitals to be compensated by service charge and government's subsidy, implementing the government's preferential policy on investment in traditional Chinese medicine hospitals (ethnic hospitals) and gradually repaying and dissolving the long-term debts of eligible public hospitals. |

**(Zhao Xuemei )**

## 17. *Opinions of the General Office of the State Council on Conducting the Consistency Evaluation of the Quality and Efficacy of Generic Drugs*

(No. 8 [2016] General Office of the State Council, February 6th, 2016)

The people's governments of all provinces, autonomous regions, and municipalities directly under the Central Government; all ministries and commissions of the State Council and all institutions directly under the State Council,

The work of conducting the consistency evaluation of the quality and efficacy of generic drugs (hereinafter referred to as the "consistency evaluation") is of great significance for promoting the national pharmaceutical industry, ensuring safety and efficacy of drugs, facilitating the upgrading and restructuring of the pharmaceutical industry and enhancing international competitiveness. In accordance with the *Opinions of the State Council on the Reform of Evaluation and Approval System for Drugs and Medical Devices* (No.44 [2015] General Office of the State Council), these *Opinions* are hereby promulgated for conducting the consistency evaluation with the approval from the State Council.

### I. Defining evaluation objects and time limit

The generic drugs, which have been approved for marketing before the implementation of the new registration classification of chemical drugs, shall be subject to the consistency evaluation provided that they have not undergone review and approval according to the principle of consistency with the quality and efficacy of original drugs. With respect to the oral solid preparations of chemical generic drugs on the *National Essential Medicine List* (2012 edition) which have obtained approval for marketing prior to October 1st, 2007, the consistency evaluation shall be completed by the end of 2018. For the varieties requiring clinical trial on efficacy and with special situations, consistency evaluation shall be completed by the end of 2021 and for those failing to complete the evaluation within the prescribed time limit, re-registration shall not be approved.

For other generic drugs which have been approved for marketing before the implementation of the new registration classification of chemical drugs, since the first variety passes consistency evaluation, the consistency evaluation for the similar variety of other pharmaceutical manufacturers shall be completed within 3 years in principle and for those failing to complete within the prescribed time limit, re-registration shall not be approved.

## II. Determining selection principles for reference preparations

For the selection of reference preparations, the original drugs shall be the preferred choice in principle, and the similar products recognized internationally may also be selected. Pharmaceutical manufacturers may select reference preparations by themselves and report to China Food and Drug Administration for filling; if China Food and Drug Administration proposes no objection within the prescribed time limit, pharmaceutical manufacturers may start relevant study. Industrial associations may also organize the pharmaceutical manufacturers of similar varieties to propose opinions on the selection of reference preparations and report to China Food and Drug Administration for review and confirmation. For controversial reference preparations, China Food and Drug Administration shall organize the experts to conduct public discussion before making selection. China Food and Drug Administration shall be responsible for timely announcing the information of reference preparations. Pharmaceutical manufacturers shall in principle select the announced reference preparations to conduct consistency evaluation.

## III. Reasonably selecting evaluation methods

Pharmaceutical manufacturers shall in principle use in vivo bioequivalence test to conduct consistency evaluation. For the varieties meeting the principle of exemption from bioequivalence test, pharmaceutical manufacturers are allowed to use in vitro dissolution test to conduct consistency evaluation. The list of specific varieties shall be announced by China Food and Drug Administration separately. When conducting in vivo bioequivalence test, pharmaceutical manufacturers shall organize the implementation in accordance with the regulations for bioequivalence test of generic drugs. For those with no reference preparations, pharmaceutical manufacturers shall conduct clinical trials on efficacy.

## IV. Implementing the primary responsibilities of enterprises

Pharmaceutical manufacturers are the subjects for consistency evaluation, who shall actively select reference preparations to conduct relevant studies and ensure the consistency in quality and efficacy between the drugs and reference preparations. After completing consistency evaluation, manufacturers may, in accordance with the procedure of supplementary application for drug registration, submit to food and drug regulatory authority the evaluation results and materials to adjust the prescription and process. For the generic drugs produced by domestic pharmaceutical manufacturers approved for marketing in European Union, United States and Japan, manufacturers may, on the basis of relevant application materials for registration overseas, apply for marketing in accordance with the new registration classification of chemical drugs, and the approval for marketing shall be regarded as equivalent of having passed consistency evaluation; and the drugs produced with the same production line and approved for marketing within the territory of China and in European Union, United States and Japan shall be regarded as equivalent of having passed consistency evaluation.

### V. Strengthening management of consistency evaluation

China Food and Drug Administration shall be responsible for issuing relevant guidelines for consistency evaluation and strengthening technical guidance for pharmaceutical manufacturers in consistency evaluation; China Food and Drug Administration shall organize experts to review the materials of reference preparations submitted by enterprises, announce, by stage and in group, the list of reference preparations reviewed and confirmed, and establish the *Directory of Reference Preparations for Generic Drugs in China*; China Food and Drug Administration shall, in a timely manner, include the drugs approved for marketing in accordance with the new standards in the *Directory of Reference Preparations* and make announcements; China Food and Drug Administration shall establish a uniform evaluation channel to review the materials of consistency evaluation and supplementary application for drug registration submitted by enterprises. China Food and Drug Administration shall approve the one-time import of the reference preparations that are purchased by pharmaceutical manufacturers themselves but not yet sold in domestic market for consistency evaluation and study.

### VI. Encouraging enterprises to conduct consistency evaluation

The drug varieties having passed consistency evaluation shall be announced to the society by China Food and Drug Administration. Pharmaceutical manufacturers may mark it in the package inserts and labels; the enterprises within the pilot areas conducting drug marketing authorization holder system may apply for being marketing authorization holder of the variety, entrust other pharmaceutical manufacturers for production and assume relevant legal responsibility after the product is marketed. The drug varieties having passed consistency evaluation shall be provided with appropriate support in medical insurance payment, and medical institutions shall give them priority in purchase and in clinical use. If there are more than three manufacturers of the similar varieties having passed consistency evaluation, the drug varieties failing to pass consistency evaluation shall not be selected in centralized procurement of drugs. For the technical transformation of pharmaceutical manufacturers having passed consistency evaluation, manufacturers may apply for financial support from central infrastructure investment and industry fund under the condition of meeting relevant requirements.

All regions and all relevant authorities shall attach great importance to, organize and guide pharmaceutical manufacturers to take active participation in, and conduct consistency evaluation related work in a scientific and standardized manner. China Food and Drug Administration shall strengthen guidance together with relevant authorities to implement relevant supportive policies and jointly promote consistency evaluation.

**(Zhao Xuemei)**

## 18. *Guiding Opinions of the General Office of the State Council on Promoting the Healthy Development of the Pharmaceutical Industry*

Office of the State Council

March 4th, 2016

The people's governments of all provinces, autonomous regions and municipalities directly under the Central Government, the ministries and commissions directly under the State Council.

Pharmaceutical industry is the important foundation for the development of medical and health undertaking and health services. Being a promising industry with huge growth potential and strong relevance with other sectors, the pharmaceutical industry is a great driving force and has played an active role in ensuring the people's livelihood and the steady social and economic growth. Vigorously developing the pharmaceutical industry is of great significance for deepening the reform of the healthcare system, promoting the construction of a healthy China and fostering the new impetus to economic development. Since the reform and opening up, China's pharmaceutical industry has made great progress with rapid growth of industrial scale and supply capacity, but it is still faced with challenges like the weak independent innovation capability, unsound industrial structure, non-standardized market order and so on. At present, the global pharmaceutical technology is developing by leaps and bounds, the pharmaceutical industry is undergoing profound adjustment and changes and the people's health needs are continuously growing. All of these pose urgent demands for transformation and upgrading of the pharmaceutical industry. In order to promote the core competitiveness and the sustainable and healthy development of China's pharmaceutical industry, the State Council puts forward the following opinions.

## I. General requirements

(1) Guiding thoughts

We shall comprehensively carry through the spirits of the 18th National Congress of the Communist Party of China (CPC) and the Third, Fourth, and Fifth Plenary Sessions of the 18th CPC Central Committee, earnestly implement the arrangements and decision of the CPC Central Committee and the State Council, firmly uphold and effectively implement the development concept of innovation, coordination, greenness, opening-up and sharing and actively embrace the new round of industrial reform. We shall optimize the environment for application, strengthen the supporting factors, adjust the industrial structure, intensify the industrial supervision, deepen the opening-up and cooperation, mobilize the innovative enthusiasm of the pharmaceutical industry, reduce the cost in the entire link from R & D to marketing of pharmaceutical products, accelerate the reform of mechanisms and systems in the fields of medical product approval, production, circulation and application, strive to make the pharmaceutical industry intelligent, service-oriented and ecology-friendly, make efforts to realize the transformation from medium and high-speed development into the medium and high-end development, and try our best to meet the multi-level and diversified health needs of the people.

(2) Basic principles.

The development of the pharmaceutical industry shall be led by the market and guided by the government. The principal position of enterprises and the market shall be strengthened with the market playing its dominant role in allocating resources and the government better excising its function. With the implementation of the relevant healthcare reform policies, we shall improve the industrial policies and supervisory system, standardize market order, boost the mutual enhancement between industrial upgrading and application, and create an environment for fair competition.

The innovation-driven, opening-up and cooperative modes shall be upheld. We shall make efforts to improve the innovation environment, promote the in-depth integration of government, enterprises, universities, R&D institutions and consumers, improve the capacity of innovating medical technology and promote the innovation in technology, products and business forms. Efforts shall also be made to accelerate the pace for docking-up the system of management, quality, standards and registration of pharmaceutical products with the world, make full use of international resources and strengthen the global industrial layout and international cooperation.

The industrial cluster shall be developed and the concept of green development shall be upheld. The formation of industrial clusters with strong environmentally sustainable capacity and favorable production supporting conditions for chemical active pharmaceutical ingredients (APIs) shall be pressed ahead. Efforts shall be made to guide the enterprises of traditional Chinese medicine and ethnic minority medicine to integrate the plantation (breeding) and processing of medicinal materials. The recycling production, recycling industrial combination and recycling industrial park transformation shall be promoted, and the green transformation and upgrading as well as the green and safe development of the pharmaceutical industry shall be boosted.

The quality shall be continuously improved and the supply shall be guaranteed. The responsibility of enterprises as the main entities shall be reinforced and the quality standards and testing system shall be improved to ensure the safety and efficacy of products. The production and supply of essential medicine shall be strengthened, the information network for medicine distribution shall be improved, and a fast-track for the examination and approval as well as the market access of innovative drugs and drugs in shortage in the market shall be established so as to improve the ability to guarantee the supply.

(3) Main objectives

By 2020, the innovation capacity of the pharmaceutical industry will be significantly improved, the capacity of guaranteeing supply will be significantly enhanced, the generic drugs of more than 90% of the major drugs with expiry patent will be available in the market, and the lack of drugs that are in shortage in clinical use will be effectively alleviated. The level of green industrial development, safety, efficiency and quality management will be significantly improved. The industrial structure will be further optimized, the system and mechanism gradually improved and the market environment significantly optimized. The scale of the pharmaceutical industry will be further expanded, the annual income growth rate of the main business will be higher than 10% and the growth of industrial added value will top the ranking among all the industries.

## II. Main tasks

(4) Technological innovation will be strengthened and the competitiveness in core areas will be improved.

The innovation capacity will be promoted. The reform of science and technology system will be intensified and the collaborative innovation system involving government, enterprises, universities, R&D institutions and consumers will be optimized. We will enhance the capacity in developing new RLD, the first generic drugs, new traditional Chinese medicine, new preparations and high-end medical equipment, optimize the allocation of scientific and technological resources, and create a scientific and technological innovation base with rational layout. The information technology like databases, computer screening and the Internet will be applied and the public service platform for R&D, industrialization, safety evaluation, clinical evaluation of pharmaceutical products and technology will be constructed. The public space for mass entrepreneurship will be actively developed, the mass entrepreneurship and innovation will be vigorously boosted, a number of innovation-oriented small and medium enterprises with special technology and high-end employees will be established, the transformation of enterprises from R & D outsourcing ones to the ones of whole-process innovation will be promoted and the ability to develop new products will be improved.

The industrialization of major drugs will be promoted. The creation of new drugs will be continuously promoted, the development of the chemical drug preparation technologies like chiral synthesis, enzyme catalysis and crystallization control will be speeded up, the R&D and engineering of the biological technologies like large-scale cell culture and purification, antibody conjugation, serum-and- protein-free medium culture will be promoted, and the capacity of making new preparations with long-acting, slow-releasing and targeting traits will be enhanced. Oriented for the clinical use, the development of drugs with targeting and highly-selective features and new functional mechanisms, and drugs treating major diseases like tumor, cardiovascular and cerebrovascular diseases, diabetes, neurodegenerative diseases, psychiatric diseases, immune diseases with high incidence, major contagious diseases and rare diseases, will be prioritized. And emphasis will also be laid on the imitation of foreign expiry patent drugs with huge market potential and urgently needed in clinical use. The R&D of new antibodies, proteins and polypeptides will be accelerated. The vaccine supply system will be improved and the much needed vaccines and adjuvants like hand-foot-mouth disease vaccine, new polio vaccine and cervical cancer vaccine will be actively developed. As for the vaccines for children, the new varieties, dosage forms and specifications that suit the children's physiological characteristics will be developed. The designated production of basic drugs that are essential in clinical use but with only a small amount needed and in shortage of market supply will be conducted and the production capacity and regular reservation of these drugs will be strengthened to meet people's needs for basic drugs.

The transformation and upgrading of medical equipment will be accelerated. Priority will be given to the development of critical components like digital detectors, superconducting magnets and high-capacity X-ray tube as well as to technologies like precise positioning and navigation surgery, data acquisition, processing and analysis, and biological three-dimensional (3D) printing. Effort will be made to develop high-performance diagnostic and treatment equipment, such as nuclear medical imaging equipment (PET-CT and PET-MRI), superconducting magnetic resonance imaging (MRI), multirow-detector helical CT (MDCT), color Doppler ultrasound, equipment for image-guided radiation therapy, proton/heavy-ion tumor therapy apparatus, medical robots and equipment for telemedicine. The industrialization of the in vitro diagnostic equipment and reagents, like the automatic biochemical analyzer, chemiluminescence immunoassay analyzer, high-throughput sequencing apparatus and five categories automatic blood cell analyzer, will be pressed ahead. Efforts will be made to develop the high-end implant and intervention products, like heart valves, pacemakers, fully degradable stents, artificial joints and vertebrae and cochlear implant, and the medium and high-end rehabilitation equipment. The medical devices based on the theory of traditional Chinese medicine will be actively explored.

The modernization of traditional Chinese medicine will be promoted. The research on the technical standards of clinical application of traditional Chinese medicine and ethnic minority medicine will be carried out, the development of technical standards for cultivating Chinese medica materia will be enhanced, the standard system of genuine regional traditional Chinese medica materia will be established, and the protection of products with geographical indications in the field of traditional Chinese medicine will be intensified. The seed (stock) breeding, modern cultivation (breeding) and the production technology promotion of traditional Chinese medica materia will be carried out, and the integrated bases with standardized cultivation (breeding) and large-scale processing will be built in the appropriate areas. The dynamic monitoring system of Chinese medica materia resources will be established, and the assessment on ecological and environmental of the utilization of wild Chinese medica materia will be conducted. The construction of the traceability system of Chinese medica materia and the processing, circulation and application of Chinese medica materia will be strengthened, and the quality and safety of traditional Chinese medicinal products will be improved. The modern extraction and purification technology of traditional Chinese medicine will be developed, R&D of preparation technology like mucosal drug delivery in line with the characteristics of traditional Chinese medicine will be conducted, and technology in quality control, automation and on-line monitoring will be applied in the processing of traditional Chinese medicine. In the field where the treatment of traditional Chinese medicine excels, the further development and application of the classic recipes will be promoted, and the traditional Chinese medicine products with definite efficacy, safety, determined effective ingredients and clear acting mechanism will be developed. The theory research on minority ethnic medicine will be strengthened, the systemic development of Tibetan medicine, Uygur medicine, Mongolian medicine, Dai medicine and so on will be promoted, and the level of preparation-making in ethnic minority medical institutions will be improved to create new varieties with superior resources and excellent efficacy.

(5) The quality upgrading will be speeded up and the green and safe development will be promoted.

The production and quality will be strictly managed. The new version of *Good Manufacturing Practices (GMP) of Pharmaceutical Products* will be comprehensively and strictly implemented and the quality management system of the whole life cycle and the whole industry chain will be improved, the quality management involving all the employees, the whole process and all the aspects will be carried out and the drug safety traceability system will be improved. The manufacturing environment standards like temperature and cleanliness will be strictly controlled, the management over documents like management standards and work standards will be strengthened, and the quality management system like quality risk prevention and control, audit of suppliers, inspection over sustainability and stability and Qualified Person will be established. The quality and safety awareness of the first responsible person in pharmaceutical enterprises will be enhanced and the main responsibility for quality will be assigned to specific person(s). The training over quality and safety will be strengthened and the strict EHS (Environment, Health and Safety) management will be exercised to improve staff quality. The production and management will be standardized to solve the main problems like placing authentication over execution and hardware over software, the supervision on quality of essential medicine will be strengthened, and pharmaceutical production enterprises will be comprehensively supervised to enhance the overall quality management level.

The quality control technology will be improved. The scientific and effective quality standards and control methods will be established, the application of advanced quality control technology will be promoted, the product design will be improved, the process route will be optimized, and the quality control system over the whole process from raw materials to finished product will be improved to effectively improve the quality of medicine. The development of technology controlling chemical impurities, solubility, solvent residues and drug polymorphism will be speeded up to improve the purity and stability of the products. The research on biological properties like biological activity, equivalence and utilization rate will be enhanced, the variability control over the biological process like fermentation and cell culture will be strengthened and priority will be given to improving the safety and effectiveness of vaccines and other biological products. The research on the material basis for the traditional Chinese medicine and ethnic minority medicine products will be intensified and the quality of the solvent will be improved to reduce the incidence of adverse reactions.

The quality standard system will be improved. The national drug standard system will be improved in line with the *Pharmacopoeia of the People's Republic of China* and the action plan for improving the standards of drugs and medical devices will be implemented. Effort will be made to upgrade the quality standards for essential medicines, high-risk medicines, pharmaceutical excipients, packaging materials and basic, universal and high-risk medical devises. The technical and quality control standards of medicinal materials and pharmaceutical products of traditional Chinese medicine and ethnic minority medicine will be optimized to improve the scientificity, rationality and operability and strengthen the authority and solemnity of the standards. The drug quality evaluation system will be further improved, and the database of drug impurities, the quality evaluation methods and the quality testing platform will be established. The methods and technical standards for evaluation on bioequivalence of generic drugs will be improved and the third-party testing and evaluation will be conducted to improve the quality of generic drugs. Priority will be given to the evaluation on quality and consistency of efficacy of the essential medicine so as to comprehensively improve the quality of the essential medicine. The risk assessment of harmful residues of traditional Chinese medicine will be carried out and the safety evaluation of traditional Chinese medicine injections will be strengthened to maintain of the quality and safety of traditional Chinese medicine product. The improvement of the public technical service platforms of metrology, standards, inspection, testing, certification, etc. will be accelerated and the construction of third-party quality and reliability evaluation platforms will be encouraged to promote the investment by enterprises and enhance the reliability of products.

The green transformation and upgrading will be carried out. The modern biotechnology will be adopted to improve the traditional production process, the alternative biological technology like genetic engineering and biocatalysis will be vigorously promoted and the bio-fermentation method will be actively used in production of active pharmaceutical substances. Efforts will be made to develop clean production technology like biotransformation, efficient extraction and purification, and the application of high-yield and low-consumption bacteria, and to strengthen the pollution prevention and control over fermentation of bulk raw materials. The application of non-toxic and harmless raw materials will be accelerated, the management of new chemical substances in outsourcing R & D enterprises will be strengthened, and the control over the source of environmental pollution will be promoted. The green factories and recycling economy parks will be constructed to promote mutual supply of raw materials, sharing of resources, better recycling of by-products, harmless treatment of wastes and comprehensive management of pollutants. The resource utilization will be strictly managed, the optimization projects of the energy system will be carried out, the technology and equipment that can save energy, water and land will be promoted, the backward process and equipment will be eliminated, the management over recycling of high-value medical supplies will be strengthened, and the utilization rate of energy and resources and the level of clean production will be improved. The control over environmental risks will be strengthened and the check-up over environmental safety hazards will be conducted to prevent unexpected environmental events.

(6) The industrial structure will be optimized and the intensive development will be enhanced.

The industrial organization and structure will be adjusted. The adjustment of enterprises' organizational structure will be strengthened, the cross-industry and cross-sector mergers and reorganizations of enterprises will be promoted, and support will be given to combination between strong pharmaceutical and chemical enterprises, between medical equipment and equipment manufacturers, between Chinese herbal medicines and proprietary Chinese medicines producers, between pharmaceutical raw materials and preparations manufactures, and between production and circulation enterprises to form an integrated corporation groups. Thus, a real solution to problems of small scale, scattered distribution, and chaotic structure will be worked out. The production of essential drugs will be concentrated in the competitive enterprises to enhance the level of intensive production and guarantee the product quality and stable supply. The leading enterprises of the pharmaceutical industry will be taken as the mainstay and be jointed with the innovative enterprises or research institutes with similar products and technology. The cooperation models like capital injection and technology appraised as capital stock will be adopted to form industrial alliances or consortium. The advantages of the key enterprises in capital, technology, etc. will be exercised, the effective integration of production factors and the reengineering of business processes will be strengthened, and the new product development, marketing and brand building will be intensified. The features of the small and medium enterprises like the closeness to the market and the flexible mechanisms will be made use of, the high-tech and high-quality complimentary products including medical media, adjuvants and packaging materials will be developed, and the win-win industrial organizational structure with labor-division and collaboration of the small, medium-sized and large enterprises will be formed.

The coordinated regional development will be developed. The regional advantages in resources will be exercised and a new pattern of coordinated development of the eastern, central and western regions will be created. The advantages of the eastern coastal areas in capital, technology and human resources will be utilized, the internationally advanced research and development centers and headquarters base will be constructed, the high value-added and low-consumption biological drugs, pharmaceutical preparations and medical equipment will be developed, and the products lacking comparative advantage will be guided to orderly transfer to other places. The geographical advantage of the middle region of connecting the east and west regions will be exercised. Taking the carrying capacity of resources and environment into consideration, the middle region will actively undertake the industrial transfer from the eastern region, carry out research and development and industrialization of high-end pharmaceutical products in its central cities and develop the labor-intensive medical devices and products like medical consumables in accordance with the local conditions. With the bounty medicinal resources and the geographical advantage of being the bordering area, the western and northeastern region will be encouraged to construct the production bases of traditional Chinese medicine and ethnic minority medicine and the export bases of special medical products to the neighboring countries.

Efforts will be made to guide the industrial agglomeration. The large-scaled and industrialized parks of pharmaceutical products will be promoted and the industrial clusters with standardized management, favorable environment, distinctive features and high degree of industrial association will be created. The competitive enterprises will be guided, in accordance with the *Good Agricultural Practices (GAP) of Chinese Medicinal Materials*, to carry out large-scaled and standardized cultivation (breeding) in the areas suitable for the growth of medicinal materials, build large-scale production and processing bases of traditional Chinese medicine in regions with rich Chinese medicinal resources, and construct production bases for ethnic minority medicines in regions inhabited by ethnic minorities. In combination with the layout adjustment and industrial transfer of chemical APIs, the advanced production bases of these chemical APIs will be constructed in the chemical pharmaceutical parks with strong environment carrying capacity, complete supporting facilities and good accessibility of raw materials and the export-oriented preparation production bases up to the international standards will be built in the border and coastal regions. In the central cities with superior human resources and technology, the high-end R & D and industrialization bases of medical devices will be established through the radiation effects of industries such as electronics, information and equipment. The areas with possible conditions will be guided to make overall use of superior local resources in medical service, traditional Chinese medicine and ecotourism and exercise the role of the tourism market. In addition, a number of integrated health tourism demonstration bases, covering the fields of old-age caring, medical service, rehabilitation and tourism will be developed and constructed and the comprehensive service system of socialized old-age caring, medical services, rehabilitation and tourism will be improved.

(7) The modern logistics will be developed and the credit system of the pharmaceutical industry will be constructed.

The modern marketing model will be established. The information system for the logistics of the enterprises will be improved, and the national drug information platform will be built by using the information obtained from the centralized drug procurement platform at the provincial level. The price, dosage, quality, circulation and other relevant information of drugs will be publicized and subjected to the supervision of the public, and the information sharing, feedback and tracing mechanism will be established. The modern medicine circulation system will be set up, the large enterprises will be encouraged to construct the drug distribution network throughout the urban and rural areas, and the network of the postal enterprises and express delivery companies will be utilized to improve the capability of drug supply and security at the community-level and in the remote areas. The specialized and professionalized development of the small and medium-sized circulation enterprises will be promoted so they can provide specialized services to meet the multi-leveled demands of the market. According to the requirements of the new version of *Good Supplying Practice (GSP) of Pharmaceutical Products*, efforts will be made to promote the chain operation of the competitive retail enterprises. The purchase and distribution, quality management, service regulation, information management and brand identity of the chain businesses will be unified to make them more standardized and large-scaled. The open system for source codes of communication protocol, fault feedback, testing and maintenance of medical equipment will be constructed, and the third parties will be encouraged to develop specialized maintenance and after-sale service teams.

The construction of the credit system will be strengthened. The integrity management mechanism of pharmaceutical products will be improved so as to optimize the market environment. The existing credit information resources will be integrated to establish the credit record files of the pharmaceutical R & D, production and circulation enterprises, and these files will be included into the unified national credit information sharing and exchange platform. The credit information will be made public in accordance with the relevant regulations on "www.creditchina.gov.cn" and the National Enterprise Credit Information Publicity System. The information collection, evaluation, and publicity mechanism will be developed and the "blacklist" of enterprises with bad credit will be established. The means like media publicity and market access will be used to jointly increase the punishment on enterprises with bad credit and to increase the cost of dishonesty. The construction of the insurance system for enterprise credit and commodity quality will be speeded up, the mandatory commercial insurance for product quality and safety will be explored and the self-discipline of the enterprises will be strengthened. The enterprises will be guided to establish credit management system, develop the evaluation system, take the initiative to carry out credit commitments and consciously accept the supervision of the public.

(8) Efforts will be made in close link with the healthcare reform to create a favorable market environment.

The medical service system will be improved. The reform of the compensation system of public hospitals will be accelerated and a scientific and reasonable system of rewards and punishments will be established. In combination with the implementation of policies like the separation of medical services and medicine sales, and the elimination of medicine markups, the management over diagnosis and treatment will be strengthened to prevent excessive and non-standardized diagnostic and treatment behaviors, and the medical expenses will be controlled. Medical institutions will write the prescriptions with the generic name of the drugs and take initiative to provide the patients with prescriptions to protect the patient's rights to choose how to purchase the drugs. The medical institutions of various types of ownerships will be pushed to share equipment and mutually recognize the examination results to reduce the repeated checkups and lessen the burden of the patients. The environment for the development of medical institutions run by social capital will be improved, the medical institutions of various kinds will be treated equally in terms of market access, designated social insurance, key specialty construction, professional title evaluation, academic status and grade evaluation, the formation of diversified models of medical services will be accelerated to give the patients more choices. The multi-site practice of doctors will be promoted, the primary health care service capacity will be enhanced, and the implementation of hierarchical diagnosis and treatment system will be accelerated.

The pricing policy and health insurance policy will be improved. The synergic reform of medical service, health insurance and medicine system will be implemented, the market mechanism will be fully exercised and the actual transaction price of drugs will be mainly regulated by the market competition. The linkage of the policies on price, health insurance, bidding and procurement will be strengthened, the payment standards of health insurance will be scientifically formulated, the comprehensive supervision over medical expenses and pricing will be enhanced, the drug price monitoring system will be improved, and the publicity of price information will be promoted. The reform over the prices of medical services will be actively and steadily pushed forward, the dynamic price adjustment mechanism based on the structural changes in cost and income will be established and the price relation of medical services will be gradually rationalized, the value of medical and technical services of the medical personnel will be effectively reflected. According to the principle of "controlling the total amount, carrying out the structural adjustment, making the price rising and falling accordingly, and putting the policies in place gradually", the price of medical service will be adjusted rationally, and the adjusted expenses will be covered by medical insurance payment and the burdens of the public will not be increased. The reform of the payment modes of health insurance will be actively promoted, the budgeting over the income and expenses of the health insurance funds will be enhanced, and a combination of payment modes including DRGs and caption payment will be adopted. According to the carrying ability of medical insurance funds, the drugs, medical equipment and medical treatment items that comply with the conditions, are of the reasonable price and are with independent intellectual property rights will be included into the payment range of medical insurance. The insurance policy for critical illnesses will be improved, the medical aid for serious and major diseases will be carried out, and the commercial health insurance will be vigorously developed to meet the diversified social needs for health insurance and pharmaceutical products.

(9) The international cooperation will be deepened and the international development space will be expanded.

The export structure will be optimized. The development of the emerging international pharmaceutical markets will be accelerated and the export structure will be adjusted. The international competitive advantages of chemical APIs will be fully exercised and the export of deep processed products such as vitamins, penicillin, erythromycin and cephalosporin will be promoted. The international strategy for pharmaceutical preparations will be vigorously implemented, the export of the preparations like the first generic drugs, recombinant protein drugs, antibody drugs and vaccines will be speeded up. The combination export of APIs and preparations will be enhanced and the well-known brands of Chinese medicine will be cultivated. The overseas sales and service system will be established and improved, the export of medical equipment like PET-CT, X-ray machine, electrocardiogram machine and B-mode ultrasound will be promoted and the added value of export will be gradually increased. The international cultural exchange of traditional Chinese medicine will be strengthened, the acceptance of traditional Chinese medicine by the international community will be improved, the influence on formulating international standards of traditional Chinese medicine will be enhanced, and the export of natural medicine and traditional Chinese medicine preparations will be boosted.

The international registration and certification will be promoted. The personnel for international pharmaceutical registration, who are familiar with overseas laws, regulations and market environment, will be introduced and cultivated to improve the capacity for international registration. The product registration in the international markets will be carried out systemically, the overseas clinical trial and registration of the patented domestic medicine will be promoted, and the international registration and certification of the brand generic drug will be speeded up. The international comparison of the medical device-related measurements will be actively carried out. In accordance with international standards, the process routes, the quality testing and analysis methods, and the EHS (Environment, Health and Safety) management system will be improved and the record management system for raw and supplement materials will be established and implemented. The international certification of production system like the one of Quality Management Practices (GMP) of Pharmaceutical Products will be speeded up, and the construction of the production line conforming to international quality standards by enterprises will be promoted. The international level of production and management will be elevated and the process of international testing and certification will be quickened. The enterprises will be encouraged to apply for overseas patents to form an effective overseas layout of patents.

The pace of international cooperation will be accelerated. The strategy of the "Belt and Road Initiative" will be implemented, the global allocation of resources will be taken into consideration, and the pace of "going out" will be quickened. Various ways of cooperation will be adopted and the competitive pharmaceutical enterprises will be encouraged to carry out overseas mergers, investment in stocks, and venture capital investment. They will also be promoted to establish overseas research and development centers, production bases, and sales and service networks, gain access to new products, key technologies, production licenses and sales channels, quicken their pace to get integrated into the international market and create a number of internationally influential brands. The enterprises will be encouraged to actively participate in international cooperation in the field of public health and continuously expand and consolidate the international market. The investment environment will be improved, the construction of supporting system will be strengthened, the efforts to "introduce needed things into China" will be enhanced, and the enterprises under specially supervised regions of the customs will be encouraged to undertake outsourcing business of bio-pharmaceuticals. The multinational companies will be promoted to build high-level pharmaceutical R & D centers, production centers and procurement centers in China, the industrial cooperation will be accelerated to extend the processing and manufacturing link to other high value-added links like R & D, design, marketing and brand cultivation, and the level of international cooperation will be elevated.

(10) New forms of business will be natured and the development of the intelligent pharmaceutical industry will be promoted.

The showcase intelligent factories will be constructed. The intelligent production process of medicine will be promoted and the demonstration of intelligent factory and digital workshop will be carried out. The application of technology and equipment like Intelligent Human Computer Interaction (IHCI) and industrial robots in the pharmaceutical production will be speeded up, and the optimization of manufacturing process simulation, the real-time information feedback and the self-adaptive control will be advanced. The technology like big data, cloud computing, the Internet and additive manufacturing will be applied and the new production models like the dynamic consumer demand perception model, crowdsourcing design and personalized customization of medical products will be established. The development of digital and intelligent medical devices will be speeded up, priority will be given to the development of mobile and auxiliary medical equipment like wearable and portable devices, and the application of new technologies such as biological three-dimensional (3D) printing technology and data chips in the implantation and intervention products will be promoted. The intelligent upgrading of pharmaceutical production equipment will be promoted, the industrial control systems, the R & D and industrialization of core technology equipment like industrial control system and intelligent sensing components will be speeded up, and the construction of intelligent pharmaceutical factories will be supported.

The intelligent medical services will be carried out. The leading role of quality medical resources will be played, the social forces will be encouraged to participate, the on-line and off-line resources will be integrated, and the management over the Internet of Things in the health field and the health care applications (APPs) will be strengthened. The online health consultation, clinic appointments, waiting time reminders, pricing and payment, inquiry of medical reports and other convenient services will be actively carried out. The integration of regional medical and health service resources will be strengthened, and the medical service institutions will be encouraged to establish medical and healthcare information platform and actively carry out on-line health care information services. The medical institutions will be guided to use information and intelligent technology and equipment to carry out telemedicine services like long-distance pathological diagnosis, imaging diagnosis, specialist consultation, monitoring guidance and surgical instructions for the community-level, remote and less-developed regions.

**III. The policy support as well as the organization and implementation will be strengthened**

(11) New financial support modes will be developed and the means like incentives, capital injection, and subsidies for demonstrative application will be used to support the projects with strong public service nature, such as the application demonstration and the construction of public service platform. The funds like industrial investment and venture capital will be utilized and guided to support the profitable and competitive projects in the sectors of R&D of new products and industrial construction. The key enterprises and industry alliances with capacity for innovative development will be assisted and the resources along the industrial chain will be integrated. The cooperation between the medical device manufacturers and financial leasing companies will be explored to provide installments for medical institutions of all types of ownerships to purchase large medical equipment. The list of the key APIs that are in shortage in China and needed to make breakthroughs will be developed, and for the listed APIs that are of clear chemical structure, conform to tariff classification rules and meet the supervisory requirements, research will be carried out to impose relatively low tax on them for a temporary period. The incentive mechanism in the links like new pharmaceutical products development, value-added service and demonstrative application will be improved. The innovative pharmaceutical enterprises with eligible conditions will be supported to finance through stock market, issue bonds and carry out mergers and reconstruction.

(12) Efforts will be made to promote the innovative products. The list of innovative and excellent drugs and medical equipment will be developed. The publicity of innovative products will be increased to enhance the clinical doctors and the public's recognition over the pharmaceutical products with independent intellectual property rights. The pilot insurance and compensation for the first (set of) major technical equipment will be carried out to facilitate the application and popularization of eligible high-end medical equipment, the application demonstration project of innovative medical devices will be continued and the piloting configuration of large medical equipment in some provinces will be carried out. The promotion of innovative medical devices will be further enhanced and the demonstrative application will be carried out at different levels of medical institutions. Pharmaceutical companies and large hospitals will be encouraged to cooperate in the construction of medical equipment application demonstration bases and training centers to form a virtuous circle of application demonstration- clinical evaluation - technological innovation - popularization.

(13) The government procurement mechanism will be improved. In accordance

with the principles of openness, transparency and fair competition, the bidding and purchasing mechanisms will be improved, and the procurement of pharmaceutical products will be gradually integrated into the public resource trading platform. The classified procurement will be conducted, review factors will be scientifically determined, and the standardized procurement coding of medicine and high-value medical consumables will be advanced to ensure the reasonable price, sufficient supply, quality and safety. The fair competition will be ensured, and the market segmentation and local protectionism of pharmaceutical products will be abolished. The two-envelope evaluation method will be further improved, and for the medicine with significantly low bidding price and possible risks in quality, the comprehensive assessment must be carried out to avoid vicious competition. The information publicity will be comprehensively advanced, the verification and dynamic adjustment mechanism for the drugs with inflated price will be established and efforts will be made to ensure that all aspects of drug procurement are done publicly. According to regional health planning, the standards for allocation of medical equipment in health institutions at all levels will be developed and improved and the purchase of unreasonably over-standard high-end equipment will be strictly controlled. The *Government Procurement Law of the People's Republic of China* will be earnestly implemented. Where the domestic drugs and medical equipment can meet the requirements, in principle, the domestic products will be purchased in the government procurement projects and the configuration of domestic equipment will be gradually increased in the public medical institutions.

(14) The reform in the review and approval will be deepened. A more scientific and efficient review and approval system for medicine and medical devices will be established. The construction of the review teams will be accelerated and the experts and scholars with experience in international review and approval will be recruited. The governmental purchasing of review services will be increased, the collaborative ability in technical review will be enhanced, and the capacity and efficiency of review and approval will be elevated. The acceptance and approval of relevant information will be done publicly to increase the transparency of the process. The review and approval of products that are oversupplied in the market, low-level redundantly developed and produced with backward process will be strictly controlled. The review and approval of innovative drugs and medical devices urgently needed in clinical use will be accelerated to guide the applicants to make orderly research and development and make scientific applications. The development of new specifications for diagnostic and clinical techniques will be accelerated. For genetic testing products that have been identified as innovative medical devices, priority will be given to their review and approval in accordance with the procedures for innovative medical devices. The entry

of innovative medical service items into the health care system will be accelerated and the clinical application of new technologies will be promoted. The pilot of Marketing Authorization Holder (MAH) will be accelerated to promote specialized division of drug research and development from drug production and to accelerate the transformation of the results of scientific research. The entrusted drug research and development and drug production will be encouraged, the restrictions on the transfer of drug approval numbers will be gradually relaxed, and the competitive enterprises will be guided to carry out mergers and reorganization so as to reduce competitive heterogeneity and waste of review resources.

(15) The nurture of human resources will be accelerated. The strategy for the priority development of human resources will be further advanced. In light of the needs like the development of new medicine, the development of core hardware and software for medical devices, the heritage of traditional Chinese medicine and the international registration of pharmaceutical products, the mechanism for human resources introduction, training and motivation will be improved to create an environment where the talents can exercise their ability to the fullest extent. The projects to attract talented people like the "thousands of talents" plan will be continued to attract high-quality individuals and teams who are capable in overseas new product development and international registration to begin innovation and entrepreneurship in China. The pharmaceutical enterprises will be encouraged to set up post-doctoral research centers.

Centering on the improvement of drug quality management and competitiveness of the enterprises, the various forms of management training for pharmaceutical enterprise will be actively carried out to cultivate a group of leading pharmaceutical entrepreneurs. The vocational education and skills training will be strengthened and the medical technology application education and training bases will be constructed so as to cultivate skilled human resources. The relevant methods for professional appraisal and post-setting in the medical institutions will be improved. The enterprises will be supported to cooperate with universities and medical institutions to cultivate medical equipment engineers and other practical technical talents.

The establishment of personnel training platforms like entrepreneurial and innovative centers will be encouraged and the collaboration in innovation will be enhanced. The building of the pharmaceutical human resources will be strengthened to enhance the service capacity of practicing pharmacists and promote safe and rational use of medicine. The mechanism for the factors like technology and skills taking part in the income distribution will be established and improved and the forms like technology being taken as capital stock will be encouraged to fully mobilize the enthusiasm and creativity of talents.

(16) The coordinated industrial supervision will be strengthened. The communication mechanism of regulatory departments, trade associations and pharmaceutical companies will be improved and the thorough supervisory network will be optimized to form the pattern of total social governance. The social groups like industrial associations will be supported to carry out monitoring and analysis over industrial operation, strategy research for industrial development and release of industrial information. The management over drugs and medical devices in the process of use will be strengthened, the monitoring of adverse drug reactions will be intensified and the responsibility for monitoring adverse reactions after the marketing of the products will be determined. The safety evaluation mechanism for the listed drugs will be improved and the drug delisting system will be established. A comprehensive evaluation system for clinical drug usage centered on basic drugs will be set up and optimized, the early warning mechanism for drug shortage will be improved, and the production situation of key enterprises will be dynamically monitored to elevate the capacity and level of supply. The construction of the system of laws and regulations for the supervision of pharmaceuticals and medical devices will be strengthened, the unannounced inspection will be intensified, and the enterprises in violation of laws and regulations will be promptly investigated and dealt with according to law. The supervision over safety and environment will be strengthened, and pharmaceutical companies failing to meet the requirements will be resolutely shut down according to law. For the chemical pharmaceutical enterprises, the analysis over response risk will be carried out, the standard design will be conducted, and the reliable and automatic control system will be equipped to enhance the level of intrinsic safety level. For the pharmaceutical enterprises using hazardous chemicals, it is necessary to establish a sound management system for hazardous chemicals, strengthen staff training and improve the capability in risk management and control. The protection of medical intellectual property rights will be strengthened, the construction of social credit system for intellectual property rights will be speeded up, the crackdown on infringement will be intensified, and a punitive damage system will be established to reduce the enterprises' cost for protecting their rights. The pharmaceutical market will be rectified and regulated, and the violations of law or regulations like production and sales of counterfeit and inferior pharmaceutical products, commercial bribery and secret manipulation of prices will be cracked down on.

All regions and relevant departments shall fully understand the importance of promoting the healthy development of the pharmaceutical industry, strengthen organization and leadership, improve the working mechanism and make joint efforts to make progress. All regions shall formulate concrete implementation plans in light of the actual situations, and meticulously organize the implementation so as to ensure that all tasks are carried out. The relevant departments shall develop complementary policies and create a good environment in accordance with the division of responsibilities. The National Development and Reform Commission shall strengthen the overall planning and coordination, work out a clear timetable for the implementation of various policies and measures, make joint efforts with relevant departments to strengthen policy guidance, supervision and inspection, and promote the sustainable and healthy development of the pharmaceutical industry.

**(Qu Yang)**

## Notice of the General Office of the State Council on Issuing *Major Task List of 2016 Concerning Deepening the Medical and Healthcare System Reform*

(No. 26 [2016] of the General Office of the State Council)

The people's governments of all provinces, autonomous regions and municipalities directly under the Central Government, and relevant departments of the State Council,

*Major Task List of 2016 Concerning Deepening the Medical and Healthcare System Reform*, as approved by the State Council, is hereby issued to you for your conscientious implementation in combination with reality.

The General Office of the State Council

April 21st, 2016

### 19. *Major Task List of 2016 Concerning Deepening the Medical and Healthcare System Reform*

Since the start of a new round of the medical and healthcare system reform, under the correct leadership of the CPC Central Committee and the State Council, all local authorities and relevant departments have worked together to promote the reform. With the top-level design constantly improved, and key and tough problems gradually tackled, the issue of the people's poor accessibility and affordability of healthcare services has been notably alleviated. Therefore the deepening of the medical and healthcare reform has yielded significant phased results. The year 2015 witnessed a life expectancy of 76.34 years, an increase of 1.51 years over 2010. In general, the people's health is better than the average level of middle- and high-income countries; personal health expenditure fell below 30% of the total health costs, the lowest level in nearly 20 years. The positive progress and achievements of the medical and healthcare system reform have laid a solid foundation for continuously deepening the reform.

A beginning year for the 13th Five-Year Plan, 2016 is also the crucial year for achieving the phased goal of deepening the medical and healthcare system reform. It is also the crucial year for achieving the goal of universal access to basic medical and healthcare services by 2020. We shall fully implement the guiding principles of the 18th National Congress of the CPC as well as the guiding principles of the Third, Fourth and Fifth Plenary Sessions of the 18th CPC Central Committee. Conscientiously implementing the decisions and arrangements of the CPC Central Committee and the State Council, we shall firmly establish and earnestly implement the development concept of innovation, coordination, green, openness and sharing. Efforts shall be made to adhere to the principles of ensuring basic medical services, bolstering support at the community level and building sound institutions, and further highlight key areas and key links to intensify the reform and innovation. The linkage of medical care, healthcare insurance and drugs shall be further promoted to intensify the integrity, systematicness and collaboration of the reform. Our capacity for the reform shall be further enhanced to promote the implementation of policies, make arrangements and steps for implementing various reform tasks set out in the medical and healthcare system reform for the 13th Five-Year Plan, and ensure greater results. Efforts shall be made to promote the establishment of a basic medical and healthcare system covering both urban and rural residents, and promote the building of a healthy China.

### I. Comprehensively deepening the reform of public hospitals

(1) Consolidate and improve the comprehensive reform of county-level public hospitals. With the classification guidance and demonstration guidance strengthened, the following cities or counties shall be selected for carrying out the demonstration work on the comprehensive reform of county-level public hospitals to promote the reform and improvement: Qidong city in Jiangsu province, Tianchang city in Anhui province, Youxi county in Fujian province and Huzhu Tu Autonomous County in Qinghai province.(The National Health and Family Planning Commission and the Ministry of Finance shall be in charge of the above task, with the participation of the State Commission Office of Public Sectors Reform, the National Development and Reform Commission, the Ministry of Human Resources and Social Security and the State Administration of Traditional Chinese Medicine. And the department ranked first is the department taking the lead, similarly hereinafter.)

(2) Expand the trials of comprehensive reform of urban public hospitals. One hundred new pilot cities shall be added, bringing the number of pilot cities nationwide to 200. The central government shall grant one-off subsidies to each new pilot city

based on the 20 million *yuan* standard; Municipal districts with public hospitals in all pilot cities shall be subsidized in line with the standard of 1 million *yuan* each. At the same time, efforts shall be made to carry out the evaluation of the effect of pilot comprehensive reform of public hospitals, and establish a mechanism to link the evaluation results with the allocation and payment of central government subsidies. Ten hospitals affiliated to the National Health and Family Planning Commission shall first participate in the comprehensive reform of local public hospitals and establish a performance appraisal mechanism. Hospitals run by state-owned enterprises shall be promoted to participate in the reform of public hospitals. Efforts shall be made to study and formulate guiding documents for military hospitals to participate in the comprehensive reform of urban public hospitals. (The National Health and Family Planning Commission, the Ministry of Finance, the State-owned Assets Supervision and Administration Commission and the Health Bureau of the Logistics Department under the Central Military Commission respectively shall be in charge of the above task, with the participation of the State Commission Office for Public Sectors Reform, the National Development and Reform Commission, the Ministry of Human Resources and Social Security and the State Administration of Traditional Chinese Medicine.)

(3) Fulfill government responsibilities. Efforts shall be made to implement the *Notice of the General Office of the State Council on Issuing the Outline for the Planning of the National Medical and Health Service System (2015-2020)* (No. 14 [2015] of the General Office of the State Council). All provinces, cities and counties shall formulate and implement standards for medical and health resources allocation (medical and health service system planning), regional health planning and county medical and health service system planning, respectively. Efforts shall be made to fully fulfill the government responsibilities for investment in public hospitals. (The National Health and Family Planning Commission, the National Development and Reform Commission and the Ministry of Finance respectively shall be in charge of the above task.)

(4) Improve the scientific compensation mechanism. Efforts shall be made to consolidate the reform results of eliminating drug markups in public hospitals, and eliminate drug markups in all public hospitals in the newly added pilot cities (excluding Chinese herbal pieces). Efforts shall be made to improve the compensation mechanisms for adjusting the price of medical services, increasing government subsidies, reforming the way hospitals pay for them, and strengthening hospitals' accounting and saving operating costs. The state policy on price adjustment for medical services shall be implemented to establish a mechanism for dynamic price adjustment of medical services on the basis of changes in the cost and income

structure. In line with the principle of "total control, structural adjustment, ups and downs and gradual implementation", the price relations between medical institutions at different levels and medical service items shall gradually be sorted out. Prices of medical services shall be further straightened out based on the steps of "making room, adjusting the structure and ensuring the connection". The cost of drugs, equipment and consumables shall be reduced through centralized procurement, cost control of healthcare insurance and standardization of medical treatment. The unreasonable cost of inspection and test shall be strictly controlled to make room for adjusting the price of medical services. Since the price of medical services shall be adjusted step by step, the price only for the elimination of drug markups shall not be adjusted, and the part of adjustment shall be included in the payment of healthcare insurance as required. Efforts shall be made to strengthen the coordinated connection of policies, such as medical service price, payment for healthcare insurance, control of medical expenditures, and hierarchical diagnosis and treatment, so as to ensure the sustainable development of medical institutions and affordability of medical insurance fund without increasing the burden on the people on the whole. The pilot cities for the reform of public hospitals shall carry out price adjustment of medical services, and the pilot provinces for comprehensive healthcare reform shall take the lead in implementing it. (The National Health and Family Planning Commission, the National Development and Reform Commission, the Ministry of Human Resources and Social Security, the Ministry of Finance and the State Administration of Traditional Chinese Medicine respectively shall be in charge of the above task.)

(5) Improve the management system of public hospitals. Efforts shall be made to formulate guiding documents for the establishment of management system for modern hospitals, and implement the autonomy of staff management, internal distribution and operations management of modern hospitals. Pilot cities shall establish and improve comprehensive performance evaluation index systems of public hospitals to introduce a third party for conducting performance evaluation. Efforts shall be made to promote professionalization and specialization for hospital presidents, and set up a mechanism for training and certification, assessment of tenure goals and responsibilities, and corresponding incentives and constraints for them. Efforts shall be made to strengthen financial budget management, implement comprehensive budget management for public hospitals, and promote the implementation of general accountant system for third-level public hospitals.(The National Health and Family Planning Commission, the National Development and Reform Commission, the Ministry of Human Resources and Social Security, the State Commission Office for Public Sectors Reform, the Ministry of Finance, the Ministry of Education and the State Administration of Traditional Chinese Medicine shall be in

charge of the above task.)

(6) Deepen the reform of the staffing system. Within the current local staffing, the staffing of public hospitals shall be rationally checked and ratified. Efforts shall be made to develop innovative ways of management for institutional staffing, and gradually implement the staffing filing system. Pilot reform of the staffing management of public hospitals shall be explored where conditions permit. In terms of post establishment, income distribution, professional title evaluation, management and use, the treatment of both internal and external staff shall be taken into full account. And the reform of old-age insurance system shall be promoted according to the regulations of the State. The employment system, the post management system and the open recruitment system shall be further improved. And high-level talents and urgently-needed talents of hospitals shall be recruited by hospitals in an examination way by rules, with the results open to public. (The State Commission Office for Public Sectors Reform, the Ministry of Human Resources and Social Security, National Health and Family Planning Commission and the Ministry of Finance respectively shall be in charge of the above task, with the participation of the State Administration of Traditional Chinese Medicine.)

(7) Establish a salary system in line with the characteristics of medical and healthcare industry. Efforts shall be made to organize and improve the pilot work of reforming the salary system of public hospitals, intensify our exploration, and promptly summarize our pilot experience. Pilot cities shall be encouraged to explore and formulate measures for evaluating the total amount of performance salary of public hospitals, and establish a distribution and incentive mechanism closely related to job responsibilities, job performance and actual contributions. Efforts shall be made to reflect the value of technical services for medical workers, standardize the pattern of income distribution, gradually improve the income and welfare of medical workers and mobilize their enthusiasm. The performance salary of the presidents of public hospitals shall be determined by government-run healthcare institutions. It shall be strictly forbidden to set any revenue target for medical staff, and medical staff's salary shall not be linked to business revenue from drugs, consumables, medical examinations and laboratory test of hospitals. (The Ministry of Human Resources and Social Security, the Ministry of Finance and the National Health and Family Planning Commission shall be in charge of the above task.)

(8) Exercise strict control over the unreasonable increase in medical expenses. Efforts shall be made to promote the implementation of the *Several Opinions on Controlling the Unreasonable Increase in Medical Expenses in Public Hospitals* by the National Health and Family Planning Commission as well as some other departments. According to the levels and growth of medical expenses in different regions, as well

as the functional positioning of different types of hospitals, each province (region and city) shall classify and determine the cost control requirements, and make dynamic adjustments. A target for increase in medical expenses nationwide shall be set. By the end of June 2016, all localities shall have reasonably determined and quantified the growth size of regional medical expenses in light of the actual situation. To strengthen supervision and inspection, regularly rank and publicize the control of medical expenses in various provinces (autonomous regions and municipalities directly under the Central Government) shall be regularly ranked and publicized. In pilot cities for the reform of public hospitals, specific lists shall be drawn up to monitor the unreasonable use of high-priced drugs, such as auxiliary drugs and nutritional drugs. Efforts shall be made to initially curb the unreasonable growth of medical expenses. (The National Health and Family Planning Commission, the National Development and Reform Commission, the Ministry of Human Resources and Social Security, the Ministry of Finance, the State Administration of Traditional Chinese Medicine and local people's governments at all levels shall be in charge of the above task.)

(9) Promote the comprehensive reform of public TCM hospitals simultaneously. Efforts shall be made to implement the preferential policies for investment in TCM hospitals, and formulate and implement differentiated price adjustment and performance appraisal policies. Efforts shall also be made to establish a new mechanism for the operation of public TCM hospitals to safeguard public welfare and highlight the advantages of TCM. The promotion and application of clinical pathways shall be strengthened to guide local governments in adjusting the price of TCM services in a scientific and reasonable manner. (The State Administration of Traditional Chinese Medicine, the National Health and Family Planning Commission, the Ministry of Finance, the Ministry of Human Resources and Social Security and the National Development and Reform Commission shall be in charge of the above task.)

(10) Vigorously improve medical services. Efforts shall be made to further implement and improve the action plan for medical services. Focus shall be put on appointment diagnosis and treatment, day surgery, information push, settlement service, pharmaceutical service, emergency treatment and quality care. Tertiary hospitals shall fully implement appointment diagnosis and treatment to enhance the level of medical service, improve the feeling of medical treatment, and enhance the people's sense of access. The pilot provinces of comprehensive medical reform shall take the lead in promoting day surgery in urban tertiary hospitals, and expand the disease range of day surgery. The project to alleviate poverty through providing health assistance shall be implemented to ensure that the population in poverty shall have access to basic medical and health services. Efforts shall be made to establish and improve a mechanism for preventing and mediating medical disputes to protect the

legitimate rights and interests of both doctors and patients in accordance with the law, and strive to build a harmonious doctor-patient relationship. (The National Health and Family Planning Commission and the State Administration of Traditional Chinese Medicine shall be in charge of the above task, with the participation of China Disabled Persons' Federation.)

(11) Specific conditions and measures shall be formulated by the people's governments at or above the county level to provide nearby public rental housing for eligible medical workers of public hospitals. (The Ministry of Housing and Urban-Rural Development, the National Development and Reform Commission, the Ministry of Finance, the Ministry of Land and Resources and the National Health and Family Planning Commission shall be in charge of the above task.)

### II. Accelerating the construction for hierarchical medical system

(1) Accelerate the trials of hierarchical medical treatment. As required by "initial visit at primary-level healthcare institutions, two-way referral, separation of chronic diseases from acute diseases, and upper and lower linkage," efforts shall be made to accelerate hierarchical medical treatment, and pilot projects shall be carried out in about 70% of prefectures and cities, with focus on the pilot provinces for comprehensive medical reform and pilot cities for comprehensive reform of public hospitals. The rate of standardized diagnosis, treatment and management for patients with hypertension or diabetes in the pilot areas shall reach 30% or above. (The National Health and Family Planning Commission, the Ministry of Human Resources and Social Security, the State Administration of Traditional Chinese Medicine and the people's governments in the pilot areas shall be in charge of the above task, with the participation of China Disabled Persons' Federation.)

(2) Expand the contracted service for family doctors. Efforts shall be made to summarize the local mature experience in promoting family doctors' contracted service, formulate policy documents on improving contracted service and management, and establish and improve the general practitioner system. Contracted service for family doctors shall be carried out in 200 pilot cities for comprehensive reform of public hospitals. And other areas where conditions permit shall be encouraged to conduct trials for contracted service. By the end of 2016, the coverage of contracted service for urban family doctors shall reach 15% or above, and that of key groups, 30% or above. Efforts shall be made to define the connotation and standards of contracted service, standardize fees for contracted service, and improve the incentive and restraint mechanism for contracted service. The contracted service fee shall be shared by the healthcare insurance fund, the basic public health service funds

and resident individuals.(The National Health and Family Planning Commission, the Ministry of Human Resources and Social Security, the Ministry of Finance, the National Development and Reform Commission and the State Administration of Traditional Chinese Medicine shall be in charge of the above task, with the participation of China Disabled Persons' Federation.)

(3) Enhance the community-level service capacity. Efforts shall be made to strengthen the capacity building of community-level healthcare institutions and county-level hospitals. With focus on the higher rate of out-of-county disease referral, the promotion of appropriate technology shall be strengthened to improve the capacity of county-level hospitals in disease diagnosis and treatment. Doctors from urban hospitals at or above the second level shall be encouraged to have multi-site practice in community-based healthcare institutions. Medical and health care resources shall be promoted to flow toward community-based healthcare institutions and rural areas. With the performance-based pay system for primary-level medical and healthcare institutions further improved, staff welfare funds and incentive funds shall be drawn from the approved balance of revenues and expenditure in accordance with the provisions of the financial system. Efforts shall be made to implement financial management measures of community-level medical and healthcare institutions for approved tasks, approved revenues and expenditures, and subsidies for performance appraisal. Strengthening performance appraisal and taking effective measures shall not only mobilize the enthusiasm of primary-level healthcare institutions and medical workers, but also prevent new profit-seeking behaviors.(The National Health and Family Planning Commission, the National Development and Reform Commission, the Ministry of Finance, the Ministry of Human Resources and Social Security, the Ministry of Science and Technology and the State Administration of Traditional Chinese Medicine shall be in charge of the above task.)

(4) Improve the supporting policies. Efforts shall be made to explore ways to establish various modes of labor division and cooperation, including medical consortia and counterpart support, and improve the policies and measures for promoting and standardizing the construction of medical consortia in cities and counties. Differentiated healthcare insurance payment policies for healthcare institutions at different levels shall be improved. The gap between the starting line and the payment ratio of healthcare institutions at different levels shall be appropriately widened. Efforts shall be made to explore community-level health institutions where patients with chronic diseases pay per person. Effective incentive guidance shall take shape for healthcare institutions to implement functional orientation and for patients to reasonably choose healthcare institutions. Relevant technical documents shall be formulated for hierarchical medical treatment of common tumors, coronary

heart disease and cerebrovascular diseases, as well as the independently established agencies for pathology, examination, imaging and hemodialysis. The standards of admission, discharge and two-way referral for common diseases shall be defined to implement the functional orientations of general hospitals at the second and third levels, and to define the standards for medical service capacities. The separation of acute diseases and chronic diseases shall be promoted. Clinical pathways of 50 diseases shall be newly designed and revised to expand the coverage of clinical pathways and improve the management quality. Efforts shall be made to carry out clinical pathway management in all tertiary hospitals and over 80% of hospitals at level II. (The National Health and Family Planning Commission, the Ministry of Human Resources and Social Security and the State Administration of Traditional Chinese Medicine shall be in charge of the above task.)

### III. Consolidating and improving the universal healthcare system

(1) Strive to establish a stable and sustainable mechanism for adjusting funding and guarantee levels. With the participation rate of basic healthcare insurance stable at 95% or above, the per capita government subsidy standard for healthcare insurance for urban and rural residents shall be raised to 420 *yuan*, and the per capita personal payment shall increase correspondingly. The new funding shall mainly be used to raise the level of basic healthcare insurance and to increase support for critical illness insurance for urban and rural residents. The reimbursement rate for hospitalization expenses within the scope of healthcare insurance policy for urban and rural residents shall become stable at around 75%. Efforts shall be made to comprehensively push forward the total amount of payments control in accordance with the budget management of the healthcare insurance fund. Efforts shall be made to accelerate the establishment and improvement of a stable and sustainable mechanism for adjusting the proportions of funding and reimbursement for basic healthcare insurance. Efforts shall be made to elevate the pooling of basic healthcare insurance to prefectural and municipal levels, and encourage eligible regions to implement provincial-level pooling. The basic healthcare insurance network and out-of-town medical settlement throughout the country shall be accelerated to set up and perfect the out-of-town settlement platform at the state level. Efforts shall be made to gradually connect with the settlement system for out-of-town medical treatment in different provinces, and basically achieve direct settlement for hospitalization expenses of retirees in different provinces. By 2017, out-of-town expenses of hospitalization that meet the requirements of referral shall be settled directly. The merger and implementation of basic healthcare insurance and maternity insurance shall be promoted. Efforts shall be

made to study and improve individual healthcare insurance accounts for employees. (The Ministry of Human Resources and Social Security, the National Health and Family Planning Commission and the Ministry of Finance respectively shall be in charge of the above task.)

(2) Promote the integration of the basic healthcare insurance system for urban and rural residents. According to the national comprehensive arrangements, by the end of June 2016, all provinces (autonomous regions and municipalities directly under the Central Government) shall complete the overall deployment of comprehensively promoting the integration of healthcare insurance system for urban and rural residents. During the year, specific implementation plans shall be formulated and implemented in all areas under the overall planning. Regions where condition permits shall be encouraged to streamline their management systems. Management shall be innovated to improve management efficiency and service level. Efforts shall be made to support qualified commercial insurance institutions and other nongovernmental organizations in participating in local basic healthcare insurance services. (The Office of the Leading Group of the State Council for Deepening the Reform of the Medical and Healthcare System, the Ministry of Human Resources and Social Security, the National Health and Family Planning Commission and People's Governments of all provinces (autonomous regions, municipalities directly under the Central Government) respectively shall be in charge of the above task, with the participation of China Insurance Regulatory Commission.)

(3) Consolidate and improve the system of critical illness insurance and medical assistance for urban and rural residents. Efforts shall be made to achieve full coverage of critical illness insurance, so that more patients with critical illnesses shall be able to reduce their burden. With critical illness insurance policy improved, the preferential payment policy shall be implemented for the urban and rural population in poverty, including the impoverished people with established cards for archives, those with five guarantees supporting and those living on minimum government subsidy, so that the scope of benefits shall be further expanded and the level of benefits shall be elevated. Provinces (autonomous regions and municipalities directly under the Central Government) shall be encouraged to reasonably determine the scope of compliance medical expenses in light of the actual situation, further reduce the burden of patients with critical diseases, and carry out provincial pooling of critical illness insurance in areas where conditions permit. Efforts shall be made to standardize the handling of critical illness insurance, strengthen supervision, inspection, examination and assessment, and fulfill the responsibilities of the main contractors. The central government shall allocate 16 billion *yuan* for medical assistance in urban and rural areas. Medical assistance for major and critical diseases shall be comprehensively

carried out to actively guide social forces to participate in medical assistance. Efforts shall be made to promote and improve coherent policies that effectively link basic healthcare insurance, critical illness insurance, medical assistance, emergency medical assistance, commercial health insurance and charitable assistance. The system of emergency assistance for diseases shall be improved to guide local authorities for standards in their work. Measures for supplementing healthcare insurance for employees shall be improved. Efforts shall be made to organize and carry out multi-level and multi-form mutual medical aid activities for staff and employees. (The Office of the Leading Group of the State Council for Deepening the Reform of Medical and Healthcare System, the Ministry of Human Resources and Social Security, the National Health and Family Planning Commission, the Ministry of Civil Affairs, China Insurance Regulatory Commission and the Ministry of Finance respectively shall be in charge of the above task, with the participation of All China Federation of Trade Union and China Disabled Persons' Federation.)

(4) Further deepen the reform of the payment way for healthcare insurance. Efforts shall be made to formulate policies and measures for deepening the reform of the payment way for healthcare insurance, accelerate the reform of the payment way, and control the unreasonable growth of medical expenses. Local successful experience shall be popularized to systematically promote the reform for multiple payment methods, such as paying per person, paying by disease, paying by bed per day, and paying by total amount in advance. The regulation of healthcare insurance on the service for healthcare institutions shall be extended to the regulation on medical service behaviors of medical workers. Efforts shall be made to perform day surgery. (The Ministry of Human Resources and Social Security, the National Health and Family Planning Commission and the Ministry of Finance shall be in charge of the above task, with the participation of the State Administration of Traditional Chinese Medicine.)

(5) Promote the development of commercial health insurance. Efforts shall be made to guide the insurance industry in strengthening product innovation, enriching health insurance products and improving service level. Trials of preferential policies for individual income tax on health insurance shall be carried out to continuously improve and optimize pilot programs. Efforts shall be made to revise the administrative measures for health insurance, improve the relevant regulatory system for health insurance, and standardize the market order of commercial health insurance.(China Insurance Regulatory Commission, the Ministry of Human Resources and Social Security, the Ministry of Finance and the National Health and Family Planning Commission shall be in charge of the above task.)

## IV. Improving the mechanism for ensuring drug supply

(1) Consolidate and improve the essential drug system. Efforts shall be made to study the catalogue, production, logo, pricing, distribution and use of essential drugs, and implement unified policies to encourage local governments to explore ahead. Efforts shall be made to study the appropriate dosage and specifications of essential drugs for children, strengthen the training on clinical application of essential drugs and dispensatory, and reinforce the assistance in pharmaceutical services for poverty-stricken areas. The consistency evaluation for the quality and efficacy of generic drugs shall be promoted to do a good job in the sampling of all essential drugs. Efforts shall be made to continue to strengthen the monitoring of adverse reactions to national essential drug varieties, and issue drug safety information to the public in a timely manner. Special inspection, flight inspection and other various forms of supervision and inspection shall be carried out to investigate and deal with on file any violation of laws and regulations in the production and operation of essential drugs. Free supply of special drugs for HIV/AIDS shall be increased. Efforts shall be made to ensure essential drug use for the elderly. (The National Health and Family Planning Commission, the Ministry of Finance, the National Development and Reform Commission, the Ministry of Science and Technology, the Ministry of Industry and Information Technology, China Food and Drug Administration and the State Administration of Traditional Chinese Medicine respectively shall be in charge of the above task.)

(2) Comprehensively promote the centralized drug procurement of public hospitals. Efforts shall be made to continue to implement the *Guiding Opinions of the General Office of the State Council on Improving the Centralized Drug Procurement of Public Hospitals* (No.7 [2015] of the General Office of the State Council). With classified procurement implemented, in principle, there shall be no more than three dosage forms for each purchased drug, and no more than two types of specifications for each dosage form. Local experience and practices shall be popularized to encourage and guide inter-provincial & cross-regional joint procurement; joint procurement between certain regions within pilot provinces of comprehensive healthcare reform shall be encouraged. The order in which drugs are purchased and sold shall be optimized to narrow the circulation link. Pilot provinces of comprehensive healthcare reform shall implement "two-invoice system" within the provinces (production enterprises shall issue invoices in circulation enterprises once, while latter shall issue invoices at healthcare institutions once). Pilot cities for the comprehensive reform of public hospitals shall be encouraged to promote the "two-invoice system". What's more, hospitals and pharmaceutical manufacturers shall be encouraged to settle drug

payments directly, and pharmaceutical manufacturers and distribution companies shall settle distribution fees, in order to narrow the intermediate link and reduce artificially high price. The pilot work of national drug price negotiation shall be summarized and evaluated to gradually increase the number of drug varieties under negotiation, and reasonably reduce the prices of patented drugs and exclusive drugs. Local experience shall be summed up to promote and improve policies and measures; centralized procurement of high-value medical consumables and open online trading shall be further promoted. Pilot provinces of comprehensive healthcare reform shall select regions to carry out centralized procurement of high-value medical consumables, and take the lead in achieving breakthroughs. Efforts shall be made to further improve the standardization of national comprehensive management information platform for drug supply and security as well as the provincial centralized procurement platform for drugs, and improve the mechanism for sharing data on drug procurement. (The National Health and Family Planning Commission, China Food and Drug Administration, the National Development and Reform Commission, the Ministry of Industry and Information Technology, the Ministry of Commerce, the Ministry of Human Resources and Social Security and people's governments of pilot provinces for the comprehensive healthcare reform shall be in charge of the above task.)

(3) Improve the mechanism for setting drug price. Efforts shall be made to further improve the mechanism for setting drug price. The regulation of drug price shall be strengthened to improve the monitoring system for drug price; price fraud and monopoly shall be investigated and punished in accordance with the law to effectively maintain the market price order for drugs. Standards for drug payment for basic healthcare insurance shall be formulated in light of relevant national policies and requirements. Efforts shall be made to promote the separation of drugs in various forms, and hospitals shall be prohibited from restricting the outflows of prescriptions. Patients shall choose to purchase drugs at the outpatient pharmacy of the hospital or at the retail pharmacy by prescription. (The National Development and Reform Commission, the National Health and Family Planning Commission and the Ministry of Human Resources and Social Security respectively shall be in charge of the above task.)

(4) Establish a new order for drug production and distribution. Efforts shall be made to further improve the policy system for the management standard of drug production quality and for the management standard of drug marketing quality, and strictly supervise its implementation. Access to pharmaceutical trading enterprises shall be strictly granted to standardize the order of drug distribution. Efforts shall be made to crack down on all violations of laws and regulations in drug purchases and

sales, and prevent and curb unhealthy trends and corruption in the procurement of drugs, medical equipment and consumables. Classified and level-to-level management of retail pharmacies shall be tried out to encourage the development of chain drugstores. Efforts shall be made to organize trials to share prescription information, healthcare insurance settlement information and retail drug consumption information in healthcare institutions, and promote separation of medical treatment from drugs. (China Food and Drug Administration and the Ministry of Commerce respectively shall be in charge of the above task, with the participation of the Ministry of Human Resources and Social Security, the National Health and Family Planning Commission and the Ministry of Industry and Information Technology.)

(5) Improve our ability to ensure drug supply. Efforts shall be made to strengthen the safeguard and early warning for the supply of drugs in shortage, and establish a mechanism for multi-sector consultation. A number of hospitals and primary-level healthcare institutions shall be selected by provincial (regional and municipal) departments as monitoring sites for the shortage of drugs to improve the information reporting system for the shortage of drugs. A comprehensive evaluation system for clinical drug use with emphasis on essential drugs shall be established. The establishment of a regular drug shortage reserve system shall be promoted. For four varieties of completed fixed-point production, public healthcare institutions shall be organized to purchase them from the designated production enterprises as required, monitor the production and supply situation of bid-winning enterprises, and solve emerging problems in time. The range of pilot varieties of designated production shall be expanded to add about five new varieties. Efforts shall be made to support the construction of production bases for small varieties. Scientific innovation shall be intensified to implement the guiding policies to promote the development of China's medical equipment and medical industry. Efforts shall be made to accelerate the self-independent innovation and industrialization of major new drugs, and accelerate the development of domestically produced and branded medical devices. Efforts shall be made to deepen the reform of the review and approval system for pharmaceutical and medical devices. Efforts shall be made to further open special channels for the review and approval of drugs for special groups, such as children and the elderly, as well as drugs for rare diseases and drugs in urgent need of clinical use, and speed up the process of registration and evaluation. Efforts shall be made to establish an appointment system for production and distribution enterprises, focus on improving the level of drug distribution management in rural and remote areas, and improve the management of drug distribution in short supply areas. (The National Health and Family Planning Commission, the Ministry of Industry and Information Technology, the National Development and Reform Commission, China Food and Drug

Administration and the Ministry of Science and Technology shall be in charge of the above task.)

(6) Establish a special working panel. Efforts shall be made to formulate policy documents for improving drug production, circulation and application, with focus on deepening the reform of the drug review and approval system, and strive to solve the problems of standardized production and distribution order of drugs. Departmental collaboration shall be intensified to support the establishment and improvement of information system, and strengthen the connectivity between different information systems. With the regulation of drug quality strengthened, the establishment of a traceability mechanism for drug ex-factory price information shall be launched. Relevant price information shall be provided to departments of price, health and family planning, industry and information technology, and healthcare insurance management. Efforts shall be made to promote the establishment of a linkage mechanism between the traceability mechanism for drug ex-factory price information, the "two-invoice system" and the incentive mechanism for medical workers, and comprehensively implement measures to reduce the inflated drug prices. Efforts shall be intensified to promote the optimization and integration of pharmaceutical production and distribution enterprises, and standardize the drug distribution order. (China Food and Drug Administration, the Ministry of Industry and Information Technology, the National Development and Reform Commission, the Ministry of Finance, the Ministry of Commerce, the National Health and Family Planning Commission and the State Administration of Traditional Chinese Medicine shall be in charge of the above task.)

(7) Formulate opinions on deepening the reform in the area of drug distribution. (The National Health and Family Planning Commission, the Ministry of Commerce and China Food and Drug Administration shall be in charge of the above task.)

### V. Establishing and improving a comprehensive regulatory system

(1) Improve the legal system for medical and health regulation. Efforts shall be made to transform government functions, and further improve the comprehensive regulatory mechanism. Regulation in the course, beforehand and afterwards shall be strengthened to organize regular supervision and inspection. Efforts shall be made to strengthen the regulation of medical quality, and reinforce the oversight and inspection of medical service charges and prices. (The National Health and Family Planning Commission, the Legislative Affairs Office of the State Council, China Food and Drug Administration, the National Development and Reform Commission and the State Administration of Traditional Chinese Medicine shall be in charge of the

above task.)

(2) Establish a mechanism for disclosure of medical expenses and other information in healthcare institutions. Efforts shall be made to strengthen the regulation of the whole healthcare industry. All healthcare institutions in the region shall be incorporated into the unified planning and regulation of the local health and family planning administrative departments. (The National Health and Family Planning Commission and the State Administration of Traditional Chinese Medicine shall be in charge of the above task.)

(3) Intensify the oversight and law enforcement in the medical and health profession. Efforts shall be made to crack down on all forms of illegal medical practices, investigate and handle any violation of laws and regulations, speed up the development of a credit system for the pharmaceutical and health industries, and promote the legal practices of various healthcare institutions. (The National Health and Family Planning Commission, China Food and Drug Administration and the State Administration of Traditional Chinese Medicine shall be in charge of the above task.)

### VI. Strengthening the team building of health professionals

(1) Continue to strengthen the training of community-level health professionals with the focus on general practitioners. Efforts shall be made to improve policies regarding the employment and contract management of free rural order and directional medical students. We shall continue to do a good job in recruiting and training free medical undergraduates, and plan to recruit about 5,000 free medical undergraduates. (The National Health and Family Planning Commission, the Ministry of Education, the Ministry of Finance and the State Administration of Traditional Chinese Medicine shall be in charge of the above task, with the participation of the Ministry of Human Resources and Social Security.)

(2) Comprehensively organize and implement standardized the training for resident physicians. A standardized training program for 70, 000 resident physicians shall be added, with a total of 190, 000 in training. Efforts shall be made to strengthen the connotation construction and dynamic management of the standardized training base for resident physicians, conduct in-depth third-party evaluation, and strictly implement the exit mechanism. Efforts shall be made to pilot a standardized training system for specialized physicians. (The National Health and Family Planning Commission, the Ministry of Finance, the National Development and Reform Commission and the State Administration of Traditional Chinese Medicine shall be in charge of the above task, with the participation of the Ministry of Human Resources

and Social Security.)

(3) Support eligible medical colleges and universities in strengthening the training of pediatrics, psychiatrics and midwifery that are urgently needed. Efforts shall be made to adopt measures for promoting the training of pediatric talents in colleges and universities, the standardized training and enrollment of resident physicians to incline to pediatric specialty, the training of county-and city-level pediatricians on job transfer, and the increasing of the general practitioners' pediatric professional skills training and other measures, and strengthen the construction of pediatric staff team. As required by the number of graduates and job requirements, 5,000 pediatric residents shall be trained in a standardized way. The training of professionals in geriatric medicine, rehabilitation and health management shall be intensified. Efforts shall be made to improve the training mechanism for high-level medical professionals. (The National Health and Family Planning Commission, the Ministry of Education, the Ministry of Finance, the State Administration of Traditional Chinese Medicine and China Disabled Persons' Federation shall be in charge of the above task.)

(4) All provinces, autonomous regions and municipalities directly under the Central Government shall formulate detailed rules for the implementation of the review and evaluation of the professional titles for primary-level health professionals. (The people's governments of all provinces (autonomous regions, municipalities directly under the Central Government), the Ministry of Human Resources and Social Security, and the National Health and Family Planning Commission shall be in charge of the above task.)

(5) Continue to pilot special posts for general practitioners. Efforts shall be made to carry out supervision and inspection of the implementation of major policy measures for building a contingent of rural doctors, and promote the implementation of the policies. A pilot program shall be launched to test the qualification of rural general practitioners as assistant physicians. Vocational training for hospital presidents shall be strengthened. Efforts shall be made to continue to promote the talent project of inheriting and innovating traditional Chinese medicine. (The National Health and Family Planning Commission, the Ministry of Human Resources and Social Security, the Ministry of Finance, the State Administration of Traditional Chinese Medicine and the people's governments of pilot regions shall be in charge of the above task.)

### VII. Steadily improving the system of equal access to basic public health services

(1) Raise the per capita financial subsidy for basic public health services to 45 *yuan*. Efforts shall be made to optimize the existing service projects to expand the

service coverage. (The Ministry of Finance, the National Health and Family Planning Commission and the State Administration of Traditional Chinese Medicine shall be in charge of the above task.)

(2) Improve the mechanism of labor division and coordination, and implement the operational management and guidance of specialized public health institutions in implementing basic public health services to primary-level healthcare institutions. Efforts shall be made to strengthen the project performance appraisal, improve the assessment methods, strengthen the county and district level appraisal, and link the assessment results to the appropriation of funds. The monitoring and evaluation of project progress shall be strengthened to improve the management and payment methods of project funds, and allocate funds according to the quantity and quality of services provided. Efforts shall be made to carry out comprehensive supervision and inspection for the implementation of basic public health service projects. (The National Health and Family Planning Commission, the Ministry of Finance and the State Administration of Traditional Chinese Medicine shall be in charge of the above task.)

(3) Strengthen the work of health promotion and formulate guiding documents on strengthening health promotion and education. Efforts shall be made to implement major public health services such as the action plan for maternal and child health. Comprehensive prevention and control of birth defects shall be further reinforced to continue to implement the national free pre-pregnancy health examination program for eugenics. An action plan for promoting the health of shifting population shall be launched to comprehensively promote equal access to basic public health and family planning services for shifting population. Efforts shall be made to provide basic medical and healthcare services covering the whole process of childbirth, from premarital check-up and pre-pregnancy examination to healthcare during pregnancy and childbirth and children's health care. (The National Health and Family Planning Commission, the State Administration of Traditional Chinese Medicine and China Disabled Persons' Federation shall be in charge of the above task.)

(4) Promote the integration of primary-level family planning service organizations and women's and children's organizations. (The National Health and Family Planning Commission and the State Commission Office of Public Sectors Reform shall be in charge of the above task.)

### VIII. Promoting the construction of health information

(1) Comprehensively promote the development of a population health information platform at the national, provincial, municipal and county levels. Efforts

shall be made to speed up the development of information systems for the application of business in public health, family planning, medical care services, medical security, drug management and comprehensive management, and achieve connectivity. Efforts shall be made to promote the continuous recording of electronic health records and electronic medical records, and the licensing of information between different levels and types of medical institutions. (The National Health and Family Planning Commission, the National Development and Reform Commission, the Ministry of Finance and the State Administration of Traditional Chinese Medicine shall be in charge of the above task, with the participation of the Ministry of Industry and Information Technology, the Office of the Central Cyberspace Affairs Commission and the National Bureau of Statistics.)

(2) Select eligible regions and fields to be the first to advance the pilot application of big data in healthcare. Efforts shall be made to integrate health management and medical information resources to promote online services such as appointment diagnosis and treatment, online payment, online follow-up and online query of inspection results. Telemedicine, disease management, pharmaceutical services and other business applications shall be actively developed. Efforts shall be made to strengthen the application and development of big data in clinical medicine. (The National Health and Family Planning Commission, the National Development and Reform Commission, the Ministry of Finance and the State Administration of Traditional Chinese Medicine shall be in charge of the above task, with the participation of the Ministry of Industry and Information Technology, the Office of the Central Cyberspace Affairs Commission and the National Bureau of Statistics.)

(3) Select some provinces (cities) to carry out pilot work on electronic licenses of healthcare institutions, doctors and nurses. (The National Health and Family Planning Commission, the State Administration of Traditional Chinese Medicine and the people's governments of pilot provinces (cities) shall be in charge of the above task.)

### IX. Speeding up the Development of Healthcare Industry

(1) Implement the policy for nongovernmental hospitals. Efforts shall be made to conduct supervision and inspection of the *Notice of the General Office of the State Council on Issuing Policy Measures to Accelerate the Development of Nongovernmental Hospitals* (No. 45 [2015] of the General Office of the State Council.) (The National Development and Reform Commission and the National Health and Family Planning Commission shall be in charge of the above task. with the participation of the Ministry of Commerce and the State Administration of Traditional Chinese Medicine.)

(2) Steadily promote and standardize the multi-site practice of physicians. Efforts

shall be made to accelerate the transformation of government functions, soften terms, simplify procedures, and improve the policy environment for multi-sited practice of physicians. Efforts shall be made to give play to the "catfish effect" to enliven the employment mechanism. Doctors shall be encouraged to practice in community-level healthcare institutions, remote areas, areas where medical resources are scarce and other healthcare institutions in need, and promote the formation of a tiered medical system. Doctors and the first practice site in healthcare institutions shall sign a contract of employment (labor) on the basis of consensus to define the personnel (labor) relations, the rights and obligations, and participate in social insurance in accordance with relevant provisions of the state. The first practice site in healthcare institutions shall support doctors in multi-sited practice and improve internal management. Efforts shall be made to allow physicians working or retired in public hospitals to practice or establish workshops in community-level healthcare institutions on a pilot basis. (The National Health and Family Planning Commission and the State Administration of Traditional Chinese Medicine shall be in charge of the above task, with the participation of the Ministry of Human Resources and Social Security.)

(3) Implement the *Notice of the State Council on Issuing the Outline of the Development Strategy Plan for Traditional Chinese Medicine (2016-2030)* (No.15 [2016] of the State Council and the *Notice of the General Office of the State Council on Issuing the Development Plan for the Health Service of Traditional Chinese Medicine (2015-2020)* (No. 32 [2015] of the General Office of the State Council. Efforts shall be made to actively develop traditional Chinese medicine and ethnic minority medicine, and vigorously develop TCM health services. (The State Administration of Traditional Chinese Medicine, the National Development and Reform Commission and the National Health and Family Planning Commission shall be in charge of the above task.)

(4) Implement the *Notice Forwarded by the General Office of the State Council Concerning the Guiding Opinions on Promoting the Combination of Health Care and Elderly Care Service Issued by the National Health and Family Planning Commission and Other Departments* (No.84 [2015] of the General Office of the State Council). Efforts shall be made to establish and improve a collaboration mechanism between healthcare institutions and pension institutions, and promote the integration of traditional Chinese medicine and old-age care services. Nongovernmental organizations shall be encouraged to set up integrated medical and nursing institutions as well as specialized healthcare institutions for the rehabilitation and nursing of the aged. Efforts shall be made to promote the extension of healthcare services to communities and families. (The National Health and Family Planning Commission, the Ministry of Civil Affairs, the National Development and Reform Commission, the Ministry of Finance, the Ministry of Human Resources and Social Security and the State Administration of Traditional

Chinese Medicine shall be in charge of the above task, with the participation of the Ministry of Commerce.)

(5) Improve policy measures to promote the development of medical care tourism. (The National Health and Family Planning Commission and the State Administration of Traditional Chinese Medicine shall be in charge of the above task.)

### X. Strengthening Organization and Implementation

(1) Establish and improve a strong leadership system and work promotion mechanism for the healthcare reform organization. Deepening healthcare reform is a complicated and systematic project. As the current reform is going into the deep-water zone and the critical stage, all localities and departments concerned shall keep in mind the overall situation, actively participate in and support healthcare reform, take comprehensive measures, and form a cohesive force to overcome tough problems. Efforts shall be made to further strengthen organizational leadership, give full play to the coordinating role of the leading group on healthcare reform, and support and encourage the establishment of a unified management system for medical care, healthcare insurance and drugs. The responsibilities of government leadership, security, management and supervision shall be implemented. A restrictive mechanism shall be established to include healthcare reform in the assessment requirements of local governments. Efforts shall be made to adhere to the reform goals, refine work plans, strengthen policy implementation, clarify the responsibilities of local governments at all levels and relevant departments, set a timetable and route map, and promote the implementation of the reform policies and tasks. Efforts shall be made to strengthen the supervision and guidance, and reinforce supervision and accountability if the work is ineffective or progress is slow. (The National Health and Family Planning Commission and the local people's governments at all levels shall be in charge of the above tasks.)

(2) Further sum up and popularize the experience and practice of the pilot provinces for comprehensive healthcare reform. Efforts shall be made to sum up and improve the reform practice and experience of Sanming City in Fujian province, and promote it in Anhui, Fujian and other pilot provinces for comprehensive healthcare reform. A number of new pilot provinces for comprehensive healthcare reform shall be added, and comprehensive reform shall be carried out in a regionally coordinated way to further enhance the integrity, systematization and synergy of the reform. (The National Health and Family Planning Commission, the Ministry of Finance and the people's governments of the pilot cities for comprehensive healthcare reform shall be in charge of the above task.)

(3) Intensify efforts to promote healthcare reform. Efforts shall be made to adhere

to the correct orientation of public opinion, reinforce the interpretation and positive publicity of healthcare reform policies, eliminate doubt and confusion in a timely manner, respond to social concerns, and guide the people's reasonable expectations and medical treatment. Mature experience of primary-level organizations shall be summarized in a timely manner. Each province (region, city) shall combine the actual situation, strengthen the experience summary, and try to refine the replicable reform model for promotion. Efforts shall be made to strengthen the research on major policy issues such as the linkage between the tripartite healthcare institutions and public health. Efforts shall be made to promote the synergy between science and technology and medical care, further improve the layout of the national center for clinical medicine research and the collaborative research network for major diseases, and strengthen scientific and technological support for healthcare reform. (The National Health and Family Planning Commission, the Propaganda Department of the CPC Central Committee, the Ministry of Science and Technology and the people's governments of all provinces (autonomous regions, municipalities directly under the Central Government) shall be in charge of the above tasks.)

Appendix: The Divisions of Some Major Tasks and Scheduling

Appendix:The Divisions of Some Major Tasks and Scheduling

| No. | Tasks | Departments in Charge | Time Schedule |
|---|---|---|---|
| 1 | To formulate the healthcare reform plan in the 13th Five-Year Plan period | The Office of the Leading Group of the State Council for Deepening the Reform of the Medical and Health System | To be completed by the end of June 2016 |
| 2 | To launch the expansion of trials of comprehensive reform of urban public hospitals and increase provincial-level trials of comprehensive healthcare reform | The Office of the Leading Group of the State Council for Deepening the Reform of the Medical and Health System | To be completed by the end of May 2016 |
| 3 | To formulate guiding documents on establishing a management system for modern hospitals | The National Health and Family Planning Commission | To be completed by the end of Sept. 2016 |
| 4 | To formulate policy measures to deepen the reform of healthcare insurance payment methods | The Ministry of Human Resources and Social Security, the National Health and Family Planning Commission and the Ministry of Finance | To be completed by the end of June 2016 |
| 5 | To revise the administrative measures for health insurance | China Insurance Regulatory Commission | To be completed by the end of Oct. 2016 |
| 6 | To formulate policy documents on improving the contracted service and management for family doctors | The Office of the Leading Group of the State Council for Deepening the Reform of the Medical and Health System | To be completed by the end of Oct. 2016 |

*Continued*

| No. | Tasks | Departments in Charge | Time Schedule |
|---|---|---|---|
| 7 | To improve policy measures to promote and standardize the construction of medical unions in cities and counties | The National Health and Family Planning Commission | To be completed by the end of Sept. 2016 |
| 8 | To study and formulate policy documents on improving the production, distribution and use of drugs, with focus on deepening the reform of drug review and approval system | China Food and Drug Administration, the National Development and Reform Commission, the Ministry of Industry and Information Technology, the Ministry of Commerce and the National Health and Family Planning Commission | To be completed by the end of Dec. 2016 |
| 9 | To formulate policy measures to improve the mechanism for ensuring drug supply | The National Health and Family Planning Commission | To be completed by the end of Oct. 2016 |

**(Shan Yongxiang)**

## Notice of the General Office of the State Council on Issuing the Arrangements for Key Work on Food Safety in 2016

(No. 30 [2016] of the General Office of the State Council)

The people's governments of all provinces, autonomous regions, and municipalities directly under the Central Government; all ministries and commissions of the State Council; and all institutions directly under the State Council:

*The Arrangements for Key Work on Food Safety in 2016* has been approved by the State Council and is hereby forwarded to you for earnest implementation.

General Office of the State Council

April 27th, 2016

### 20. Arrangements for Key Work on Food Safety in 2016

In 2015, the situation of food safety remained stable and was turning for the better nationwide. However, the basis for food safety was still weak and potential risks should not be ignored. We hereby make the following arrangements for the key work on food safety in 2016 in order to implement the spirit of the CPC's 18th National Congress, the third, the fourth and the fifth plenary sessions of the 18th National Congress, the Central Committee's economic work conference and the Central Committee's agricultural work conference, implement the deployments of the State Council on food safety work and further improve the curbing capability and guarantee level of food safety work.

## I. Accelerating the improvement of food safety law and regulations

Efforts shall be made to fully publicize and implement the newly revised food safety laws and cooperate with the Standing Committee of the National People's Congress to carry out law enforcement and inspection on food safety law. (China Food and Drug Administration Food Safety Office of the State Council in conjunction with the people's governments at the provincial level shall be responsible.) Efforts shall be made to promote the enactment and revision of *Agricultural Product Quality Safety Law, Grain Law, Regulation on the Implementation of the Food Safety Law, Regulation on Pesticide Administration* and *Regulations on the Administration of the Slaughter of Livestock and Poultry etc.* (Ministry of Agriculture, China Food and Drug Administration, Legislative Affairs Office of the State Council, and State Administration of Grain shall be responsible.) Reform of food production and trading licenses shall be deepened. (China Food and Drug Administration shall be responsible.) Efforts shall be made to accelerate the enactment and revision of regulations on labeling administration, supervision and inspection, on-line food trading, registration of special food, administration of health food inventory, supervision and administration of food safety in railway operations and supervision and administration of food at national frontier ports etc. (National Health and Family Planning Commission, General Administration of Quality Supervision, Inspection and Quarantine, China Food and Drug Administration and China Railway shall be responsible.) *Implementation Outline for Building a Government Ruled by Law (2015-2020)* shall be carried out to improve the procedure of food safety administrative law enforcement, regulate law enforcement behaviors and fully implement the accountability system of administrative law enforcement. (Ministry of Agriculture and China Food and Drug Administration shall be responsible.) The investigation of food adulteration and counterfeiting and other criminal responsibility shall be intensified. (Committee of *Political and Legislative* Affairs and China Food and Drug Administration shall be responsible.)

## II. Improving standard system for food safety

National standard catalogue and local standard catalogues for food safety shall be established and published. (National Health and Family Planning Commission and Ministry of Agriculture in conjunction with all the provincial governments shall be responsible.) The enactment and revision of a batch of key standards for food safety and standards for pesticide and veterinary medicine residue shall be sped up. The publication of integrated national standards for food safety shall be sped up and other relevant standards for food shall be annulled or revised. A working mechanism for the enactment, modification and publication of the national standards of food safety shall be established, tracing evaluation strengthened and the coordination between standard enactment and law enforcement enhanced. (National Health and Family Planning Commission, Ministry of Agriculture, China Food and Drug Administration and General Administration of Quality Supervision, Inspection and Quarantine shall be responsible.) *Working Plan for Accelerating and Improving Standard System for Pesticide Residue in China (2015-2020)* shall be implemented, and new standards shall be enacted including 1,000 standards for pesticide residue, 100 standards for veterinary medicine residue and 300 sectorial standards for agriculture. (Ministry of Agriculture, National Health and Family Planning Commission and China Food and Drug Administration shall be responsible.) The national risk monitoring plan for food safety shall be implemented. (National Health and Family Planning Commission shall be responsible.)

### III. Strengthening the control over edible farm produce from the source

Such measures shall be taken as improvement of standards, formulation of conduct norms, strengthening of sample inspection and establishment of traceability systems etc., and a strict management system for the use of agricultural inputs adopted; special cracking down shall be launched on prohibited pesticides, "Three Fish Two Medicines" (the illegal use of malachite green and nitrofuran for mandarin fish, turbot and snakeheaded fish), antibacterials for animals and clenbuterol as well as the comprehensive rectification on the illegal use of antibacterials for livestock, poultry and aquatic products, with special efforts to solve the problem of residual of pesticides or veterinary medicine. The management system for the plantation of edible farm produces and the breeding of livestock, poultry and aquatic products shall be implemented to regulate the production and trading behaviors. Violations of laws and regulations shall be severely investigated and dealt with such as illegally adding illicit drugs, buying and slaughtering sick or dead livestock or poultry, and making and selling fake agricultural products. A list for the supervision of key risks and hidden dangers shall be established, inspections and supervision & spot inspections intensified and inspection and cracking down implemented coordinately. The construction of "Three Gardens and Two Fields" (standard garden for vegetable, standard garden for fruit, standard garden for tea and standard demonstration field for livestock and poultry breeding and health field for aquaculture) shall be strengthened with the advantageous regions of edible farm produces and products under "vegetable basket"(non-grain food supply) program as the key to promote the standardization production of agriculture. Safe and high-quality food products will be vigorously developed such as pollution-free food, green food, organic food, and edible farm produces with geographical indications. (The Ministry of Agriculture shall be responsible.) Environmental protection at the place of production and control from the source shall be strengthened. Control over air, water and soil pollution shall be intensified to reduce the impact of pollutant emissions on food safety. (Ministry of Environmental Protection and Ministry of Agriculture in conjunction with provincial governments shall be responsible.) Measures by the State Council on strengthening control over heavy metal pollution on grains shall be implemented. (Food Safety Office of the State Council, National Development and Reform Commission, Ministry of Science and Technology, Ministry of Finance, Ministry of Land and Resources, Ministry of Environmental Protection, Ministry of Agriculture, China Food and Drug Administration and State Administration of Grain in conjunction with relevant provincial governments shall be responsible.) Supervision and inspection on the quality safety of food from overseas sources shall be intensified, and the construction of demonstration areas for the quality safety of exported farm produces shall be further promoted. (General Administration of Quality Supervision, Inspection and Quarantine shall be responsible.) Standards for the construction and operation of cold-chain logistics for edible farm produces and food shall be improved to better the level of cold-chain logistics. (National Development and Reform Commission, Ministry of Agriculture, Ministry of Commerce, General Administration of Quality Supervision, Inspection and Quarantine and China Food and Drug Administration shall be responsible.)

## IV. Strengthening measures for risk prevention and control

Study on the division of power for administrative review and approval, random inspection and monitoring, supervision and inspection shall be carried out to improve the supervisory system with clear division of power and matching power & responsibilities. Studies shall be carried out on establishing a risk rating system and enacting measures for the tiered management of risks for food production and trading to promote the implementation of tiered supervision and administration. (China Food and Drug Administration shall be responsible.) Programs for sample inspection on the quality safety of food and edible farm produces shall be coordinated to achieve the reasonable division of labor and complete coverage between the central government and the local governments, and departments and departments so that the supervision and sample inspection shall be really carried out for the residue of pesticides and veterinary medicines, additives and heavy metal pollution in the daily consumed food. (Food Safety Office of the State Council, Ministry of Agriculture and China Food and Drug Administration shall be responsible.) The risk consulting and pre-waring & communicating mechanisms of food safety shall be improved, data from food safety risk monitoring, and supervision & sampling inspection shall be integrated with those from risk monitoring of edible farm produces and supervision & sampling inspection to intensify date analysis and improve the efficiency of data using. Emergency response shall be strengthened and an information reporting system for emergencies and a monitoring system for public opinions shall be established to expand the channels and forms of risk communication. (Food Safety Office of the State, Ministry of Agriculture, National Health and Family Planning Commission, General Administration of Quality Supervision, Inspection and Quarantine, China Food and Drug Administration, and State Administration of Grain shall be responsible.) Evaluation shall be strengthened on the quality of farm produces and food safety risks. (Ministry of Agriculture and National Health and Family Planning Commission shall be responsible.) Information publication mechanism shall be improved to publicize information on administrative licensing, supervision & sample inspection, administrative penalty and accountability etc. (China Food and Drug Administration shall be responsible.) Reform shall be launched on the inspection and supervision mechanism at ports for imported food and supervision & sample inspection system for exported food. (General Administration of Quality Supervision, Inspection and Quarantine shall be responsible.)

### V. Comprehensive rectification of prominent and key problems

Lists shall be made for hidden dangers for food safety, prominent problems and supervisory measures. Management shall be standardized for the registration of the formula of infant formula milk powder product, formula food for special medical use and health food. Supervision shall be strengthened on infant formula milk powder, infant food supplements, dairy, meat products, liquor, seasoned flour products, edible vegetable oil, food additives and other key products. (China Food and Drug Administration shall be responsible.) Such prominent problems as the illegal adding and exceeding the limits and amounts of food additives shall be especially curbed. Special inspections shall be launched on imported edible vegetable oil, aquaculture products, meat products, liquor and other key products and comprehensive inspection shall be launched for the quality safety of imported infant formula milk powder. (General Administration of Quality Supervision, Inspection and Quarantine and China Food and Drug Administration shall be responsible.) Efforts shall be made to properly handle the purchase and disposal of contaminated grain and prevent it from entering the grain market. (State Administration of Grain, National Commission of Development and Reform and Ministry of Finance, Ministry of Agriculture in conjunction with relevant provincial governments shall be responsible.) Management of food safety in rural areas shall be strengthened, collective dinning in the rural areas regulated, food safety in school dining halls or around school campuses rectified and joint supervision and examination launched in key dining areas such as tourist destinations and railway stations etc. (China Food and Drug Administration, Ministry of Education, China National Tourism Administration, and China Railway shall be responsible.) The operation of wholesale markets for edible farm produces and the on-line operation of food products shall be standardized. (China Food and Drug Administration shall be responsible.)

### VI. Strictly implementing primary responsibility of production and operation

The sense of primary responsibility for food production and operation shall be strengthened to urge the enterprises to strictly implement such manage systems as training and examination, self-inspection of risks, product recall, whole-process record and emergency handling etc. and strengthen the managing and controlling measures for food safety that cover the whole process of food production and operation. Examination and verification system shall be imposed on foreign enterprises by the food importers and registration shall be strictly implemented for foreign manufacturers of imported food. Special supervision and inspection of food related certification shall be carried out. "See-through kitchens" and tiered management for catering service enterprises shall be carried on. Efforts shall be made to promote the establishment of a normalized mechanism for interviewing on corporate responsibility. (China Food and Drug Administration and General Administration of Quality Supervision, Inspection and Quarantine shall be responsible.) Enterprises shall be urged and guided to establish by law the traceability system for meat products, vegetables, infant formula milk powder, liquor, edible vegetable oil and other key products. (Ministry of Industry and Information Technology, Ministry of Agriculture, Ministry of Commerce, Administration of Quality Supervision, Inspection and Quarantine and China Food and Drug Administration shall be responsible.) The construction of food safety credit system shall be strengthened, the campaign of food safety commitment launched and a mechanism that incents good credits and punishes cracking credits improved. (National Commission of Development and Reform, Ministry of Industry and Information Technology, State Administration for Industry

& Commerce and China Food and Drug Administration shall be responsible.) The food safety liability insurance system shall be promoted to encourage food production and operation enterprises to participate in food safety liability insurance. (Food Safety Office of the State Council, China Food and Drug Administration and China Insurance Regulatory Commission shall be responsible.)

### VII. Continuing to severely punish violations of laws

Focusing on investigating and handling such cases as frozen goods smuggling, producing edible oil with chicken waste and waste from slaughter processing, and crimes of Internet food safety etc., we shall strengthen cross-department and cross-region communication and collaboration in case transfer, supervision and handling, joint punishment and information release. Systematic analysis shall be strengthened about the clues on violation of law and case information, common problems summarized in a timely manner and the industry's "hidden rules" cracked down on according to law. Serious violations of laws shall be severely cracked down on continually, such as the illegally adding, producing and selling fake, and illegally using pesticide and veterinary medicine whose use are prohibited or limited and more about the key cases shall be exposed. (Central Committee of Political and Legislative Affairs, Ministry of Industry and Information Technology, Ministry of Public Security, Ministry of Agriculture, General Administration of Customs, State Administration for Industry and Commerce, General Administration of Quality Supervision, Inspection and Quarantine, and China Food and Drug Administration shall be responsible.)

### VIII. Strengthening the capacity building for food safety supervision

The national plan for food safety during the 13th Five-Year Plan period shall be compiled, policy support increased and supporting measures strengthened. The national medium- and long-term strategic plan for food safety shall be compiled which shall propose development goals, major tasks and comprehensive supporting measures, and implementation steps shall be clarified. (Food Safety Office of the State Council in conjunction with the members of the Food Safety Committee of the State Council shall be responsible.) The capacity building for the quality safety of edible farm produces and supervision and law enforcement of food safety shall be strengthened. The capacity building for the safety testing (monitoring) of edible farm produces and food shall be strengthened continually and the purchase of testing and inspection equipment and the renovation of laboratories shall be supported to improve the capacity of testing and inspection at the community level.

*Opinions of the General Office of the State Council on Accelerating the Advancement of the Construction of Important Product Information Traceability Systems* (No. 95 [2015], General Office of the State Council) shall be implemented to advance the development of important informationalization projects, accelerate the construction of national informationalization projects and platform for food safety supervision, advance the construction of information platform for the traceability management of edible farm produces' quality safety, so that with unified standards and connectivity and communication, food safety information shall be interconnected and shared soon. (National Commission of Development and Reform, Ministry of Industry and Information Technology, Ministry of Agriculture, Ministry of Commerce, National Health and Family Planning Commission, State Administration of Industry and Commerce, General Administration of Quality Supervision, Inspection and Quarantine, China Food and Drug Administration and General Administration of Quality Supervision, Inspection and Quarantine and State Administration of Grain shall be responsible.) Regulations shall be enacted on the construction and management of quality and safety supervision stations at the township level for farm produces and exploration shall be made to establish the system of certified supervisors at the township level. (Ministry of Agriculture shall be responsible.) Risk monitoring, supervision & law enforcement and training of technical personnel shall be intensified, and the capacity building for food safety risk monitoring shall be strengthened as well as the standardization building of basic law enforcement equipment for food supervision to improve the level of equipment and ensure the responsibility, posts, personnel and methods of risk monitoring and supervision at the community level. (National Commission of Development and Reform, Ministry of Finance, National Health and Family Planning Commission and China Food and Drug Administration in conjunction with all the provincial governments shall be responsible.) Supervision and law enforcement behaviors at the community level shall be regulated, the gridding of supervision at the community level, the charting of on-site inspection and the opening of persons responsible for supervision promoted, and the on-site inspection capacity of community-level supervisory departments strengthened for breeding, production, processing, marketing and catering enterprises. (Ministry of Agriculture and China Food and Drug Administration shall be responsible.) The building of designated ports for imported food in inland areas shall be pushed forward and a big data platform for the supervision of the safety of imported and exported food shall be established. (General Administration of Quality Supervision, Inspection and Quarantine shall be responsible.)

## IX. Implementing responsibility system for food safety

Responsibility system for food safety shall be strengthened, methods for the evaluation of food safety work formulated, and supervision and evaluation of food safety further intensified; the quality of edible farm produces and food safety shall be fully included in the scope of the performance evaluation and comprehensive social management evaluation for the local governments, and the results of the evaluations shall be the important basis for the comprehensive evaluation of the leading bodies and relevant leaders. Efforts shall be made to urge the local governments to establish and improve the smooth connecting mechanism between "origin permits" system and "market access" system for farm produces and enact methods for the management of the small workshops of food production and trading, peddlers and small catering businesses. Efforts shall be made to urge the supervisory departments to effectively fulfill their responsibility of daily inspection and supervision & sample inspection. Efforts shall be made to urge local governments to appraise and evaluate the food and drug regulatory departments at the same levels and other relevant departments on food safety supervision and management. (Food Safety Office of the State Council, Legislative Affairs Office of the State Council, Ministry of Agriculture and China Food and Drug Administration in conjunction with all the provincial governments shall be responsible.) Pilot program on the construction of food safety cities and quality safety counties of farm produces shall be carried forward, and experience on the pilot shall be summarized and spread in a timely manner. (Food Safety Office of the State Council, Ministry of Agriculture and China Food and Drug Administration in conjunction with relevant provincial governments shall be responsible.) Negative list, power list and responsibility list shall be compiled and implemented. Responsibility system for food safety shall be improved at all levels and accountability system for food safety shall be formulated. Accountability for food safety shall be strictly carried out and those responsible for dereliction of duty or malfeasance shall be severely punished. (China Food and Drug Administration and Ministry of Supervision shall be responsible.)

## X. Promoting social collaborative governance for food safety

The capacity building for complaining and reporting system shall be strengthened and the channel for complaining and reporting shall be kept open. National Publicity Week for Food Safety shall be launched. Radios, televisions, newspapers, magazines and web portals shall be encouraged to set up columns on food safety and new media like "WeChat", "Weibo" and mobile client shall be used to enhance the publicity of public welfare and popular science on food safety. (Member entities of Food Safety Committee of the State Council and all the provincial governments shall be responsible.) Risk warning or consumption tips on food safety shall be announced to protect the rights of the consumers in an effective manner. (State Administration of Industry and Commerce, General Administration of Quality Supervision, Inspection and Quarantine and China Food and Drug Administration shall be responsible.) Efforts shall be made to promote food industry associations to strengthen self-discipline of the industry, guide and urge food producers and operators to produce and operate by law strictly and publicize and popularize food safety knowledge. (Ministry of Industry and Information Technology, Ministry of Commerce and China Food and Drug Administration shall be responsible.) Efforts shall be made to promote the merge and reorganization of infant formula milt powder enterprises. (Ministry of Industry and Information Technology in conjunction with National Development and Reform Commission, Ministry of Finance and China Food and Drug Administration shall be responsible.) Efforts shall be made to organize research on the key technology of food safety, establish shared database for food safety and promote the new development of Internet Plus food safety inspection and testing. Innovation project for food safety shall be implemented and demonstration of technological innovation shall be launched. (Ministry of Science and Technology shall be responsible.) Food safety education shall be included in relevant courses in primary and middle schools. (Ministry of Education shall be responsible.) Social forces shall be mobilized to participate in food safety supervision, the team of food safety informants and coordinators at the community level shall be given full play to and trade unions, the communist youth league and women's federations at all levels shall take food safety supervision as a part of the voluntary service work. (Food Safety Office of the State Council, China Food and Drug Administration, All China Federation of Trade Union, the Central Committee of Communist Youth League and the All-China Women's Federation shall be responsible.)

### XI. Improving unified and authoritative supervision system

The improvement of the unified and authoritative supervision system and institution shall be accelerated to render food safety supervision more professional and systematic. Opinions shall be formulated on improving the unified and authoritative food and drug supervision system. (Food Safety Office of the State Council, China Food and Drug Administration and State Commission Office for Public Sector Reform shall be responsible.) A professional inspection team shall be established to strengthen the inspection force. (China Food and Drug Administration,

State Commission Office for Public Sector Reform and Ministry of Human Resources and Social Security shall be responsible.) The technical position system shall be researched on that is suitable for the characteristics of food safety supervision. (China Food and Drug Administration and Ministry of Human Resources and Social Security shall be responsible.) Supervisory approaches with on-site inspection as the main approach shall be implemented to lead the supervisory forces down to the community level. (China Food and Drug Administration shall be responsible.) Food safety offices at all levels shall play their role of making overall planning and coordinating & urging to the full, and strengthen the coordination & cooperation in information notification, publicity & education, hidden danger screening and combating crimes. Efforts shall be made to clarify the assignment of responsibility among member entities of food safety committees, and improve the situation consultation, risk communication, emergency handling, coordination & cooperation and other working mechanisms. (Food Safety Office of the State Council shall be responsible.)

**(Zhao Xuemei)**

## 21. Plan for the Pilot Program of the System of the Drug Marketing Authorization Holders

In accordance with *the Decision of the Standing Committee of the National People's Congress on Authorizing the State Council to Conduct the Pilot Program of the System of the Drug Marketing Authorization Holders in Certain Areas and the Relevant Issues*, the pilot program of the system of the drug marketing authorization holders is to be conducted in ten provinces (cities), namely, Beijing, Tianjin, Hebei, Shanghai, Jiangsu, Zhejiang, Fujian, Shandong, Guangdong and Sichuan. The following plan is hereby made for effectively conducting the pilot work.

### I. Contents of the pilot program

The drug research and development institutions and scientific research personnel within pilot administrative regions may file drug clinical trial applications and drug marketing applications as drug registration applicants (hereinafter referred to as "applicants"), and the applicants that obtain drug marketing licenses and drug approval numbers are eligible as the drug marketing authorization holders (hereinafter referred to as "holders"). The relevant legal liabilities for drug clinical trials and drug production and marketing as prescribed in laws and regulations shall be undertaken by the applicants and holders.

The holder that does not possess the corresponding qualification shall entrust a qualified drug production enterprise (hereinafter referred to as an "entrusted production enterprise") within the pilot administrative region to produce the drug approved to be marketed. Where a holder possesses the corresponding production qualification, it may conduct production by itself or authorize an entrusted production enterprise to conduct production.

During the period of review and approval or after the approval of a drug registration application, an applicant or holder may file a supplementary application for the modification of the applicant, holder or entrusted production enterprise.

### II. Scope of pilot drugs

(1) New drugs approved to be marketed after the implementation of this Plan, including: 1) chemical drugs of Class I through Class IV and Class V (only limited to targeting preparations, sustained released preparations and controlled released preparations) declared according to registration classification in the current *Measures for the Administration of Drug Registration*, traditional Chinese medicines and natural medicines of Class I through Class VI, biological products for curative uses of Class I and Class VII and biosimilars; and 2)chemical drugs of Class I and Class II declared according to the new chemical drug registration classification (hereinafter referred to as "new registration classification") after the reform of the chemical drug registration classification).

(2) Generic drug approved to be marketed according to the new standards consistent with those for the quality and efficacy of reference listed drugs, including chemical drugs of Class III and Class IV declared according to the new chemical drug registration classification after the reform of the chemical drug registration classification.

(3) Certain drugs that have been approved to be marketed before the implementation of this Plan, including: 1) drugs that have passed the quality and efficacy consistency evaluation; and 2) the drugs whose drug approval numbers are held by the drug production enterprises which are relocated in their entirety or are relocated in their entirety after they are merged within the pilot administrative regions.

Narcotic drugs, psychotropic substances, toxic drugs for medical treatment, radioactive drugs, preventive biological products and blood products are not included in the scope of pilot drugs.

### III. Conditions for applicants and holders

To be eligible as applicants and holders, drug research and development institutions or scientific research personnel shall meet the following conditions:

(1) Basic conditions.

1) They fall within the scope of the drug research and development, institutions that are legally formed within the pilot administrative regions and are capable of assuming liabilities independently, or the scientific research personnel who work within the pilot administrative regions and are of the nationality of the People's Republic of China.

2) They are capable of assuming liabilities of drug quality safety.

(2) Application dossiers:

1) Qualification dossiers.

A) Drug research and development institutions shall submit photocopies of legal registration certificates (business licenses, etc.).

B) Scientific research personnel shall submit photocopies of their resident identity cards, personal credit reports, work resumes (including education background, work experience of drug research and development, etc.) and letters of integrity commitment.

2) Relevant dossiers on the capability of assuming liability of drug quality safety.

A) Scientific research personnel who apply for drug clinical trials shall submit responsibility letters of drug clinical trial risks, promising to submit to the drug regulatory department of the province, in which the drug manufacturer is located, the warrants they sign with warrantors or the insurance contracts they sign with the insurance agencies before conducting the clinical trials.

B) Drug research and development institutions or scientific research personnel who apply to be holders shall submit responsibility letters of drug quality safety, promising to submit to the drug regulatory department of the province, in which the drug manufacturer is located, the warrants signed with warrantors or the insurance contracts signed with the insurance agencies before the drug is marketed; as for injectable drugs, they shall promise to submit insurance contracts before the drug is marketed.

### IV. Conditions for entrusted production enterprises

The entrusted production enterprises shall be drug manufacturers that are legally formed within the pilot administrative regions and hold the *Drug Production License* of the corresponding scope of drug production and *Good Manufacturing Practice for Pharmaceutical Products* (GMP) certificates.

### V. Obligations and liabilities of applicants and holders

(1) The applicants of drug registration and drug production enterprises shall

fulfill the obligations prescribed by *the Drug Administration Law of the People's Republic of China* and other laws and regulations on drug research and development registration, production, distribution, and monitoring and evaluation etc. and assume corresponding legal liabilities.

(2) The holders shall sign contracts and quality agreement with entrusted production enterprises to stipulate the rights, obligations and liabilities of both parties.

(3) The holders shall entrust the entrusted production enterprise or eligible drug trading enterprises to sell the drugs on their behalf, agree on sales requirements, urge them to abide by relevant laws and regulations and assume the liabilities of drug traceability management.

(4) The holders shall, through the Internet, actively disclose the approval information of the drug marketing license, the package inserts of drugs, the information of rational drug use etc. to facilitate inquiry for the society.

(5) Where personal injury is caused by the drug approved of marketing, the victim may claim compensation from the holders, or from the entrusted production enterprises or the distributors. Where the holders compensate for what is the liability of the entrusted production enterprises or distributors, the holders are entitled to claim compensation from the entrusted production enterprises or the distributors; where the entrusted production enterprises or distributors compensate for what is the holders' liability, the entrusted production enterprises or distributors are entitled to claim compensation from the holders. The implementation shall be in line with the specific provisions of *the Tort Law of the People's Republic of China*.

### VI. Obligations and Liabilities of the Entrusted Production Enterprises

(1) The entrusted production enterprises shall fulfill the obligations in respect of drug production as prescribed by *the Drug Administration Law* and other laws and regulations and assume corresponding legal liabilities.

(2) The entrusted production enterprises shall fulfill relevant obligations agreed with the holders in accordance with the laws and assume corresponding legal liabilities.

### VII. Holders' application

(1) Newly registered drugs

While filing application of drug clinical trials or application of drug marketing, the applicant may apply to be the holder of newly registered drugs after the implementation of this Plan that is eligible for the pilot program.

The applicant may submit supplementary application to be the holder of drug eligible for the pilot program whose clinical trial application or marketing application has be accepted but not approved before the implementation of this Plan.

While filing marketing application or supplementary application, the applicant who intends to entrust entrusted production enterprise to conduct production shall submit information of the entrusted production enterprise simultaneously.

(2) Drugs approved to be marketed

While filing supplementary application, the applicant may apply to be the holder of drug that has been approved to be marketed before the implementation of the Plan and is eligible for the pilot program.

(3) Modifying application

The holder may file supplementary application to modify the holder or entrusted production enterprise after his application for drug to be marketed is approved. The holder may file supplementary application to modify the holder or entrusted production enterprise during the period when clinical trial application or marketing application has been accepted but not approved yet.

Where the holder or the applicant is modified, both the transferor and transferee shall file application to the provincial drug supervisory department where the transferee is located for the provincial drug supervisory department to submit to China Food and Drug Administration for approval; where the entrusted production enterprise is modified, the holder or applicant shall file application to the provincial drug supervisory department where the transferee is located for the provincial drug supervisory department to submit to China Food and Drug Administration for approval.

(4) Other requirements

The approval certification of the drug varieties under the pilot program shall contain the relevant information of the holder, the entrusted production enterprise and so on, and also indicate that the holder shall, in accordance with the relevant requirements, submit to the provincial drug supervisory department where the holder is located the warrant signed with warrantors or the insurance contract signed with the insurance agency. The package inserts and package labels of the drug varieties under the pilot program shall contain information of the holder, the entrusted production enterprise and so on. The approval number of the drug issued during the period of the pilot shall remain valid for the period of validity specified in the drug registration approval document after the expiration of the pilot period.

## VIII. Supervision and administration

(1) Post-marketing supervision and administration

The provincial drug supervisory department where the holder is located shall be responsible for the supervision and administration of the holder and the drug approved to be marketed, and, in conjunction with the provincial drug supervisory department where the entrusted production enterprise is located, for the extended supervision and administration of the entrusted production enterprise which is not within the administrative region. The provincial drug supervisory department shall strengthen the supervision and administration of the holder's fulfillment of obligations such as ensuring the quality of drugs, marketing and service, drug monitoring and evaluation, and drug recall etc., and urge the holder to establish a strict quality management system to ensure the fulfillment of responsibility.

The provincial drug supervisory department where the entrusted production enterprise is located shall strengthen supervision and inspection of the drug manufacturers to conduct production under the conditions of GMP and take control measure in a timely manner if risks are found in production or operation.

Where drugs approved to be marketed are found to have quality risks, drug supervisory and administrative departments shall, according to the actual conditions, take risk control measures against holders and relevant entities such as interviewing, sending warning letters, making rectification within a prescribed time limit, revising drug package inserts, restricting use, recalling drugs under supervision, revoking drug approval certifications as well as suspending research and development, production, sales and use etc.

Where the holders and entrusted production enterprises violate *Drug Administration Law* and other laws and regulations or the relevant provisions of this Plan, the provincial drug supervisory department where the holder is located shall investigate and deal with the violations by law and investigate the liability of those responsible.

(2) Information disclosing

China Food and Drug Administration shall, in accordance with regulations, disclose the acceptance, evaluation, approval, post-marketing modification and other relevant information about the drug varieties under the pilot program. The provincial food and drug supervisory and administrative departments shall actively disclose the supervisory and administrative information about the holders' fulfillment of obligations, routine supervision and inspection and administrative penalty etc.

**IX. Others**

This Plan shall be implemented from the date of issue till November 4, 2018. The drug production enterprises within the pilot administrative regions shall refer to the relevant regulations of this Plan.

China Food and Drug Administration shall be responsible for the interpretation of this *Plan*.

**(Zhao Xuemei)**

## 22. Guiding Opinions of the General Office of the State Council on Promoting and Regulating the Application and Development of Big Data in Health and Medical Care

(No. 47 [2016] of the General Office of the State Council)

The people's governments of all provinces, autonomous regions, and municipalities directly under the Central Government, all ministries and commissions of the State Council, and all institutions directly under the State Council:

Big data in health and medical care is the important, fundamental and strategic resource of the state. The application and development of big data in health and medical care is to bring profound changes to the mode of health and medical care, which is helpful to trigger and deepen the motivation and vigor for the reform of the medicine and health system, improve the efficiency and quality of health and medical care service, expand resource supply, and constantly satisfy the multiple-layer, and the diversified needs of the people for health. It is also helpful to foster new business types and economic growth points. For the purpose of implementing the requirement of the *Notice of the State Council on Issuing the Action Plan for Promoting the Development of Big Data* (No. 50 [2015] by the State Council), following the development trend of emerging information technology, and regulating and promoting the integration, sharing and opening application of big data in health and medical care, with the approval of the State Council, the following opinions are hereby offered.

### I. Guiding ideology, basic principles and development goals

(1) Guiding ideology. The spirit of the 18th National Congress of the Communist Party of China (CPC) and the Third, Fourth, and Fifth Plenary Sessions of the 18th CPC Central Committee shall be implemented in depth, the concept of innovative, coordinated, green, open and sharing development shall be firmly developed and practically implemented. According to the decisions and arrangements of the CPC Central Committee and the State Council, the decisive role of the market in resource allocation shall be made full use of, and the role of the government be made better use of. Beginning with the guarantee of the whole people's heath, the top design shall be strengthened, community-level foundation be consolidated, the policy system

improved, innovation in the working mechanism conducted, the interconnection, integration, opening and sharing of the government's health and medical care information system and the public health and medical care data vigorously promoted. Information isolated islands shall be eliminated, a development environment to promote the safety, regulation and innovative application of big data in health and medical care be vigorously created. Through the "Internet plus health and medical care," new service modes shall be developed, the new business types be fostered, and the medical care and health undertaking satisfying the people vigorously developed, so as to provide powerful support to the building of a healthy China, comprehensively finish the building of a moderately prosperous society, and realize Chinese Dream of the great rejuvenation of Chinese nation.

(2) Basic principles. Adhering to the people-oriented values and the driving-force innovation. The application and development of big data in health and medical care shall be incorporated into the state strategic arrangement of big data, the joint and collaborative innovation of politics, industry, academics, research and application be advanced, the basic research and the core technology development strengthened, and the key fields and the key parts of health and medical care highlighted. The big data shall be used to expand service channels, extend and enrich service contents, and better satisfy the needs of the people for health and medical care.

Adhering to regulation, order, safety and controllability. Regulation, order, safety and controllability shall be adhered to. Rules and systems for the opening up and protection of big data in health and medical care shall be established and improved to enhance the construction of the standards and safety system, the security management responsibility, the relationship between application and development, security guarantee, and the ability in technical safety support, so as to effectively protect personal privacy and information safety.

Adhering to the publicity, integration, joint construction and sharing. The cooperation between government and the social forces shall be encouraged with the overall planning, the combination of the short-term and the long-term targets, and the demonstration and leading. The priority shall be given to the revitalization and the integration of the existing resources in order to promote a favorable situation for the vigorous development in which all parties support and open up in accordance with the law, and provide convenience and benefit for the people by fully releasing data dividends, and triggering the vigor for the entrepreneurship and the innovation among all the people.

(3) Development goals. By the end of 2017, the interconnection between the state and provincial-level population health information platforms and national medicine biding and procurement business application platform shall be realized to basically

form the pattern of sharing and jointly using the cross-departmental health and medical care data resources. By 2020, a state medical care and health information rating and open application platform shall be developed to realize cross-departmental and cross-regional sharing of the resources about population, legal persons, space, geography, and other basic data, and significant achievement in the integration and application of data in all the relevant fields of medical care, medicine, medical insurance and health shall be made. The regional distribution shall be arranged in an overall-planning way, and 100 regional clinical medicine data demonstration centers be established based on the existing resources. Therefore, it shall be basically realized that urban and rural residents have standardized electronic health archives and health cards with complete functions. Policies, regulations, safety and protection, and application standard systems with regard to big data in health and medical care shall be constantly improved, the mode of the application and development of big data in health and medical care suitable for the state actuality be basically developed, and the system of the industry of big data in health and medical care initially formed so that the new business types shall thrive, and the people shall obtain more tangible benefits.

## II. Key tasks and significant projects

(1) Consolidating the foundation of the application of big data in health and medical care

1) Accelerating the building of a unified, authoritative and interconnected population health information platform. An information project on national health protection in accordance with the principle of safety first and privacy protection shall be implemented. Fully relying on the national e-government network and the unified data sharing and exchanging platform, the existing facilities and resources should be expanded and improved, and a national, provincial, municipal and county level population health information platform that is accessible and shared be comprehensively built. Data collection, integrated sharing and business collaboration in the use of information systems for public health, family planning, medical services, medical security, drug supply and comprehensive management shall be strengthened. The management models shall be innovated to promote the online registration of births. Data barriers shall be removed to unimpeded data sharing channels between departments, regions and industries, explore the communication mechanism for social health care data, and promote the aggregation of health and medical care data, the handling of business matters, and the support of government's decision-making on the platform.

2) Promoting the sharing and opening of big data resources in health care. All types of medical care and health institutions shall be encouraged to advance the

collection and storage of big data in health and medical care, strengthen application support and technical guarantee for the operation and maintenance, and open up the sharing channel of data resources. The development and improvement of the basic core database with residents' electronic health archives, electronic medical history, electronic prescription, etc. shall be accelerated. The close interdepartmental cooperation, the unified and centralized health and medical care data sharing mechanism for health and family planning, traditional Chinese medicine and education, science and technology, and ministries or departments of industry and informatization, public security, civil affairs, human resources and social security, environmental protection, agriculture, commerce, safety supervision, inspection and quarantine, food and drug administration, sports, statistics, tourism, climate, insurance supervision, and federation for disabled persons shall be established. The access to the population health information platform shall be explored and promoted for data resource specifications of wearable devices, smart health electronic products and mobile applications of health care. A national data resource catalog system of health and medical care shall be established, policies and standards on the open application of big data in health and medical care by category, rating, and region be developed, and the opening-up of big data in health and medical care steadily promoted.

(2) Comprehensively deepening the application of big data in health and medical care

3) Promoting the application of big data governance in health care industry. The monitoring and evaluation of the reform of medical and health system will be deepened and the accurate statistics and forecast evaluation of important data, such as the health status of the residents be strengthened to give the strong support to the construction planning and decision-making of a healthy China. The integrated use of health and medical care data resources and information technology will be made, the hospital evaluation system be improved, the deepening of the reform of public hospitals promoted, and the system of modern hospital management improved so as to layout the optimization of medical and health resources. The supervision of medical institutions shall be strengthened, monitoring mechanism for the income formation and the changing trends of medical treatment, medicines, consumables and others be perfected. The coordination among medical service prices, medical insurance payments, drug bidding and procurement, drug use and other business information shall be made to push forward the coordinated reform of medical treatment, medical insurance and medicines.

4) Promoting the application of big data in clinical and scientific research of health care. With the existing resources, a number of demonstration centers of clinical medical data, such as cardiovascular and cerebrovascular, tumor, senile diseases and pediatrics,

are built to integrate the national medical big data resources such as genomics and proteomics and establish a clinical decision support system. The application of gene chip and sequencing technology in the diagnosis of hereditary diseases, early diagnosis of cancer and disease prevention and detection shall be promoted, the safety management of population genetic information strengthened and the development of the precision of medical technology promoted. Centering on the needs of clinical drug development for major diseases and the common key technologies for drug industrialization, a mechanism for the side effect prediction of drugs, and the data fusion and sharing for innovative drug research and development shall be established. The advantageous resources shall be made full use of to optimize the distribution of biomedical big data. Relying on the national clinical medicine research center and collaborative research network, the integration and sharing of clinical and scientific data resources shall be strengthened, the efficiency of medical research and application be enhanced, and the development of smart medical treatment promoted.

5) Promoting the application of big data on public health. The building of an information system for public health service shall be strengthened, the application functions of information systems such as national immunization planning, direct online reporting, network first aid, occupational disease prevention and control, the early warning and decision-making of port public health risks, and mobile emergency response platforms be improved, the information sharing and business collaboration between medical institutions, public health institutions and port inspection and quarantine institutions promoted, and the capacity of public health monitoring, evaluation and decision-making and management comprehensively enhanced. Social network of public information resources shall be integrated to improve the early warning mechanism for disease sensitive information, the disease trend of the whole crowd and the global outbreak of infectious diseases information such as international public health risks be timely grasped and the dynamic analysis made in order to improve the ability to warn and respond to public health emergencies. The monitoring data of environmental sanitation, drinking water, health hazard factors, port medical media biology and nuclear biochemistry shall be integrated to effectively evaluate the social factors affecting health. The medical biological monitoring on the key infectious and occupational diseases, port input medium of sexually transmitted diseases shall be carried out to integrate the multi-source monitoring data of infectious diseases and occupational diseases, set up the quick identification network system of laboratory pathogen detection results, and effectively prevent and control major diseases. The monitoring and evaluation of disease risk factors and the intelligent application of maternal and child health care, elderly health care and international travel health care shall be promoted to popularize healthy lifestyles.

6) Cultivating new business model of big data application of health care. Key technologies such as strengthening health care massive data storage and cleaning, analysis and mining, security and privacy protection shall be tackled. Social forces to innovate and develop health care services shall be actively encouraged to promote in-depth integration of health care services and big data technologies, accelerate the construction of the health care big data industry chain, and continue to promote the coordinated development of health care, good health maintenance, old-age care, housekeeping and other services. Home health information services shall be developed, the online pharmacies and medicine of the third-party logistics and distribution services be standardized to promote good health maintenance by means of traditional Chinese medicine, keeping in good health for the aged, and health management, health advice, health and culture, and keeping fitness by sports, healthy medical tourism, health environment, healthy diet and other industrial development.

7) Developing and popularizing the intelligent equipment for digital health care. The development of the artificial intelligence technology related with health care, biological three-dimensional (3D) printing technology, medical robot, large medical equipment, auxiliary equipment, wearable health and rehabilitation equipment and the related micro sensor shall be supported. The transformation of the research achievements shall be accelerated, and the digital medical equipment, Internet equipment, intelligent health products, functional status of traditional Chinese medicine examination and health care equipment manufacturing level be improved to promote the industrial upgrading of health intelligent equipment.

(3) Standardizing and promoting "Internet + health care" services.

8) Developing smart and healthy medical services for the benefit of the people. A leading role of excellent medical resources shall be given a play to encourage social forces to participate in the integration of online and offline resources, medical networking and health application (APP) management be regulated to vigorously promote the application of Internet health consultation, online appointment booking, mobile payment, inspection result query and follow-up tracking, optimize the formation of a standardized, shared and trusted diagnosis and treatment process, and explore the Internet health care service model. Basing on the signing service of the family doctor, the application integration of the residents' health card and the social security card shall be promoted to activate the application of residents' electronic health records and promote integrated electronic health services covering the whole life cycle of prevention, treatment, rehabilitation and health management.

9) Establishing a comprehensive telemedicine application system. The cloud service plan of healthy China shall be implemented to build an integrated platform for health and medical services, provide remote consultation, remote imaging,

remote pathology and remote electrocardiogram diagnosis services, and improve the mechanism for mutual recognition and sharing of the inspection results. The data resource sharing and business collaboration shall be promoted among large hospital and community-level health institutions, general practitioners and specialists, the information system for hierarchical diagnosis and treatment based on the Internet and big data technology be improved, the service capacity of medical and health institutions expanded and enlarged to make the targeted promotion of "the center moving down, and the resources sinking".

10) Promoting the application of education training in health care. The establishment of an education training cloud platform based on the open university for health care and supported by China education MOOC alliance of health care shall be supported to encourage the development of MOOC medical and health training materials and explore new Internet teaching models and methods. The high-quality teachers shall be organized to promote the application of the open sharing and online interaction of education resources, remote training, remote operation demonstration and teaching, learning effect evaluation so as to make it convenient for medical personnel to take education for life and improve medical and health service capacity at the community level.

(4) Strengthening the big data security system of health care

11) Strengthening the building of a system of regulations and standards. The laws and regulations to improve the application and development of big data in health and medical care shall be formulated, the standard management of residents' health information services be strengthened, the right to use information clarified, and the legitimate rights and interests of all parties concerned effectively protected. The service supporting system for data opening and sharing shall be improved and a management system of "hierarchical authorization, classified application, and consistent authority and responsibility" be established. The access standards for big data applications in health care shall be standardized, the integrity mechanism and exit mechanism of big data application be established, and the development, mining and application of big data strictly standardized. The unified standards for disease diagnosis coding, clinical medical terminology, examination and test specifications, drug application coding, information data interface and transmission protocol shall be established so as to promote standardization of health care big data products and service processes.

12) Promoting the development of a network credibility system. The digital identity management of medical and health care must be intensified, and a nationwide unified identification system for medical and health personnel and medical and health institutions with trusted medical digital identities, electronic real-name authentication and data access control information systems be established, the application of

electronic signature actively promoted, and a new model of health care management that can trace service management gradually established so as to ensure the safe operation of health and medical care data, and participate in multi-party cooperation.

13) Enhancing the security of medical data. The development of a health and medical care data security system shall be accelerated, a responsibility system for data security management be established, and the rules for labeling, scientific classification, risk classification and safety review formulated. The population health information security plan shall be formulated to strengthen the technical capacity of national and regional population health information engineering, and the importance to content security and technical security be attached to so as to ensure the independent, controllable and stable security of the country's key information infrastructure and core systems. The reliability, controllability and security evaluation of big data platforms and service providers, as well as the application security evaluation and risk assessment shall be conducted. The software evaluation and security review systems for security protection, system interconnection and sharing, and civil privacy protection shall be established. The security of big data monitoring and early warning shall be improved, a linkage mechanism for security information notification and emergency response, and the service safety working mechanism of "Internet + health care" be established and improved so as to improve measures to address and respond to risks and hidden dangers, strengthen protection of important information concerning national interests, public security, patient privacy and trade secrets and intensify the security precautions in medical schools and scientific research institutions.

14) Strengthening the building of a comprehensive talent pool based on health care informatization. National health information talent development plan shall be implemented, the development of medical informatics and the cultivation of "digital doctors" be strengthened, the cultivation of high-level and comprehensive research and development talents and scientific research teams focused on, and a group of internationally influential professionals, academic leaders and industry leaders cultivated.

### III. Strengthening organization and implementation

(1) Strengthening the overall planning. A working pattern for multi-party participation of the Party and government leaders, resource sharing and collaborative promotion shall be established. National Health and Family Planning Commission should comprehensively coordinate and intensify its implementation, and all the relevant departments should cooperate closely and work together to implement the key tasks. All regions should attach importance to the application and development of big

data in health and medical care, effectively carry out the overall planning, infrastructure construction and safety supervision, and ensure the implementation of all tasks and measures. The integration of big data in health and medical care between the military and the people, and the standardization, connectivity, sharing, and the collaborative application of the military and the local health care data should be promoted. The guidance of health and medical care data application and development, and the overall coordination of technology research and development, the construction of new businesses, and the application and promotion of technology should be strengthened. Expert committees should be studied and established to organize the research and formulate the development strategies and the relevant policies, regulations and standards.

(2) Focusing on breakthroughs. Starting from where the urgent needs of the people locate, the online appointment and referral, the remote medical treatment, and the sharing and mutual recognition of examination and test results, which is convenient for the people and benefits the people should be focused on. The nationwide networking of basic medical insurance and settlement of medical treatment in different places shall be accelerated. The development of smart medical devices and smart wearable devices shall be supported and the research on key issues such as difficult diseases be strengthened. A number of regions and fields with good basic conditions, high work enthusiasm and guaranteed privacy and security protection shall be selected to carry out the pilot application of big data in health and medical care, summarize experience and make steady and orderly progress.

(3) Increasing policy support. The support policies of government shall be formulated and the necessary support be given to the development of big data in health and medical care from fiscal, taxation, investment and innovation. The use of the public-private partnership (PPP) model shall be promoted to encourage and guide social capital to participate in the infrastructure and the application development and operation services of big data in health care. The government should be encouraged to cooperate with enterprises and social institutions to explore ways to integrate government applications and social applications in the field of big data in health and medical care through government procurement and social crowdsourcing. The related investment fund has been given full play to fully stimulate the enthusiasm of social capital and private capital to participate, encourage innovation in diversified investment mechanisms, improve risk prevention and regulation systems, and support the application and development of big data in health care.

(4) Enhancing publicity and popularization of policies. Policy interpretation on the application and development of big data in health and medical care shall be strengthened, the significance and prospects of the application and development be vigorously promoted to respond to social concerns and foster a favorable social

atmosphere. The medical and health institutions and social forces should be guided to actively carry out various forms of popular science activities, popularize health and medical care data application knowledge, encourage the development of simple and easy-to-use digital medical tools and constantly improve people's ability to master the relevant applications and the public health literacy.

(5) Promoting international exchanges and cooperation. The exchanges and cooperation of the application and development of big data in health and medical care technology should be promoted in an orderly manner. The relevant enterprises and the institutions of scientific research should be encouraged to introduce, digest, absorb and re-innovate the internationally advanced technologies, and promote the simultaneous development of China's independent technology and the world at large. The efforts should be increased to track, evaluate and transform international standards for the application of big data in health and medical care, and actively participate in the formulation of international standards and enhance the voice of the relevant rules. The principle of self-reliance, strengthening oversight and ensuring security shall be adhered to so as to steadily explore new models of international cooperation on the application and development of big data in health and medical care, and continue to improve the application level, core competitiveness and internationalization level of China's big data in health and medical care.

(Ji Chenglian)

## 23. Circular of the General Office of the State Council on Adjusting the Composition of the Leading Group for Deepening the Medical and Health Care System Reform under the State Council

(No. 75 [2016] of the General Office the State Council)
October 21st, 2016

The people's governments of all provinces, autonomous regions and municipalities directly under the Central Government; the ministries and commissions, and the departments directly under the State Council,

The State Council has decided to adjust the composition of the leading group for deepening the medical and health care system reform under the State Council (hereinafter referred to as the Leading Group), according to the needs of the work and changes in personnel.

The Leader:

Liu Yandong, the Vice Premier of the State Council

The Deputy Leader:

Li Bin, the Director of Health and Family Planning Commission

Xu Shaoshi, the Director of Reforms Development Commission

Lou Jiwei, the Finance Minister

Yin Weimin, the Minister of Department of Human Resource and Social Security

Jiang Xiaojuan, the Deputy Secretary-general of the State Council

Members:

Guo Weimin, the Deputy Director of Information Office

Li Xiaoquan, the Deputy Director of the State Commission Office of Public Sectors Reform

Zhuang Rongwen, the Deputy Director of the Office of the Central Leading Group for Cyberspace Affairs

Wang Xiaotao, the Deputy Director of National Development and Reform Commission

Lin Huiqing, the Deputy Minister of Education

Xu Nanping, the Deputy Minister of Science and Technology

Xin Guobin, the Deputy Minister of Industry and Information Technology

Gong Puguang, the Deputy Minister of Civil Affairs

Yu Weiping, the Deputy Minister of Finance

You Jun, the Deputy Minister of Human Resources and Social Security

Fang Aiqing, the Deputy Minister of Commerce

Wang Hesheng, the Deputy Director of Health and Family Planning Commission

Meng Jianmin, the Deputy Director of State-owned Assets Supervision and Administration Commission

Wu Zhen, the Deputy Minister of Food and Drug Administration

Yuan Hongshu, the Deputy Director of Legal Affairs Office

Han Wenxiu, the Deputy Director of Research Office of the State Council

Huang Hong, the Vice Chairman of China Insurance Regulatory Commission

Ma Jianzhong, the Deputy Director General of Administration of Traditional Chinese Medicine

Jiao Kaihe, the Vice Chairman of All China Federation of Trade Union

Li Qingjie, the Director General of the Health Bureau of Logistics Department under Central Military Commission

Jia Yong, the Vice Chairman of China Disabled Persons' Federation

Wang Hesheng is also the Director of the Leading Group Office. Wang Xiaotao, Yu Weiping, You Jun are also the Deputy Director of the Leading Group Office. Liang Wannian, the Director of the Structural Reform Division of Health and Family Planning Commission, is the Full-time Deputy Director of the Leading Group Office.

**(Wang Ruisi)**

**1. Analyze the Situation and Make Clear the Train of Thought to Ensure the Good Opening of the Reform and Development of Health and Family Planning in the 13th Five-Year Plan Period**

(Li Bin, January 7th, 2016, Beijing)

The CPC Central Committee and the State Council attach great importance to safeguarding the people's health and the reform and development of health and family planning. Prime Minister Li Keqiang addressed the meeting and made important instructions. He pointed out that in 2015, the national health and family planning system conscientiously implemented the decisions and arrangements of the CPC Central Committee and the State Council, achieved new breakthroughs in deepening the medical reform, and made new achievements in major health emergencies, family planning services and management, upgrading the ability of pharmaceutical services and other work. He also encouraged the leaders and workers of the national health and family planning system to firmly establish a new concept of development, to scientifically plan and promote the reform and development of the health and family planning cause during the 13th Five-Year Plan period, to grasp the key and difficult issues and conquer them, to promote the medical reform to achieve more obvious results, to effectively reduce the burden of patients to seek medical care with the full coverage of major illness insurance, to implement the universal two-child policy in a sound and orderly manner, to further improve the quality of medical services and the equalization of public health services, and to make greater contributions to promoting the construction of a healthy China. On the afternoon of January 6, Vice Premier Liu Yandong attended the forum on health and family planning and medical reform, and delivered an important speech, fully affirming the outstanding achievements made in the reform and development of health and family planning during the 12th Five-Year Plan period. She listened to the opinions and suggestions from all sides and put forward clear requirements for the work during the 13th Five-Year Plan period and the work of 2016. The important instructions of Prime Minister Li Keqiang and the important speech of Vice Premier Liu Yandong are encouragement to the workers of health and family planning in China. We must conscientiously study and understand them and implement them in an all-round way.

## I. Development effects of health and family planning reform in 2015

(1) Breakthroughs were made and remarkable results were achieved in deepening medical reform.

More than 20 policies and documents on deepening the medical reform were issued at state level, laying out better top-level designs and clearer implementation paths. At the provincial level, significant progress was made in four provinces of Jiangsu, Anhui, Fujian and Qinghai. With the policy of "Two Comprehensive Reforms, Two Comprehensive Implementations" as the main thread, the reform was advanced to depth with firm determination all over the country. The working mechanism was established for the leaders of the National Health and Family Planning Commission to focus on the provincial medical reform and the departmental directors were stationed at community-level for supervision to guarantee the implementation of the major reform policies and measures.

1) The reform of public hospitals was accelerated. Special trainings on public hospital reform were organized and more than 2600 administrative staff and directors of public hospitals were trained successively, so as to unify the thoughts and make clear the operational requirements. All localities closely focus on the three key sections of breaking up compensating medical cost with drug sale, innovating system mechanism and mobilizing the enthusiasm of medical personnel, implemented the government responsibilities, strengthened the public welfare and promoted the reform as a whole. The comprehensive reform of county-level public hospitals was fully advanced, and a scientific and reasonable compensation mechanism and a new mechanism of running through the top to bottom were being established. The number of pilot cities for comprehensive reform of public hospitals was increased to 100, the increase in medical expenses of public hospitals in the pilot cities dropped markedly, and the rising trend of medical expenses nationwide was initially contained.

2) The universal medical insurance system was further improved. The basic medical insurance coverage rate was stable at more than 95 percent, the per capita government subsidy standard for urban residents' medical insurance and the New Rural Cooperative Medical Scheme was raised to 380 *yuan*, and the proportion of outpatient and inpatient expenses paid within the policy scope reached 50 percent and 75 percent, respectively. The insurance for major illness of urban and rural residents was fully implemented, covering more than 1 billion urban and rural residents, with no less than 50% reimbursement. Emergency medical assistance was delivered to 140 thousand person-times, medical assistance for major diseases was carried out in an all-round manner, and the medical aid system was further improved. The management of basic health insurance service was steadily improved, 21 provincial information platforms for the

New Rural Cooperative Medical Scheme were connected to the national platform, the pilot work of cross-provincial medical expenses verification and reporting was started, and the reform of health insurance payment mode was actively promoted. According to the "Six Unifications", the documents for the management system of the basic medical insurance for urban and rural residents were formulated and integrated. Commercial health insurance developed rapidly, with an estimated annual premium income of more than 230 billion *yuan*, an increase of 50% over the same period last year, and meeting the needs of people for diversified health insurance.

3) New steps were taken in the reform of the drug supply guarantee mechanism. A new round of centralized drug procurement in public hospitals was fully implemented. Important results were achieved in the pilot work of national drug price negotiation. The state administration of the catalogue of essential drugs was promulgated to ensure the supply of scarce and low-cost medicines, to strengthen the protection of drug use for children and the elderly and to successfully complete the pilot work of the first batch of designated production of essential drugs. The comprehensive drug management information platform portal was officially opened and interlinked with the provincial platforms. In cooperation with the relevant departments, the reform of drug price classification was pushed forward, and the standard of payment for medical insurance drugs was studied and formulated.

4) New progress was made in the construction of tiered diagnosis and treatment system. The planning outline of health care service system was implemented. All localities strictly controlled public hospital construction projects and bed number, and promoted the scientific and rational allocation of resources. The pilot of tiered diagnosis and treatment was pushed forward with the improvement of the service ability at primary level as the key point, common diseases, frequent diseases and chronic diseases as the breakthrough point. Twenty-four provinces issued documents on tiered diagnosis and treatment, and all the pilot cities for the reform of public hospitals started the tiered diagnosis and treatment work, and more than 50 percent of the counties (county-level cities and districts) carried out the pilot system of first-visit responsibility at the primary level. Good experience and good practices of tiered diagnosis and treatment in some provinces and cities were promoted throughout the country.

5) The comprehensive reform at primary level was continuously consolidated and deepened. The connotation construction of primary medical and health care institutions was strengthened, the management of community health services was standardized, and the first batch of 1,300 "Township Health Centers Satisfied by the masses" was selected. The team of rural doctors was stabilized and optimized, and 26 provinces issued implementation plans to strengthen the construction of rural doctors. The key contact points of comprehensive reform of national medical and health institutions at primary-

level covered 34 counties in 17 provinces and accumulated experience in perfecting the personnel distribution system, performance appraisal, service mode transformation and so on. The public health service projects were continuously implemented, the per capita standard of subsidy for basic public health services was increased to 40 *yuan*, all new funds in rural areas were used for village doctors, and the management of funds was further standardized. The major public health service projects was progressed favorably with remarkable effect of implementation.

6) The information construction of population health was accelerated. The plan of action for information benefiting people was implemented, the pilot work on the application of resident health cards was carried out in 29 provinces. Provincial and municipal health information platforms were set up in 126 cities of 14 provinces and cities, achieving regional interconnection in varying degrees. Hospitals used network technology to improve their services, actively developed telemedicine, and promoted the use of high quality medical resources at primary level .

7) The building of talent teams and the work of scientific research were strengthened. The cooperation of medicine and education was deepened, the program of resident physician standardized training enrolled 120,000 students in total, the dynamic management of the training base was strengthened, and the specialist standardized training pilot was started. More than 173,000 general practitioners were trained in various ways, and more than 1,000 pilot general practitioners in special posts went to the post to work. The pediatrics specialty was resumed, the enrollment of psychiatry was increased, and, by taking incentives, nearly 3,600 people passed the examination for the qualification of pediatric doctors. Positive progress was made in the reform of the health science and technology system, a number of new achievements were achieved in the two major special projects of "New Drug Creation" and "Prevention and Control of Infectious Diseases", which entered the national pilot projects of science and technology reform, thus winning an opportunity for the scientific innovation and development in medicine and drugs. The biosafety was promoted to become a national security strategy. The measures for the management of stem cell clinical research was issued and the construction of key scientific research bases was pushed forward steadily.

8) Health services were booming. We implemented equal treatment, removed the policy obstacles that hindered the development of nongovernmental hospitals, implemented the "License before Certificate" policy, encouraged social forces to run a health service industry, and guided doctors to conduct multi-practice in hospitals at the primary level. Private hospitals accounted for more than 51 percent of the total number of hospitals, with the number of outpatients accounting for 22% the total number of outpatients in the country. The pattern of diversified medical services was initially formed. Investment in fixed assets in social health was expected to exceed 390

billion *yuan*, 24% increase from a year earlier, a bright spot for steady growth under the new normal situation. The selection of excellent national equipment catalogue was carried out and the development and application of domestic equipment was accelerated. The combination of medical treatment and care for the aged was actively promoted to meet the needs of health care for the aged in various forms.

(2) New and important progress was made in the work of family planning.

1) The universal two-child policy was actively studied and deployed. All localities steadily implemented the separate two-child policy, released some of the potential energy for bearing children, accumulated experience, and laid the foundation for the implementation of the universal two-child policy. A working group was set up to gradually adjust and improve the fertility policies, to implement the requirements of the important instructions and directives of central leadership, to calculate the population change trend under the conditions of a universal two-child policy in various ways, and to assess comprehensively its impact on the economic, social, and resource environment. The supporting policies and measures were researched and put forward to provide an important basis for the central scientific decision-making. After the central authorities made the universal two-child policy decision, we actively did a good job of propaganda and guidance, accurately interpreted the policy, and made timely arrangements for the implementation of the policy.

2) The management of family planning services was continuously improved. With the reform of the birth service card system as a starting point, the implementation of the commitment system, online processing and other convenient measures were carried out to solve the basic problem of "Difficult in Obtaining Certificates". The collection and management of social alimony was more standardized. The reform of electronic marriage and childbearing certificates for migrating population was carried out in an all-round way, and the level of equalization service was continuously improved. The special action to rectify the "Two Illegal Acts" was implemented deeply, the sex rate at the birth dropped by a large margin, and the target task of the 12th Five-Year Plan was successfully completed. The first batch of 32 national demonstration cities for creating happy families was established. The family award and support policy for family planning was improved, and the support and care for special families carrying out family planning was continuously increased.

3) The maternal and child health work achieved remarkable results. The State Council held a symposium on the 20th anniversary of the implementation of the Maternal and Child Health Law. 100 national quality service demonstration counties (county-level cities, districts) were elected, and more than 7000 baby-friendly hospitals were reviewed. The standardized construction and management of maternal and child health care institutions was actively promoted. The integration

of resources was steadily implemented, and the new maternal and child health care and family planning services network was being developed. More than 11 million planned pregnant couples received free pre-pregnancy eugenic health examination services, and the prevention of mother-to-child transmission of HIV / AIDS, syphilis and hepatitis B covered all counties (county-level cities and districts), so that the World Health Organization rated our country as a country with high performance in women's and children's health.

(3) Public health, food safety and health emergency response were constantly strengthened.

1) Significant results were achieved in the health emergency response to major emergencies. We successfully completed the tasks of preventing and controlling Ebola haemorrhagic fever in China and helping Africa to fight the epidemics, with the results of "Zero Input and Zero Infection". The State Council solemnly commended advanced collectives and individuals for the prevention and control work, and General Secretary Xi Jinping gave important instructions. Effective and orderly emergency medical rescues were performed well for such emergencies as Middle East Respiratory Syndrome, Sinking of "Oriental Star" passenger ship, Fire and Explosion in Tianjin Port and other emergencies, so as to effectively protect people's lives, health and safety.

2) The ability to prevent and control major diseases improved significantly. The State Council integrated 9 mechanisms for the prevention and control of single diseases, set up a joint inter-ministerial meeting mechanism for the prevention and control of major diseases, convened a forum on public health and prevention and control of infectious diseases, and made clear its key tasks. Hepatitis B and poliomyelitis immunization strategy was improved, the prevalence rate of hepatitis B surface antigen in children under 5 years of age was reduced to 0.322, the incidence of tuberculosis decreased steadily and the control of the transmission was achieved in all schistosomiasis endemic counties. The funds for social organizations to participate in AIDS prevention and control were established, and more than 750 projects of social organizations were funded. The overall AIDS epidemic was controlled under the low prevalence level. The epidemic situation of key infectious diseases such as dengue fever, hand, foot and mouth disease and other major infectious diseases of social concerns was decreased significantly. Construction of the third batch of national comprehensive prevention and control demonstration zone for chronic diseases was finished and the three-year action plan for cancer registration management practices and cancer control was implemented. The national mental health work plan was issued and 4.77 million patients with severe mental disorders were comprehensively treated and managed. The pilot project on comprehensive control of echinococcosis in Shiqu County, Sichuan Province was launched. The *Measures for the Administration of Occupational Health Inspection* was issued,

and the monitoring of major occupational diseases covered all cities. The State Council held a national patriotic health work conference, launched a new round of urban and rural environmental hygiene action, the guidance and evaluation index system were formulated for healthy city construction, and a dynamic management and exit mechanism for health towns were established.

3) The food safety standard system and the risk monitoring network were continuously improved. The integration of food safety standards was completed comprehensively, 614 national standards on food safety were considered, and the capability of risk monitoring and assessment, food-borne disease monitoring report and traceability analysis was further improved.

(4) The quality and level of medical services were continuously improved.

The management of medical quality and safety was strengthened. The quality control indicators for 6 specialties like anesthesia were released, and the clinical pathways for 102 kinds of diseases of 16 specialties were formulated and revised. By implementing the national strategy of curbing bacterial resistance, the utilization rate of antimicrobial drugs in inpatients was decreased by 8 percentage points. Blood nucleic acid detection in blood stations achieved full coverage and effectively prevented the risk of clinical blood safety. The donation and transplantation of human organs were advanced steadily. The donation after the death of citizens became the main source of transplant organs. The action plan to further improve medical services was implemented. We implemented the appointment to visit a doctor, optimized the process, improved the environment, popularized the high quality nursing service, made great efforts to alleviate the "wartime" state of the big hospitals, improved the order of seeking medical treatment obviously, enhanced the people's sense of obtaining benefit, and constantly improved the doctor-patient relationship. The counterpart support was developed to depth to promote the comprehensive ability of county hospitals. The annual operation volume in county hospitals was increased by 35% compared with that before the reform, and the number of intensive medical departments was increased by 38%. The county-level medical imaging centers were built in the pilot project, more than 13,000 medical personnel of tertiary hospitals were sent to work in county hospitals, and the medical attendance rate in the county areas was further improved. We formulated a the implementation plan of poverty relief work for health and family planning, dispatched "national medical teams" to go round visiting patients in former revolutionary base areas, areas inhabited by minority nationalities , remote and border areas and poverty-stricken areas of 14 provinces. During the week of large-scale free medical consultation, a total of 12 million people were served. In conjunction with the Organization Department of the Central Committee of the CPC, the work of "Group Type" to assist Tibet was carried out. The medical security task for military parade in the 70th anniversary of the victory of the Chinese People's War of Resistance against Japan and the World Anti-Fascist War was successfully completed. The "combined boxing" of prevention and treatment of medical disputes achieved effect. The National People's Congress formally incorporated the medical related crimes into the scope of criminal law control, which provided a powerful legal guarantee for cracking down on medicine-related crimes and "hospital-disturbing" behaviors. Medical institutions participating in medical liability insurance increased by 11 thousand, presenting a good situation in which the success rate of people's mediation rose, and the number of illegal and criminal cases and medical disputes decreased.

(5) The characteristic advantages of traditional Chinese medicine were brought into play.

The reform of traditional Chinese medicine was deepened and the construction of the national pilot area for comprehensive reform of traditional Chinese medicine was speeded up. The project of upgrading the service capacity of traditional Chinese medicine at primary level was completed, and the quantity and quality of traditional Chinese medicine service at primary level were both greatly improved. The State Council's deployment on the development of health services of traditional Chinese medicine was implemented, and the new industry forms of health tourism, health care for the aged and others through traditional Chinese medicine were accelerated to develop. The health project of "Preventive Treatment" and the inheritance and innovation project were fully implemented to innovate the mechanism and the mode of foreign exchange and cooperation of traditional Chinese medicine. Researcher Tu Youyou was awarded Nobel Prize in Physiology or Medicine of 2015, breaking the fact that Chinese scientists had won no Nobel Prize and marking a new peak of the scientific and technological development of traditional Chinese medicine.

(6) Solid promotion was made in plan guidance, law construction, investment guarantee and propaganda work.

1) We organized to research and work out the key and special programs for the 13th Five-Year Plan. The major and special projects were studied in the early stage of planning formulation, the key planning drafts were being studied and demonstrated, and the formulation of Beijing, Tianjin and Hebei medical and health coordinated development plans was accelerated.

2) We adhered to the administration by law. By cooperation with the NPC, we completed the annual research task of the *Basic Medical and Health Law*. The NPC Standing Committee amended the *Population and Family Planning Law* and the *Traditional Chinese Medicine Law (draft)* and submitted them to the NPC Standing Committee for deliberation. We cleaned up and standardized the intermediary

services for administrative examination and approval, and the administrative examination and approval items set by the central authorities for the local governments to implement, and we also focus on the supervision during and after the event. The comprehensive supervision on the administrative law was further strengthened, the special supervision and inspection for the implementation of laws and regulations such as the blood donation law and mental health law, and for the infectious disease prevention and control was carried out, and the special rectification of radiation health technical service institutions was conducted. The 2nd Health and Family Planning Supervision Skills Competition was successfully held.

3) Investment in health and family planning was continuously increased. In 2015, the central government allocated 255.9 billion *yuan* to local health and family planning funds. The central government was arranged to invest 22.8 billion *yuan* to support 35,000 projects to speed up the improvement of health and family planning service conditions. The management of funds and the supervision were strengthened, the performance appraisal was implemented and the efficiency of the use of funds was improved.

4)The propaganda work was in full swing. The correct guidance of public opinion was adhered to, and new ideas, new initiatives and new achievements of reform and development were publicized and interpreted in depth. Comprehensive publicity and reporting of the results and experience of medical reform was well done to achieve the full coverage of reporting activities of advanced typical deeds. The social concerns were positively responded, the social opinions were correctly guided, and the public opinions showed a positive trend. The creation of literary and artistic works on the subject of health and family planning was more prosperous. The healthy lifestyle of the whole people covered 80% of the districts and counties, and the self-care awareness and health literacy of the people were further improved.

(7) China's international health influence was prominent.

We participated deeply in the high-level humanity exchanges between China and the United States, China and the United Kingdom, China and Russia and China and France, and organized such activities as the China-US Ebola Forum and the Global Health Forum, Health Policy Dialogue, AIDS Prevention and Control, and so on. The Conference on Health Cooperation between China and Central and Eastern European countries, and China and Central African countries was successfully held in the Czech Republic and South Africa, and the 26th Executive Committee Conference of the South-South Cooperation Organization on population and development, the China-Arab Health Cooperation Forum and other international conferences were successfully held in China, and the exchanges and cooperation with such international organizations as the World Health Organization and the World Bank were consolidated and deepened in the fields of medical reform, prevention and control of major diseases, health emergencies and others.

The year 2015 was the closing year of the 12th Five-Year Plan. All in all, the 12th Five-Year Plan period was a five-year period in which the reform of Health and Family Planning Undertakings in China was vigorous, the development was fast and people benefited more. In these five years, a new round of reform took substantial steps, breakthroughs were made in important areas and key sections, and the reform dividends continued to release. In these five years, the basic medical and health service system covering urban and rural areas was basically built up, the total amount of resources increased, the structure improved, and the ability to prevent and treat major diseases and health emergency capacity were significantly enhanced. The availability and quality of basic medical and public health services were constantly improved. In these five years, the guarantee of medical and health care was continuously strengthened, and the guarantee system of the basic medical insurance, insurance for major illness, medical assistance, emergency relief for diseases, charitable assistance and commercial insurance was established, with the proportion of personal health expenditure of residents in the total health expenditure dropping to 30%, the lowest level in recent 20 years. In these five years, governments at all levels increased their investment and the fiscal expenditure on health and family planning increased rapidly, which provided strong support for the development of the cause and the deepening of the medical reform. In these five years, we carefully planned, carefully studied, steadily and orderly carried out the adjustment and improvement of the fertility policy, and realized the historic transformation of the family planning policy in three steps of "two children for a couple who both are the only child in their respective families, two children for a couple with either the husband or the wife being a single child, and two children for all couples". These five years were of special significance to the health and family planning system. We experienced a major test of institutional reform, the two teams were integrated into one and worked hand in hand, the supporting roles of governance by law, talents, science and technology, information, publicity, international cooperation and others were more powerful, and the modernization level of the governance system and governance capacity leapt to a new level.

Over the past five years, the health level of people had increased significantly, and the life expectancy per capita was expected to increase by more than one year compared with that of 2010. The maternal mortality rate dropped from 30/10 million in 2010 to 21.7/10 million in 2014, and the infant mortality rate fell from 13.1 per thousand in 2010 to 8.9 per thousand in 2014, both achieving in advance the 12th Five-Year Plan and the United Nations' Millennium Development goals. The health level of residents was generally at the average level of the middle and high income countries, which laid a solid health foundation for ensuring the overall construction of a well-off society.

## II. Task of health and family planning reform and development in 2016 and in the coming period

The 13th Five-Year Plan period is the decisive stage of building a well-off society in an all-round way and is also the decisive stage to establish and improve the basic medical and health system covering urban and rural residents. China's resident consumption structure transformation and upgrading, population aging, the acceleration of new-type urbanization, the coexistence of multiple disease threats, the increased threat of new and sudden outbreaks of infectious diseases, and a variety of health factors intertwined all put forward a new challenge to the safety of public health. The people's new expectations for health are more prominent and urgent. Deepening medical reform into the deep water area and tackling key problems involves more complicated adjustment of interest relations. It is urgent to put forward a comprehensive solution to the global, fundamental and long-term problems of national health improvement from the perspective of national strategy. The CPC Central Committee and the State Council have placed the work of health and family planning in the important position of the "Four Comprehensives" strategic layout, and deepened the breakthroughs in the key areas of medical reform, which have even more condensed our confidence in our determination to fight and win. Under the new normal, structural reforms on the supply side further release the multilayered and diversified health needs of people, and the reform and development environment is more favorable. On the whole, the development opportunity of the health and family planning reform is greater than the challenges, and it is still in a period of great strategic opportunity.

In the next five years, we will resolutely implement the Central Committee's decision and plan on "Promoting the Construction of a Healthy China" and the requirements of the *Decision on Implementing the Universal Two-child Policy Reform and Improving the Management of Family Planning Services*, regard the maintenance and protection of the people's health as the highest mission, comply with the new trend of the world health development, insist on providing the basic medical and health system as a public product to the whole people, consciously carry out the concept of innovation, coordination, green, open and shared development to the whole process and every section of reform and development, put the mechanism construction in a more prominent position to ensure basic medical services, bolster support at the community level, complement the weak parts and speed up the reform of medical and health system, and promote the basic medical and health system with Chinese characteristics to be more mature and more established. We should adhere to the basic national policy of family planning, implement the universal two-child policy in a steady and orderly manner, reform and improve the management of family planning services, improve the quality of the population, and promote the balanced development of the population. Efforts will be made to establish a more perfect system of public health, medical services, medical security, drug supply security and service supervision, as well as a more perfect management system and operational mechanism for medical and health institutions. We will promote the transition of health care from "Disease-centered" to "Health-centered", further meet the new expectations for the people's health, and achieve universal access to basic medical and health services.

(1) Scientifically compiling and implementing the 13th Five-Year Plan

We should focus our efforts on the compiling and implementing the *Outline of the Healthy China 2030 Plan*, the *"13th Five-Year Plan" on Sanitation and Health*, and the *"13th Five-Year Plan" for Deepening the Reform of the Medical and Health Care System*, guide the plan formulation with the five major development concepts, accurately grasp the plan orientation. We should not only base ourselves on the current situation, but also plan for the long term, and, from the height of great health and hygiene, break through the thinking of departments and give prominence to the macro, comprehensive and strategic aspects of the plans. In particular, it is necessary to properly handle the relationship between the overall outline and the five-year plan, the reform plan and the development plan, so as to focus on each other and link up with each other. It is necessary to scientifically set goals and targets for planning, and plan well for major policies, major projects and major projects. We must persist in seeking advice and needs from the public, drawing on collective wisdom and absorbing all useful ideas in compiling the plans in an open form. All localities should also study and compile the local plans for the reform and development of health and family planning in accordance with the uniform requirements, do a good job of in connecting with the national plans, and ensure that all of them are issued within the year.

(2) Speeding up the deepening of the reform of the medical and health system

1) We will comprehensively deepen the reform of public hospitals. We will consolidate, expand and improve the three-tier pilot work, and strive to establish a modern hospital management system. The comprehensive reform of county-level public hospitals will be consolidated and the classified guidance and demonstration be strengthened. The state has selected one county in each of the 4 pilot provinces to further improve the reform measures, sum up experience and set up a model. All localities should also focus on the demonstration, take the middle, promote the backward, consolidate the effectiveness of reform, and make new progress every year. The pilot cities of comprehensive reform of urban public hospitals will be expanded to 200 and the provincial pilot of comprehensive reform of health care reform will be broadened to transform the deepening of the medical reform from "One City, One Place" pilot to the overall regional promotion, so as to give play to the combined

driving effect. Taking the speeding up the construction of a new mechanism for the operation of public hospitals as the core, we will straighten out the pharmaceutical price system, establish a salary system in line with the characteristics of the industry, and build a modern hospital management system framework. The key to build a mechanism lies in the "joint reform of medical service, medicine supply and medical insurance", and the governments at all levels should strengthen unified leadership and give full play to the organizing and leading role of the medical reform leading groups and the coordinating and promoting role of the medical reform offices. Public hospital reform is a typical supply-side reform, and all levels of health and family planning departments are duty-bound and must fully promote it.

2) We will further improve the medical insurance system for all people. Efforts will be made precisely in the "Protecting the Focus, Grasping the Integration, and Promoting the Reform". The Central Government attaches great importance to improving the people's livelihood and continues to raise the standard of per capita financial assistance for basic medical insurance for urban and rural residents. We will pay special attention to the insurance against major diseases, achieve a level of raising funds per capita of no less than 30 *yuan*, and effectively lighten the burden of people who suffer major diseases. It is necessary to stabilize the proportion of reimbursement for hospital expenses, ensure that the proportion of reimbursement within the scope of the policy is not lower than 75, and stabilize the level of reimbursement for outpatient expenses, chronic diseases and special diseases. We will further improve the basic medical insurance management services and continue to promote the cross provincial medical expenses check and report work for the New Rural Cooperative Medical Scheme (NRCMS). All provinces (autonomous regions, municipalities directly under the Central Government) are encouraged to expand the scope of compliant medical expenses based on the practical appropriateness and explore the preferential policies for the poor. The seamless connection with such systems as the medical aid, the disease emergency aid and charity aid should be strengthened to prevent the incidents which impinge the bottom line of social morality. The integration of the basic medical insurance system for urban residents and the NRCMS should be promoted to realize the "Six Unification". The implementation of health insurance payment reform will be speeded up, which is a powerful lever to guide and regulate medical behavior, and control the unreasonable growth of the expenses. Practice proves that where this lever is used well, the role of institutional innovation is obvious. On the other hand, if this lever is immobile or moves too slow, the role of medical insurance in promoting the reform will be greatly diminished. The reform of the payment system is a major task this year, and all localities should pay close attention to it.

3) We will speed up the promotion of hierarchical diagnosis and treatment. The implementation of hierarchical diagnosis and treatment is a basic system design that

fundamentally alleviates the difficulty of seeing a doctor and the high expenses for seeing a doctor, which is related to the success or failure of medical reform. We will conscientiously implement the requirements of the State Office's *"Guiding Opinions on Promoting the Construction of the Hierarchical Diagnosis and Treatment System,"* and carry out pilot trials of hierarchical diagnosis and treatment in about 70% of the localities. We should take comprehensive measures, define the functional orientation, mobilize the initiative and enthusiasm of the large hospitals in urban areas to carry out hierarchical diagnosis and treatment, and truly assume the role of large hospitals of the guidance of emergency and serious illness treatment, personnel training, scientific research, and so on, and link up and down in such ways as establishment of medical consortia and others. With common diseases, frequently-occurring diseases, chronic diseases as the starting point, we will gradually expand the pilot diseases for hierarchical diagnosis and treatment and implement the practice of separate treatment for acute and chronic diseases. By taking the measures of contract service, price control and convenience and benefit to the people, we should guide the first consultation at the community level, so that the urban and rural residents can really feel the convenience and change their concepts of seeking medical treatment. This year, the increase in the financial subsidy standard for the per capita expenditure of basic public health services has been completely used in contracted services of general practitioners (village doctors) to assist in hierarchical diagnosis and treatment. We will further improve the service purchase management of the basic public health service programs, and deeply and extensively carry out the activities of "Township Health Centers to the Satisfaction of People" and the national community-level health skills competition to continuously strengthen the primary units.

4) We will continue to improve the guarantee mechanism for drug supply. We will adapt to the new situation of zero difference rate of drug sales after the reform, study and formulate the policies and measures to improve the degree of essential drug system, and further improve the timely distribution and use of essential drugs. We will conscientiously implement the State Office's the *Guiding Opinions on Improving the Centralized Procurement of Drugs in Public Hospitals*, and meticulously organize the centralized procurement work. We will encourage and guide joint procurement across regions to effectively reduce the false high drug prices. Step by step, we will expand the scope of the state drug price negotiations and the number of varieties, and effectively reduce the prices of patented drugs and exclusive varieties. We should make full use of the national information platform for comprehensive management of drug supply, strengthen monitoring and analysis, and establish a drug shortage warning mechanism.

5) We will vigorously develop the health service industry. The social-run medical policy environment will be further optimized to promote the same treatment of non-profit private hospitals and public hospitals. We will strengthen the supervision of

industry management, promote the quality improvement and healthy development of social-run hospitals, carry out the healthy aging projects, start the trial pilot of the combination of medical treatment and health care for the aged, vigorously develop the life service industry, such as health care for the aged, promote the development of nursing care, rehabilitation, hospice care and other extended services, and improve the policies and measures to actively promote the development of medical tourism.

6) The construction of health informatization will be speeded up. The construction of application of information systems for public health, family planning, medical services, medical security, drug management and integrated management will be accelerated to realize the interconnection, and the electronic health archives, electronic medical continuous records and information authorization to use will be implemented. The network business applications such as telemedicine and disease management should be actively developed, the health care management and medical information resources be integrated, and the services like clinical reservation services, online payment, online follow-up and online query of examination results be promoted. The pilot demonstration work on the application and development of health care big data will be carried out, the "Internet + Health Care" services be actively implemented, and to amplify people's sense of acquisition by means of information technology. We will strengthen the supervision, promote the orderly development of online health services, and crack down on bad practices such as online fraud.

(3) Implementing the universal two-child policy in a sound, down-to-earth and orderly manner

1) We will study and implement the central decision-making and deployment in-depth. It is necessary to carry out the study and training at various levels, strengthen the publicity and advocacy, comprehensively grasp the spiritual essence of the *Decision*, fully affirm the historical achievements of family planning work, and make clear the target tasks of planning and fertility work in the new period, and unify the thoughts and actions into the spirit of the *Decision*. We should guide all localities to scientifically formulate a plan for the implementation of the universal two-child policy, timely revise the local relevant laws and regulations on the rules of population, family planning and others, perfect the supporting policies, and safeguard the legitimate rights and interests of people.

2) We will reform and improve the management of family planning services. The birth registration service system will be implemented, and the birth of two children will no longer be examined and approved. The services of maternal health care, child health care, vaccination, family planning and others will be integrated, and the pilot on the use of mother and child health manual will be expanded. We will promote the national information connection of birth and medical certificate and the network

remote inquiry for mobile population marriage and childbearing information. We will carry out nationwide monitoring of the birth population, improve the statistical monitoring of the mobile population, adhere to and improve the responsibility system for the management of family planning objectives.

3) We will improve the maternal and child health service capacity. The demonstration project for quality maternal and child health services should be promoted, the guiding opinions be studied and formulated, the construction of the maternal and child health service system and children's hospitals (specialties) be strengthened, the capacity of obstetrical and pediatric services be improved, and the supervision of baby-friendly hospitals be strengthened. The coverage of free pre-pregnancy eugenic health examination will be expanded and the full range of pregnancy and childbirth services be implemented. Cities and counties with large population should complete the task of building the capacity of maternal and neonatal emergency and critical care, and universally establish referral channels to ensure the safety of mothers and infants.

4) We will promote the family development of family planning and services for the mobile population. We will improve the reward and support policy of family for family planning and do a good job in providing special support and care for the families abiding by the family planning policy with special difficulties. We should deeply carry out the action of caring for girls and intensify the efforts to combat the "Two Illegal Actions". We will fully develop the projects to create a happy family and a "New Family Plan", do a good job in the pilot work of scientific child-rearing in families, adolescent health development and care for the aged, strengthen the equalization of basic public services of health and family planning for the mobile population, and promote the social integration of the mobile population.

(4) Consolidating and upgrading the quality and level of medical services

1) The medical service system and capacity-building will be strengthened. All localities should follow the requirements of the *Planning Outline of National Medical and Health Service System (2015-2020)*, issue the plans at provincial, prefectural and county levels within the year, and carry out special supervision and inspection on the actual use of the plans to promote their implementation. In view of the weak aspects, we will continue to improve the county hospital service capacity.

2) The supervision of medical services should be strengthened to ensure medical safety. The *Measures for Medical Quality Management* will be formulated, and a long-term mechanism of medical quality control will be established. The clinical pathway application will be accelerated, The suitable clinical pathways will be selected and be promoted to implement in tertiary hospitals and county hospitals, and the training of clinical pathway management be strengthened to improve the coverage and

management quality of diseases. We will perform the standardized management of diagnosis and treatment of major diseases like cancer, and revise the *Measures for the Management of Clinical Application of Medical Technology*. We will also strengthen the clinical pharmacy management, strengthen the joint prevention and control, continue to implement the national strategy to contain drug resistance of bacteria, consolidate the complete coverage of blood nucleic acid detection in blood stations, promote the rational clinical use of blood, and ensure the blood supply.

3) We will further improve the medical services. The year 2016 is the second year of the three-year action plan. All localities should further refine and implement the specific plans, work hard to do several practical things, resolve the outstanding contradictions and problems by starting from where people are dissatisfied, and improve their services. It's not about fineness, it's about effectiveness. The tertiary hospitals should fully implement pre-registered medical services, gradually develop daytime surgery, and continue to promote quality nursing services. The "Three Mediations and One Insurance" medical dispute prevention and treatment mechanism should be improved to promote a harmonious relationship between doctors and patients. The meticulous management should be strengthened, and the guiding principles of hospital constitutions, the post responsibility and work system of medical institutions should be formulated. The performance evaluation of public hospitals should be strengthened, and promote the online opening to the public of registration information of medical institutions, doctors and nurses. We will actively and steadily push forward the reform of doctor qualification examination and launch a pilot for rural assistant physician qualification examination for general practice.

(5) Implementing the Health Poverty Alleviation Projects

It is an important political task entrusted by the Central Committee in the 13th Five-Year Plan period to carry out the health poverty alleviation projects and effectively prevent poverty due to illnesses. Health and family planning departments at all levels should attach great importance to it, make great efforts to promote it and improve the level of precise poverty alleviation. We will establish health cards system for the poor in rural areas, carry out contracted services, and implement the policy of "Two Increases and Two Decreases" for the poor population covered by the archive and cards, that is, to increase the reimbursement level of NCMS outpatient service, to increase the proportion of reimbursement within the scope of the policy with the increasing rate no less than 5 percentage points; to decrease the starting line of reimbursement for sick and disabled children, severely disabled people and major illness insurance, and decrease the personal actual expenditure of the poor population for major illnesses. We will implement the mechanism of providing counterpart assistance, implement the "Group-type" assistance provided steadily and constantly by the tertiary hospitals all over the country to the county-level hospitals of the poor counties, so as to ensure that the level and appearance of hospitals in the poor counties are upgraded and changed and basically meet the basic medical service needs of the residents in the counties. We will carry out poverty alleviation policies and measures as a whole, strengthen the efforts to prevent and cure infectious and local diseases in key areas, adopt various policies and measures to gradually change the production and living conditions and living customs in poverty-stricken areas, and allow the rural poor people to step into a well-off society hand in hand with the people of the whole country.

(6) Raising the level of public health, food safety and health emergency response

1) We will conduct the prevention and control by focusing on major diseases. We will continue to implement the national basic and major public health service projects, strengthen immunization, promote the replacement by using bivalent poliomyelitis attenuated live vaccines, and push forward the insurance pilot for the vaccination abnormal response compensation. Social organizations will be encouraged to participate in AIDS prevention and control fund projects and the supervision and management and the effectiveness evaluation be strengthened. The pilot projects of comprehensive prevention and treatment of tuberculosis and comprehensive management of mental health will be expanded, the free supply of special drugs for the treatment of such diseases as HIV/AIDS, tuberculosis and severe mental disorders be increased, and explore ways to reduce the financial burden of patients with major diseases like tuberculosis and serious mental disorders through out-patient coordination. The population iodine nutrition monitoring will be carried out in 1/3counties of China. We will step up efforts to prevent and treat pneumoconiosis among migrant workers. A new version of the dietary guidelines for Chinese residents will be released. We will launch the second-phase action of the national healthy lifestyle, promote the patriotic health movement in depth, comprehensively open up the construction of healthy cities, and promote the reform of latrines in rural areas. Attention should be paid to the effects of drinking water and air pollution on the health of urban and rural residents and the surveillance of vector organisms. We will further strengthen the construction of the disease control system, promote the implementation of the guidelines of the organization of the CDC and the opinions on the safety and protection of personnel involved in the prevention and control of infectious diseases, lose no time to issue the plan for adjusting the subsidy for health and epidemic prevention, and carry out standardized training for public health physicians.

2) We will strengthen the construction of food safety standards and risk monitoring. We should implement the *Food Safety Law*, revise and improve the implementing regulations and supporting documents, speed up the formulation and revision of food safety standards in key fields, comprehensively implement the

annual national food safety risk monitoring plan, and strengthen food-borne disease surveillance report and traceability building.

3) We will enhance the core ability of health emergencies. We will formulate the guidance to support the professionalization of health emergency response teams at primary level, improve the joint command and coordination mechanism, promote the comprehensive monitoring, risk assessment and timely early warning of public health emergencies, start the construction of a three-dimensional emergency medical rescue network for land, sea and air, and do a good job in health emergency for public health emergencies and disasters.

(7) Improving the policies and mechanisms for the development of traditional Chinese medicine

We will conscientiously implement the spirit of the important instructions of General Secretary Xi Jinping and Premier Li Keqiang on the development of traditional Chinese medicine, seize the favorable opportunities to speed up the development of the cause of traditional Chinese medicine. The *Outline of Strategic Planning for the Development of Traditional Chinese Medicine (2015—2030)* will be formulated and implemented to promote the reform of traditional Chinese medicine hospitals, improve the differentiated reform policy, and increase the comprehensive service capacity of county-level traditional Chinese medicine hospitals. We will promote the development and upgrading of traditional Chinese medicine health industry, deepen the reform of the science and technology system of traditional Chinese medicine and the reform of education in traditional Chinese medicine institutions, strengthen the construction of the national clinical research base of traditional Chinese medicine and provincial research institutes of traditional Chinese medicine. The fourth General Survey of Traditional Chinese Medicine (TCM) will be carried out. We will strengthen the construction of experimental areas for comprehensive reform of traditional Chinese medicine and promote the construction of overseas centers for traditional Chinese medicine.

(8) Promoting the innovation of medical science and technology and the construction of qualified personnel

We will implement the national strategy of innovation-driven development, make great efforts to build a scientific and technological innovation system for the health of the population, and promote the preparation for construction of the national laboratory for major diseases. We will continue to implement the two major scientific and technological projects, launch the implementation of key national R & D projects such as precision medicine and birth defects intervention, establish a national coordination mechanism for bio-safety work, strengthen the supervision of laboratory bio-safety, optimize the layout of key scientific research bases, construct the management system of clinical research of new medical technology, and push forward the technology evaluation and promotion. We will also establish a convergence mechanism of medical talent training and talent demand of health and family planning industry, strengthen the construction of talent training base, improve the quality of standardized training for physicians, and carry out pilot projects of standardized training for specialists. The training of general practitioners will be strengthened. Taking the rural primary units in less developed areas as the focus, the pilot training of "3 + 2" assistant general practitioners will be launched, and the special post program for general practitioners expanded to 20 provinces. We will further reform and improve the evaluation of professional titles of health personnel at primary level, highlight the performance of medical services with no more emphasis on papers, foreign languages, computers and other requirements.

(9) Coordinating and advancing all key tasks

1) The building of the rules of law and comprehensive supervision will be strengthened. We will actively cooperate with the National people's Congress in completing the drafting and administrative examination and approval of the *Basic Medical and Health Law* (draft). We will continue to clean up the items of administrative examination and approval, complete the adjustment of the management mode of large equipment, push forward the "One Window" service mode, carry out the opinions of the six departments, integrate the administrative law enforcement resources of health and family planning, further strengthen the comprehensive supervision work, try out the "Double Random" inspection mechanism, and use the means of credit supervision to strengthen the combination of release and management. We will carry out the special supervision and inspection on the implementation of laws and regulations like the *Law on Population and Family Planning* and the *Law on the Prevention and Treatment of Occupational Diseases*, as well as on the clinical application of stem cells, and conduct the special rectification involving medical safety and the strong problems reflected by the people. We should make supervision information public and strengthen social supervision.

2) We should strengthen the publicity and guidance and health promotion. The professional spirit of health and family planning should be vigorously carried forward and practiced to encourage the vast number of health care workers to take the advanced collectives in Ebola hemorrhagic fever epidemic prevention and control, Tu Youyou and other advanced models as examples and wholeheartedly serve for the people's health. We will improve the pertinence and timeliness of publicity work, play the role of mainstream media, and, by using the language people can understand and remember, explain the policies thoroughly and the target task, measures for reform and progress effectiveness clearly and the benefits of people understandable. We will improve the mechanism of information release, timely grasp the dynamics of public opinions to keep present in major issues and not silent at critical moments,

so as to win the understanding, support and participation of the whole society. We should carry out healthy China activities, firmly promote the pilot projects of health promotion into counties (districts), guide people to improve their health literacy and self-care awareness, and continue to do a good job in tobacco control performance. We will prepare well for the Ninth Global Health Promotion Conference.

3) We will actively participate in the global health and population cooperation. We will take the initiative to serve the overall interests of diplomacy, promote the implementation of the 2030 sustainable development agenda, and consolidate and expand the cooperation with international organizations such as the World Health Organization and the Partnership of South-South Cooperation on population and development at the platform of major cooperation mechanisms. With "Belt and Road" as the starting point, the Forum on Health Cooperation with ASEAN and Central and Eastern European Countries will be held, and the joint projects of China, Japan and South Korea, the Mekong Sub-region and the China-Arab countries will be implemented. We will implement new measures for health cooperation between China and Africa, strengthen the management innovation of foreign aid medical teams, help construct the capacity of African countries' health systems, and continuously enhance our right to speak to the outside world. We will practically promote medical and health cooperation with Hong Kong, Macao and Taiwan.

**(Chen Ying)**

## 2. Scientifically Plan the Routes and Key Tasks of Disease Prevention and Control in the 13th Five-Year Plan Period

(Li Bin, January 29$^{th}$, 2016, Beijing)

### I. Achievement of disease control and prevention during the 12th Five-Year Plan period

**(1) The prevention and control policy mechanism has been constantly innovated and improved.** *Law of the People's Republic of China on Prevention and Control of Infectious Diseases* and *Mental Health Law of the People's Republic of China* have been issued and amended at the national level. Important policy documents have been issued such as the opinions on strengthening the safety protection of infectious disease prevention and control personnel, the three-year action plan for cancer prevention and control, and mental health planning. The State Council has integrated nine single disease prevention and treatment mechanisms and established an inter-ministerial joint conference system for the prevention and treatment of major diseases. Fund projects have been established for social organizations to participate in AIDS prevention and treatment. Comprehensive prevention and treatment zones for chronic diseases have been established in 265 counties. Pilot projects on comprehensive mental health management have been carried out. Social stability and harmony have been promoted.

(2) **Significant progress has been made in the prevention and control of major diseases.** The policies suitable for the diseases have been adhered to. The prevention and control strategies of major diseases have been constantly improved. Immunizations have been intensified. China has stopped to be one of the countries with high incidence of hepatitis B. The incidence of infectious diseases most vaccines can prevent has hit a historical low. The impoverished patients and rural patients have received free treatment of tuberculosis, thus achieving one of the UN millennium development goals five years ahead of schedule. Through the implementation of the measures such as the "Four Frees and One Care" policy, the full coverage of blood nucleic acid testing at blood stations, and the expansion of maternal and child blockade, overall AIDS epidemic has been of low prevalence. The monitoring of key occupational diseases has covered all cities and has effectively protected the health of workers. The pilot program of echinococcosis prevention and control has been launched. The prevention and treatment of endemic diseases such as schistosomiasis have made remarkable achievement.

(3) **The epidemic prevention of major emergencies has been orderly and effective.** The tasks at the two fronts—domestic prevention and control of the Ebola hemorrhagic fever epidemic and medical aid to Africa against epidemics—have been accomplished. "Zero Input, Zero Infection" has been achieved, which has been widely praised by domestic and international parties, and highly recognized by the Party Central Committee and the State Council. There has been successful emergency treatment of cases such as the imported case of the Middle East Respiratory Syndrome and outbreaks of dengue fever in some areas. There has been no major post-disaster epidemic in Lushan, Sichuan province, Ludian, Yunnan province and other earthquake-stricken areas, effectively protecting the lives, health and safety of the people. The tasks of epidemic prevention and security for major events have been fulfilled such as the Nanjing Youth Olympic Games and the Beijing APEC Conference. New contributions have been made to the overall service.

(4) **The disease prevention and control capacity has been consolidated and improved.** Annual deployment, quarterly scheduling, monthly assessment, and weekly analysis have been implemented. Infectious disease monitoring and early warning have reached the international advanced level. The monitoring coverage of health hazards such as major diseases, common diseases, key occupational diseases, air pollution, rural environmental sanitation, and urban and rural drinking water has been continuously expanded. The characteristics and development trends of major

chronic diseases such as cancer have been basically mastered. The per capita financial subsidy standard of basic public health service has been raised to 40 *yuan*. The service projects have been extended to 12 categories and 45 items, which has basically covered the entire life-cycle of residents. The service quality and level have been significantly improved. The major public health service projects have covered nearly 200 million people. The general public have noticed the new changes and new benefits brought about by the improvement of public health services.

(5) **The patriotic health movement has achieved development and upgrade.** The State Council has issued a programmatic document to strengthen patriotic health in the new era, intensified comprehensive environmental management, and launched a new round of urban and rural environmental sanitation and clean-up actions. The urban and rural environmental health has been improved significantly. A number of national healthy cities and healthy towns (counties) have been established. Management and exit mechanisms have been established. Dynamic management has been implemented and guidelines for the construction of healthy cities and evaluation indicators have been formulated. The national healthy lifestyle action has covered 80% of the counties (regions) in the country. The awareness of disease prevention and the quality of civilized health have been enhanced. There has been remarkable improvement in some aspects.

### II. Profound analysis of the situation and clear ideas of work

The "13th Five-Year Plan" period is the decisive stage for the comprehensive construction of a moderately prosperous society in all respects. It is also the decisive stage of establishing and improving the basic medical and health system covering urban and rural residents. China's residents' consumption structure has undergone transformation and upgrade. There has been new urbanization. Population ageing has been accelerated. Multiple diseases have coexisted. The double burden of infectious diseases and chronic diseases has been larger and larger. People's new expectations for health have been more prominent and more urgent. It requires the simultaneous growth of service resources and health needs to ensure that all citizens have equal access to basic medical and public health services, and strive for less illness, late illness, and no major illness. The level of physical and mental health is compatible with and suitable for the level of a moderately prosperous society in all respects. With the deepening of China's opening up to the outside world, a large number of cross-border and cross-region people, commodities, etc. are rapidly circulating. By means of modern transportation, disease vectors can spread at an unprecedented rate. If prevention and control were made improperly and diseases were mistakenly responded to, it would pose a serious threat to national public health security, but also become a major issue affecting politics, economy and diplomacy. It requires the state to comprehensively strengthen public health at the strategic level, continuously improve national health to make overall and long-term institutional arrangements and provide coordinated solutions.

The 5th Plenary Session of the Eighteenth Central Committee of the Communist Party of China made major decision-making arrangements for "promoting healthy China's construction" on the basis of the strategic layout of "four comprehensives" and pointed out the direction for public health work in the new era. From the point of "big health and great health", the development concept of innovation, coordination, green development, openness and sharing should be firmly established. Our institutional advantages and organizational advantages should be given full play to. Health should be included into various economic and social policies. Prevention should be given priority to. Combination of prevention and control, joint prevention and joint control, group prevention and group control should be adhered to. Efforts should be made to achieve a transition from "disease-centered" to "health-centered" to ensure that there will be a comprehensive public health service system with clear division of labor, information exchange, resource sharing, coordination and interaction, and efficient operation by 2020. Efforts should be made in the following 4 aspects:

**(1) Saving against a rainy day and establishing and improving disease monitoring and early warning system**

Stable, continuous, comprehensive and accurate population health monitoring data is an important prerequisite for scientific decision-making in disease prevention and treatment, and it is also the key to taking the initiative of prevention and treatment. It has been basic experience in several decades of disease prevention and treatment, and many campaigns against major epidemics. The first is to improve the disease surveillance network. It is necessary to further integrate monitoring networks such as infectious diseases, chronic diseases, foodborne diseases, causes of death, and health hazards, optimize information sharing mechanisms, and form disease monitoring, risk assessment and early warning platforms to truly reflect the status of diseases and health hazards, and to make early detection of the prevalence of major epidemics. The second is to enhance the ability of monitoring and early warning. It is necessary to gradually extend the monitoring content and improve the quality of monitoring. Nowadays, people often go to hospitals instead of disease control agencies. It is necessary to improve the knowledge and ability of personnel of community medical institutions to discover and control infectious diseases, and effectively monitor the role of monitoring as outposts to achieve early detection, early reporting, early diagnosis and early treatment. To have more time for dealing with the epidemic, there must not be any delay. The third is to strengthen the construction of disease control information. At the national level, a top-level design should be made to improve the disease control information system as soon as possible and promote interconnection in combination with the overall construction of population health information. It is necessary to adhere to giving priority to standards, strengthening business synergy, improving the universality of information and the timeliness of reporting and feedback, and guiding the community-level institutions to effectively carry out prevention and control.

**(2) Innovating institutional mechanisms to promote closer integration of public health policies and deepening medical reform measures**

Improving the function of the service system and continuously improving the service capacity are not only important goals for deepening medical reform, but also important conditions for smooth medical reform. All medical reform policies and measures must fully consider the internal development rules and requirements of public health undertakings. The two should promote each other and complement each other. In promoting the construction of a hierarchical diagnosis and treatment system, and with infectious diseases such as hypertension, diabetes, and other common diseases, frequently-occurring diseases, chronic diseases, and tuberculosis as starting points, the pilot diseases of hierarchical diagnosis and treatment should be gradually extended. Rapid division of treatment of acute and chronic diseases should be implemented. The level of management intervention should be raised. In terms of improving the basic medical insurance system, it is necessary to explore disease-based payment for diseases such as AIDS, tuberculosis, and severe mental disorders, and to solve the medical security problems of the poor with such major diseases through basic medical insurance, major illness insurance, and medical assistance, etc. In addition, it is necessary to reform the outpatient reimbursement method so that the expenses of these infectious diseases can be reasonably reimbursed in outpatient treatment to reduce the burden on patients, and effectively control the spread of infectious diseases. In controlling the unreasonable growth of medical expenses, it is necessary to establish a health management consortium, calculate large accounts, calculate general ledgers, and reform some reimbursement methods to save medical insurance expenses and mass medical expenses in an overall way to find a win-win solution. In terms of information construction, it is necessary to encourage the "Internet + public health" pilot programs, promote the deep integration of information technology and public health services such as big data, and improve public literacy of disease prevention and public access to health services.

**(3) Collaboration of teaching of and research on medical prevention and intellectual support for disease prevention and control**

It is necessary to strengthen the combination of prevention and control, and further clarify the responsibilities of disease prevention and control, medical services, primary health care and health supervision agencies in the prevention and treatment of infectious diseases. Some major diseases should be gradually taken over by medical institutions, especially designated medical institutions; The public health departments in the primary health care institutions should be responsible for patient community health management, follow-up services and health education, etc., which must enter the service package of the contract service; It is necessary to further strengthen epidemic monitoring, analysis, research and determination, epidemiological investigation, epidemic disposal, laboratory test, monitoring and evaluation, supervision and inspection, etc., and lead the establishment of a collaborative mechanism. The incentive and restraint mechanism for medical personnel to engage in public health services should be improved. The construction of designated hospitals for the clinical treatment of major infectious diseases at the provincial, prefectural and municipal levels should be accelerated. The synergistic treatment model with Chinese and Western medicine should be explored.

It is necessary to strengthen the coordination of medical education. It is necessary to take the initiative to join the education sector, strengthen the training of talented professionals of public health, improve the quality of training, and gradually reach the balance between supply and demand in the training of public health professionals. It is necessary to strengthen the theory and skill assessment of infectious disease prevention and control in resident standardized training courses. This year, standardized training for public health doctors will be carried out. The third is to enhance the ability of independent innovation. The important opportunity of the country to implement the innovation-driven development strategy should be seized to strengthen scientific research on major disease prevention and control, and strive to make a breakthrough in localizing vaccines, drugs, diagnostic reagents, new technologies for the treatment with Chinese and Western medicine, key equipment of diagnosis and medical treatment, etc. National laboratories are the key carrier of achieving technological innovation. The National Health and Family Planning Commission will promote the construction of national laboratories for major disease research, especially the construction of the P4 laboratory of the China CDC. It is necessary to implement innovation projects of medical and health science and technology, adhere to high-starting-point layout, and form a moderate-scale and highly efficient and coordinated network of national disease prevention and control laboratories. Each province should have a third-level biological safety laboratory to improve laboratory testing capabilities and strive to become a member of the national reference laboratories and technology network, and play a role in the detection of epidemics and the diagnosis of diseases.

**(4) Strengthening community-level institutions, compensating for the insufficient and paying close attention to the weak links in prevention and control work**

It is necessary to coordinate the overall situation, optimize and adjust the layout of public health resources, highlight the weak links and lagging areas, focus on high-risk areas and vulnerable groups, focus on tackling key problems, and make up for the insufficient to prevent risks. It is necessary to pay attention to the health of the student group. With focus on rural boarding secondary schools, early screening and patient treatment management of tuberculosis should be strengthened, and school communication flow should be curbed. With focus on university students, interventions should be innovated, and communication of AIDS should be reduced. At the same time, eye health care and the prevention of oral diseases should be ensured. Disease prevention and control in poor areas should be paid attention to. All localities should adopt a counterpart poverty alleviation approach and increase assistance to poverty-stricken counties at the national level. The state should pay special attention to some poverty-stricken counties and raise the level of precision poverty alleviation. The public health problems highly concerned by the masses and arousing public attention should be effectively solved. A variety of rescue channels or assistance measures for helping children with abnormal reactions to vaccination should be explored. The problems such as compensation, follow-up rehabilitation, assistance and enrollment should be solved. The prevention and control of migrant workers' pneumoconiosis should be intensified. The occupational health examination of migrant workers, the diagnosis, identification and treatment of pneumoconiosis should be promoted. The rights and interests of occupational health should be earnestly safeguarded. The monitoring and evaluation of the impacts of air pollution, drinking water, etc. on the health of the population should be strengthened. The implementation of interventions to reduce the harm to the health of the people should be promoted.

(Excerpt from the speech at the National Symposium on Disease Prevention and Control)

**(Wang Guimin)**

### 3. Conscientiously Understand the Important Instructions on Learning and Education of "Party Building Studies" and Do a Good Job in Implementing Them

Li Bin, April 15th, 2016, Beijing

**I. Profoundly understanding the significance of Learning and Education of "Party Building Studies"**

**(1) Carrying out learning and education of "Party Building Studies" is an inevitable requirement for the party to be strictly governed in an all-round way.**

Since the 18th National Congress of the Communist Party of China (CPC), the

Central Committee of the Party with Comrade Xi Jinping as its general secretary has made a series of major decisions and arrangements for comprehensively enforcing strict party discipline, and significant results have been achieved in solving the problems of governing the party with leniency and softness. At the same time, it is important to see clearly that at present, the results achieved in governing the party are periodic; Problems such as weakening party leadership, lack of party building, and inadequate strict governance of the party still exist to varying degrees. To solve these problems, we should not only focus on the "key minority", but also on the vast majority. General secretary Xi Jinping made it clear that we need to extend the party's strict governance to the community level. To carry out the learning and education of "Party Building Studies" is to promote inner-party education from leading cadres to broad masses of party members and to the general public, from centralized education to regular education, and it is to implement the strict requirements on every branch and every party member.

(2) **Carrying out learning and education of "Party Building Studies" is an important arrangement for strengthening theoretical armed forces and strengthening ideological and political construction.**

Since the 18th National Congress of the Communist Party of China (CPC), the Central Committee of the Party with comrade Xi Jinping as its general secretary has attached great importance to the building of the party's ideology and made great efforts to consolidate the ideological foundation for strictly governing the party, and the ideological and political quality of party members and cadres has been improved. At the same time, we should also see that there are still some problems among some party members and cadres, and we need to work hard on education regularly. To carry out the learning and education of "Party Building Studies" is to base on the principle of frequently doing, paying attention to details and doing for a long time, integrating ideological and political development into the daily political life of the party and arming all party members with the latest theoretical achievements of adapting Marxism to China; it is also to further solve the problems of party members in thinking, organization, style of work and discipline through "learning" and "doing" so as to lay a solid foundation for the whole party to maintain highly consistent with the central committee of the party with comrade Xi Jinping as its general secretary and ensure that the party remains the core of strong leadership in the cause of socialism with Chinese characteristics.

(3) **Carrying out learning and education of "Party Building Studies" is an urgent need to promote the reform and development in health and family planning.**

At present, the national health and family planning system is deepening the reform of the medical and health system and the reform of the management of family planning services, which is pushing forward the construction of a healthy China. To carry out the learning and education of "Party Building Studies is to guide all party members to further study and implement the important speeches of general secretary Xi Jinping, especially the important discourse spirit on health and family planning work; it is to promote the full implementation of the party's main responsibility of comprehensive strict governance, and give full play to the role of community-level party organizations as battlefields and the role of party members as vanguards and models; it is also to find problems, purge discipline, make use of forced reform and promote development in accordance with the relevant requirements of the ongoing special inspection tour of the central government. Thus we can lay a solid foundation and provide a powerful guarantee for health and family planning career so that it may have a good start in the 13th Five-year Period.

### II. Laying a solid foundation, grasping the key and making solid progress in learning and education of "Party Building Studies"

The foundation of "Party Building Studies" is to learn. The Party Constitution is the fundamental law of the Party. It is the general rule of governing the party and the common code of conduct that the whole party must observe. Party discipline is the extension and concretization of the party constitution, which clearly stipulates the discipline and rules that party members should strictly observe. A series of important speeches by general secretary Xi Jinping have profoundly answered a suite of major theoretical and practical problems which arose in the career development of the party and our country in the new historical conditions, further enriched and developed the party's theory, guidelines and policies, and proposed new requirements with more characteristic of the times for all the party members and cadres. The party constitution and rules are closely related to the general secretary's series of important speeches and they come down in one continuous line. They must be learned through the link and understood through unity.

For all party members, learning the party constitution and rules means that they should read the party constitution thoroughly, read the principles of integrity and self-discipline, the regulations on disciplinary punishment and the regulations on safeguarding the rights of party members so as to further clarify the criteria for becoming qualified party members, and raise the consciousness of respecting, revering and abiding party constitution. Learning Xi Jinping's series of important speeches is mainly to learn to grasp their fundamental spirit, learn to grasp the basic content of the new concepts, new ideas and new strategy of the CPC central committee in governing the country, understand and grasp the fundamental requirements of enhancing party spirit breeding, practicing the concept of purpose and cultivating moral character, and really use the spirit of the general secretary's series of important speeches to unify our thinking, improve our understanding and profoundly grasp the responsibilities and missions of party members in the new situation.

For the leading cadres of party members at or above the county level, they should not only be familiar with the content that all party members should learn and master, but also master the regulations and requirements closely related to the performance of their duties. To learn the general secretary's series of important speeches is to grasp the rich connotation and the core idea, master Marxist standpoint, viewpoint and method throughout it, understand the firm belief in the faith, historical responsibility, sincere feelings for the people and pragmatic ideology. In particular, it is important to understand the new concepts, new ideas and new strategies of governing the country which are implied in the important speeches of the general secretary. For us, we should also focus on the general secretary Xi Jinping's important speech and indicative spirit on health and family planning, further clarify working ideas and objectives, and study and propose specific measures to strengthen and improve work.

The key point of "party building studies" is to do. That is, to be a qualified communist party member. The most fundamental thing is to strengthen political consciousness, overall consciousness, core consciousness and sense of unity. We must implement the practical action of keeping up with the CPC central committee, and make it mandatory.

The learning and education program issued by the central government has put forward the standard of "Four Principles and Four Requirements" for qualified party members in the new situation.

What stressing on politics and having faith emphasizes is political qualification. It is to be loyal to the party and have ideal and belief. We should speak for the party while in the party, worry about the party while in the party, work for the party while in the party and love the party while in the party. What stressing on rules and having discipline emphasizes is the implementation of discipline is qualified. That is, we must strictly observe the party's political discipline and rules and regulations, strengthen the concept of organization, obey organizational decisions, and know how to respect, draw the line and observe rules. What stressing on moral and having good behavior emphasizes is morality is qualified. That is, we need to uphold morality, public morality and private morality, inherit the party's fine style of work, promote traditional Chinese virtues, live up to the socialist core values and uphold the lofty ideals of the communist party. What stressing on dedication and having achievement emphasizes is playing a role is qualified. That is, we must live up to the party's purpose, remain true to the people, be responsible and responsible, and serve as a pacesetter and model in advancing reform, development and stability. Every party member should measure himself and examine himself with "Four Principles and Four Requirements", and set up the communist party member's vanguard image.

### III. Conscientiously fulfilling the entity responsibility to ensure that learning and education of "Party Building Studies" is effective.

#### (1) Strengthening organizational leadership and fulfilling responsibilities at all levels

The learning and education of "party building studies" of the party committee of the organs directly under the CPC Central Committee is carried out under the leadership of the leading party group of the CPC Central Committee. As secretary of the leading party group, I take the lead. All the members of leading party group of the CPC Central Committee take charge of the implementation according to the work they are in charge of. The main comrades who are in charge of each unit shall assume the responsibilities of the first person in charge to examine and approve the work plan personally, to deploy the important task personally and do a great job of learning and education strictly in the light of practical situation. Party organization secretaries at all levels should build up awareness of the construction of party member team and shoulder the responsibilities, bring the situation of learning and education into the assessment and appraisal about the report on party building at the primary level, strengthen specific guidance for learning and education of the whole system and study and put forward suggestions on strengthening industry guidance. The members of leading party group of the CPC Central Committee shall do a good job of guidance according to the division of work and the contact points of medical reform. Each division should combine business work and the finished annual key work to give good guidance.

#### (2) Persisting in asking leaders to take the lead and set a good example for others

Leading cadres of party members, the "key minority", should be good examples, take it, guide it, play the role of model and take the lead so as to form the overall effect of the interaction between the upper and lower levels and the whole. The members of leading party group of the CPC Central Committee and the leading cadres at the departmental level shall strictly implement the system of dual organizational life, participate in the activities of their branches as ordinary party members,take the lead in participating in study and discussion, take the lead in talking about experience, giving party lessons, making reports and making contributions in their own posts of duty. Before July 1$^{st}$, the secretaries of party organizations in various units should concentrate on party lessons in conjunction with the activities to commemorate the 95th anniversary of the founding of the party.

**(3) Strengthening the Issue-oriented approach in order to achieve actual effect**

Party organizations and party members at all levels under the organs directly under the CPC Central Committee should, in light of their respective realities, conduct in-depth investigations and make detailed investigation to solve such problems as party members' vague ideals and beliefs, party members' weak consciousness, weak sense of purpose, low spirits, and moral misconduct. They shall find out the specific manifestation of the problems, study the specific measures to improve and solve them so that they can make changes while learning and make changes right after they know. It should be closely combined with the rectification of problems discovered by special inspection tour of the central committee. They shall seriously reflect on the problems reflected in the inspection tour, so as to grasp implementation and rectification with the spirit of driving nails.

**(4) Giving prominence to regular education and strengthening the building of community-level organizations**

The party branch shall be taken as the basic unit, and the specific task, working measure and method carriers that the party branch should have for carrying out learning and education shall be explicated. It is necessary to take the organizational life of the party as the basic form to hold meetings of small party groups well, organize meetings of party branch members well, give party lectures well, and hold organizational activity meetings with special topic well; We shall take the implementation of the system of education and democratic evaluation of party members according to the regulations, and deal with unqualified party members steadily and orderly. It is necessary to conscientiously strengthen community-level party building, improve the daily education management of party members, and focus on solving the problems of educating and managing mobile party members, "pocket" party members and missing party members. Nearly 800 party organization secretaries directly under the central government shall be trained.

**(5) Persisting in highlighting the characteristics and giving full play to the initiative and creativity of all units**

All the departments and bureaus of the CPC Central Committee should set a benchmark, demonstrate, take the lead in learning well, doing a good job, and solving their own problems. All directly affiliated and contact units should combine their own characteristics, embody the characteristics of the industry, and show the spiritual outlook of the party members and cadres of health and family planning. Such window units as the ones which provide medical service, public health service and family planning service should, in combination with the action plan for further improvement of medical service, raise awareness of the masses, awareness of service and awareness of quality, and do everything possible to solve the actual difficulties of the masses. For retired cadre party members and worker party members, feasible ways and means should be adopted. The party committees at all levels of the organs directly under the CPC Central Committee shall provide on-the-spot guidance to all the party branches under their jurisdiction throughout the whole process. The steering group should put the emphasis of supervision and guidance on community level and party branch, thoroughly understand the development and actual results of learning and education, timely summarize and popularize the good experience and good practices created at the community level, and identify and correct the tendentious problems and the ones that are just emerging.

**(6) Strengthening overall planning of work and adhering to the principle of "grasping with two hands and promoting with two hands"**

It is necessary to combine learning and education of "Party Building Studies" with doing a good job in various aspects of the current reform and development of health and family planning, with accomplishing the annual key work of this unit, and with the party members' and cadres' performing their duties with due diligence. Party members and cadres should be guided to set up five major development concepts. Main work should be promoted; and the reform and development of health and family planning undertakings should be carried forward to achieve a good start of the 13th Five-year Plan. Attention should be paid to making good use of the cadres' "baton." It is necessary to recommend to the CPC and the State Organs Work Committee of the CPC that we should commend "Two Excellent One First" in combination with the commemoration of the 95th anniversary of the founding of the CPC. We should do a good job in propaganda and guidance and create a good atmosphere.

(Excerpt from the speech delivered at the mobilization and deployment meeting about learning and education of "Party Building Studies" held by the organs directly under the CPC Central Committee)

**(Tong Yanlong)**

## 4. Do a Good Job in Building a Clean and Honest Government in the Health and Family Planning System

(Li Bin, in Beijing, April 15<sup>th</sup>, 2016)

### I. Significant results of the construction of the health and family planning system in 2015

(1) Innovating leadership mechanism, and apparently enhancing the sense of responsibility of the main body of the Party, and the construction of clean and honest

government

National Health and Family Planning Commission (NHFPC) renamed the former leading group for the system construction of punishing and preventing corruption the leading group for building a clean and honest government, and anti-corruption of the NHFPC. The opinions and measures on the implementation of the requirements for strict Party control with layer upon layer responsibility transmission are printed and distributed. Most provincial health and family planning committees have set up leading groups for building a clean government and anti-corruption. The tasks of building a clean and honest Party style should be timely decomposed and the relevant safeguard system and responsibility list for the implementation of the principal responsibility be formulated. The inspection and assessment, interview and reminding, and responsibility and integrity report should be carried out. Those who fail to perform their duties properly shall be held accountable for their actions. The implementation of "three turns" by discipline inspection and inspection authorities should be strongly supported, and the organization construction for discipline inspection and supervision be strengthened to timely report typical cases of violation of discipline and law. Therefore, the initiative and self-consciousness of the Party organizations at all levels to implement the principal responsibility must be continuously strengthened.

(2) New progress in the combination of discharge and management by cleaning up the items of administrative approval, simplifying administrative affairs and promoting decentralization

National Health and Family Planning Commission focuses on strengthening the supervision in and after the events, effectively streamlines administration and delegates power with the combination of discharge and management, the changes of government functions, and the strengthened supervision responsibility. Ten items requiring delegated administrative approval have been cancelled and the intermediary services for administrative approval been cleaned up. *Opinions on Strengthening Supervision in and after the Event of Administrative Approval* is printed and distributed to make the overall arrangements for the elimination of the administrative approval delegated to lower levels with "double random" checking mechanism. Provincial health and family planning commissions will continue to deepen the reform of the administrative examination and approval system, complete the liquidation of administrative approval items, refine service guidelines, review working rules, and improve administrative approval. A list of administrative powers, a negative list, and a responsibility list have been formulated to make administrative approval public, implement online approval, and actively and consciously accept social supervision.

(3) Preliminary results in steadily carrying out the special topic education and

consciously practicing the "Three Stricts and Three Steadies"

The achievements have been obtained after National Health and Family Planning Commission deepened the Party's public line education practice and launched the special topic education of "Three Stricts and Three Steadies". The Party members take the lead in giving Party lectures, and carrying out serious criticism and self-criticism to clarify the direction and measures of rectification. Leading bodies of provincial health and family planning commission take the lead in implementing the "Three Stricts and Three Steadies", strengthening supervision and inspection, and further changing the work style. Departments of health and family planning at all levels earnestly put discipline and rules ahead, and widely publicize the *Code of Integrity and Self-discipline* and *Disciplinary Ordinance* of the Communist Party of China (CPC). Positive and negative aspects of typical education have been carried out to let the Party members and cadres know the reverence, the bottom line, and the vigilance. Through the special topic education, practical results in deepening the "Four Winds" regulation, creating a loyal, clean and responsible image, respecting discipline and obeying rules, building a good political environment, earnestly implementing and promoting reform and development have been achieved by health and family planning departments at all levels. The practical results in abiding by the rules and building a good political environment and the initial results in making the real efforts to promote reform and development have been achieved.

(4) Persevering in the implementation of the spirit of the eight regulations of the Central Committee and strengthening discipline constraints

The Party group of National Health and Family Planning Commission has carried out the major surveys on health and family planning, and the special supervision and inspection on medical reform in order to help the communities to solve the problems arising from the reform and development, summarized and refined the effective experience to guide the work on the surface, seize the important node, focus on the acts violating the spirit of the eight regulations of the Central Committee with serious investigation on the use of official vehicles, traveling with public funds, eating, drinking and giving gifts with public funds, and releasing the signal that the further you go, the more serious punishment you will get. The provincial health and family planning committees at all levels have continuously step up the investigation and punishment of the problems of violating the spirit of the eight regulations of the Central Committee by means of secret spot inspection, centralized supervision and inspection, and disclosing the names to the public. Health and family planning departments at all levels insist on catching early and catching small, warning early, preventing early, and preventing minor mistakes from becoming big ones.

(5) New achievements in health industry discipline with better construction of

medical and health practices of "Nine Prohibitions"

National Health and Family Planning Commission printed and distributed *Opinions on the Implementation of Strengthening the Construction of Medical Health Practice* to define tasks and responsibilities. The cases involving industrial practices will be investigated and handled, and such problems as receiving "kickbacks" and "red envelopes" be thoroughly dealt with. The health and family planning commissions from fourteen provinces (cities) carried out 880 times of special style rectification, promptly investigated and dealt with any violation of the "Nine Prohibitions", revoked the qualifications of the medical personnel concerned in a timely manner, and timely reported the typical cases of violation of discipline and laws. The health and family planning commission of Guangxi Zhuang Autonomous Region has launched a special campaign against problems existing in the new rural cooperative fund, and the health and family planning commission of Jiangxi Province has made solid efforts to tackle the problem of receiving "red envelopes". Some of the provincial health and family planning commissions have carried out special campaigns targeting at the prominent problems of commercial bribery and kickbacks in key areas such as pharmaceuticals, high-value consumables, equipment procurement and infrastructure construction, and the significant results have been achieved.

(6) New breakthroughs in strengthening intra-Party and trade supervision with comprehensive conduction of inspections

The Party group of National Health and Family Planning Commission attaches great importance to the inspection and made 3 rounds of inspections in 18 directly affiliated and the related units throughout the year. Inspection and rectification are vigorously promoted. The leading group of the CPC on building a clean and honest government and anti-corruption was briefed on the inspection and rectification of the inspected units and the relevant departments so as to ensure that every rectification is in place. The budget management of the entrusted hospitals should be supervised and twelve entrusted hospitals were inspected. The implementation of the *Blood Donation Law* and other five laws and regulations are supervised, and the special renovation is carried out to improve the institutions providing technical service for radiological health. The oversight of the budget management of the entrusted hospitals is strengthened, and ten province-level health and family planning commissions carried out the inspection on units directly under their control. 130 large-scale hospitals are inspected by health and family planning commissions from 26 provinces (autonomous regions, municipalities directly under the Central Government). Health and family planning commissions across the country will continue to step up their oversight of medical institutions, public places and illegal medical advertisements, punish illegal activities and safeguard people's health rights and interests.

## II. Deeply understanding the severe and complex situation that the health and family planning system faces in building a clean and honest government and fighting against corruption

(1) Frequent occurrence of illegal and criminal problems. In recent years, crimes in the health and family planning system are still serious and corruption cases have occurred from the top of National Health and Family Planning Commission to the bottom of township hospitals. Corruption of the persons in charge of community-level medical institutions is a serious problem, which is mainly manifested in the purchase of medical equipment, the purchase and sale of drugs, the construction of projects and the acceptance of bribes by electing and appointing officials. Simultaneously, there are many nest cases and series of cases, and some medical institutions are involved in commercial rebate cases, usually from the hospital presidents to the department directors, doctors, nurses and so on. In the current anti-corruption struggle under the high pressure, the individual Party cadres of the system are still do not restrain or hold back. The task of the health and family planning system to reduce the corruption stock and curb the increase of corruption remains arduous. The profound lessons of the series of cases of illegal vaccine business in Jinan, Shandong Province have exposed illegal and criminal acts in the field of vaccine circulation, the loopholes and hidden dangers in the supervision of vaccine circulation and use, the weak awareness of compliance by individual vaccination units and the institutions of disease control center and vaccination at the community level, non-standardized daily management, poor management of individual vaccination units, and the lax supervision from administrative department of health and family planning.

(2) Frequent violations of six disciplines. The violations of six disciplines were highlighted in health and family planning system. Some Party members and cadres do not have a strong sense of discipline, do not observe discipline, do not observe rules, they step on the "red line", "the bottom line", and hit the "minefield", instead. Some Party members and cadres are unorganized, do not ask for reports on major matters, and seriously violate the organizational discipline. Some Party members and cadres violate the integrity and discipline by receiving gifts and money from subordinate units and management service objects during the inspection and assessment. Other Party members and cadres at community level violate public discipline, and the violations of the interests of the masses have occurred from time to time. Still other Party members and cadres violate the discipline of work and lack responsibility. They are unwilling to undertake or do not conscientiously fulfill the overall responsibility of exercising strict control over the Party. Still others do not conscientiously study and implement the Guidelines and Regulations so we still have a long way to go to build a high level of integrity and uphold the bottom line of discipline.

(3) Repeated violations of the spirit of the eight regulations of the Central Committee. Although the Central Committee has given repeated orders and injunctions, but still some Party members and leading cadres are unscrupulous and do things their own way. In 2015, National Health and Family Planning Commission and most provincial health and family planning commissions investigated and dealt with violations of the spirit of the eight regulations of the Central Committee. The Ministry of Discipline Inspection of the Central Commission reported on its website the cases of the violations of the spirit of the eight regulations of the Central Committee, and the health and family planning system accounts for a certain proportion of the cases. The violations are such problems as eating with public funds, traveling with public funds, illegal handling of wedding, funeral and other issues, and there are also illegal receiving and sending of gift money, illegal distribution of subsidies and other issues. All these show that serious problems exist in the "Four Winds". To consolidate and implement the achievements of the spirit of the eight regulations of the Central Commission, we still need to work hard for a long time.

(4) Bad effects of the violations of the "Nine Prohibitions". Over the past two years or so, the health and family planning departments at all levels have investigated and dealt with a number of violations of the "Nine Prohibitions", which has played an effective and deterrent role. But malpractice and corruption in the field of medical health remain the focus of public concern. Problems such as prescribing order commissions, excessive examinations, illegal fees and accepting donations from social donors can hardly be prohibited in some medical and health institutions. Individual medical and health workers are accustomed to receiving "red envelopes", and even worse, some openly ask for the "red envelopes", so the public is quite indignant. Some medical and health institutions have been lenient and soft in punishing those who violate the "Nine Prohibitions". The violations of the "Nine Prohibitions" damage the vital interests at the expense of ordinary people, gnaw at the sense of gain of the public, and squander the people's trust in the Party at the community level. To these people and things like "a rat excrement spoiled a pot of soup", we must never condone, and must investigate and punish in accordance with the law. Those who have repeatedly broken the forbidden shall be held accountable to the hospital director in accordance with the law. If the circumstances are especially serious, the hospital director shall be held accountable.

### III. Implementation of the Central Commission's requirement to comprehensively enforce strict governance of the Party and earnestly strengthen the building of a clean and honest Party style in the health and family planning system

(1) Strict enforcement of the Party's discipline and consolidation of the

responsibilities for managing and governing the Party

The Party organizations at all levels of the health and family planning system shall bear the principal requirements responsibility, bear all the requirements in mind, put them on shoulder and grasp them in hand in the whole process of strictly governing the Party. First of all, we should earnestly enhance the awareness and discipline awareness of the Party cadres. The success of medical reform and the comprehensive implementation of the family planning policy must depend on the leadership of the Party. In particular, the leading cadres of the Party members must speak for the Party, care for the Party, and strive for the Party as the Party members. Education should be effectively strengthened and the Party officials should be organized to study the *CPC's Code of Integrity and Self-discipline* and *Regulations for Disciplinary Punishment* to clarify the high standards pursued by the Party members and the rules managing and governing the Party.

We should launch the careful study and the education of "Two Learns and One Action" so as to educate and guide the Party members to respect the Party rules and regulations. With the series of the important speech spirit of General Secretary Xi Jinping in arming our minds, guiding our practice and promoting our work, we must strive to solve the problems existing in Party members' thinking, organization, style of work and discipline, make efforts to strengthen the Party members' political consciousness, overall situation consciousness, core consciousness and sense of unity, firm their ideals and beliefs, maintain their loyalty to the Party, build a clean and upright spirit and dare to take responsibility for what is done, and give full play to the role of the pioneers and models.

Taking political discipline and organizational discipline seriously. Leading cadres at all levels of the health and family planning system should be good at looking at problems politically, stand firmly, keep the right direction, consciously maintain a high degree of ideological and political agreement with the Central government in faithfully implementing the Central government's decisions and arrangements on promoting the building of a healthy China, deepening medical reform and implementing the universal two-child policy. The health and family planning departments at higher level should know more about the practical work at the community level and listen to more opinions and suggestions, while the health and family planning departments at the lower levels shall, in a practical and realistic manner, report the working conditions and existing problems to the higher authorities, provide true figures, and make serious and responsible opinions and suggestions. For major problems, the request for instructions shall be submitted in a timely manner, and the report shall be reported on time basis, and shall not be concealed from being reported or handled by oneself.

We must put discipline ahead, take "Six Disciplines" as the ruler, dare to bear responsibility, dare to compare truth, dare to fight, and firmly maintain the seriousness of the Party discipline with the intolerance of a little mistake. It shall be normal to raise one's collar and pull one's sleeve, and make one in red face and sweating while locating a problem. If the problem is serious, the organizational processing shall be treated by the organization, and the disciplinary punishment shall be taken. With the accountability as an important gripper, we shall comprehensively and rigorously exercise the governing of the Party, adhere to "a case with double check", form the normalized accountability system, and make the governing of the Party truly from wide, loose, and soft degree to strict, tight, and hard degree.

(2) Carrying out patrol inspections, and patrol examinations and rectifications, and effectively strengthening the oversight within the Party

The leading bodies of the administrative departments of health and family planning at all levels shall consciously accept the supervision of the discipline inspection unit assigned and strengthen the supervision of the discipline inspection committee over the Party committees at the same level. At present, the Party group of National Health and Family Planning Commission is receiving the special patrol inspection of the patrol inspection group. According to the feedback of patrol inspection group, the Party Committee and the Party group will study and formulate a comprehensive rectification work plan, define the rectification target and responsibility subjects, and complete the rectification work comprehensively. In the near future, the first round of inspection tour of the Party committee and the Party group in 2016 will be launched, and the inspection tour of directly affiliated units will be fully covered within the year. Each provincial health and family planning commission should continue to strengthen the inspection of units directly under its jurisdiction, and explore and accumulate the experience. The relevant units shall be urged to make a prompt implementation of the rectification. Those who make perfunctory rectification or fail to implement the responsibilities must be seized as the typical and their accountability be taken seriously. We will continue to carry out the patrol inspections in large-scale hospitals, implement the scheme for 2015-2017 annual inspections, focus on the problems existing in the large-scale hospitals, innovate the way of patrol inspection, deepen, refine and implement the inspection work, and promote the improved medical service and operation management in the large-scale hospitals.

(3) Deepening the building of the work style and letting the spirit of the eight regulations of the Central Committee take root

We will implement the eight regulations of the Central Committee, which is to be deepened in the course of persistence, and persisted in the course of deepening. With the constant efforts of swallows in building their nests, the tenacity of ants in gnawing their bones, and the tenacity of old cattle in climbing the hills, we should persevere to overcome difficulties, improve ourselves constantly and achieve good results. We shall adhere to style construction, the Party's ideological construction, organization construction, system construction, and the construction of fighting corruption and building a clean and honest government, rely on a firm ideals and beliefs, reliable institutional guarantees, strong and effective efforts to punish corruption, and ensure the achievements of our work style construction. We should regard the implementation of the code of integrity and self-discipline as an important tool to improve the work style, which guides the Party members and cadres to cultivate noble moral sentiments and resist unhealthy practices. We should attach importance to the cultivation and shaping of the positive atmosphere of the new wind and explore a long-term mechanism to consolidate and improve the achievements of the construction of the work style. We should start from small points, continue to correct the style of writing and reform the rules of the meetings, and solve the problems that the public strongly reflect, and let the people see our changes bit by bit and enhance their confidence. We need to implement the requirements for stricter discipline in the future, pay closer attention to the new trend and performance of the unhealthy wind, and seriously investigate the "Four Winds" of hidden variation.

(4) Highlighting the key points of punishment and continuing to maintain a high pressure to curb corruption

The leading cadres of the Party members, who failed to hold back, and had serious problems and to whom the public has reacted strongly should be put in the most important place after the eighteenth national congress of the Party. We will resolutely prevent promotion with illness and taking up the post with disease, hold tight to discipline and keep it as a yardstick, catch early and catch little, carry out the "Four Forms" throughout the whole process of supervision, discipline and accountability. According to the principle of "learning from the past mistakes and avoid the future ones, curing diseases and saving life", we should further reduce stock and suppress increment, and achieve political and social effect by punishing a few and educating the most. We will intensify efforts to rectify, investigate and deal with irregularities and corruption at the community level that infringe upon the interests of the people. The investigation on the malpractice and corruption against the interests of the people by the health and family planning institutions at the community level, which is incompatible with the public welfare nature of the health and family planning undertaking and is hated the most by the public, must be resolutely carried out. These irregularities must not be allowed to persist or stand in the way of medical reform. The obstinate diseases that the masses revile or the fort that can not be attacked for a long time, or the indulgence that is even encouraged, the persons on-the-job and off-duty, and both units and individuals must be investigated with discipline violations and corruption, so that the corruption at the community level can not be evaded.

(5) Cleaning up industry discipline and building a strong contingent of health and family planning officials

In general, all sectors of society and the people highly commend and admire the hard work, dedication and perseverance of the Party members and medical workers in the system. The more such, the more the vast majority of medical workers consciously maintain the image of "White Angel". The professional spirit of "being fearless of hardship, willing to sacrifice, saving the dying, supporting the wounded, and offering boundless love" must be vigorously promoted, and a number of advanced models be introduced. Good spirit and fashion should be set up in the whole system to observe discipline by focusing on moral conduct, and remaining good spirit of reputation. The ideological dynamics and work performance of the health and family planning cadres should be paid attention to so as to timely guide and correct any problems found. The methods of assessment, evaluation and selection need to be improved to value the ability and character, political achievements and moral values so that the virtuous cadres can receive praise and put in important positions and the cadres of inferior conduct are warned and disciplined. "Nine Prohibitions" is the iron discipline and the untouchable bottom line of medical and health industry. The discipline inspection commission of medical and health institutions and the higher discipline inspection commission shall take the investigation and punishment of any violation of the "Nine Prohibitions" as their main responsibility. As for the possible future violations of the "Nine Prohibitions", we must deal with them strictly and seriously, and resolutely expel the black sheep from the medical and health teams.

(6) Intensifying our responsibility to fight corruption and building a clean government to safeguard reform and development

1) Breaking through barriers of interest and pushing the deepening of the reform. The reform involves the adjustment of the old pattern of interest relations, which inevitably moves the "cheese" of the vested interests and may involve various corruption problems. We should take a highly responsible attitude towards people's health, take responsibility, comprehensively deepen medical reform, and remove from mechanism the soil on which corruption and malpractice live. In 2016, the comprehensive reform of county-level public hospitals should be consolidated by abolishing the drug bonus in all public hospitals of the pilot areas, establishing a scientific compensation mechanism and speeding up the establishment of a personnel compensation system that conforms to the characteristics of the industry. The centralized procurement of medicines in public hospitals and online procurement of high-value medical consumables are fully implemented, the quantity of medicines is increased by national drug price negotiations and the inflated drug price effectively lowered.

2) Strengthening the oversight and management in the middle and after the incidents. Administrative departments of health and family planning at all levels should further streamline administration and delegate power truly to increase the weight of power, strengthen the effectiveness of regulation by means of true management and highlight service initiatives. The "double random and one publicity" regulation should be comprehensively pushed forward to strengthen the integrated online and offline supervision. All kinds of "exotic" proofs, the unnecessary, and over elaborate formalities should be cut off so as to make the procedures easier and faster for the masses to do things. Regular supervision and inspection of laws, regulations and the implementation of major decisions and arrangements by the Central Committee shall be carried out, and inspection teams be timely dispatched to inspect at irregular intervals.

3) Focusing on daily supervision. The supervision should be focused on the followings: the over-examination, over-medication and over-treatment, the acts of participating in marketing activities such as medical products and health care products, and the arbitrary charges or hitchhiking charges in the management of family planning services for the floating population. We should draw lessons from a series of cases concerning illegal vaccine business in Jinan, Shandong Province, and formulate the *Opinions on Further Strengthening the Administration of Vaccine Circulation and Vaccination* with the relevant departments. And in accordance with the newly revised *Regulations on the Administration of Vaccine Circulation and Vaccination*, we will further improve the long-term mechanism for vaccine management and strengthen the management, close loopholes, increase penalties and accountability, and effectively prevent such cases from happening again.

(Speech at the 2016 Conference on the Construction of Upright Party and Clean Government in National Health and Family Planning System)

**(Ji Chenglian)**

## 5. Take Practical Measures to Improve the Accuracy of Poverty Alleviation

(Li Bin, July 5th, 2016, Lanzhou, Gansu)

The CPC Central Committee and the State Council attach great importance to the work of aiding the poor in health. The central government convened a conference on poverty alleviation and development as it entered the decisive stage of building a moderately prosperous society in all respects to make comprehensive arrangements for overcoming poverty and tackling key problems, including healthy poverty alleviation. It shows that the central government attaches great importance to the work of aiding the poor and is firmly determined to do so. On April 24th, 2016, when General Secretary Xi Jinping visited Jinzhai County in Anhui Province, he pointed out that the problems of poverty caused by illness and returning to poverty due to illness often occur, and that the poverty alleviation mechanism should further improve the underwriting measures. More support should be provided for medical insurance and the new rural cooperative medical care system. Premier Li Keqiang personally studied, personally coordinated, and decided to raise the per capita financial subsidy standard of basic medical insurance for urban and rural residents by another 40 *yuan*, 10 *yuan* of which was used for serious illness insurance, despite the very tight financial situation in those years. It calls for the implementation of tendentious payment policies for the rural poor to enhance the accuracy of serious illness insurance and poverty alleviation in health. Vice Premier Liu Yandong conducted two surveys in poverty-stricken areas this year and chaired a meeting of the State Council's leading Group on Health Reform to specially study the work of helping the poor in health. Prior to this meeting, she made important instructions pointing out that poverty caused by illness and returning to poverty due to illness are important factors causing poverty, and that all localities and departments should give full play to their political and institutional advantages and take practical measures to improve the accuracy of poverty alleviation so as to provide health protection for the rural poor and the people of the whole country to step into a comprehensive well-off society. Vice Premier Wang Yang issued an important directive to the meeting, calling for adhering to accurate poverty alleviation, precise poverty eradication, ensuring realization of the goal of "basic health care is guaranteed," and providing strong support for winning the tough fight against poverty. We should conscientiously study and understand it, and do a good job in implementing it.

### I. Enhancing the sense of responsibility and mission of implementing the project of helping the poor in health

(abbreviated)

### II. Adopting a precise and effective strategy to promote the implementation of the project of health poverty alleviation for substantial results

The period between now and 2020 is a crucial stage for winning the tough fight against poverty. We must resolutely implement the basic strategy of the central authorities for precisely helping the poor and extricating themselves from poverty, take extraordinary measures, come up with excellent measures, adopt different strategies for different people in different places, and administer classified treatment for different diseases. We must achieve "six accuracies" to effectively improve the pertinence and effectiveness of poverty alleviation. The "six accuracies" are: accurate objects of poverty alleviation, accurate project arrangements, accurate use of funds, accurate measures to households, accurate dispatch of people because of villages and accurate anti-poverty effectiveness.

According to the central government's deployment requirements for anti-poverty work, 13 departments including the National Health and Family Planning Commission, the Poverty Alleviation Office of the State Council, together with the State Development and Reform Commission, the Ministry of Civil Affairs, the Ministry of Finance, the Ministry of Human Resources and Social Security, and the Logistics Department of the Central Military Commission, studied and drafted *Guidance on the Implementation of the Project of Health Poverty Alleviation* on the basis of a large amount of field research and sufficient solicitation of the opinions of local and social parties concerned. It has been issued with the approval of the state council. All localities and departments should conscientiously implement and organize the implementation in the light of actual conditions. We will focus on five tasks:

**(1) Improving the universal medical insurance system and further enhancing the ability to prevent serious diseases and drive around the bottom line.**

We shall continue to raise the per capita government subsidy standard for the new rural cooperative medical system, form a sustainable financing mechanism commensurate with the level of economic development and the income situation of residents and further increase the actual reimbursement rate for outpatient and inpatient expenses. The basic medical insurance system should give more support to the rural poor, and a linkage mechanism with such systems as serious illness insurance, medical assistance and commercial health insurance shall be established so as to realize "three coverages, two tilts, two amplifications and one window". They are synergistic and complementary and form safeguard resultant force. The "three coverages" means that the new rural cooperative medical insurance system, the insurance system for serious diseases, and the medical assistance system for serious and extraordinarily serious diseases will fully cover the rural poor population.

The rural poor population's individual contribution part of the new rural cooperative medical insurance system is subsidized by the finance according to the regulations. The newly increased financing for the new rural cooperative medical insurance system will increase its support for the serious illness insurance and extend the scope of medical assistance to all the rural poor people with serious and extraordinarily serious diseases. We will ensure that the rural poor receive basic medical insurance, improve the underwriting security mechanism, further raise the level of relief, and never allow any rural poor person to fail to receive timely medical treatment because of medical expenses.

"Two tilts" means the preferential policies of the new rural cooperative medical insurance system and the serious disease insurance for the rural poor population. We should take the lead in carrying out the overall out-patient planning in poverty-stricken areas, improve the level of overall planning and reimbursement level of outpatient service and effectively solve the problem of reimbursement of long-term outpatient treatment expenses for the patients with chronic diseases. We shall increase the proportion of reimbursement for hospitalization expenses within the scope of the policy for the new rural cooperative medical insurance, by more than 5 percentage points this year. By reducing the limit to start to pay for serious illness insurance and increasing the proportion of reimbursement and other measures, we can effectively reduce the burden of medical expenditure on the rural poor patients with serious illness.

"Two amplifications" is to increase support for health poverty alleviation through commercial health insurance and temporary assistance. Commercial insurance institutions will be encouraged to develop insurance products related to poverty alleviation in health. Governments in poor areas will be urged to purchase supplementary commercial health insurance for the rural poor population. We will increase the intensity of temporary assistance for those patients who are temporarily unable to get family support for a major sudden illness and who are trapped in their basic lives, and actively mobilize social assistance through commonweal organizations and charitable organizations.

"One window" means setting up a comprehensive service window in designated medical institutions to realize "one-stop" information docking and real time settlement of such medical assistance as basic medical insurance, serious illness insurance and emergency medical assistance. Indigent patients are only required to pay for their own medical expenses at the time of discharge. All departments should strengthen cooperation to implement this policy well and should not increase the burden on medical institutions in poverty-stricken areas because of the implementation of this project for the benefit of the people. At the same time, it is necessary to establish a health card for the rural poor people so that it will have the functions of supporting contract signing, one-card medical treatment, pay after treatment, "one-stop" settlement and telemedicine so as to facilitate the masses to seek medical treatment, settle accounts and enhance the sense of gain.

The above precise measures are the core tasks of the project of health poverty alleviation and also the underwriting safeguard measures. All localities must implement them well and see actual results.

**(2) Implementing classified treatment to help the poor people recover their productive and living capacity as soon as possible**

1) Getting the right guy. We shall further check and approve the situation of the

families suffering from poverty due to illness and returning to poverty for illness on the basis of the data on the established files and cards so that the diseases that cause poverty could be found out and a file could be established for each household. This is prerequisite and basic work that must be done in a down-to-earth manner. In April, the National Health and Family Planning Commission, together with the Ministry of Human Resources and Social Security and the Poverty Alleviation Office of the State Council, issued a survey plan. All provinces (autonomous regions and municipalities directly under the Central Government) are expected to complete the investigation by July 15th, analyze and evaluate according to the verification results, and formulate specific plans for implementing classified policies.

2) Measures must be precise. Classified treatment should be carried out for indigent patients with severe diseases. Those who can be cured at once shall be treated with concentrated efforts; those who need maintenance treatment shall be treated for a long period of time; and those who require long-term treatment and health management shall be treated by hospitals in cooperation with primary medical and health institutions. It is also necessary to carry out light project to provide treatment for the poor patients with cataract in rural areas. From this year on, it is necessary to organize and carry out special treatment for major diseases in rural poor families. We shall select patients with nine major diseases including acute lymphocytic leukemia in children, end-stage renal disease to receive concentrated treatment. These patients should be the ones who have heavier disease burden, a clear diagnosis and treatment path, and definite curative effect. We shall do a good job in the calculation of expenses, clarify the proportion of joint reimbursement, and effectively reduce the burden on the expenses of indigent patients with serious diseases.

3) See to it that actual results are achieved. Classified treatment should be carried out on a wall map. We shall mobilize and organize the strength of medical and health institutions and medical personnel at all levels, give prominence to key populations and key types of diseases, and carry out key treatments. The National Health and Family Planning Commission and the Poverty Alleviation Office of the State Council will set up a dynamic information management system to carry out dynamic monitoring and strengthen coordination.

**(3) Enhancing the capacity of medical and health service in poverty-stricken areas to basically prevent visits to doctors outside the county**

1) We will improve the capacity of medical and health service in poverty-stricken areas, enable the rural poor population to obtain timely and convenient basic medical and health service in close proximity, and strive to increase the visiting rate to about 90 percent in the counties of poverty-stricken areas by 2020, basically preventing visits to doctors outside the county.

2) Strengthening the construction of the medical and health service system in poverty-stricken areas. During the 13th Five-Year Plan period, the National Health and Family Planning Commission, in conjunction with the National Development and Reform Commission, will strengthen the construction of 1000 county-level hospitals and 2000 township health centers in poverty-stricken areas in accordance with the principle of promoting and thoroughly improving the entire county. A number of turnover dormitories will be built for township hospitals as supporting facility and township hospitals will be equipped with emergency transport vehicles; in accordance with the principle of completion, we will strengthen the construction of more than 400 county-level women's and children's health care facilities and more than 300 county-level centers for disease control and prevention in order to strengthen prevention and control of infectious diseases and endemic diseases in poor areas. Governments at all levels should also increase their investment to ensure that each county has at least one county-level public hospital, that each township has one standardized health center, that each administrative village has one clinic, and that a network of health and family planning service is firmly built.

3) Strengthening the comprehensive training of talents. We will strengthen the coordination between medical treatment and medical education and rationally determine the enrollment plan for medical colleges and medical specialties in the region. We will train more and better medical and health personnel for the poor areas through standardized raining for residents, training for assistant general practitioners, free training for order orientation, and special post plans for general practitioners and specialists, etc. Three to four years is needed to complete the rotation of rural doctors training. We should strengthen the construction of clinical specialties for common and frequently-occurring diseases in counties, establish demonstration bases, and constantly improve the level of diagnosis and treatment of primary medical and health personnel. In order to encourage more good doctors to go to the community level, we should give proper preference to the primary health care personnel in the promotion of professional titles, education and training and also salary and treatment. We need to try our best to retain and make good use of talents.

4) Implementing stable and continuous "group type" counterpart assistance in tertiary hospitals. Competent tertiary hospitals should be selected to help the hospitals in the poor counties in order to achieve one-to-one assistance. A president or vice president and at least 5 medical personnel shall be stationed at county-level hospitals in poverty-stricken areas. The key is to strengthen the construction of the specialties in the top 5 to 10 diseases transferred out of the county in the first three years. We will focus on the promotion of medical technology suitable for county-level hospitals and have the technology, system and style of the supporting hospitals "transplanted with soil" to the

recipient county hospitals. The "hemopoietic function" of the assisted hospitals should be strengthened. At the same time, we will promote one-to-one assistance between tertiary hospitals and county-level hospitals in poverty-stricken counties and establish a stable cooperative relationship of telemedicine service. By 2020, at least one hospital in every poverty-stricken county will have met the standard of secondary hospital. At least one hospital in a poor county with a population of more than 300,000 will have reached second-class A level so that the medical treatment, education, science and management level of the county hospital could be comprehensively improved, its face changed, and its leading role could be better played. We will take the implementation of counterpart support task as an important content of performance appraisal in tertiary hospitals. The Committee is studying and developing assessment methods and mechanism to supervise the implementation of the task.

**(4) Taking deepening the medical reform as the motive force to increase the endogenous motive force of medical service in the poverty-stricken areas**

1) Speeding up the construction of a hierarchical diagnosis and treatment system. We should establish a division of labor and cooperation mechanism for medical and health institutions in the county of a poor area, adhere to the first primary treatment at the primary level, establish a team of family doctors, and give priority to providing three-dimensional and continuous health management and basic medical service for rural poor people. We will explore ways to build a medical consortium that shares interests and risks and promote the integrated management of counties, townships and villages so as to increase the degree of integration of people, goods and materials. Thus, an inter-hospital referral can become an in-hospital referral. This can significantly improve the overall efficiency of the regional medical service system and extend the reach of the resources of good quality.

2) Pushing forward the reform of payment methods. We will strengthen the budget management of the fund, implement more accurate payment policies, and, in combination with the implementation of clinical approaches, implement a composite payment method that combines payment by person, payment by disease, payment by bed day, and total amount prepaid. Thus, we will increase the benefits of health insurance funds and the benefits of the poor people.

3) Accelerating the comprehensive reform of public hospitals.

We should eliminate the mechanism of compensating for doctor's salary through drug-selling profits, improve the compensation mechanism of public hospitals and improve the scientific, detailed and informational level of hospital management. We will gradually adjust the prices of medical service and strictly control unreasonable increases in medical expenses. We will establish a system of remuneration in line with the characteristics of the medical industry and an incentive mechanism for the performance of the units responsible for poverty alleviation so that the labor value of medical personnel can be fully embodied.

**(5) Strengthening public health work in poverty-stricken areas and improving the health level of the rural poverty-stricken population**

1) Intensifying efforts to prevent and control infectious diseases, endemic diseases and chronic diseases in poverty-stricken areas. We will expand the coverage of cancer screening and early diagnosis and treatment, strengthen screening, registration, treatment and assistance for patients with severe mental disorders in poverty-stricken areas and management of service. We will also comprehensively prevent and treat Kaschin-Beck disease and Keshan disease and other key endemic diseases and strengthen the prevention and control of zoonoses so that echinococcosis in the western agricultural and pastoral areas could be basically controlled and the spread of brucellosis could be effectively contained.

2) Improving women's and children's health service in poor areas in an all-round way. Such projects as free pre-pregnancy health check-ups, folic acid supplementation for rural women to prevent neural tube defects, screening for "two cancers" in rural women, nutrition improvement for children and screening for neonatal diseases will be fully implemented in poor areas to promote comprehensive prevention and treatment of birth defects. We will strengthen capacity building in poor areas for the treatment of pregnant women and infants in acute and severe cases and strengthen rural women's health care during pregnancy and childbirth to ensure maternal and child safety. We will establish a system of rehabilitation and assistance for disabled children.

3) Deepening patriotic health campaigns in poverty-stricken areas. We will strengthen the creation of health towns and cities and implement efforts to improve the living environment in poor rural areas so that the quality of the living environment in poor areas could be effectively improved. We will combine the renovation of rural toilets with the renovation of dilapidated buildings in rural areas to speed up the construction of sanitary toilets in rural areas. We will strengthen monitoring, investigation and evaluation of rural drinking water and environmental sanitation, carry out projects to consolidate and improve the safety of rural drinking water, promote treatment of rural garbage and sewage, and comprehensively address such environmental pollution problems as atmospheric pollution and surface water pollution. We will strengthen health promotion and health education so as to improve health awareness of the rural poor people, make them form good health habits and healthy lifestyles, and strive to reduce illnesses and serious illnesses.

Here I would like to stress once again that all localities should step up efforts to help special families with family planning and do a good job in their life care, old-age security, treatment of serious diseases and spiritual consolation. We will increase support to the poor families with family planning, improve their ability to develop, and ensure that they have priority in enjoying the fruits of reform and development.

(Excerpt from the speech at the National Conference on Health and Poverty Alleviation)

**(Tong Yanlong)**

## 6. Promote the Implementation of Key Policies and Measures on Health and Family Planning

(Li Bin, in Guiyang, Guizhou, July 14th, 2016)

### I. Major progress in the first half of the year

The CPC Central Committee and the State Council have always been attaching great importance to developing health and family planning and safeguarding people's health. Since 2016, General Secretary Xi Jinping has issued important instructions on health and family planning, chaired the meetings of leading group of the Central Committee on comprehensive deepening of the reform, dedicated to listening to the report on medical reform in Sanming City of Fujian Province, and studied and deployed the reform and development of children's medical and health services and the contract services of family doctors. During the 32nd collective study of the Political Bureau of the CPC Central Committee, General Secretary Xi Jinping once again placed the emphasis on promoting the integration of medical care and health care, and achieving healthy ageing. Premier Li Keqiang put forward in this year's *Government Work Report* that the reform of medical treatment, medical insurance, and medical pharmaceutical linkage should be coordinated to improve the universal two-child policy. He has also presided over many executive meetings of the State Council to discuss and review the important medical reform documents. Vice Premier Liu Yandong has guided, investigated and coordinated the resolution of major health and family planning problems and promoted the key work, all of which have provided basic guidelines for doing good work.

(1) Key breakthroughs in the key areas of deepening medical reform

1) Obvious results of comprehensive reform in pilot provinces. Four of the first pilot provinces of comprehensive medical reform in Jiangsu, Anhui, Fujian and Qinghai have made bold exploration and created a lot of duplicable and scalable experience with pioneering innovation. In 2016, seven provinces, including Shanghai, Zhejiang, Hunan, Chongqing, Sichuan, Shaanxi and Ningxia, were added as the

second batch of pilot provinces of comprehensive medical reform, and a situation of regional synergy is formed. We will adhere to the system of linking key provinces with the leadership of the CPC in medical reform and guide the implementation of medical reform tasks in different regions.

2) Comprehensively deepened reform of public hospitals. Qidong City of Jiangsu Province, Tianchang City of Anhui Province, Youxi County of Fujian Province and the mutual aid county of Qinghai Province have been established as the benchmark counties, and the demonstration of the comprehensive reform led by example has been carried out. The number of comprehensive reform pilots of urban public hospitals has been expanded from 100 to 200. The comprehensive reform experience of public hospitals in cities such as Sanming, Fujian Province has been vigorously promoted by holding the on-site meetings and carrying out trainings to develop the reform in depth. The evaluation and assessment of the comprehensive reform of public hospitals have been comprehensively carried out, and the assessment results will be linked to the central government's financial subsidies. The affiliated hospitals to commissions in Shanghai, Changsha and other prefectures have been coordinated to participate in the comprehensive reform of local public hospitals.

3) Progress in building a system of hierarchical diagnosis and treatment. 312 prefecture-level and above cities have declared pilot programs for hierarchical diagnosis and treatment of nearly 90% coverage. Contract services of family doctors are actively promoted. *Suggestions on Further Strengthening the Team Construction of Rural Doctors* has been carried out and a pilot program to test the qualification of rural general practitioners as assistant physicians been launched. The basic standards and recommendation standards of medical service capacity of county hospitals have been formulated to lay a foundation for hierarchical diagnosis and treatment.

4) The further improved basic medical insurance system. The per capita financial subsidy for basic medical insurance in urban and rural areas was increased to 420 *yuan* and the proportion of outpatient and inpatient expenses paid within the policy range was about 50% and 75% respectively. The insurance system for major diseases was consolidated, benefiting more than 4.5 million patients. 13 provinces have completed the integration of basic medical insurance systems for urban and rural residents. The *National Plan for the Settlement and Reporting of New Rural Cooperative Medical Service* was printed and distributed jointly with Ministry of Finance in different places to expand pilots for cross-provincial medical verification and reporting. The 15 counties and cities were identified as the connection points of the reform of the new rural cooperative compound payment method, which has played a radiation-driving role.

5) The further improved mechanism for ensuring drug supply. The new round of centralized procurement of medicines has been comprehensively promoted and 16

provinces have completed two-envelope open tender procurement with drug prices dropping by an average of 15% to 20%. 30 provinces (except Tibet) have launched direct online procurement. Important progress was made in the negotiations on national drug prices, with the prices of patented drugs and exclusive drugs dropping by more than 50% on average. A monitoring and reporting system on a pilot basis of the second batch of targeted production of medicines that were clinically necessary, small in quantities and short in supply on the market, were launched.

6) The expanded supply of medical and health services for children. The new recruitment of 5,000 pediatric resident physicians for standardized training has been completed. And we have coordinated with Ministry of Education to support the resumption of the undergraduate enrollment in pediatrics department in 8 universities. The *First Encouraged Research and Declaration Lists of the Medicines for Children* is formulated to ensure medications for children. The construction of national children's medical center and the homogeneity of pediatric services among regions are promoted.

7) The accelerated development of health services. *Guidance on Promoting and Standardizing the Application and Development of Big Data in Health Care* by the State Council has been carried out and the interconnection between the information platform of provincial population health, affiliated hospitals of the Ministry, and national platforms been coordinated and promoted. The reform of the approval system for the allocation of large medical equipment has been accelerated. To strengthen licensing of medical and nursing service institutions, the first 50 state-level pilot units for the combination of medical and nursing care to develop TCM health and old-age care services were selected. Medical services provided by social forces should be actively supported by revising the *Implementation Rules of the Regulations on the Administration of Medical Institutions* and shortening the bidding time of the organizations. Basic standards and management standards for the four kinds of independent medical institutions, like the center of blood purification, pathological diagnosis, medical test laboratory, and medical imaging diagnostic center should be formulated to expand the area of social capital investment.

(2) The steady progress in the reform of family planning service management

General Secretary Xi Jinping and Premier Li Keqiang have issued important instructions for the 8th national congress of the China family planning association to emphasize that the basic state policy of family planning must be upheld for a long time. The decision of the CPC and the opinions of General Office of the CPC Central Committee and the State Council should be implemented and the principal responsibility system for the management of the family planning goals of the Party committee and the government be carried out. There are 29 provinces (autonomous regions, municipalities directly under the Central Government) in the country that have deliberated and passed the newly revised local population and family planning regulations. And the implementation of the system of fertility registration services in the 15 provinces (autonomous regions, municipalities directly under the Central Government) of Beijing, Hebei, and so on, and the overall development of the two-child policy are progressing well. The basic work of family planning at the community should be strengthened and a new round of activities to create advanced units with quality family planning services across the country be launched. *Opinions on Further Improving the Input Mechanism of Family Planning* was printed and distributed by Ministry of Finance to increase support and care for special families of the family planning. The healthy family initiative and the happy family campaign were launched. The intensive care and caring activities were carried out for the migrant population, the number of pilot cities for social integration of the migrant population is increased to 22, and the dynamic monitoring and survey of the migrant population was carried out.

The further improved health services for women and children. The evaluation criteria for health institutions of women and children were formulated, the establishment of a baby-friendly hospital in children's hospitals was launched, and the establishment of a demonstration base for the early development of children was promoted. The optimization and integration of health care for women and children, and the technical services for family planning have been steadily promoted, and the three-level integration of eight provinces has been basically in place. The pilot health care manual for women and children was carried out and the "one book in hand, enjoying the whole service" was realized. Free pre-pregnancy health checks for 3 million families have been provided. The fifth child physical development survey was completed, and the results showed that the physical development of children in China has significantly improved, exceeding the standards issued by World Health Organization.

(3) The strengthened health emergencies and public health

1) New results in health emergency work. The role of the joint prevention and control mechanism has been given full play so as to respond promptly to and deal with the imported Zika virus and yellow fever. Teams were sent to Hubei, Anhui and Hunan to guide health emergency against floods. The national health emergency team construction project on schedule was completed, and the national health emergency response force has taken initial shape. Shanghai international emergency medical team has been certified by WHO as one of the first international emergency medical teams.

2) Disease prevention and control in all directions. The per capita subsidy for basic public health services increased to 45 *yuan*, major public health services were steadily implemented, and the level of equalization was further raised. The cases of illegal vaccine business should be properly handled with the relevant departments by revising the *Regulations on the Administration of Vaccine Circulation and Vaccination*.

The polio vaccine immunization strategy adjustment was completed, so were the AIDS free antiviral treatment standard adjustment and extension. The *Administrative Measures for the Construction of National Demonstration Areas for the Comprehensive Prevention and Control of Chronic Diseases* were revised, a set of best practice cases for the comprehensive prevention and control of chronic diseases compiled, and the pilot work for the comprehensive management of mental health carried out. The prevention and control of pneumoconiosis among rural migrant workers shall be strengthened and their rights and interests be ensured. The monitoring of common diseases and iodine deficiency disorders in schools shall be organized and the early warning of public health be strengthened.

3) Carrying out the patriotic health campaigns. A plenary session of the national patriotic health association was convened to organize the spring patriotic health campaign. In 2015, the evaluation on national health city (district) and national health county (township) was completed and the guidelines for the construction of healthy cities and towns were formulated. We will carry out pilot evaluation in 24 cities and strive to build a number of healthy cities and villages with exemplary characteristics.

(4) The constantly improved quality and level of medical services

Vice Premier Liu Yandong discussed with the representatives of nursing workers and made request for comprehensive improvement of nursing work. *Administrative Measures on Clinical Application of Medical Technology* and 15 key technical management standards were printed and distributed to enhance the management of clinical application. 50 clinical pathways were issued to strengthen the standardized diagnosis and treatment management of tumors and other diseases. A green channel for human donated organs was set up jointly with 6 departments to win time for saving lives. In Beijing, Tianjin and Hebei, pilot work on electronic licenses for medical institutions, doctors and nurses has been carried out to promote the registration in one district and use of electronic licenses in all districts. Key medical cases (matters) shall be supervised and handled together with the relevant departments to maintain normal medical order and the safety of doctors and patients.

(5) The advancement of the rule of law construction, comprehensive supervision and food safety

1) Accelerating the legislations on health and family planning. We will actively cooperate with the NPC in its legislative work of *Basic Medical and Health Law* and *Law of Traditional Chinese Medicine*, promulgate *Provisions on the Prohibition of Sex Determination of Fetuses for Non-medical Purposes and the Selection of Sex for Artificial Termination of Pregnancy*, and promote the revision of many other laws and regulations.

2) Strengthening the comprehensive supervision of health and family planning.

The supervision and inspection of the implementation of the *Law of Occupational Disease Prevention and Treatment* and the activities of supervision and inspection of the relevant laws and regulations by means of "looking back" will be carried out. The 2016 national supervision and sampling inspection plan is formulated, the sampling inspection of public health and disinfection products and vaccination of Class II vaccines and the special supervision and inspection on administrative law enforcement of family planning are carried out. *Code of Investigation and Punishment for Unlicensed Medical Practice* is printed and distributed, and a campaign to crack down on "drug traffickers" and "online medical care providers" is launched.

3) Ensuring food security. The sanitation and food business license of catering service places have been integrated and adjusted by cancelling 11 intermediary services. 1,992 food safety standards were cleaned up and integrated, the problems of contradiction, crossing and duplication among standards solved, and the good risk monitoring and foodborne disease reporting were well done.

(6) Further developing the characteristics and advantages of traditional Chinese medicine

*Outline of Strategic Planning for the Development of Traditional Chinese Medicine (2016-2030)* was issued by the State Council. Some suggestions on strengthening the inheritance and innovation of TCM theories were printed and distributed, and the education training program for outstanding doctors (TCM) was implemented. More than 5,700 items have been registered for the protection of the knowledge of traditional Chinese medicine and medication. The development plans for the "One Belt and One Road" initiative of traditional Chinese medicine and medication were formulated to support the construction of 10 overseas TCM centers in countries along the belt and road. The forum for the development of traditional Chinese medicine of four places on both sides of the Straits (Hong Kong) was held, so was the seminar on the development and cooperation of traditional Chinese medicine across Taiwan straits. Therefore, the overseas influence of traditional Chinese medicine is expanding.

(7) Positive results in planning and construction, education in science and technology, health and poverty alleviation, and press and publicity

The preparation of *Outline of the Healthy China 2030 Plan*, the "13th Five-year Plan" for medical reform, medical and health care planning and other work is progressing smoothly. The Central Committee allocated 22.24 billion *yuan* to support the construction of 3,297 health and family planning institutions, which further improved the service conditions. A mechanism of "science and technology cooperation" has been established by strengthening scientific and technological innovation. The recruitment of standardized training for resident physicians in 2016 was completed so as to launch the standardized training of assistant general practitioners and solve the problem of insufficient community general practitioners step by step. We will work with the poverty relief office of the State Council and other 15 departments to implement the healthy poverty alleviation project, complete the survey on the return of rural poor to poverty due to illness, and thoroughly make clear of the situations from house to house, from person to person, and from illness to illness, which lays the foundation for the future health poverty alleviation. 889 hospitals of Grade Three were organized to support 1,149 county hospitals in 834 poverty-stricken counties. With the focus on positive publicity, General Secretary Xi Jinping presented awards to Jia Liqun, a doctor from Beijing Children's Hospital, at the 95th anniversary of the founding of the communist Party of China (CPC). We cooperated with China Central Television to shoot series documentaries such as "Looking for the Most Beautiful Doctor" and "Chinese Medicine". The advanced typical was deeply excavated in each place, the typical recommendation reported, and the report tour within the provinces by the report group organized.

(8) Extensive and in-depth international exchanges and cooperation

The 69th effective session of the world health assembly has been successfully completed, Taiwan-related issues been addressed and China's achievements in health reform and development publicized by means of the multilateral arena. *China-WHO Nation Cooperation Strategy (2016-2020)* was issued to steadily implement the "One Belt and One Road" health cooperation program. The Second Minister of Health Forum of China-Central and Eastern European Countries was successfully held to deepen people-to-people and the cultural exchanges at higher levels, including China-the United States, China-Russia, China-Germany and China-Israel. In accordance with *Beijing Action Plan*, the south-south cooperation in the field of population and development has yielded remarkable results, the establishment of a steering committee on the south-south cooperation on population and development has been facilitated, and the cooperation is being deepened.

(9) Solid progress in learning and education on "Two Learnings and One Becoming"

The whole system has carefully studied and implemented the important speech delivered by General Secretary Xi Jinping at the congress to mark the 95th anniversary of the founding of the CPC, firmly establish four consciousness, firmly respect the *Constitution of the Party*, resolutely implement the spirit of General Secretary Xi Jinping's major speeches and the important instructions on health and family planning, strengthen the building of community-level Party organizations, promote the development of the undertaking, and emphasize the principal responsibility of the "key minority" of the Party members and the leading cadres. We will continue to promote the reform through learning and promote development through the reform, combine the learning and education on "Two Learnings and One Becoming" with the inspection and rectification of the Central Committee, and effectively solve problems that are strongly reflected by the public. We will strengthen the oversight and the control over key posts and key links, pay attention to the building of long-term mechanisms, and guard against the risks of clean and honest government.

### II. Key work arrangements for the second half of the year

(1) Doing a good job in implementing the spirit of the "Sanitation and Health Conference", and the "One Outline and Two Plans". The Central Committee decided to hold the first national sanitation and health conference ever since the new century in the first year of the decisive stage in building a moderately prosperous society in all respects. After the meeting, *Outline of the Healthy China 2030 Plan* will be issued to promote the building of a healthy China and chart the course for the reform and development of our undertaking, which demonstrates that, as a milestone, the Central Government attaches great importance to sanitation and health undertakings. The State Council will also issue the *"13th Five-year Plan" for Medical Reform* and the *"13th Five-year Plan for Sanitation and Health Planning*. We need to seize the opportunity, build and condense consensus, learn and understand deeply, and ensure that the decisions and arrangements of the Central Committee and the "One Outline and Two Plans" are implemented. All regions should closely integrate with reality and proceed from the height of "Mass Health and Great Health". Simultaneously, we will continue to implement the *Outline of National Plan for Medical and Health Service System (2015-2020)* to ensure that the three levels of the planning of provinces, cities and counties will be formulated and issued within the year.

(2) Promoting and carrying out the tasks related to the deepening of medical reform

1) Ensuring the implementation of the pilot reform in 100 new urban public hospitals. The key is to abolish the profit-seeking mechanism, synchronously establish and improve the multi-party shared compensation mechanism of the adjustment of medical service price, increase of government subsidies and the reform of payment, the strengthened hospital accounting, and the saving of running cost. In accordance with the principle of "total volume control, structural adjustment, price rising, falling and gradually putting in place", the price comparison relationship between medical institutions at different levels and medical service projects is gradually straightened out. Among them, the price adjustment should be carried out in accordance with the steps of "vacating space, adjusting structure and ensuring cohesion". In recent years, several ministries and commissions have issued opinions on price reform, and local governments

need to further elaborate and implement them. Meanwhile, government input should be ensured. Price adjustment is a dynamic process. We need to learn from the experience of pilot regions, combine the local reality, and do a good job in the basic work.

2) Ensuring the contract signing services provided by family doctors. Contract signing service of family doctors is an important basic job in building a hierarchical medical system. The core is to transform the basic medical and health service mode, strengthen the function of service network, and guide the focus of medical and health work to move down, and the resources to sink so that a health "gatekeeper" system can be really established. Pilot cities for comprehensive reform should take the lead in providing contract services of family doctors and the pilot trials in other areas where conditions permit will be encouraged actively. The elderly people with chronic diseases, people with severe mental disorders, pregnant and parturient women, children and disabled persons should be taken as the key groups for the contract signing services, which will be gradually expanded to the general population. By the end of the year, the contracted service coverage of urban family doctors should reach more than 15%, covering more than 30% of the key population. This is a very detailed job for the masses and we need to conscientiously organize and do our best to make it the closest to the masses.

3) Ensuring the implementation of the "two invoice system" in the field of drug purchase and marketing. Implementing the "two invoice system" and promoting transparency in the price adding process will not only reduce the circulation links of drugs and costs, but also improve efficiency and help to reduce the artificially high drug prices, crack down on ticket money laundering, and purify the circulation environment, which, in the long run, is conducive to increasing concentration of pharmaceutical enterprises, accelerating the establishment of modern pharmaceutical logistics, and improving competitiveness, and is a key step to improve the drug supply guarantee mechanism. At present, to improve the procurement mechanism, the pilot provinces of comprehensive medical reform should comprehensively promote the centralized procurement of drugs in public hospitals. We will encourage 200 pilot cities to implement the "two invoice system" and direct settlement of expenses between hospitals and production enterprises, production enterprises and distribution enterprises to lower the artificially high drug prices. We will integrate the storage and transportation resources of pharmaceutical trading enterprises, encourage the integration between urban and rural areas in regional drug distribution, and provide basic conditions for advancing the "two invoice system".

4) Ensuring the integration of medical insurance in urban and rural areas and the settlement in different places. According to the requirements of "six unifications" of covering scope, financing policy, guaranteeing treatment, medical insurance catalogue,

designated management and fund management, the specific implementation plans will be formulated and implemented within the year in order to comprehensively integrate the medical insurance system for urban and rural residents, actively explore effective management forms such as medical insurance fund management center, and give full play to the leverage of medical insurance. Qualified commercial insurance institutions will be supported to participate in the handling of basic medical insurance. The basic medical insurance network and the off-site medical settlement throughout the country should be accelerated by means of establishing and improving national off-site medical settlement platform for the off-site medical treatment, gradually docking with the provincial settlement system for the full implementation of settlement at different places within the province. Each province should conduct pilot cross-regional referral settlement for hospitalized patients, which is the livelihood that people pay close attention to, and we must do it well.

5) Ensuring the implementation of the reform and development policies for children's medical and health services. Strong measures will be taken to improve the network of medical and health services for children and increase the supply of the resources. Through "training a batch, transferring a batch, and improving a batch", the number of medical staff can be increased, and the overall quality of the team and the quality of service be improved. We will rationally adjust the price of pediatric medical services, improve the remuneration and treatment of pediatric personnel, improve the incentive policies, and make pediatric positions more attractive. We will also take care of and protect rural left-behind children and poor children, and strengthen health care services, monitoring and evaluation, mandatory reporting and medical assistance.

At the same time, the concept of "three linkages of medicine" will be carried out and the reforms be pushed forward in an overall way. In medical field, National Health and Family Planning Commission will formulate the guidance documents for modern hospital management system, the implementation of the pilot program of remuneration system in public hospitals, and the conduction of the performance assessment in the entrusted and the affiliated hospitals of the commissions and ministries. All regions should continue to consolidate and improve the comprehensive reform of county-level public hospitals, give full play to the demonstration effect of the reform in "model county", strengthen guidance and demonstration on classifications, and consolidate and enhance the results of reform by taking a case of excellence as an example for the rest of the whole lot to follow. The training and treatment for resident physicians will be implemented, the standardized training, examination and evaluation of the resident physicians be carried out, and a pilot program of the standardized training for specialized physicians performed to expand the scope of pilot projects for special posts of the general practitioners. The pilots will be released so that doctors above attending physicians in public hospitals shall set up workshops at the community level, and they are also encouraged to practice in communities, remote areas and areas where medical resources are scarce. The reform of the evaluation of professional titles of the community-level health professionals should be accelerated and improved so that the equal treatment can be implemented, and the social forces to set up non-profit medical institutions, the integrated medical and nursing institutions, and the institutions of rehabilitation and nursing for the aged encouraged. Demonstrations of telemedicine services will be carried out and the construction of information technology and the application of big data be promoted. The unreasonable growth of medical expenses in public hospitals should be strictly controlled. All localities should reasonably determine the annual growth range of medical expenses in their respective regions and the target of fee control should be decomposed into local prefectures (county cities) and public hospitals step by step.

In terms of medical insurance, we should improve the level of medical insurance, and actively promote the improvement of the pooling level of basic medical insurance and strive to increase the reimbursement rate for hospitalization expenses within the scope of the new rural cooperative medical insurance policy. The compound payment method should be actively implemented. In 2016, the pilot urban public hospitals will comprehensively promote the reform of payment by disease. The management of verification and the report of disease emergency rescue fund, and the performance appraisal should be strengthened, and a joint system between major illness insurance and medical assistance be formed and put in place to expand the benefits of major disease insurance and reduce the cost of medical treatment for serious chronic diseases in a variety of ways.

In the field of medicine, we will continue to do a good job of national drug price negotiations, gradually increase the number of drug varieties, reasonably lower the price of patented drugs and exclusive drugs, effectively coordinate the state's centralized procurement of medicines and the payment of medical insurance, and implement classified procurement. We will strengthen the support and the early warning for the supply of medicines in short supply, organize production at designated points, and actively promote pilot security to ensure the full supply of essential drugs. We will continue to promote the development and application of domestic medical equipment and the application of "Internet + health care" services. The medical reform offices at all levels should coordinate comprehensively to monitor and evaluate the progress of medical reform.

(3) Continuously deepening the reform of family planning services

1) Implementing the universal two-child policy. We will promote and guide the local governments in formulating and implementing opinions on the comprehensive

implementation of the Central Commission's Decision, and cooperate with the Office of the Central Commission and the Office of the State Council in special supervision and inspection of the implementation of the policies. All localities should adhere to and improve the responsibility system for the management of family planning goals, further improve the monitoring mechanism for birth population, and evaluate the implementation effect of the universal two-child policy. Simultaneously, the rational allocation of infant and young child care, policy recommendations on public service resources such as education in pre-school and primary and secondary schools should be studied and put forward to make more families in line with the policy able to afford the reproduction, have the ability to reproduce and reproduce healthy babies.

2) Improving the management of family planning services. We will implement a birth registration service system to further streamline the administration for the convenience of the people, stabilize and strengthen the network at the community level and properly address the issues of treatment and security. We will intensify our efforts to deal with "Two Illegal Acts", and improve the sex ratio of the population at birth, further equalize the basic public services for health and family planning of the migrant population, improve family development policies such as family support, child care and old-age care, especially the care of the families who have lost their only child, and carry out new family planning and activities to create happy families.

3) Strengthening capacity building for woman and child health services. A "one-stop" service for women's and children's health should be promoted to implement free pre-pregnancy checkups, give pre-pregnancy guidance to the elderly couples, and comprehensively prevent and treat birth defects. The building of a contingent of midwifery technicians and the training in reproductive technology should be strengthened. A demonstration project on quality services for women's and children's health shall be built continuously, and the use of the manuals for women and children's health be summarized and promoted. The number of maternity and pediatric beds will be increased, the capacity of rescuing the critically ill pregnant women and the newborns be strengthened for the treatment, and make every effort to ensure the safety of mothers and babies.

(4) Earnestly strengthening public health and health emergency

*National Basic Public Health Service Standards (2016 Edition)* is printed and distributed to enhance the performance appraisal of the service projects. All regions must strengthen the comprehensive prevention and control of major diseases, continue to focus on the prevention and control of infectious diseases such as dengue fever and influenza, promote the hierarchical diagnosis and treatment of tuberculosis and the service mode for the comprehensive pilot prevention and control, perfect supervision and management, and evaluation mechanism of social organizations participating in the funding for AIDS prevention and control, make good disposal of the comprehensive project of echinococcosis prevention and control and the construction of a demonstration area for the comprehensive prevention and control of chronic diseases, and promote actions of a healthy lifestyle for all. The management of patients with severe mental disorders and the guidance of mental health services in accordance with the requirements of the Central Commission should be strengthened. The supervision and inspection of clean and tidy environmental sanitation in urban and rural areas should be carried out and the construction of healthy cities, healthy villages and healthy towns be promoted. The important instructions of garbage "going to the mountainous areas and settling in the countryside" made by General Secretary Xi Jinping must be implemented to give full play to the advantages of patriotic health committees at all levels in coordinating and mobilizing the public for the implementation of the centralized regulation of the rural garbage. Sudden acute infectious disease prevention and control such as, disease of Zika Virus and yellow fever will be done continuously, the building of emergency command centers for public health emergencies be strengthened, the connectivity at the national, provincial and prefectural levels intensified in order to move the post-implementation report forward to prior risk monitoring and assessment. The development of a three-dimensional emergency medical rescue network for land, sea and air should be promoted, the construction, operation and maintenance of health emergency response teams be improved to push forward medical emergency rescue in a whole chain, throughout the whole process and in all directions. China has entered the main flood season and floods occur in many places. Disaster situation is an order. All efforts should be made to make emergency preparations for flood control and drought relief, prevent diseases from invading public health, deal with injuries and help patients, and provide psychological assistance, so as to ensure that there is no major epidemic after a major disaster. At the same time, we should promptly plan the rehabilitation and reconstruction of health and family planning institutions after disasters.

Here, I would like to highlight the work of vaccination. After the promulgation and implementation of the newly revised *Regulations on the Administration of Vaccine Circulation and Vaccination* under the State Council, at the beginning of June, National Health and Family Planning Commission and the General Administration of Food and Drug issued a notice on the implementation of the *Regulations* and put forward clear requirements. The key is the implementation. We should conscientiously summarize and draw lessons from the "series of cases concerning illegal vaccine business in Jinan, Shandong Province", and firmly establish the objective sense of serving the people wholeheartedly. We need to adhere to the problem-oriented approach. In view of the current charging standard, cold chain distribution, platform construction and other problems in the supply of the second-class vaccines, we will earnestly study and solve the problems, and safeguard people's health rights and interests and the safety of their lives. We must firmly grasp the main contradiction, which at present is to make every effort to meet the needs of the public for vaccination. All places must take the initiative from a political perspective and take immediate measures to ensure the implementation of vaccine, especially rabies vaccine. It must not be delayed because of the late procurement, which results in a shortage of vaccines, or out of stock, and affects the vaccination. In accordance with the requirements of the "six specifications", the preventive vaccination service should be strengthened to ensure the safety of vaccination. Simultaneously, the initiative must be taken to communicate with the media, respond to the concerns of the public in a timely manner, and guide the public opinion correctly. Recently, National Health and Family Planning Commission has worked in conjunction with the relevant departments to further clarify the requirements for the work in the transitional period, and jointly supervise and inspect the implementation of the local responsibilities together with other departments such as General Administration of Food and Drug Administration. We must take it seriously for those who "do not act in a political way" that affects the supply and vaccination of vaccines, cause public dissatisfaction and even affect social stability.

(5) Further enhancing the capacity of medical and health service

1) The action plan to improve medical services should be implemented continuously to promote the mature experience, and focus on the diagnosis and treatment by appointment, ambulatory surgery, information push service, pharmaceutical service, emergent first aid and rescue, quality care and other work, which emphasizes the enhancement of people's sense of access. Hospitals of Grade Three should fully implement the appointment diagnosis and treatment, and improve the scientific, refined and informatization management of hospitals.

2) Medical quality management will be strengthened by printing and distributing *Medical Quality Management Measures*, and issuing normative documents on the management of electronic medical records. Local governments should strengthen supervision over the clinical application of medical technology, carry out special remediation on the establishment and approval of medical institutions as required, promote the authorized use of electronic medical records and electronic health records among various medical institutions at all levels, fully implement the "national plan of action to curb bacterial drug resistance", strengthen pharmaceutical services and nursing management, consolidate the complete coverage of nucleic acid testing in blood stations, establish a clinical evaluation system for blood use, and strengthen the management of medical waste according to law in order to prevent loss. At the same time, we will expand the coverage and management quality of the clinical pathway

and strive for over 80% coverage in all hospitals of Grade Three. Secondary hospitals will carry out clinical pathway management.

3) The ability construction of community-level medical institutions and hospitals at the county level should be enhanced continuously, activities for building township health centers and projects for improving community health services that satisfy the public be organized and implemented, and a national health post training and skill contest at the community level carried out.

4) Continuous establishment of the "Peace Hospital". A few days ago, National Health and Family Planning Commission, together with 8 departments, launched a year-long crackdown on medical crimes. All localities should conscientiously organize and carry out the special operations in accordance with the requirements of the plan, earnestly form a joint force of strict fighting and prevention, and effectively curb the occurrence of violent injuries of medical workers. Simultaneously, we will improve the system of "Three Mediations and One Insurance" to ensure that medical institutions continue to improve the order of medical treatment.

5) We will formulate the guiding opinions on Party building in public hospitals, convene a symposium on exchange of experience, earnestly strengthen Party building in public hospitals, give full play to the role of leading and exemplary Party cadres, and provide quality services to the public.

(6) Promoting the development of traditional Chinese medicine

The relevant guiding opinions on accelerating the innovation system construction of science and technology of traditional Chinese medicine, and the reform and development of the education of traditional Chinese medicine deepened in cooperation with medicine and education are printed and distributed, the *Outline of the Strategic Planning for the Development of Traditional Chinese Medicine (2016-2030)* and the implementation plan for promoting the health culture of traditional Chinese medicine formulated, and the launching of the third "master of traditional Chinese medicine" and "national famous Chinese medicine" awards will be discussed. All localities should implement the relevant opinions, plans and other requirements, promote the inclusion of all public TCM hospitals in the reform of public hospitals, enhance their service capabilities at the community level, and organize the inspections of large-scale TCM hospitals. The pilot TCM health tourism will be explored and promoted and a number of TCM health tourism demonstration areas be identified. Scientific and technological innovation in traditional Chinese medicine will be promoted and a number of national clinical research bases for traditional Chinese medicine be established. The construction of the national experimental area for comprehensive reform of traditional Chinese medicine will be deepened continuously, and the innovative pilots of TCM diagnosis and treatment models and national standardization of traditional Chinese medicine be promoted. At the same time, the long-term development plan of "One Belt and One Road" for traditional Chinese medicine is formulated and implemented, and the pace of traditional Chinese medicine "going out to the world" is accelerated.

(7) Strengthening the rule of law and the relevant standards for health and family planning

The legislation on the Basic Medical and Health Law, the *Law on Traditional Chinese Medicine and the Regulations Governing Smoking in Public Places* must be accelerated, the legislation of large medical equipment configuration license be completed, and the approval and the reform of the "three new foods" coordinated. In accordance with the requirements for streamlining administration, delegating power to lower-level governments, and improving services, all places should make innovations in the way of supervision and strengthen the oversight in the middle and after the implementation of delegated approval. All regions should also focus on improving the system, integrate supervision resources, improve supervision mechanisms and speed up the establishment of a comprehensive supervision system. *Population and Family Planning Law* and *Regulations on the Health Administration in Public Places* must be carried out, the supervision and inspection on school health, medical and health institutions, and the activities of "looking back" be launched. Special supervision on *Regulations on the Administration of Vaccine Circulation and Vaccination* and *Standard of Vaccination* must be implemented to improve the long-term mechanisms, plug loopholes and strengthen management. At the same time, we will monitor food safety risks and report foodborne diseases, and strengthen standard management and coordination.

(8) Carrying out all key tasks in a whole planned way

We should do good preparations for major medical and health exchanges between China and Asian, China and the central Africa, China and the United States, and actively participate in cultural and people-to-people exchanges between China and the United Kingdom. We shall prepare for the 9th world health promotion conference and take this world-class health event as a stage to show China's achievements in health development and effectively transform it into a driving force for domestic health promotion. *Plan for National Health Protection Project Construction* is printed and distributed to improve the basic infrastructure of health and family planning institutions. A national conference on innovation in health and health science and technology should be convened to formulate guidelines and implement key tasks for innovation-driven development. The measures for the administration of clinical research on new medical technologies should be formulated, and major projects on clinical science and technology be organized and implemented continuously. We need to take various forms, interpret the reform policies and measures in a timely, accurate and incisive manner, respond positively to social concerns and people's voices, and guide social expectations in a reasonable way. We must do a good job in reducing poverty through health. All places must carry out the requirements of national work conference on poverty alleviation by health, and strive for the implementation of various tasks. The six accuracies of poverty alleviation targets, project arrangements, the use of funds, measures to reach households, deploying people by villages, and the results of lifting people out of poverty must be implemented. We will accomplish the glorious tasks that the Central government has assigned to the health and family planning system.

(Speech at the Seminar on the Implementation of the Health and Family Planning Policy in 2016)

**(Ji Chenglian)**

## 7. Make Solid Efforts for "Group" Assistance to Tibet and Xinjiang

(Li Bin, in Lhasa, Tibet, August 1$^{st}$, 2016)

### I. Progress in "group" assistance to Tibet and Xinjiang

The implementation of "group" assistance to Tibet and Xinjiang is an important measure and institutional innovation of the CPC Central Committee and the State Council to safeguard the health of the people in Tibet and Xinjiang, and to support the development of medical and health services in ethnic minority areas and border areas, which is fully recognized by Yu Zhengsheng, Chairman of National Committee of the Chinese People's Political Consultative Conference (CPPCC) and other leading comrades in the Central Committee. Under the coordination of the Central Organization Department, National Health and Family Planning Commission jointly with Ministry of Human Resources and Social Security, and Ministry of Education have successively sent more than 300 outstanding medical personnel from the affiliated hospitals to commissions, affiliated hospitals to universities, and 11 provinces and cities, forming 16 medical teams to enter Tibet and Xinjiang. The team members overcame all kinds of difficulties and worked hand in hand with the comrades in the hospitals to push forward the work of support.

The important periodic results of "group" assistance to Tibet have been achieved. Beijing Concorde Hospital, Peking University Hospital, People's Hospital of Peking University, the Third Hospital of Beijing, and 7 provinces (cities) of Beijing, Shanghai, Chongqing, Anhui, Guangdong, Liaoning, and Shaanxi provide the paring support to the people's hospitals of the autonomous region and 7 people's hospitals in prefectures. In the past year, the management level of recipient hospitals has been significantly improved. Through grafting management method, rules and regulations, and working standard have been perfected, service flow been optimized, and the management refined. With the significant improvement in medical quality and technology, people's hospitals in Linzhi City and Changdu City were turned into the comprehensive hospitals of "Class B". The people's hospital in Ali District has passed the preliminary review of "Class A, Grade Two". Recipient hospitals have carried out nearly 350 items of new technology and some difficult surgeries of high level. Many operations were performed for the first time in the recipient region or even the whole autonomous region. Radiofrequency ablation of myocardial infarction and other 50 major diseases can be treated within the autonomous region, and more than 300 kinds of diseases of minor severe can be treated within the prefectures. The autonomous region has set up the "group" training centers and bases for medical professionals so that the ability of local health workers was improved significantly. In order to help Tibet, nearly 150 experts have been invited to Tibet for the exchanges and 100 medical personnel were selected to study and train in supporting hospitals to improve their technical ability and business confidence.

Good beginning of "group" assistance to Xinjiang. In April 2016, seven provinces (municipalities directly under the Central Government) of Tianjin, Liaoning, Shanghai, Jiangsu, Zhejiang, Hunan and Guangdong provided the paring support to 8 prefecture-level and city-level hospitals and regiment-division level hospitals. The accuracy of the support shall be improved to promote the development of key disciplines such as urology and pediatrics, guide the development of invasive arterial monitoring and other new technologies, and promote the new projects. The first international certification of the first aid training base has been established in the First Hospital of Kashgar in Southern Xinjiang, and the First Eye-Light Center of the People's Hospital been set up in Aksu District of Southern Xinjiang. Focusing on strengthening the construction of talent team, the Second Hospital of Kashgar cooperated with the provinces and cities offering the assistance on the "on-the-job graduate student training project". People's Hospital of Kezhou organized the staff members to form the relationship of teachers and apprentices or working partners with the aid experts for the further close business contacts and the obtaining of the real scriptures. By focusing on the development of remote medical service, exploring remote diagnosis, remote pathology, remote training, demonstration support technologies such as remote surgery, frontier patients can directly receive high level services in large cities, win treatment time and reduce economic burden.

## II. Pioneering in innovation and achieving the tangible results in the "group" assistance to Tibet and Xinjiang

Because of natural conditions and historical reasons, some regions in Tibet and Xinjiang have scarce health resources and weak medical service capabilities, which make it difficult to meet the needs of local people for medical services. This has also become an important reason for some people to return to poverty due to illness. On the basis of summarizing the successful experience of assistance to Tibet and Xinjiang in the past few decades, the "group" assistance has been taken to provide all-round assistance to recipient hospitals, comprehensively improve the level of medical treatment, teaching, service and management, and greatly expanded the connotation of assistance to Tibet and Xinjiang in the new era. Practice has proved that this is a practical and dynamic system.

(1) Keeping eyes on the target, combining the near and far and constantly pushing forward. We proposed the goal of "two drops, one improvement and three stays" of medical assistance to Tibet and Xinjiang. Among them, the reduction of maternal and infant mortality and the improvement of life expectancy are the comprehensive reflection of the health of the people and the development of medical and health undertakings, which requires us to make unremitting efforts for a long time. By 2020, the goal of "serious disease treatment in the autonomous region, minor serious disease treatment in the prefecture and the ailment treatment in the county" will have basically been achieved in the next five years, which will involve scientific support planning to clarify the directory of "serious disease", "minor serious disease" and "ailment" , break down the tasks to each team, department and doctor of medical assistance, clarify the responsibilities of the work, and do it again and again to ensure the timely implementation.

(2) Focusing on key programs and diseases. The dual orientation of problems and demands should be adhered to, and the key diseases the local residents went out to seek medical treatment be sorted out to improve the ability of diagnosis and treatment of key disciplines in hospitals receiving assistance and actively create hierarchical hospitals. We will implement the system of leading experts for "group" assistance to Tibet and Xinjiang by forming groups, implement special funds, and policies and measures, and give full play to the role of the leading experts in discipline building and personnel training. We will make full use of informatization technology to build a remote diagnosis and treatment platform between the hospitals offering assistance and the ones receiving assistance, improve the model of telemedicine cooperation, and give full play to the strong supporting role of high-quality resources in the mainland.

(3) Exploring and improving the system of "teaching man to fish". The training

for the medical personnel in recipient areas should be a long-term initiative and the focus of work. Starting from the training law of clinical medical personnel, the training mechanism of "one-to-one" and "one-to-many" should be improved. By means of experts teaching the backbones and masters teaching the apprentices, the whole process of learning can be achieved to train a group of trusted and competent medical personnel who can stay in the local places.

(4) Mobilizing the enthusiasm of the recipient areas. To promote the scientific development of medical and health undertaking in Tibet and Xinjiang, our own efforts are the internal factors and the assistance is the external ones. Both factors are important while the internal factors play a decisive role. Under the guidance of the team of medical assistance, the recipient should not only learn from the advantages of technology and management and improve their own service ability, but also strengthen the subject consciousness, promote ownership, combine receiving assistance with self-reliance, "blood transfusion" with "blood making", continuously strengthen the endogenous power, and form a benign mechanism to promote the development of the undertaking.

### III. Strengthening management and further implementing organizational safeguards

(1) Improving the working mechanism. We should focus on the two basic points of "organizing a group" and "precision", sort out and improve the relevant supporting policies, clarify the relationship between power and responsibility, and ensure the implementation of policies. In accordance with the requirements of "synchronous rotation" and "stubble handover", the team members of the previous and the latter batches can fully communicate with each other so as to keep talents on file, the work going on, and the experience being passed on.

(2) Doing a good job in logistics. The hospitals offering the assistance must implement the relevant treatment of allowance subsidies, visiting relatives on leave, promotion, title assessment, etc. and help the supporting experts to solve practical difficulties, and remove troubles back at home. The units receiving assistance should do a good job in life and other services and provide necessary conditions for the comrades to work energetically.

(3) Conducting performance appraisal. In accordance with the principle with "scientific, reasonable, achievable, sustainable and evaluable characteristics", we should establish and improve the assessment system and indicator system, and comprehensively and objectively evaluate the supporting work and the implementation effect.

(4) Strengthening publicity and guidance. The achievements of the "group" assistance to Tibet and Xinjiang have been obtained, the advanced typical medical personnel and the outstanding deeds have been publicized, the positive energy has been spread to the whole society, and the clean and upright industry has been shaped.

(Speech at the Promotion Conference on "Group" Assistance of Medical Professionals)

**(Ji Chenglian)**

## 8. Place Scientific and Technological Innovation at the Center of Health Services

(Li Bin, November 13th, 2016, Beijing)

### I. Have a deep understanding of the important role of scientific and technological innovation in promoting the construction of Healthy China

Since the founding of new China, we have given full play to our institutional strengths, concentrated our efforts on scientific research and achieved a series of world-class achievements in medical technology innovations. In 1996, the National Conference on Health Work explicitly defined "relying on science, technology and education" as one of the party's health work guidelines in the new era, firmly establishing the idea of relying on scientific and technological progress to develop health services. At the National Conference on Sanitation and Health held in 2016, general secretary Xi Jinping defined the party's guiding principle of health work under the new situation, clearly put forward "reform and innovation as the driving force" and stressed that we should try out best to push forward theoretical innovation, institutional innovation, management innovation and technological innovation, so as to ensure people's health in all aspects and throughout the whole cycle.

Since the 18th National Congress of the Communist Party of China, the overall strength of science and technology in China's health sector has been continuously improved. The innovation environment has been continuously optimized. Major innovations have been constantly emerging and their transformation into clinical applications has been sped up significantly. The number of talents force has been growing and our international influence has been improving constantly. Tu youyou won the 2015 Nobel Prize in physiology or medicine. Wu Mengchao, Wang Zhongcheng and Wang Zhenyi won the national highest science and technology awards. In the 12th Five-year Plan period, 194 national awards for science and technology were conferred to the health sector.

In terms of prevention and control of major diseases, breakthroughs were made in key technologies for the prevention and control of major infectious diseases such as

AIDS, and the "three diseases and two rates" were effectively reduced. The diagnosis and treatment technical specifications and the prevention and control strategies for hundreds of major diseases were formulated and promoted, and good results were achieved. The direct network reporting system for infectious diseases and public health emergencies is at the world leading level. Eight world leading achievements, including pathogen diagnosis, were made while handling the influenza A (H1N1) epidemic. In the field of new drug development, 24 Class-I innovative drugs were approved for production, and a number of cutting-edge technologically innovative drugs were approved for clinical trials. In terms of research and development of medical devices, the monopoly of foreign countries over brain pacemakers, orthopedic robots and other medical equipment was broken. In the field of traditional Chinese medicine, theoretical researches on traditional Chinese medicines have been continuously advanced. A number of traditional Chinese medicines have been reinvented and the process of internationalization has been accelerated. In terms of innovation system construction, a collaborative innovation system for health, which combines "the knowledge and technological innovation of universities and R&D institutions, the technical innovation of enterprises and the transformation and innovation of medical and health institutions", was basically established. In terms of management over scientific research, regulations on laboratory biosafety management and clinical research management of stem cells have been issued in succession. The system has become increasingly sound and the management has become more standardized.

The development of science and technology of health services is changing from strengthening the foundation to improving the quality, from key breakthroughs to comprehensive improvements, from "follower" to "racer" and "leader".

**II. Create a new situation for science and technology innovation in the health sector**

(1) The development of major innovation projects will be strengthened.

The health ensuring project aiming for the goals of 2030 will be organized and implemented. Focusing on the key needs of building a Healthy China, we will strengthen top-level design, innovate implementation mechanism, make breakthroughs in a number of key technologies in the prevention and control of major diseases, the health maintenance of key populations, the development of the pharmaceutical industry and the national bio-safety, develop a number of urgently needed products, and transform and apply a number of important achievements.

The national key science and technology projects will be organized and implemented. Taking the landmark achievements as the lead, we will make centralized configuration of scientific and technological resources, improve the supporting measures, strengthen the fulfillment of responsibilities, and make final efforts to complete the major projects of new drug development and infectious disease prevention and control. We will continue to promote the implementation of national key research and development projects and strive for launching a number of other key projects.

The "Innovation Project of Medical and Health Technology" of the Chinese Academy of Medical Sciences will be organized and implemented. We will further innovate mechanisms, strengthen performance appraisal, highlight industrial characteristics, adhere to problem-orientated approaches, focus on the combination of basic researches and clinical practices, and strive to produce a number of internationally leading achievements.

The inheritance and innovation of Chinese traditional medicines will be organized and implemented. We should tap deep into the treasure house of Chinese traditional medicines for better innovations and creations so as to occupy the highest point in competition. The compilation of the Collection of Chinese Medicines will be organized and the ancient books of traditional Chinese medicines, traditional knowledge and special diagnosis and treatment technologies will be systematically explored and collated. We will improve the technology system for the preventive treatment of diseases by Chinese medicines and strengthen researches on the prevention and treatment of major and difficult diseases by traditional Chinese medicine. We will strengthen the development of classic Chinese medicines and the development of new drugs, implement the action plan for standardization of traditional Chinese medicines, lead the transformation and upgrading of the industry and promote the overseas development of traditional Chinese medicine.

(2) The transfer and transformation of innovation results will be strengthened.

The main role of medical innovations in medical and health institutions and technicians will be given full play. Medical and health institutions at all levels, especially large public hospitals, shoulder the dual missions of saving the sick and the dying and innovating science and technology. Medical and health institutions are at the junction of innovation chain, industrial chain and application chain, playing an irreplaceable role in the demand link, research and development link and application link of scientific and technological innovations.

A reasonable profit distribution and incentive mechanism will be established and improved. The medical and health institutions and their technical personnel are an important part of scientific and technological innovations, and they equally enjoy the country's various incentive policies for technological innovations. The performance appraisal system will be established and improved, and classified evaluation and incentive policies will be carried out for scientific and technological talents in different fields. The incentives for the transfer and transformation of scientific and technological achievements and methods for profit distribution will be formulated, and all proceeds should be retained to the institutions. The management system for scientific research funds will be reformed and the rewards to those who contribute will be highlighted.

The promotion and application of appropriate health technologies will be enhanced. The fundamental purpose of scientific and technological innovations is the people's health, which should always be remembered. Research papers should be written in the practice of disease prevention and control. Demonstration bases for the promotion and application of appropriate health technologies will be built. Low-cost, high-quality and inclusive technologies for preventing and controlling diseases and ensuring health should be vigorously developed, and service costs should be reduced. The health and family planning departments at all levels should take it as an important part in deepening the reform of public hospitals, alleviating poverty in terms of health and conducting continuing medical education.

The awareness of intellectual property protection should be enhanced, and greater importance should be attached to formulation of standards. Great emphasis should also be laid on the researches over evaluation methods and standard systems. An information platform for national health science and technology achievements will be built to promote technology trading and intellectual property protection.

(3) The construction of important scientific and technological innovation platforms will be strengthened.

A number of laboratory platforms at the national level will be built. Aiming at the forefront of science and technology, focusing on strategic competition, relying on superior innovation units, we will make plans for the construction of national laboratories. The building of the branches of the Chinese Academy of Medical Sciences will be strengthened. We will continue to promote the construction of national key laboratories and engineering technology centers. The functional orientation and key directions of the key laboratories at the commission level will be clearly defined and the layout of the construction will be optimized.

A number of technical platforms for clinical medical research will be built. The construction of clinical research centers and their collaborative research networks will be strengthened. Efforts will be made to establish a stable support mechanism, and promote the full coverage of major clinical disciplines. Five national transformation medical centers will be established. The coordination between the central and local governments will be strengthened and a number of regional scientific and technological innovation centers will be built.

A number of resource-based supportive technology platforms will be built. Efforts will be made to actively prepare the construction of the national engineering laboratory for health care big data application technologies and clinical medical data demonstration center. The construction of high-level bio-safety laboratory networks, bacteria (viruses) species preservation centers, and the National Human Genetic Resources Center will be advanced. Under the premise of ensuring national bio-safety, the sharing of scientific research platform resources, data, and achievements will be steadily pushed forward.

(4) The construction of the collaborative innovation system will be strengthened.

The mechanism of "coordinating science and health care" will be improved and perfected. The National Health and Family Planning Commission will work with the Ministry of Science and Technology to strengthen top-level design of science and technology innovation in the health sector, study and formulate innovative plans, coordinate resource allocation, and make plans for implementing major science and technology projects and programs. The local health and family planning administrative departments should also work closely with the competent science and technology departments.

The innovation mechanism of "coordinating medical and health institutions, scientific research institutions and enterprises" will be improved and perfected. The basic rule of organizing scientific and technological innovation activities in the field of health is to take clinical as the main body, to take the application as the guide, and to coordinate medical and health institutions, scientific research institutions and enterprises. Medical and health institutions should pay attention to health needs and organize the implementation of applied researches. Scientific research institutions should be demand-oriented and make breakthroughs in key and core technologies. Enterprises should play a major role in technological innovations and improve their own market competitiveness. The government should establish a classified supervision system to strengthen the clinical research, access, and application management of new technologies.

(5) The construction of innovation talent team will be strengthened.

High-level innovative talents will be cultivated and introduced. On the basis of the national talent cultivation plans, platforms and projects, efforts will be made to foster and gather a number of high-level talents. The overseas intelligence bases will be established and the introduction of overseas talents in weak and scarce areas. The selection of "young and middle-aged experts with outstanding contributions" will be conducted and the project of cultivating young talents for technological innovations will be speeded up. Emphasis will be laid on strengthening the cultivation of clinical or public health research talents, senior research technical talents, interdisciplinary innovation talents and professional management talents.

The mechanism of "coordinating hospitals and universities" will be pushed forward, and talents will be cultivated constantly. Efforts will be made to improve the education system in medical colleges, adjust the scale, optimize the structure, and strengthen clinical practice and scientific research literacy. The scientific research consciousness training and skill training will be taken as important contents of clinical medical talents cultivation.

Services and incentives for the talents will be ensured. The autonomy of the employers will be enhanced in terms of talent selection, employment, professional title appraisal and performance evaluation. The reform of the professional title system will be deepened and the reform of talent evaluation mechanism will be pushed forward. The reform of the salary system will be steadily pushed forward and an income distribution system and a stable growth mechanism that are guided by the increase of knowledge value and are consistent with job responsibilities will be established. Measures of the Central Committee on the Administration of Funds for Scientific Research Projects will be comprehensively implemented. The administration of the teaching and scientific research personnel in the institutions directly under or administrated by the National Health and Family Planning Commission and units under the management of the Commission who go abroad temporarily on business will be improved.

Attention will be paid to the construction of ethics and morality of science and technology. The innovative culture of "contribution and research" will be carried forward and an innovative atmosphere of "dare to be first, dare to question and tolerate failure" will be created. The bottom line of professional ethics in scientific researches will be strictly observed, strengthen the construction of credit system, ethical supervision will be strengthened, and a positive academic atmosphere will be fostered.

(6) The popularization and education of health science will be promoted.

The popularization and education of health science should be oriented to the community level, close to reality, close to life, close to the masses. It should also be included in the contract services of family doctors. The health issues that are of wide social concerns will be selected and disseminated in a way that is easy for the public to understand, accept and participate in. The popularization and education of health science should be well targeted. For key populations such as children, pregnant women, elderly people, and chronic disease patients, health science popularization needs to be selected at a suitable place, at a suitable time, and in a suitable manner. Health science popularization should be standardized, and it should not provide communication channels and platforms for false health education activities. The training of health science popularization skills for medical and health personnel should be strengthened, and scientific knowledge should be communicated in a plain and easy way for the public to understand, listen and follow. The public should be helped to develop health concepts, adopt healthy behaviors, master health skills and improve health literacy.

(From the Speech at the National Conference on Health Science and Technology Innovation )

**(Zhou Dan)**

# Part III

# Deepening the Reform of the Medical and Health System

## 1. Overview of Deepening the Reform of the Medical and Health Care System in 2016

In 2016, important matters in deepening the reform of health care happened one after another and all tasks were comprehensively completed. In August 2016, the first national conference on health and health in the new century was held and it was clearly required to focus on construction of five systems, namely, hierarchical diagnosis and treatment, modern hospital management system, all-people medical insurance, drug supply guarantee and comprehensive supervision. The *Outline of the Healthy China 2030 Plan* , the *"13th Five-year" Health and Health Plan* and the *"13th Five-year" Plan for Deepening Reform of the Medical and Health System* were issued and implemented, clarifying the goal, direction, task and path of deepening health care reform in the next 5 to 15 years. General secretary Xi Jinping chaired five meetings of the central leading group on comprehensively deepening reform, specially listened to the report on medical reform in Sanming City, Fujian Province, and studied and deployed the reform and development of medical and health service for children, household doctors' signing service, further promoted the experience of deepening medical reform and improved the policy of drug production and circulation. In his *Government Work Report*, Premier Li Keqiang called for coordinated reform of medical care, medical insurance and medicine. He presided over several executive meetings of the State Council to deliberate important documents on health care reform, requiring we should resolve to break through the difficulties such as overall medical insurance, hierarchical diagnosis and treatment, inflated drug prices and public hospital reform. Yu Zhengsheng, chairman of the National Committee of the Chinese People's Political Consultative Conference(CPPCC), presided over a special consultation on health care reform, calling for strengthening leadership over the work, encouraging local governments to practice boldly, and concentrating on solving the problems of compensating for doctor's salary through drug-selling profits. Liu Yandong presided over meetings and symposiums of the leading group on health care reform of the State Council to personally guide and coordinate the solution of major medical reform issues and promote key work.

Under the leadership of the CPC Central Committee and the State Council, various localities and departments concerned paid close attention to system innovation, target implementation, mechanism guarantee and tracking and insurance of effectiveness. The organization and leadership of medical reform was significantly strengthened, with five provincial party committees and the main governmental responsible people of 19 provinces serving as the head of the medical reform leading group. There was a marked increase in the consensus on health care reform, and the departments concerned formed a joint force for reform. Medical and health institutions and medical personnel took the initiative to participate in the medical reform, and the majority of the people understood the medical reform, cared about the medical reform, and their call for the promotion of health care reform was getting louder and louder. Comprehensive reform efforts were significantly increased, with 11 pilot provinces carrying out comprehensive medical reform. The reform was pushed forward from local pilot projects in one city and one place to regional pilot projects to form an overall effect. The implementation capacity of medical reform was significantly enhanced. Strong and effective promotion mechanism of medical reform was established and improved everywhere. Schedules and route diagrams were detailed and supervision and guidance intensified.

### I. Efforts were made to continue to deepen the comprehensive reform of public hospitals

The achievement of comprehensive reform of all the county-level public hospitals was further consolidated. Qidong City in Jiangsu Province, Tianchang City in Anhui Province, Youxi County in Fujian Province and Huzhu County in Qinghai Province were established as demonstration cities or demonstration counties. The number of pilot cities increased from 100 to 200, accounting for 60 percent of all cities at or above the prefectural level. 1568 city hospitals abolished medicine markups. The synchronous implementation of comprehensive reform in hospitals of traditional Chinese medicine was promoted; participation of military hospitals in the comprehensive reform of urban public hospitals was encouraged and the reform of medical institutions run by state-owned enterprises was deepened. The hospitals affiliated to the National Health and Family Planning Commission were coordinated and guided to participate in the comprehensive reform of territorial public hospitals. The corporate governance structure of public hospitals was improved; the mechanism of compensating for doctor's salary through drug-selling profits was gradually broken down; enthusiasm of medical staff was mobilized; and the unreasonable rise of medical expenses was controlled.

## II. Construction of hierarchical diagnosis and treatment system was promoted in an orderly manner.

Trying to enhance the ability of primary medical service was taken as the key point; carrying out hierarchical diagnosis and treatment of common diseases, frequently-occurring diseases and chronic diseases was taken as a breakthrough; and high-quality medical resources was gradually guided to go down. Guidance documents were issued in 31 provinces and trials of hierarchical diagnosis and treatment were carried out in 80% of the cities and 50% of the counties. The capacity of primary medical and health service was effectively improved and more than 80% of the residents could reach the nearest medical center within 15 minutes. The signing rate of family doctors reached 22% and that of key population reached 38.8%. The proportion of diagnosis and treatment in primary medical and health institutions in 19 provinces was on the rise, with some provinces exceeding 60%. The supporting policies for hierarchical diagnosis and treatment were being gradually improved. Development of a compact medical consortium was encouraged. Thus, a rational order for treatment in which "minor diseases were treated at the community level, major diseases in hospitals, patients' recovery at the community level" would soon come into being.

## III. The universal healthcare system was further improved.

Per capita financial subsidies for basic medical insurance for urban and rural residents were raised to 420 *yuan*. The integration of the medical insurance system for urban and rural residents was promoted; the direct settlement of in-patient medical expenses of the retirees in different places across provinces was started; the national network of basic medical insurance and direct settlement for remote medical treatment were steadily promoted. The coverage of basic medical insurance was expanded and the adjustment of the list of medicine was completed. Reform of the payment system was deepened; the mechanism for guaranteeing major and extraordinary major diseases was gradually improved; full coverage of the major diseases insurance system for urban and rural residents was consolidated, benefiting more than 10 million people. Emergency medical assistance benefited 130,000 people. We promoted special treatment for rural poor patients with major diseases in eight provinces and regions, and the actual compensation proportion of poor people who were hospitalized was nearly 12 percentage points higher than in 2015. The medical assistance system was continuously improved, and 93% of the regions had achieved the "one-stop" settlement of medical assistance and medical insurance expenses. Commercial health insurance developed rapidly, with the annual premium income of 404.25 billion *yuan*, up 67.71 percent from the same period last year.

### IV. The drug supply guarantee mechanism was further improved

From such key links as production, circulation and use, the drug supply guarantee mechanism was improved. With the exception of narcotic drugs and psychotropic substances of category I, the prices of drugs previously set by the government was abolished. On the basis of the first batch of 4 designated drug varieties like methimazole, 3 new designated drug varieties in short supply were added. The method for centralized procurement of medicines and high-value medical consumables in public hospitals was reformed and improved and the "two-invoice system" was implemented, in which one invoice was issued from production to circulation and one from circulation to medical institutions. 31 provinces (autonomous regions and municipalities directly under the Central Government) launched online direct procurement of generic drugs, urgent (emergency) rescue drugs, and commonly used low-cost drugs for women and children's specialties; 19 provinces (autonomous regions and municipalities directly under the Central Government) completed public bidding in two envelopes, reducing prices by an average of about 15%. Twenty-eight provinces (autonomous regions and municipalities directly under the Central Government) had implemented "sunshine procurement" for all or part of high-value medical consumables. A national price negotiation strategy was adopted for some patented drugs and exclusively manufactured drugs. The first three patented drugs had a price reduction of more than 50%. The qualification rate of Chinese patent medicine, chemical medicine and biological product was kept above 97%.

### V. Various reforms in the medical sector were promoted as a whole

Twelve categories of basic public health services were provided to all residents free of charge, and per capita subsidy for basic public health services was increased to 45 *yuan*. Major public health service projects continued to advance. The construction of health talent team was further strengthened. The standardized training for general medical residents enrolled 10,300 people and 5,636 rural medical students were enrolled for free on orders. Eight universities were supported to carry out the training of pediatric undergraduates and Beijing and Shanghai were supported to explore and carry out the pilot project of comprehensive education reform for postgraduates majoring in clinical medicine doctor of 5+3+X. Social medical and health services continued to develop; non-public hospitals account for 52% and the number of outpatients accounts for 22% of the total number of outpatients in China. We launched the first batch of national pilot projects to build health and medical big data centers and industrial parks. Medical reform experience of Sanming City was promoted in Anhui and Fujian provinces with World Bank loans.

In general, in 2016, the leadership system and working mechanism for deepening medical reform were further improved; the top-level design was improved continuously; the organization was further strengthened; and the deepening of medical reform reached a new level. The burden of the masses experienced "one optimization and two drops". That was, the income structure of hospitals was continuously optimized, and the proportion of drugs in public hospitals dropped from 46.33% in 2010 to about 40%; The rapid growth of medical expenses was initially curbed, with the increase in the income of government-run medical institutions falling to about 10% from 18.97% in 2010. Residents' burden of medical treatment was reduced and the proportion of personal health expenditure in total health expenditure dropped to below 30%, the lowest level in nearly 20 years. People's health level achieved "one rise and two falls", that was, the average life expectancy continued to increase, from 74.83 years in 2010 to 76.34 years, up by 1.51 years. The maternal mortality rate dropped from 31.9 per 100,000 to 19.9 per 100,000 and the infant mortality rate from 13.8 per 1,000 to 7.5 per 1,000. People's health level was better than the average level of middle and high income countries on the whole, with less investment to achieve higher health performance. According to the World Bank and the World Health Organization, China had made rapid progress in achieving universal health coverage, and its reform achievements had attracted worldwide attention.

(Tong Yanlong)

## 2. Formulating and Issuing the *Plan for Deepening Reform of the Medical and Health System in the 13th Five-year Plan Period*

On December 27<sup>th</sup>, 2016, the State Council issued the *Plan for Deepening Reform of the Medical and Health System in the 13th Fie-year Plan Period*, putting forward the guiding ideology, basic principles, main objectives, key tasks and safeguard measures for deepening medical reform in the 13th Five-year Plan period. Breakthrough would be made in construction of five Systems: ①Establishing a scientific and rational grading diagnosis and treatment system. We would establish and improve the family doctor contract service system and promote construction of medical consortia. By 2020, we would basically establish a hierarchical medical treatment system in line with China's national conditions, and a new medical order featuring first treatment at the community level, two-way referral, separately treating acute and chronic diseases, and linkage of upper and lower levels will take shape. ②Establishing scientific and effective modern hospital management system. We would deepen the comprehensive reform of county-level public hospitals and accelerate the comprehensive reform of urban public hospitals. By 2020, a modern hospital management system with clear rights and responsibilities, scientific management, sound governance, efficient operation and effective supervision and with Chinese characteristics would be established. ③Establishing a universal health care system that can operate efficiently. We would improve the mechanism for adjusting the proportion of financing and reimbursement, deepen the reform of the payment method for medical insurance, improve the accuracy of the payment of major medical insurance to the needy, and improve the mechanism for connecting various types of medical insurance. By 2017, the direct settlement of expenses for long-distance medical treatment and hospitalization that meet the referral requirements would be basically achieved. ④Establishing a standardized and orderly drug supply safeguard system. We would carry out the reform of the whole process of drug production, distribution and use, build a national drug policy system that is in line with China's national conditions, rationalize drug prices, and ensure that drugs are safe, effective, reasonably priced and adequately supplied. ⑤Establishing a strict and standard comprehensive supervision system. We would deepen reform of "relinquishing, management and service", build a diversified regulatory system, strengthen comprehensive regulation of the entire industry, and guide and standardize third-party evaluation and industry self-discipline.

**(Tong Yanlong)**

### 3. Formulating and Issuing *Summary of Efforts to Deepen the Reform of the Medical and Health System in 2015* and *Key Tasks for Deepening the Reform of the Medical and Health System in 2016*

On April 21st, 2016, the General Office of the State Council issued *Key Tasks for Deepening the Reform of the Medical and Health System in 2016,* putting forward 50 reform tasks in 10 aspects. They were: comprehensively deepening the reform of public hospitals, consolidating and perfecting universal health care system, accelerating construction of the hierarchical diagnosis and treatment system, improving drug supply security mechanism, establishing and improving the comprehensive supervision system, strengthening construction of health talent team, consolidating the system of equalizing basic public health services, advancing construction of health informatization, promoting the development of health services, strengthening organization and leadership. The task leading department and time schedule were clearly defined so as to achieve traceability, assessment and accountability.

On April 27th, 2016, the State Council's Leading Group on Health Care Reform held a teleconference on national health care reform in 2016. On the basis of a comprehensive summary of the achievements made in deepening medical reform during the 12th Five-year Plan period, vice premier Liu Yandong profoundly analyzed the new situation and new requirements in deepening medical reform and made comprehensive arrangements for deepening medical reform in 2016. She emphasized that we should take the new development concept as guideline, overcome difficulties, accelerate the progress of key reforms and make new breakthroughs so as to make a good start and take a good step in implementing the medical reform during the 13th Five-year Plan period. On May 5th, 2016, the Medical Reform Office of the State Council issued *Summary of Efforts to Deepen the Reform of the Medical and Health System in 2015*, pointing out that in 2015, the leadership system and working mechanism for deepening the medical reform had been continuously improved, and that the top-level design was improved, and that the concerted efforts of various departments had been further strengthened, and that the consensus of all sectors of society on reform had been further condensed , and that deepening medical reform had stepped to a new level.

(Tong Yanlong)

## 4. Formulating and Issuing *Opinions on Integrating the Basic Medical Insurance System for Urban and Rural Residents*

On January 3rd, 2016, the State Council issued the Opinion, putting forward that in accordance with the "six unified" requirements of unified coverage, unified financing policy, unified guarantee for treatment, unified medical insurance catalogue, unified fixed-point management and unified fund management, the basic system and policies should be integrated, the management system should be encouraged to be straightened out, agencies should be integrated and management should be innovated. At the same time, it was required to improve service efficiency, improve overall planning level, perfect information system, improve payment method and strengthen medical service supervision. By the end of June 2016, all provinces (autonomous regions and municipalities directly under the Central Government) should have made plans and arrangements for the integration of urban and rural residents' health insurance, and made clear the timetable and route diagram. Specific implementation plans should have been issued by the end of December 2016 in all regions.

**(Tong Yanlong)**

## 5. Strengthening the Publicity of Medical Reform

On October 21st, 2016, the General Office of the State Council issued *Notification on Adjusting the Personnel of the Leading Group of the State Council for Deepening the Reform of Medical and Health System* incorporating the Network Information Office of the Central Government into its member units. All regions integrated the local network information departments into their member units of medical reform leading groups at the same level with the national practice as reference. The Institutional Reform Division of the National Health and Family Planning Commission set up an information publicity department to strengthen communication with the Propaganda Department of the Central Committee of the CPC, the Network Information Office of the Central Government and the Central Reform Office. The provincial health insurance offices made it clear that $1-2$ persons as liaison were responsible for the daily work of health care publicity, and experts such as members of the Experts Advisory Committee of the Medical Reform Leading Group of the State Council were actively involved in health care publicity. Two training courses on medical reform publicity were held to improve the media literacy and publicity ability of medical reform staff. Cooperation mechanism was established with nearly 10 media, such as live broadcasting, medical reform column and video program production; carriers such as "Weibo", "WeChat" and mobile client were enriched; medical reform coverage with all media features took shape. We adhered to the correct guidance of public opinion and increased the interpretation and positive publicity of medical reform policies. We organized and held more than 10 press conferences and media communication meetings to further summarize and promote the mature experience of local medical reform, condense consensus among all parties in the society, respond to social concerns in a timely manner and guide the rational expectations of the masses.

**(Tong Yanlong)**

## 6. Formulating and Issuing Guidance Documents to Further Promote the Experience of Deepening Medical Reform

Since the launch of a new round of deepening the reform of the medical and health system, in order to sum up the experience of the pilot provinces of comprehensive medical reform, formulate documents for deepening the reform of the medical and health system, and give better play to the leading role of advanced and typical models, on November 8<sup>th</sup>, 2016, examined and approved by the Central Leading Group for Comprehensively Deepening Reform at the 27th conference, *Opinions on Promoting the Experience in Deepening the Reform of Medical and Health System* by the Leading Group of the State Council for Deepening the Reform of Medical and Health System was forwarded by the General Office of the CPC Central Committee and the General Office of the State Council, popularizing 24 successful experience in 8 aspects. On December 8<sup>th</sup>, the Leading Group of the State Council for Deepening the Reform of the Medical and Health System issued the *Typical Cases of Deepening the Reform of the Medical and Health System,* popularizing 15 typical cases including Fujian Province so that all localities had examples to learn from and had common templates to follow.

(Tong Yanlong)

## 7. Formulating and Issuing *Guidance on Promoting Family Doctors' Signing Services*

On May 25<sup>th</sup>, 2016, examined and approved by the Central Leading Group for Comprehensively deepening Reform at the 23rd conference, the *Guidance on Promoting Family Doctors' Signing Services* was jointly issued by the State Council Medical Reform Office, the National Health and Family Planning Commission, the National Development and Reform Commission, the Ministry of Civil Affairs, the Ministry of Finance, the Ministry of Human Resources and Social Security and the State administration of Traditional Chinese Medicine. Centering on the establishment of long-term stable contracted service relationship between family doctors and residents, the *Guidance* clarified the goal and main measures of contracted service and made great efforts to strengthen the construction of system and mechanism so as to mobilize the enthusiasm of both the supply and demand sides for signing service. It put forward that by 2016, family doctor signing service should have been carried out in 200 pilot cities for comprehensive reform of public hospitals, with emphasis on the breakthroughs in the ways, content, charge and payment, assessment and incentive mechanism of signing service. Priority should be given to the elderly, pregnant and parturient women, children and the disabled, as well as to patients with chronic diseases such as hypertension, diabetes and tuberculosis and to the patients with severe mental disorders. By 2017, the coverage rate of family doctor contracted service would have been over 30% and that of key groups over 60%. By 2020, we should strive to expand contract service to the whole population to form a long-term and stable contract service relationship, and basically achieve the full coverage of the family doctor contract service system.

(Tong Yanlong)

## 8. Pushing forward the Joint Study of "Three Parties and Five Departments" in Deepening Health Care reform

With the approval of the State Council, the Ministry of Finance, the National Health and Family Planning Commission and the Ministry of Human Resources and Social Security have assisted the World Bank and the World Health Organization in conducting a joint study on deepening the reform of China's medical and health system since December 2014. By carrying out a large amount of investigation and research, the project research team compiled and completed the policy summary of *Deepening the Reform of China's Medical and Health System and Building A Quality Service Delivery System Based on Value,* and held a release conference about the research results in Beijing on July 22nd, 2016. The report affirmed the remarkable progress made in China's health care reform, saying that China had made rapid progress in achieving universal health coverage, and that the accessibility and affordability of basic medical and health services had been improved, and that high health performance had been achieved at a lower cost and the achievements of the reform had attracted the attention of the world.

(Tong Yanlong)

## 9. Formulating and Issuing the Guidance Document for the Performance Assessment of the Hospitals Affiliated to and Managed by the National Health and Family Planning Commission

On March 3rd, 2017, the National Health and Family Planning Commission issued the *Notification on Carrying out the Comprehensive Performance Assessment of the Hospitals Affiliated to and Managed by the National Health and Family Planning Commission,* which insisted on the public interest orientation of the comprehensive performance assessment and made it clear that the assessment would cover social benefits, the provision of medical services, economic efficiency and sustainable development. By conducting quantitative and qualitative assessment, self-examination and self-assessment, non-on-site online comprehensive assessment in the whole-process and on-site spot check and review of key issues, the performance of the hospitals affiliated to and managed by the National Health and Family Planning Commission was comprehensively assessed. There were 63 items in 6 categories of index for evaluating and scoring. The final score was calculated on a percentage basis. Hospitals with unqualified results or outstanding problems would be notified for rectification within a time limit. At the same time, the application of the assessment results should be strengthened as an important basis for financial subsidies, planning formulation, major project initiation and establishment of key disciplines, as well as the principal basis for the assessment of the dean.

(Tong Yanlong)

## 10. Promoting the Work of Pilot Provinces on Comprehensive Health Care Reform

The National Health and Family Planning Commission, through in-depth investigation and research, promoted the successful experience of Jiangsu, Anhui, Fujian and Qinghai, the first four pilot provinces of comprehensive health care reform in 2016. It guided the 7 provinces (autonomous regions and municipalities directly under the Central Government), Shanghai, Zhejiang, Hunan, Sichuan, Chongqing, Shanxi and Ningxia to improve the pilot program, reported to the Medical Reform Leading Group of the State Council for reviewing and issuing *the Letter on Adding Shanghai and the Other Seven Provinces (Autonomous Regions and Municipalities directly under the Central Government) to the Pilot Program to Carry out the Comprehensive Medical Reform* so as to launch the second batch of pilot program of comprehensive medical reform. It guided relevant provinces to improve pilot programs and cultivated the third batch of pilot provinces of comprehensive medical reform. Eighteen liaison officers were selected from 11 contact units directly under the National Health and Family Planning Commission and assigned to the pilot provinces in batches for carrying out the work. The Commission selected 22 liaison experts for 11 pilot provinces in order to intensify efforts in policy consulting, supervision and evaluation, publicity and training in the pilot provinces. On November 13th, 2016, an exchange meeting on the comprehensive health care reform of Shanghai, Jiangsu, Zhejiang, Anhui and Fujian provinces (autonomous regions, municipalities directly under the Central Government) was held.

Li Bin, minister of the National Health and Family Planning Commission, attended and delivered a speech at the meeting. Wang Hesheng, vice minister of the National Health and Family Planning Commission and director of the Medical Reform Office of the State Council, presided over the meeting. At the meeting, the system of joint conference for comprehensive reform in the four provinces and one city,

Shanghai, Jiangsu, Zhejiang, Anhui and Fujian, was established and an agreement was signed.

(Tong Yanlong)

## 11. The Leaders of the National Health and Family Planning Commission Focused on the Work of the Key Provinces Carrying out Health Care Reform

*Notification on the Division of Labor of the Leaders of the National Health and Family Planning Commission in Focusing on the Work of the Key Provinces Carrying out Health Care Reform in 2016* and *Notification on Adjusting the Work of the Leaders of the National Health and Family Planning Commission in Focusing on the Health Care Reform of the Key Provinces* were issued, in which division of responsibility and specific work requirements of the leaders of the National Health and Family Planning Commission in the key provinces in which health care reform was carried out and bureau liaison officer system were clarified. The leaders of the Commission should provide guidance and support to the provincial governments, conduct research and inspection on medical reform in the provinces, and fully understand the progress and existing problems of the local medical reform.

(Tong Yanlong)

## 12. China Health Care Reform Promotion Project with the World Bank

According to the consensus reached between the Chinese government and the World Bank and the *Alternative Project Plan for 2016-2018 Loan by International Financial Organization*, the World Bank planned to invest $600 million to support the promotion of Sanming medical reform experience in Anhui and Fujian Provinces and promote faster and better realization of comprehensive medical reform goals in the two provinces. The Medical Reform Office of the State Council took the lead in establishing a Joint Working Group of World Bank Loan Projects composed of the State Development and Reform Commission, the Ministry of Finance and the National Health and Family Planning Commission, conducting research on project areas, coverage, funding arrangements and requirements for organization and implementation, drafting and forming a program of project activities at the central level, strengthening coordination and guidance for project provinces, cooperating with the World Bank in carrying out appraisal and technical review and preparing for project implementation.

(Tong Yanlong)

## 13. Implementing the "Two-invoice System" for Drug Purchase

On December 30$^{th}$, 2016, the Medical Reform Office of the State Council issued the *Implementation Opinions (Trial) on the Practice of "Two-invoice System" in Drug Purchase of Public Medical Institutions*. It is required to implement the "two-invoice system" in the procurement of drugs in public medical institutions. That is, an invoice should be issued once from manufacturing enterprises to circulation enterprises and once from circulation enterprises to medical institutions, so as to compress the circulation of drugs, make the intermediate price increase transparent, promote the reduction of the inflated price of drugs, and reduce the burden of medication on the public.

(Tong Yanlong)

## 14. Conducting Research and Supervision on Deepening Reform of the Medical and Health Care System

In 2016, it was required by the Central Reform Office to sort out the documents of health and family planning reform, formulate a supervision plan for implementing the measures of health and family planning reform, and report to the Central Reform Office for the record. In May, investigation and supervision were organized and the teams were led respectively by all the leaders of the National Health and Family Planning Commission and the people in charge of the relevant departments and bureaus to carry out field investigation and supervision on the deepening of medical reform in 31 provinces (autonomous regions and municipalities directly under the Central Government). In early June, according to the investigation and supervision sub-reports provided by the inspection teams and the self-inspection reports of various provinces, the investigation and supervision reports were researched and drafted, and reported to the Central Reform Office and the State Office of Supervision. At the same time, the feedback to the investigation and supervision situation was also provided to the provinces respectively to push the medical reform further.

(Tong Yanlong)

## 15. Monitoring on Medical Reform

In order to grasp the progress of the key work of medical reform in various regions and supervise and urge the implementation of the annual tasks about medical reform, the Medical Reform Department of the State Council stepped up the monitoring of medical reform. The monitoring indicators in 2016 were divided into annual monitoring indicators (170) and quarterly monitoring indicators (31), totaling 201. The monitoring results showed that the key tasks of medical reform had been well implemented and significant progress was made: (1) the reform of public hospitals was comprehensively deepened. Evaluation of the pilot results of comprehensive reform of public hospitals was carried out in 190 cities, and modern hospital management systems such as the legal person governance structure of public hospitals and the chief accountant system were constantly established and improved. (2) The construction of hierarchical medical system was progressing constantly. Trials of hierarchical diagnosis and treatment were carried out in 87% of counties (county-level cities and districts), and trials of primary diagnosis and treatment responsibility system at the community level were carried out in 83.1% of counties (county-level cities and districts). The coverage rate of family doctor signing contracts in 187 cities reached more than 15%. (3) The universal healthcare system was consolidated and improved. The number of people participating in three basic medical insurance programs reached 1.34 billion, and the rate of participating in three basic medical insurance programs reached 98.8%. The annual task of stabilizing the participation rate above 95% for five consecutive years was completed. (4) The drug supply guarantee mechanism was continuously improved. Standards for the payment of drugs for basic medical insurance were set in seven provinces (autonomous regions and municipalities directly under the Central Government); a drug price monitoring system was established in 178 cities; the two-invoice system was introduced in 69 cities. (5) The construction of health talent team was strengthened continuously. The number of standardized training for general practitioners reached 7,932; the number of transferred training for general practitioners reached 7,092; the number of standardized training for residents reached 72,556; the average government subsidy for rural doctors in 2016 was 23.8 thousand per person per year.

**(Tong Yanlong)**

## 16. Comprehensive Reform of Public Hospitals

For deepening comprehensive reform of public hospitals at the county level and strengthening classified guidance and demonstration, in 2016, the National Health and Family Planning Commission determined to carry out demonstration work in Tianchang City of Anhui Province, Youxi County of Fujian Province, Qidong City of Jiangsu Province and Huzhu County of Qinghai Province. 167 model counties (county-level cities, districts) were determined in 28 provinces (autonomous regions and municipalities directly under the Central Government) and Xinjiang Production and Construction Corps. The practice of prepayment of medical insurance by the medical community in Tianchang City, Anhui Province was popularized. The pilot program for comprehensive reform of urban public hospitals was expanded, and the number of the pilot cities in the whole country reached 200, covering nearly two-thirds of the country's cities. The hospitals affiliated to (managed by) the National Health and Family Planning Commission and the State Administration of Traditional Chinese Medicine were urged to take part in the comprehensive reform of the territorial public hospitals. Reform was launched in 17 hospitals affiliated to (managed by) the National Health and Family Planning Commission and the State Administration of Traditional Chinese Medicine in 6 pilot cities. Financial input was increased. In 2016, a total of 8.422 billion *yuan* was allocated to support and promote the comprehensive reform of public hospitals. Efforts were made to strengthen assessment and incentive, organize and carry out evaluation and assessment of the effect of the comprehensive reform of public hospitals in 2015, and provide encouragement and support to the areas where the comprehensive reform of public hospitals had achieved obvious results. Efforts were also made to control the unreasonable growth of medical expenses, urge provinces (autonomous regions and municipalities directly under the Central Government) to determine the quantitative growth rate of annual medical expenses, rank and report the growth rate of medical expenses in each province. On the whole, the comprehensive reform of public hospitals continued to expand and deepen; the responsibility of the government for medical treatment was advanced and implemented; a scientific compensation mechanism for public hospitals was initially established; significant progress was made in the key areas and key links of reform, such as personnel remuneration, hierarchical diagnosis and treatment, and cost control; the level of medical services was effectively improved; and a multiparty-win situation was taking shape among the government, hospitals, medical personnel, and the masses who sought medical treatment.

(Tong Yanlong)

## 17. Evaluation on the Effect of the Comprehensive Reform in Public Hospitals for the First Time

In 2016, the Medical Reform Office of the State Council, together with the National Health and Family Planning Commission, the Ministry of Finance, the Central Compilation Office, the National Development and Reform Commission, and the Ministry of Human Resources and Social Security, carried out the evaluation and assessment of the effect of the comprehensive reform in public hospitals in 2015, covering 1,977 counties (county-level cities) and 100 pilot cities in 31 provinces (autonomous regions and municipalities directly under the Central Government) and Xinjiang Production and Construction Corps. On the basis of the self-evaluation of each province, 169 county-level public hospitals and 67 urban public hospitals were selected for random inspection, and a questionnaire survey was conducted among 5,451 medical personnel and 5,470 patients. The results of evaluation and assessment were linked to the special financial subsidies of the central government, rewarding the advanced and punishing the backward. An effective incentive and accountability mechanism was established.

**(Tong Yanlong)**

## 18. Training on the Policies for the Comprehensive Reform of Public Hospitals

In 2016, four training courses on the comprehensive reform of urban public hospitals were held, training more than 800 people, including the people in charge of the related departments and offices of the Health and Family Planning Commission and the Medical Reform Office and the heads of public hospitals in all the provinces and 100 newly added pilot cities. We organized and convened an on-site meeting on comprehensive reform demonstration work of the county-level public hospitals, an on-the-spot meeting on the comprehensive reform of public hospitals in the new pilot cities, and an on-site meeting on the reform of the hospitals affiliated to (managed by) the National Health and Family Planning Commission and the State Administration of Traditional Chinese Medicine, etc. A total of over 940 people in charge of the Medical Reform Offices, the Health and Family Planning Commissions and the public hospitals at all levels were trained. Four regional symposiums on the comprehensive reform of public hospitals were held to exchange reform progress and highlight experience in various regions.

**(Tong Yanlong)**

# Part IV
# Professional Work in Health and Family Planning

## ▌Chapter I   Development Planning and Information Statistics

**1. *Outline of the Healthy China 2030 Plan* Was Issued by CPC Central Committee and the State Council**

On October 25th, 2016, *Outline of the Healthy China 2030 Plan* (hereinafter referred to as the *Outline*) was jointly issued by the CPC Central Committee and the State Council. This *Outline* was the first middle to long-term strategic planning in the health field formulated at the national level. The important strategic decision to advance the construction of a healthy China was made at the Fifth Plenary Session of the 18th CPC Central Committee. According to the deployment of the Central Committee, the Leading Group of Healthcare Reform of the State Council led the formulation of the *Outline*, including the basic framework and the main contents. In addition, in March of 2016, the working group for the outline formulation was set up, with vice premier Liu Yandong as the team leader, the chiefs from the National Health and Family Planning Commission, the National Development and Reform Commission, the Ministry of Finance, the Ministry of Human Resources and Social Security, the General Administration of Sports of China and other commissions and ministries as vice team leaders, and other 21 departments like the Ministry of Ecology and Environment of the People's Republic of China and the State Food and Drug Administration as the members. An expert team in the relevant field was also formed. During the formulation, the opinions from scholars, local governments, enterprises, public institutions and social societies were solicited. On August 19th-20th, the opinions from the delegates of the National Health Conference were asked. On August 27th, the *Outline* was deliberated and approved at the conference of the CPC Central Committee.

The *Outline* clearly defined the general strategy for advancing the construction of a healthy China. In the *Outline*, it was pointed out that the principle of putting people first should be adhered to, the new development concepts should be upheld and implemented, and the right health policies should be carried out. In addition, the enhancement of people's health should be put at the center, the reform and innovation of the systems and mechanisms should be taken as the drive, and health should be integrated into all the policies. What's more, the transformation of development modes in the health field should be accelerated and the all-round cradle-to-grave maintenance and guarantee of people's health should be realized. Finally, the health level should be greatly elevated and the equal access to health service should be significantly improved. To "contribute and share to build a healthy nation" was the theme of the Health China Strategy. Centering on "building an all-round moderately prosperous society" and the realization of the "two centenary goals", the *Outline* well linked up the objectives in different phases of economic and social development, actively fulfilled China's commitment to world made in UN's 2030 Agenda for Sustainable Development and put forth the three-step strategic goals, i.e. main health indicators ranking top in upper middle-income countries in 2020, main health indicators being equal to high-income countries in 2030 and building a healthy China complemented with a modernized socialist country in 2050. Taking the health influence factors into consideration and in the order from the internal to the external and from the main body to the environment, the *Outline* put forward the major tasks in the following 5 aspects: healthy living for all, optimizing healthcare services, improving health security, building a healthy environment, and developing healthcare industry.

**(Qu Yang)**

## 2. The State Council Issued the *"13th Five-Year Plan"* on Public Health

On December 27th, 2016, the State Council issued the *"13th Five-Year Plan" on Public Health*, which was one of the national key special plans approved by the State Council. The preparation work lasted for more than one year. In accordance with the State Council's deployment, the National Health and Family Planning Commission and the relevant departments carried out research on the medical and healthcare development, population strategy and policy for aging population, and also conducted 31 major and special research projects for the "Thirteenth Five-Year Plan". Opinions and suggestions were solicited from all sectors by the means of field research, experts discussions, public collections, etc.. During the period, the State Council's Healthcare Reform Leading Group conducted several studies. On December

21$^{st}$, the State Council executive meeting reviewed and approved the *"13th Five-Year Plan" on Public Health*.

The overall thinking of the *"13th Five-Year Plan" on Public Health* was to address the outstanding problems faced by the people's health needs and career development, to maintain and promote health as the central task, to provide the whole population with the cradle-to-grave health services. In terms of contents, the main body was the development of the health and family planning industry, and it extended to areas closely related to health such as environmental protection, physical fitness, and food and medicine. The *"13th Five-Year Plan" on Public Health* proposed that by 2020, the basic medical and healthcare system covering urban and rural residents should be established gradually to achieve basic medical and health services for all, and the life expectancy per capita would increase by one year on the basis of 2015. The *"13th Five-Year Plan" on Public Health* clearly assigned 10 tasks, namely, strengthening the prevention and control of major diseases, promoting patriotic health campaigns and health promotion, enhancing maternal and child health care and reproductive services, developing elderly health care services, promoting the health of key groups such as the poor, improving family planning policies, improving medical service levels, promoting the inheritance and innovation of traditional Chinese medicine, strengthening comprehensive supervision and law enforcement and monitoring food and drug safety, and accelerating the development of the health industry. It also put forward 10 categories of 34 projects and 5 major projects in special columns. At the same time, division of tasks was clarified in the department to ensure and promote the smooth implementation of the *"13th Five-Year Plan" on Public Health*.

**(Zhang Nan)**

# Chapter II    Health Emergency Response

## 1. Overview of Health Emergency Response in 2016

### I. Efforts made in doing well the top-level design, putting forward development ideas and highlighting key tasks

(1) The development idea of "One Body Two Wings" was put forward. During the special research at the beginning of 2016, the Party Leadership Group of the National Health and Family Planning Commission put forward the development idea of "One Body Two Wings", with the system and core capacity building as the "Body", and the prevention and control of acute infectious diseases as well as the construction of medical emergency rescue as the "Two Wings".

(2) "Two *Plans*" and one *Guiding Opinions* were issued. *The 13th Five-Year Plan for the Prevention and Control of Acute Infectious Diseases (2016-2020)* and *the 13th Five-Year Plan for Medical Emergency Rescue (2016-2020)* were the special plans issued for the first time in the area of health emergency. They put forward the overall development goals and key tasks for the areas of both the prevention and control of acute infectious diseases and medical emergency rescue. In addition, the main tasks and construction projects of the two *Plans* have already been brought into relevant plans of the state. The issuance of the *Guiding Opinions on Strengthening the Standardization Construction of Health Emergency Work* will strongly promote the continuous improvement of health emergency management and the capacity to deal with health emergencies.

(3) Local governments actively drew up local plans. Twenty-four provinces (autonomous regions, municipalities directly under the Central Government) and 97 sub-branches at city level are drawing up or are about to draw up overall and special plans as well as implementation plans for health emergency.

### II. Progress in team building and drilling

(1) Team building. Twelve national teams were added into the construction, which will achieve a universal coverage of national teams for all provinces upon the completion of construction. The funds for daily operation and maintenance of the teams were put to use. Moreover, efforts were made to launch the construction of the national mobile disposal center for health emergency. What's more, with the promotion of "going global" for the national health emergency teams, the national medical emergency rescue team organized by Shanghai became one of the world's

first international health emergency teams upon the certification of the WHO.

(2) The team role. In 2016, the national teams of provinces of Jiangsu, Hubei, Hunan, Shaanxi and Shandong played important roles in health emergency response. All local governments paid attention to the integration of daily routine and emergencies. Thereinto, the national medical emergency rescue team organized by Hunan province participated in the national free clinic week in Ruijin of Jiangxi province, which was fully affirmed by vice premier Liu Yandong.

(3) The state made policies to subsidize the temporary work of epidemic prevention and control personnel. With the consent of the State Council, the Ministry of Human Resources and Social Security and the Ministry of Finance jointly issued a document to establish a temporary work subsidy for epidemic prevention and control personnel. This was the first time since the founding of the People's Republic of China that China has issued a subsidy policy for those involved in the emergency response of public health emergencies at home and abroad.

(4) Local team building. Chongqing and Guangxi took the lead nationwide in exploring the building of a professional marine (aquatic) medical emergency rescue team. Twenty-five medical emergency rescue teams at the provincial level were set up in Fujian province. Daily operation and maintenance management of the teams were regulated in the provinces of Shaanxi, Sichuan and Yunnan.

(5) Drill work. Joint drills were organized in Beijing, Tianjin, Hebei, Guangdong, Guangxi, Jiangsu, Shandong, Sichuan, Chongqing, Guizhou, Shanxi, Shaanxi and Henan, respectively, with natural disasters, accident disasters and outbreak of acute infectious diseases as the scenes. In Liaoning, Jilin, Heilongjiang and Xinjiang Production & Construction Corps, joint military, police and local exercises were carried out. And the training and exercises for the national health emergency teams were organized in Shanghai, Inner Mongolia, Shaanxi, Henan, Hubei, Fujian and Hainan.

### III. Health emergency work in various localities

(1) Regional cooperation. The signing of cooperation agreements among neighboring districts and counties were promoted in Beijing-Tianjin-Hebei Region. The cooperation agreements for health emergency were signed in the provinces of Jiangsu, Anhui, Shandong and Henan. Started with the drills, the teams' long-distance mobility and on-site cooperative handling capacities were exercised and tested in Guangdong, Guangxi, Shanxi, Shaanxi, Henan, Jiangsu, Shandong, Sichuan, Chongqing and Guizhou.

(2) Legal and institutional construction. Formulated in Gansu province, the

*Regulations on Plague Prevention and Control* was listed as the first local regulations of Gansu in 2016. Tianjin city innovatively introduced quality control concept to establish the first provincial quality control center for health emergency nationwide. The information reporting system for medical emergency rescue was improved in Shandong, Shanxi and Hunan. The county's (banner's) implementation plans and construction standards of health emergency standards were formulated in Jiangsu and Inner Mongolia, which promoted the standardization of health emergency response from the demonstration on the point to the standards on the surface.

(3) Aero-medical rescue. Efforts were made to actively explore aero-medical rescue in Beijing, Shanghai, Hubei and Sichuan. The provincial health and family planning departments and healthcare institutions in Tianjin, Hebei, Fujian signed cooperation agreements with general aviation (GA) enterprises. Hunan and Shanxi provincial health and family planning commissions cooperated with provincial armed police force.

(4) Social involvement. Jiangsu and Liaoning took the lead in the project of improving universal self-rescue and mutual aid literacy. Emergency knowledge and skills were popularized in Shanghai, Jiangsu, Chongqing and Tianjin. In Chongqing, Zhejiang, Shaanxi, and Qinghai, experts were organized to go into the communities and rural areas at community level.

### IV. Health emergency response to various emergency incidents

(1) Scientific and orderly response to the outbreak of acute infectious diseases. In the face of the overseas outbreak of Zika virus, we promptly organized evaluation, study and judgment, launched the joint prevention and control mechanism, and preceded the WHO in making arrangements for the prevention and control of the virus. Twenty-four cases of imported Zika virus were found and successfully treated in Jiangxi, Zhejiang, Beijing and Henan provinces. In the face of the rare outbreak of imported rift valley fever (RVF), Beijing experts played a decisive role in recognizing the virus as RVF through pathogen screening, which saved precious time for effective case treatment and epidemic prevention and control. In addition, 11 cases of yellow fever were detected and effectively treated in time in Beijing, Shanghai, and Fujian without any outbreak spread. A case of Bubonic plague was found and successfully treated in time in Yunnan province. In Qinghai, Xinjiang, Gansu, Tibet and Inner Mongolia, efforts were made to strengthen the monitoring and disposal of plague in animals, which effectively prevented the outbreak of plague in humans. Public health experts were sent to Angola to guide the management of local yellow fever and other diseases, and arrangements were made to guide the prevention and control of tropical

diseases such as Zika in Guyana.

(2) Medical emergency rescue for natural disasters. In the face of tornado and hailstorm in Jiangsu, 55 ambulances were dispatched within 12 hours to transfer 846 injured people to 35 hospitals for effective treatment. Furthermore, 35 national and provincial experts arrived in the area within 20 hours to reinforce the treatment of the wounded. Faced with the most devastating floods since 1998, Anhui, Hebei, Hubei, Hunan and other 11 disaster-hit provinces (autonomous regions, municipalities directly under the Central Government) earnestly implemented the measures of "health care for floods, flood victims and rescue teams in place" in medical treatment and "disease prevention and control, environment renovation for patriotic health environmental, and publicity of disease prevention being kept pace" in epidemic prevention. They also strengthened the comprehensive treatment of "six synchronizations" to achieve the situation of post-disaster epidemic free.

**(Jing Ran)**

# Chapter III    Disease Prevention and Control

## 1. Overview of National Disease Prevention and Control and Patriotic Health Work in 2016

### I. Improving the policies and mechanisms

The 1st plenary session of inter-ministerial joint conference of the State Council on the prevention and treatment of major diseases was held and issued detailed working rules. The General Office of the State Council issued plans for the prevention and treatment of AIDS, tuberculosis, chronic diseases and occupational diseases. Many sectors jointly issued plans for the prevention and control of key parasitic diseases such as endemic diseases, schistosomiasis and echinococcosis, and defined the objectives, tasks and key measures for the prevention and control of major diseases during the "13th Five-Year Plan".

### II. Enhancing the overall ability of the disease control team

The implementation of the guidelines on the standards for staffing quotas of disease prevention and control centers was promoted by the State Commission Office of Public Sectors Reform and the other two departments. The pilot program for standardized training of public health physicians was formulated. Public health physician training was incorporated into the standardized resident training program. The comprehensive evaluation of the standardized construction of provincial-level CDCs was organized. The implementation of relevant policies such as staffing, post setting, infrastructure, and funding guarantee was promoted. The *Opinions of the General Office of the State Council on Strengthening the Safety Protection of Infectious Disease Prevention and Control Personnel* was implemented. Temporary work subsidies for infectious disease prevention and control personnel were established. The adjustment of health and epidemic prevention allowances was promoted. The Ministry of Human Resources and Social Security was invited to initiate the research.

### III. Laying solid foundation for national immunization planning

The series of illegally operated vaccines in Jinan, Shandong province was properly disposed of. The *Regulation on the Administration of Circulation and Vaccination of Vaccines* was amended. The General Office of the State Council issued the *Opinions on Further Strengthening Vaccine Circulation and Vaccination Management.* The revision of the *National Immunization Program for Children's Immunization Procedures* and the *Working Rules for Vaccination* was organized to further standardize vaccination and establish a long-term management mechanism. The immunization strategy conversion of polio vaccine was implemented. One dose of polio inactivated vaccine and three doses of 2-valent polio attenuated live vaccine were inoculated to replace the trivalent polio attenuated live vaccine (sugar pellet). The work experience of compensation insurance pilots for abnormal response was accumulated.

### IV. Remarkable achievement in infectious disease prevention and treatment

Joint prevention and joint control were strengthened. The import of Zika virus disease, yellow fever and Rift Valley fever was effectively disposed of and there was no local epidemic spread. The import of infectious diseases such as Middle East respiratory syndrome and Ebola hemorrhagic fever were successfully prevented. The monitoring of epidemic situation in flood-hit areas was strengthened. The post-disaster health and epidemic prevention was guided. There was no major epidemic after major disasters. In 2016, the epidemic situation of infectious diseases in China was generally stable, and no large-scale epidemic occurred. The active detection of AIDS was strengthened. The comprehensive intervention of high-risk groups was strengthened. The standards of anti-viral treatment were adjusted. The tax exemption policy for the anti-viral AIDS treatment drugs of the "13th Five-Year Plan" was determined. In 2016, there were 125,000 newly reported infected people and 116,000 additional patients receiving anti-viral treatment, an increase of 7.9% and 8.2% respectively over the previous year. The linkage mechanism between drug treatment and compulsory isolation detoxification, community detoxification and community rehabilitation was determined together with the Ministry of Public Security and the Ministry of Justice. The pilot scope of prevention and control work of institutions of higher learning was extended together with the Ministry of Education. The establishment of the anti-AIDS fund of institutions of higher learning was supported. The social organizations' participation cycle in the AIDS prevention and control fund project was adjusted to two years. The supervision and evaluation method was formulated. The notice on further strengthening the prevention and treatment of tuberculosis was issued. The pilot program for hierarchical diagnosis and treatment of tuberculosis and integrated prevention and treatment services was launched. Survey on the incidence of multidrug-resistant tuberculosis was conducted. The base of the epidemic was found out. Inter-provincial cross-inspection of key work on tuberculosis was organized and carried out. In 2016, there were 811,000 newly reported cases of tuberculosis in China, 5.8% lower than the previous year, and the patient cure rate remained at above 90%.

### V. Consolidation of achievements in the prevention and control of key parasitic disease and endemic disease

The four provinces (autonomous regions)—Zhejiang province, Fujian Province, Guangdong province and Guangxi Zhuang Autonomous Region— were reviewed and found to have attained the goal of eliminating schistosomiasis. Supervision was carried out in Hunan, Hubei, Jiangxi, and Anhui provinces, and post-disaster schistosomiasis prevention was strengthened. The 6th National Parasitic Disease Control Technology Competition was held to further improve community-level prevention and control. The pilot project for comprehensive prevention and control of echinococcosis was guided in Shiqu County, Sichuan province and remarkable achievements were achieved. Supervision was carried out together with the United Front Department and the experience of prevention and control of echinococcosis in Tibetan areas was accumulated. Survey on the prevalence of echinococcosis was carried out in 70 districts (counties) in 17 counterpart provinces assisting Tibet. Revision of *Regulations on Elimination of Iodine Deficiency through Salt with Iodine* was organized. The iodine deficiency monitoring program was revised. Iodine nutrition monitoring was implemented in one-third of the counties in China.

### VI. Advancement in the prevention and treatment of chronic diseases

The construction management method for the demonstration zones of comprehensive national chronic disease prevention and control was revised and issued. The construction of the fourth batch of demonstration zones and the review of the first batch of demonstration zones were initiated. The first phase of the National Healthy Lifestyle Action with the theme of "10,000 steps per day, balance between eating and moving" was accomplished. The professional edition and the popular science edition of 2016 version of the China Dietary Guide were released. The comprehensive prevention and treatment work plan for stroke was issued together with the State Administration of Traditional Chinese Medicine. Tumor registration covered approximately 340 million people in all provinces. The 4th epidemiological survey on national oral health status was conducted.

### VII. Innovative development of mental health work

The National Health and Family Planning Commission, together with the Publicity

Department of the Central Committee of the CPC and the Office of the Comprehensive Administration of Public Security Commission under the Central Committee, issued guidelines on strengthening mental health services. The pilot program for comprehensive mental health management was promoted. Remarkable achievements were made in improving the comprehensive management mechanism, "one-stop" service for patients' treatment and assistance, and community rehabilitation services, etc. Six departments jointly issued opinions on the implementation of the policy of awards in place of subsidies and the implementation of the custody responsibility for patients with severe mental disorders. Management services were well provided such as reporting and registration of and follow-up visits to patients with severe mental disorders. By the end of 2016, there were 5.4 million registered patients with severe mental disorders in China, with a management rate of 88.7%, an increase of 480,000 cases and 3.2% respectively over the previous year. The general hospitals were guided to set up mental (psychological) departments. Institutions of higher learning were guided to begin to offer mental health programs.

### VIII. Quality improvement in the "Four Major Health Fields"

Opinions on strengthening the prevention and control of pneumoconiosis among migrant workers were issued together with 10 departments. The system construction was strengthened and the service network was improved. There were 17 new occupational health check-up institutions and 23 occupational disease diagnosis and treatment institutions in China. 20 provinces (autonomous regions and municipalities directly under the Central Government) achieved full coverage of prefecture-level occupational disease diagnosis institutions, and 9 provinces achieved full coverage of county-level occupational health check-up institutions. The prefecture (municipality) coverage ratios of key occupational diseases, occupational radioactive diseases and medical radiation protection in China reached 84%, 78% and 75% respectively.

The scope of environmental health impact monitoring was further extended. By the end of 2016, national urban and rural drinking water monitoring covered all prefectures, counties and 80% of townships. The monitoring of air pollution impact on population health covered 126 monitoring sites in 60 cities. The monitoring of health risk factors in public places, students' common diseases and health risk factors was initiated nationwide. The plan for conducting survey on national soil pollution was made and special surveys were conducted in 16 provinces and cities. Research on, determination of and emergency response to impacts of severe air pollution, drinking water pollution and other environmental pollution on the health of the population were guided and carried out.

## IX. New achievement in patriotic health work

With the approval of the State Council, the National Patriotic Health Association issued guidelines on the development of healthy cities and healthy rural townships and villages, and comprehensively launched the construction of healthy cities and healthy villages and townships. Thirty-eight national healthy cities (districts) were chosen to be the first pilot zones for the construction of healthy cities in China. A third-party assessment of healthy city construction of 247 national healthy cities (districts) was organized. The healthy city mayor forum of the 9th Global Conference on Health Promotion 2016 and the first China-US healthy city forum were successfully held. The *Shanghai Consensus on Healthy Cities* and *China-US Declaration on Health Promotion* were released. Urban and rural environmental sanitation and clean-up actions were further promoted in China. In 2016, the national village garbage disposal rate reached 60%; the proportion of administrative villages that treated sewage in China reached 22%, 4 percent higher than the previous year; rural drinking water security level was further improved and the rate of rural sanitary toilets steadily increased. The *National Vector Monitoring Program* was revised and issued. The spring patriotic health campaign with the theme of "Clean Home, Anti-mosquito and Disease Prevention" was organized nationwide to effectively control the occurrence of mosquito-borne diseases. In 2016, the incidence of dengue epidemic fell by 47% compared with the previous year.

**(Wang Guimin)**

# Chapter IV  Medical Administration

## 1. Overview of Medical Administration in 2016

### I. Centering on medical reform, breakthroughs were made in innovation in the important fields of medical administration

The construction of tiered diagnosis and treatment system was steadily promoted. In 2016, focused on chronic diseases like hypertension, diabetes and etc., with medical treatment alliance and day surgery as the breakthrough points, pilot work was carried out in hierarchical diagnosis and treatment. By the end of 2016, thirty-one provinces (autonomous regions, municipalities directly under the Central Government) nationwide issued guidelines on hierarchical diagnosis and treatment, with 80% of cities and 50% of towns launched pilot projects in hierarchical diagnosis and treatment.

Great achievements were made in implementing the medical service improvement action plan. "Action Plan to Further Improve Medical Service" was promoted. By the end of the year 2016, tertiary hospitals nationwide fully carried out appointment diagnosis and treatment and excellent nursing services and in 3,329 medical institutions, period-division appointment diagnosis and treatment was carried out; mobile payment and settlement service was provided in 1,378 medical institutions, being 710 more than that in 2015; day surgery accounted for 11% of elective surgery, which effectively enhanced the medical service efficiency; the telemedicine service was carried out by over 6,800 medical institutions, covering 1,330 counties. Nearly 70,000 medical institutions subscribed medical liability insurance and medical risk mutual funds, and the function of the mechanism "Three Mediations and One Insurance" for preventing and dealing with medical disputes was increasingly obvious.

Progress was made in "Decentralization-Management-Service" reform. Reform of "License First, Certificate Later" was comprehensively carried out, multi-site practice of doctors was promoted, and regional registration and other ways were explored. The development of hospitals run by social capitals was promoted in accordance with law to ensure the orderly and healthy development of these hospitals. By the end of 2016, the number of doctors practicing at multiple sites reached 61.3 thousand, with 43.4% serving in the hospitals run by social capitals and 66.3% serving in community-level medical institutions. The total number of private hospitals reached 16,000, which accounted for 55.7% of the total number of hospitals nationwide, initially forming a healthy pattern of coordinated development between private and public hospitals.

## II. Medical service capacity was elevated

The medical service system and ability building was continuously enhanced. The guiding principles on medical institution installation planning (the year 2016-2020) and the installation plan of the National Medical Center as well as regional medical centers were formulated, the top-level design of medical service systems was optimized and the appropriate distribution and balanced development of medical resources were promoted. A number of 889 tertiary hospitals were arranged to help 1,149 counterpart county hospitals in 834 impoverished counties. Fifteen hospitals under the National Health and Family Planning Commission and 15 national medical teams were sent to make medical tours around remote and poverty-stricken areas. Cooperation with the related ministries and commissions was carried out to print and distribute "Recommendations on Reinforcing the Reform and Development of Medical Service for Children" and promote the sustainable and healthy development of medical and health care for children. The establishment of Children's National Medical Center and National Children's Regional Medical Center was organized and launched and the pediatric system construction was actively promoted.

"Assistance Provided in way of a Group" to Xinjiang and Tibet was carried out. Equal importance was attached to "blood transfusion" and "hematopoiesis". Compared with the same period in the year of 2015, the number of outpatient and emergency treatments in 8 autonomous region and prefectural hospitals in Tibet increased by 14.3%, with in-patient number rising by 12.2% and the operation number growing by 14.8%, and 476 items of new business and new technology were developed. A good start for group assistance for Xinjiang was made and a good trend of development was seen in many areas like key subject construction and personnel training.

The connotation of medical institutions was reinforced. Clinical diagnosis and treatment was standardized and 574 clinical paths were formulated, making the total number of clinical paths 1,010. The clinical path management was implemented in 88% of public hospitals. Rational drug use in clinical practice was promoted, the National Action Plan for Curbing Bacterial Resistance was jointly issued by 14 ministries and commissions, and the inter-ministry "mechanism for joint prevention and control of bacterial resistance" was set up. In 2016, the usage rate of antimicrobial agents for inpatients nationwide decreased to 37.5%; the use intensity of antimicrobial agents of inpatients fell to 49.6 DDD; the usage rate of antimicrobial agents prescribed in outpatient clinics declined to 8.7%; the detectable rate of major drug-resistance bacteria showed a downward trend.

The professional ethics construction in healthcare industries and the party construction in public hospitals were further consolidated. Guiding opinions for professional ethics construction in health and family planning system was formulated, "special rectification of malpractices in the purchase and sale of medicines and in medical services" was promoted, the institutional construction centered around "Nine Prohibitions" was strengthened and the supervisory measures was reinforced. The inspection in large-scale hospitals was continuously carried out, with the total number of problems discovered reaching 990 and 706 rectification opinions as well as suggestions presented. The guiding opinions on strengthening and improving party construction work in public hospitals were formulated and the public hospitals were guided to implement tight policy for disciplining party conducts.

The development of nursing industry was accelerated. The development plan of nursing care during the 13th Five-Year period was issued, effort was made to comprehensively promote high-quality nursing service promoted and the nursing human resources were continuously developed.

### III. The security line for the quality of medical care was continuous improved.

The medical care quality was improved. "Administrative Measures for Monitoring Medical Care Quality" was issued, and the assessment system of medical care quality management was perfected. Special work to enhance medical care quality for the year 2016-2017 was carried out, and a new pattern of multi-party co-governance with government supervision, institutional autonomy, self-regulation and social supervision was gradually formed. The 2016 security report on national medical service and quality was formulated.

Medical safety was strengthened. In 2016, the sum of medical disputes nationwide saw a year-on-year decrease of 6.7%. The management over medical advertising was strengthened, more efforts were exerted to fight against false and illegal medical advertisements. The monitoring on nosocomial infection was intensified, special supervision over the management of nosocomial infection and medical waste treatment was carried out in 72 basic medical institutions in 12 provinces (autonomous regions, municipalities directly under the Central Government). The implementation of pilot monitoring programs on information of nosocomial infection was accelerated in the 14 provinces (autonomous regions, municipalities directly under the Central Government).

Blood safety was effectively guaranteed. The full coverage of nucleic acid detection in blood station was achieved, publicity was made over the national awarding activity for free blood donation in 2014-2015 and over the promotion activities of World Blood Donor Day, and a good social atmosphere was created for free blood donation. Compared with last year, the number of volunteers for unpaid blood donation and the total amount of blood collection in 2016 witnessed a rise of 6.1% and 6.2% respectively, the highest growth since the year of 2011.

### IV. The core work of medical management was advanced and the management level over the access to medical industry was further improved

The "Reform Program for Medical Qualification Examination" was issued, which streamlined the training and registration mechanism of medical practitioners. Pilot work for qualification examination of rural assistant doctor of general practice was launched and over 7,200 examinees passed the exams, which effectively alleviated the shortage of rural health workers.

The management over medical technology was strengthened. The requirements of the State Council for reforming administrative review and approval system were implemented and the monitoring on clinical application of medical techniques in the course and afterwards was reinforced. The Administrative Measures for the Clinical Application of Medical Techniques and 15 management regulations of restrictive medical techniques as well as quality control indicators were revised and improved, and the medical institutions were guided to standardize the clinical application of related medical techniques to guarantee the medical quality and safety. The supervision of human organ donation and transplantation was enhanced, and the "Administrative Measures on Doctor Training and Registration for Human Organ Transplantation (trial version) was issued. There were 4,128 organ donation cases in 2016, increasing by 50% compared with the former year, and the number of organ transplantation operations reached 13.2 thousand, making China rank the second around the world in terms of organ donation and transplantation, which hit the record high.

The hospital evaluation system was established and optimized. The work of disease diagnosis related groups (DRGs) was advanced, the implementation plan was formulated, grouping and nomenclature principles of DRGs were standardized, the basic grouping scheme and supporting document system of DRGs was formed, and the "Four-Unification" of medical terms, i.e. the unification of primarily realize the writing convention for the first page of medical record, disease classification coding, an medical operation coding was primarily realized. The hospital evaluation system was optimized, unified evaluation criteria were developed, hospital evaluation criteria were revised, and hospitals were guided to strengthen quality management.

## V. The people's demand for medical service was effectively guaranteed

The medical order was effectively maintained. The construction of "Safe Hospital" was advanced, the work of "Three Mediations and One Insurance" was promoted, a harmonious doctor-patient relationship was forged, and the typical experience like "Jiangxi Pattern", "Tianjing Pattern", "Fujian Solution", etc. was formed all over the nation. In 2016, the total number of medical disputes and medical crimes saw a year-on-year decrease of 6.7% and 14.1% respectively, keeping the positive trend of "Decrease in Double Indicators" for three consecutive years. The diversified mechanisms for resolving medical disputes were gradually developed, the principal channel for resolving medical disputes through people's mediation was formed, and the number of resolved medical disputes reached over 60,000, with the resolution rate hitting 60%. Over 8,000 new medical institutions of medical liability insurance were built, among which 90% were primary health care institutions.

The availability of medical service to key groups like the impoverished and the elderly was continuously improved. The program of "Special Medical Rescue for Rural Patients with Critical Illnesses" was initiated and promoted in eight provinces (autonomous regions, municipalities directly under the Central Government). The management over emergency medical assistance was strengthened and the funds were allocated to the areas in "real urgent needs". In 2016, the total number of patients assisted reached 130,000 nationwide. The large-scale activity of "Free Consultation Week" was organized and carried out all over the country, and over this time period, 19.6 million patients were diagnosed and treated by medical workers. The cataract surgery rate (CSR) was further elevated, and compared with the year 2015, the CSR in China in 2016 rose by 18%, reaching 1,782 per million. The national eye health program for the "13th Five-Year Plan" period was formulated and issued.

(Wang Qinghua)

# Chapter V    The Health Work at the Community Level

## 1. Overview of Health Work at the Community Level in 2016

### I. Making greater efforts to ensure basic services

(1) Contract signing services of family doctors were promoted and the on-site training courses on contract signing services were held with medical reform office explaining the policy of contract signing. Shanghai, Hangzhou of Zhejiang and Dafeng of Jiangsu promoted contract services of family doctors with various methods to promote the dual implementations of basic medical care and basic public health functions so that the urban and rural residents could increase the utilization rate of community-level services.

(2) Improving the equalization of national basic public health service project. In 2016, the national per capita basic public health service funding standard reached 46.8 *yuan*. We organized and carried out project performance appraisal, standardized capital management, and improved the quantity and quality of the services together with Ministry of Finance.

(3) Consolidating and improving the new rural cooperative medical system. In 2016, the subsidies provided by governments at all levels were raised to 420 *yuan*, the proportions of outpatient and inpatient expenses paid within the policy range were stable at around 50% and 75%, and the per capita funding for the new rural cooperative medical insurance increased to about 30 *yuan*. Nationwide online settlement and reporting of new rural cooperative medical services in different places were sped up, 8 provinces (autonomous regions and municipalities directly under the Central Government), including Liaoning and Jilin were organized to sign the agreements of inter-provincial medical network reporting service, and the reform of the new rural cooperative payment system was actively promoted.

### II. Improving and strengthening the community level health care

(1) Strengthening the capacity building at the community level. Township health centers and community health services that satisfy the public were built. In 2006, a total of 3,370 township health centers of public satisfaction were selected, and 100 demonstration community health institutions were elected according to the appraisal.

(2) Carrying out the post training activities. We launched "National Basic Health Posts Training and Skills Competition" with the Federation of Trade Union, covering

340,000 community-level institutions, more than 1.5 million community-level medical workers and 516,000 participants. It was a large-scale activity with the broadest coverage and the largest number of community-level participants.

(3) Stabilizing the ranks of rural doctors and keeping the rural health net intact. We urged all localities to continue to implement the *Implementation Opinions on Further Strengthening Team Construction of Rural Doctors* issued by the Office of the State Council, focused on strengthening policies and measures related to rural doctors' income and treatment, and improved the old-age care policies for rural doctors. We, jointly with the medical administration and the hospital management authorities, launched pilot programs in 9 provinces to test the qualification of rural general practitioners as assistant physicians. More than 20,000 rural doctors were among the first to take the exam and those who passed the examination were qualified as assistant doctors of rural general practitioners. In this way, we were exploring the career development path of village doctors.

### III. Deepening the reform and constructing mechanism

We summarized the experience of all parts of the country in advancing community-level health reform and pushed forward the local reforms in compensation mechanisms, personnel systems and distribution systems. Anhui Province improved the financial compensation methods, abolished the management of the two lines of revenue and expenditure, and fully implemented the prescribed financial subsidies. Documents were issued in Fujian, Chongqing, Jiangsu and Zhejiang provinces and a number of measures were taken to establish and improve the incentive distribution mechanism. Sanming City would take 80% of medical business savings as performance increment wages.

**(Ji Chenglian)**

# Chapter VI    Maternal and Child Health Service

## 1. Overview of Maternal and Child Health Service of 2016

### I. Maternal and child health development program was launched

In the first year of the "Thirteenth Five-year Plan" period, in order to comprehensively accelerate the construction of maternal and child health service system, entirely carry forward the good-quality services for women and children, strengthen the human resource cultivation and innovate in the service mode and the management mechanism, major policies, projects and programs were scientifically planned, associated with the compilation of "One Outline and Two Plans", namely, the *Outline of the "Healthy China 2030" Plan*, the *13th Five-year Plan on Public Health* and the *13th Five-year Plan on Deepening the Healthcare Reform*. The goals, tasks and measures of maternal and child health in the new period were clarified.

### II. The implementation of the universal two-child policy was guaranteed

After the implementation of the universal two-child policy, *Opinions on Maternal Management and Clinical Treatment for Women of Advanced Reproductive Age* was printed and distributed, which required that the maternal and newborn health should be the priority and all supporting measures should be fully implemented. Fertility service counseling and special management of high-risk pregnant women was strengthened. Referral network for intensive and emergency case was improved. Coordination and collaboration mechanism should be established. Obstetric safety management office should be set up in midwifery institutions so as to strengthen the clinical treatment for intensive and severe cases. Medical institutions tapped their own potential to explore file-building grading system and made the high-quality maternal and child health service more accessible to the general public. Through cultivation of urgently-needed talents and other measures, service resources have been enlarged. The problem of "difficult access to a bed" was relieved in some places, thus, the safety of mothers and infants could be ensured. Counter measures were taken actively based on actual conditions of various places. More than 1,000 beds were added to obstetrics department by turning special wards into general wards within the hospital. In Beijing, more than 800 midwifery personnel were added by means of stabilizing the existing obstetric staff, attracting the certificate holders back, conducting designated training, adjusting the entry quotas, etc. In Sichuan, Shanxi, Fujian and other provinces, the guidance of maternal fertility for older mothers was strengthened and the grading management of pregnancy was promoted actively. In Jiangsu, Qinghai and other provinces, maternal and child health service alliance was set up in order to make high-quality service more accessible to the general public and effectively improved the service capacity of community-level institutions

### III. The capacity of women and children health services was improved

Actively coordinated with the National Development and Reform Commission, investment in maternal and child health care institutions' construction was further increased so as to improve infrastructure at the community-level. In 2016, the central government invested 2.91 billion *yuan* to support the construction of 45 municipal and 202 county-level maternal and child health care institutions. The investment scale increased significantly compared with that in the "Twelfth Five-Year Plan" period. Investment and construction efforts were also increased in all the localities to build, renovate and expand maternity and child health care institutions. The standards and rules for the evaluation of maternal and child health hospital was printed and distributed. A scientific, standard and normative accreditation and evaluation system was gradually built up. The standardized management and connotation construction of maternal and child health care institutions was enhanced. The integration of maternal and child health and family planning service resources was accelerated and the deep integration of personnel, management and services was also promoted. In Shandong Province, the improvement of the maternal and child health service system was pushed forward by expanding 20 maternal and child health care centers and building 19 new ones. In Chongqing, the reform of "Four Business Departments" in maternal and child health care institutions was carried out in half of the districts and counties to clarify the function setting, operation mechanism and safeguard measures, which exerted the characteristics and advantages, namely, the combination of prevention and treatment, of maternal and child health service institutions.

### IV. A new mechanism of whole-process health care services was established

The National Development and Reform Commission, Ministry of Human Resources and Social Security and other 3 ministries and commissions issued *Several Opinions on Strengthening the Basic Health Care Services for the Whole Process of Reproduction*, requiring that maternal and child health service resources should be adjusted and expanded as soon as possible to promote the downward flow of high-quality resources. The work of linking a complete set of whole-process health care service policy should be intensified and the service model and operation mechanism should be improved. High-quality whole-process reproductive service was enhanced and the level of maternal and child health service was improved. The mother and child health manual pilots were conducted in 15 counties (county-level cities, districts), which integrated pre-pregnancy care, pregnancy care, hospital delivery, child healthcare, vaccination and family planning services to achieve "one manual in hand, whole-process service around". Remarkable results were obtained. Whole-process reproductive service was implemented in Guizhou province, in the course of which high-quality service for the maternal and child health was comprehensively promoted. In Zhejiang province, four distinctive modes of the application of the mother and child health manual was explored, which reflected the idea of centering on the women and children's health.

### V. The application of information technology in maternal and child health was promoted

Taking the national birth certificate management information system interconnection as the starting point, efforts were made to strengthen the classification guidance, conduct supervision and research on the slow-moving provinces (autonomous regions and municipalities directly under the Central Government), and promote the information construction of maternal and child health. In 2016, the birth certificate management information system was linked to the national platform in 30 provinces (autonomous regions and municipalities directly under the Central Government). At the same time, the convenient "Internet plus maternal and child health" service and public-benefiting measures were promoted in various localities. Using Internet plus technology, regional telemedicine and consultation system for maternal and child health was built, tiered diagnosis and treatment was carried forward and service capacity of community-level hospitals was improved. Maternal and child health information system was re-developed in Guangxi Province. The birth certificate information system could be shared by the police department in Jilin Province, achieving the goal of cracking down on forged certificates and making information run errands but not the people. Many maternal and child health care institutions in Guangdong established a whole-process service WeChat platform to provide convenient services such as online appointments, waiting time reminders, payment service, results inquiries, etc., effectively improving the patients' experience.

At the same time, services for the second pregnancy were actively promoted. Prevention and treatment measures of birth defects were improved. High quality maternal and child service demonstration project and the construction of early childhood development bases were continuously carried forward.

In 2016, the national maternal mortality rate dropped to 19.9/100,000, and the mortality rate of infants and children under five dropped to 7.5‰ and 10.2‰ respectively. Maternal and child safety should be ensured in order to prevent rebounding of the maternal mortality.

**(Zhang Nan)**

## 1. Overview of Work in Food Safety Standards and Monitoring & Assessment in 2016

### I. Implementing policies and measures to stabilize growth and render food safety standards more complete, scientific and practical

The improvement of food safety standard system was accelerated, with the focus on addressing inadequacies and improving the level of standard research. Nearly 5,000 standards were sorted through and integrated and a batch of key and urgent standards of grains and vegetable oil etc. were formulated or revised in accordance with the needs of supervision. A cumulative total of 979 national standards were formulated and promulgated (296 new ones in 2016), with nearly 20,000 indicators involved covering all kinds of daily consumption food. We participated in international activities on food standards, which comprehensively enhance our influence and voice on international standards.

### II. Improving monitoring system for food safety risks

The monitoring network for food safety risks covered 94 percent of the county level administrative regions and was extended to regions under the county level; one billion *yuan* was invested to configure monitoring equipment for the prefecture-level disease control institutions to improve monitoring capacity. Monitoring work during the 12th Five-Year-Plan period was summarized systematically; in 2016, 130,000 pieces of food in 27 categories were monitored, the results of consultation and monitoring were notified to relevant departments to enhance the handling and prevention & control of risks, and 3,737 outbreaks of foodborne diseases were monitored, outbreaks of rhabdomyolysis syndrome caused by crayfish in multiple provinces were detected in time and handled properly. Seven risk assessments including dietary rare earth exposure and iodine nutritional status were finished, among which the assessment of rare earth filled international gap and surveys of consumption of cereals, potatoes, etc. were conducted in 15 provinces, which provided a basis for relevant risk assessment and standard development.

### III. Promoting the reform of management on "Three New Foods"

The leaders of the Commission reported to the leaders of the NPC, the State

Council and the State Commission Office for Public Sector Reform and guided the reform of the "Three New Foods". Six special investigations were organized to solicit opinions from the localities and enterprises; the reform idea of cancelling examination and approval managing in accordance with standards was proposed; repeated communication and coordination were made to vigorously promote the implementation of the "Three New Foods" reform; at present, the reform plan has passed the examination by the expert of the State Council Review and Reform Office. Meanwhile, strict and prudent reviews of the "Three New Foods" were carried out in accordance with the law and the approvals of a total of 115 "Three New Foods" products in 9 batches were announced.

### IV. Fulfilling duties legally, normatively and effectively, formulating and improving the management system, and improving the long-term working mechanism

We assisted in law enforcement inspection by the NPC and the revision of the *Regulations on the Implementation of the Food Safety Law*. Supporting rules and regulations were formulated in accordance with the law, *A list of Diseases That Interfere with Food Safety* was issued and relevant systems were formulated to strengthen the management of food safety standards and standardize the monitoring reports of foodborne diseases. The cooperative mechanism was innovated and improved with China Food and Drug Administration, the Ministry of Agriculture and the Standardization Administration of China to promote the development of standards to be more standardized and effective.

### V. Strengthening guidance on system work and serving the localities, communities and the public

*The 13th Five-Year Plan for Food Safety Standards and Monitoring Evaluation* was printed and issued, *National Nutrition Program* was formulated and special investigations on the current situation of food nutrition safety in poor areas were finished. *Guidance on the Food Safety Work for Community-level Institutions of Health and Family Planning* was formulated to serve the public for the Last Kilometer

**(Zhao Xuemei)**

# Chapter VIII　The Integrated Supervision

## 1. Overview of the Integrated Supervision in 2016

I. In order to implement The *Decision of the State Council on Integrating and Adjusting Public Health Permit and Food Business License in Catering Service*, the National Health and Family Planning Commission jointly with the State Food and Drug Administration printed and distributed the notice, made specific arrangements for implementing the requirements and carried out supervision on the implementation work in local areas. The integration and adjustment of 4 kinds of catering service place permit had been finished, and 238,000 catering service places, with their health permits formerly issued by health and family planning departments, were taken over, given permits and supervised by the food and drug administration departments.

II. The supervision over vaccine procurement and use was reinforced. Efforts were made to participate in the investigation into series of cases on illegal vaccine sale in Ji'nan City of Shandong Province and inspection work was carried out in the involved 14 provinces (autonomous regions, municipalities directly under the Central Government). Special supervision and inspection on the involved vaccines was conducted, a total number of 88,000 disease control institutions and vaccination entities were examined, 1835 illegal cases were discovered and tackled, and 795 entities were given a warning. In the second-half of 2016, special supervision and inspection was carried out on vaccination, a total number of 71,000 disease control and prevention institutions and vaccination entities were examined, 1,000 illegal cases were discovered dealt with, and 685 entities were given a warning.

III. Specific rectification activities on "scalpers" and "on-line hospital scalpers" as well as special supervision and inspection on legal practice of medical institutions were carried out. Centering on the issues of social focus, the special rectification aimed at curbing "scalpers" and "net hospital scalpers" was conducted together with eight departments, these illegal acts were strictly tackled, and unannounced investigation and supervision on these acts were made in the targeted provinces (autonomous regions, municipalities directly under the Central Government). In Beijing, Shanghai, Sichuan and other provinces (autonomous regions, municipalities directly under the Central Government), 1,510 scalpers were arrested. Meanwhile, strictly monitoring and screening on the harmful online information about "scalpers" was carried out. Through the specialized regulation and monitoring, the medical service order seriously disturbed by the organized, internally and externally collusive gang crimes was effectively curbed. The National Health and Family Planning Commission, in cooperation with the State Administration of Traditional Chinese Medicine, carried out a one-year special supervision and inspection on legal practice of medical institutions.

IV. The supervision and inspection on the implementation of the *Law of Occupational Disease Prevention and Treatment and The Law of Population and Birth Control* was smoothly completed.

The all-round supervision and inspection on the implementation of the *Law of Occupational Disease Prevention and Treatment* was carried out in all the localities, a sample check of 3,475 occupational health organizations and 10,000 radiology clinics was made, the base number and the existing 3 categories of 21 problems were figured out, and 4,590 entities were instructed to rectify and reform. The specific supervision and inspection on the implementation of *The Law of Population and Birth Control* was conducted in 18 provinces (autonomous regions, municipalities directly under the Central Government), and the special research on the overall implantation of the universal two-child policy was carried out, providing evidence for future revision and improvement of the relevant laws, regulations and policies.

V. New methods for supervision and inspection were invented. Efforts were made to implement the requirements of "Decentralization Management Service" issued by the State Council and the "doubly randomized" sampling information system was developed. In the national sampling supervision in 2016, "doubly randomized" sampling mechanism was trialed in the four selected provinces, with a total number of 50,000 task lists extracted in these provinces (autonomous regions, municipalities directly under the Central Government), which accounted for over 80% of market supervision and law enforcement cases carried out by the health department. The pilot work of comprehensive evaluation on classified supervision of the infectious disease prevention and control in medical and health institutions in 12 provinces (autonomous regions, municipalities directly under the Central Government) was carried out to enhance the regulatory levels.

VI. The construction of supervisory system was promoted. Efforts were made to guide and urge the localities to implement the *Guidance on Further Strengthening Comprehensive Supervision and Administrative Law Enforcement in Health and Family Planning Sector*, which was jointly issued by six departments. Twenty-three provinces (autonomous regions and municipalities directly under the Central Government) had issued the documents to implement the *Guidance* and practiced according to the documents. The system construction had achieved the preliminary results. The on-the-spot meeting on national family planning supervision was held, and the experience in integrating health and family planning resources at community level and strengthening supervision system construction was generalized. The law enforcement behaviors were standardized, the *Norm on the Investigation and Handling of Medical Practice without Legal Permission* was printed and distributed, the special supervision and inspection on law enforcement of family planning administration was carried out, the recording system of the whole process of supervision and law enforcement was improved and the training of supervisory personnel was strengthened. The supervisory and safeguarding capabilities was enhanced, the supervisory expenses were covered by subsidy funds of 2016 for major public health services, the construction of provincial and prefecture-level supervision institutions was included in the *Construction Planning on Health Care for All*. The "13th Five-Year" supervision plan was formulated, research work on comprehensive supervision system construction was conducted, and the industry-wide regulation was promoted. In 2016, the Supervisory Bureau rigorously clarified the entity responsibility and supervisory responsibility for construction of the Party conduct and of an honest and clean government, and the within-bureau task division plan was formulated for the construction of the Party conduct and of an honest and clean government and for the work of checking unhealthy tendencies as well as malpractices. "Two Studies, One Action" activities were actively conducted, the "Blue Shield Spirit" for Party branch work was summarized, and the education of clean politics was included in the content of professional training and was deployed and implemented at the same time with professional work.

**(Wang Qinghua)**

# Chapter IX  Drug Policies and the Essential Medicine System

## 1. Overview of Work on Drug Policies and Essential Medicine System in 2016

### I. Classified procurement of drugs was advanced and supervision over the implementation of the document requirements was conducted

In accordance with the requirements of *Guiding Opinions of the General Office of the State Council on Improving the Centralized Drug Procurement for Public Hospitals* and *Circular of the National Health and Family Planning Commission on Implementing and Improving the Guiding Opinions on Centralized Drug Procurement for Public Hospitals*, the local governments were guided to carry forward a new round of centralized drug procurement. Four training courses on the procurement policies of medicines and high-value medical consumables were held in Zhejiang, Hebei, Gansu and Guangxi provinces. The responsible persons of provincial pharmaceutical administration and drug procurement departments, prefectural and municipal pharmaceutical administration departments, and medical institutions were trained for over 400 times. Researches and evaluations of centralized drug procurement in public hospitals were carried out nationwide. Classified procurement of drugs in public hospitals was orderly pushed forward. Implementation of the results of the national drug price negotiations was accelerated. Local experience and good practices were summarized and exchanged.

### II. Organization and coordination were strengthened and the implementation of the results of the national drug price negotiations was pushed forward

Approved by the State Council, an inter-ministerial joint conference system for drug price negotiations attended by 16 departments including the Health and Family Planning Commission, the National Development and Reform Commission and the Ministry of Human Resources and Social Security was established. After rounds of negotiations, the procurement prices of three types of drugs, namely, Tenofovir disoproxil fumarate (TDF), Icotinib, and Gefitinib, decreased by 67%, 54%, and 55%, respectively. The National Health and Family Planning Commission printed and issued the *Circular on Doing Well the Centralized Procurement of Drugs of National Negotiation* in conjunction with seven other departments, including the National Development and Reform Commission, the Ministry of Human Resources and Social Security, etc. and published the results of the national drug price negotiations to the public. The commission also printed and issued the *Circular on Linking up Policies for National Negotiated Drugs and New Rural Cooperative Medical Reimbursement*, required local governments to link negotiated drugs to local health insurance policies actively and publicized the negotiation results on the centralized provincial drug procurement platform in time.

### III. The work on securing the supply of children's medicines was pushed forward

The National Health and Family Planning Commission formulated and issued the *Task Division Plan on Effective Measures to Securing the Supply of Medicines for Children* in conjunction with six other departments, including the National Development and Reform Commission, defined 12 specific tasks and their time limits, reported the progress of the work to the State Council and guided the local governments to secure the supply of medicines for children. To implement the key task requirements of the Office of the Central Leading Group for Comprehensively Deepening Reform, the National Health and Family Planning Commission organized experts to study and sort out drugs which were listed abroad but in lack of suitable dosage forms and specifications for domestic children and drugs which had been in long-tern shortage in clinical practice in conjunction with the Ministry of Industry and Information Technology, the China Food and Drug Administration, etc. and formulated and issued *The List of the First Batch of Children's Drugs Whose Development and Application Will Be Encouraged*. Legislative preparations for children's drug use were launched and a preliminary draft of regulations on securing the supply of children's drug use was formed. The function of the Expert Committee on the Use of Drugs for Children would be continuously excised, pilot studies on clinical comprehensive evaluation of children's drug use were pushed forward, children's medication guidelines and expert consensus were compiled and researched, regulations on the administration of children drugs were studied, and training on drug policy for pharmaceutical personnel in children's hospitals nationwide was conducted. The National Health and Family Planning Commission printed and issued the *Opinions on Prioritizing the Review and Approval to Solve the Problem of Backlog of Drug Registration Applications* in conjunction with the China Food and Drug Administration and further ensured that the review and approval process for children's drugs could be accelerated. Coordinating with industry and information, science and technology departments and other departments, the National Health and Family Planning Commission increased investment in production, research and development. Children's drugs would be supported to be listed in the major tasks of the special action of "Three Products" in the consumer goods industry and major special task deployment of new drugs. Development and creation of new drugs for children would be encouraged.

### IV. Designated production for medicines in shortage was gradually expanded

The National Health and Family Planning Commission urged all localities to continue to organize the production and supply of the first batch of four designated varieties such as deslanoside, which had already been a designated produced drug, guided all localities to carry out their procurement work and monitored and coordinated production supply and use so as to secure supply. We expanded the range of pilot varieties which had been designated produced and promoted designated production of drugs with low dosage, clinical necessity and shortage of market supply. In combination with the centralized procurement price setting, on the basis of the completion of the bidding evaluations and on-line publicity of the companies which had designated produced Digoxin oral solution and other 2 varieties, we coordinated and promoted production and supply actively in conjunction with the Ministry of Industry and Information, the Food and Drug Administration, the National Development and Reform Commission and etc. and guided local procurement and use.

### V. Platform construction was standardized and the monitoring, early warning and classification of drugs in shortage were strengthened

The National Health and Family Planning Commission, together with the National Development and Reform Commission, the Ministry of Industry and Information Technology, the Ministry of Commerce and the China Food and Drug Administration, formulated a report on the establishment and improvement of monitoring, early warning and grouping response systems for drugs in shortage and submitted it to the State Council. The *Circular on the Establishment of Pilot Systems for Monitoring and Reporting Drugs in Shortage* was printed and issued. More than 15 public medical and health institutions were identified as monitoring sites for drugs in shortage in various provinces (autonomous regions and municipalities directly under the Central Government). They carried out monitoring and early warning of drugs in shortage, and uploaded the results monthly to the national drug control platform via the provincial level centralized drug procurement platforms. Information of the drugs in shortage reported by the local governments was summarized and sorted out. Further researches and analyses on the classification, trend, causes and countermeasures of the drug shortage were carried out. The *Circular on the Promotion of Connection and Standardization of Centralized Drug Procurement Platforms* was printed and issued. All localities were required to use uniform drug codes and medical and health institutions (organizations) codes.

### VI. Sunshine procurement was pushed forward and new procurement mode for high value medical consumables was explored

Twenty-six provinces (autonomous regions and municipalities directly under the Central Government), including Tianjin, Hebei, Anhui, Sichuan, made transparent procurement for all or part of high value medical consumables. Among them, 12 provinces (autonomous regions and municipalities directly under the Central Government) such as Jiangsu carried out pilot work of bidding and procurement. Standardization of procurement codes for high value medical consumables was also carried out. Some high value medical consumables were selected for the pilot work and the unified national procurement coding rules were formulated. The pilot of cooperation between Shanghai and Hong Kong to purchase high value medical consumables was actively promoted and the implementation plans were studied and formulated.

### VII. The essential medicine system was consolidated and improved and the use of essential medicines in medical institutions at all levels was comprehensively evaluated.

The construction of the clinical comprehensive evaluation system for drugs was accelerated and pushed forward, the *Overall Plan for the Construction of a Clinical Comprehensive Drug Evaluation System (Draft)* was formulated, relevant institutions were commissioned to carry out pilot studies on the comprehensive evaluations over clinical application of essential medicines and children's medicines, and the criteria and indicators for evaluating base construction were initially formed. Researches on improving the level of essential medicines supplies were carried out. Report on improving essential medicines supplies for the treatment of severe mental illness, tuberculosis, hypertension and diabetes was completed. Training on rational use of essential medicines and training of community-level pharmacy personnel were organized and conducted, and special support was given to six poverty-stricken cities and prefectures in the Lüliang region to conduct training on rational use of essential medicines. A total of more than 1,100 provincial teachers were trained.

### VIII. The drug policies were consolidated and improved.

The National Health and Family Planning Commission (NHFPC) studied, drafted and promoted the deliberation and adoption of the resolution *Promoting Innovation and Access to Quality, Safe, Efficacious and Affordable Medicines for Children* at the 69th World Health Assembly. NHFPC studied policies and measures to secure the supply of drugs for the elderly, and organized and convened the preparatory meeting for the expert committee of the commission on drug use for the elderly. NHFPC carried out information construction of drug supply and the related work, and supervised and surveyed the construction of electronic drug (vaccine) regulatory system in medical and health institutions. NHFPC conducted the formulation of the Law of the People's Republic of China on Pharmacists and completed the main framework and main contents. In combination with the key tasks of the year, NHFPC entrusted China University of Political Science and Law China Pharmaceutical University, etc. to carry out extensive researches on drug policies.

**(Zhou Dan)**

# Chapter X  Guidance for Family Planning at Community Level

## 1. Overview of Guidance for Family Planning at Community Level in 2016

### I. Progress in implementing the universal two-child policy

**Increasing coordination in a whole-planned way and doing a good job in top-level design.** The State Council convened a national teleconference on family planning work to fully implement the two-child policy. National Health and Family Planning Commission (NHFPC) set up a working group to steadily and orderly implement the two-child policy by issuing and implementing the *Decision of the State Council of the CPC Central Committee on Implementing the Universal Two-child Policy Reform and Improving the Management of Family Planning Service* so as to guide provinces (autonomous regions, municipalities directly under the Central Government) to formulate comprehensive implementation plans for the two-child policy, revise the regulations on population and family planning, strengthen policy coordination, and do a good job in filing.

**Actively publicizing and training, and guiding public opinions.** National Health and Family Planning Commission has formulated the plans for the study and the implementation, and the publicity outline, issued guidance on strengthening family planning publicity, compiled and printed the *Reading Books of Universal Two-child Policy*, organized the series of publicities and reports, popularized the significance of adjusting and perfecting the fertility policy, expounded the goal and task of promoting the long-term balanced development of population, which shows the masses' "sense of gain" brought by the universal two-child policy. Special press conferences and press conferences have been held on many occasions to comprehensively and deeply interpret policies and respond to social concerns in a timely manner.

**Strengthening the research and supervision, and ensuring the implementation of the work.** National Health and Family Planning Commission formed 11 research teams to conduct survey and research in 31 provinces (autonomous regions and municipalities directly under the Central Government) to guide local governments to improve supporting policies and measures, and coordinate policies. The symposiums on the implementation of the universal two-child policy were held in different regions to call on all localities to further implement the Central spirit, study and judge the situation of the population at birth, perfect the supporting policies and measures, and make steady progress in policy implementation. Many special meetings have been held to urge the implementation of all work. The relevant departments are invited in regular consultation requests to summarize the progress of the implementation of the universal two-child policy and report to the Party Central Committee and the State Council.

**Coordinating and improving the supporting policies based on people's concerns.** The Office of the Central Committee and the Office of the State Office printed and distributed the related work plan for universal two-child policy implementation, and National Health and Family Planning Commission formulates the internal division of labor among departments and ministries, and improves the relevant supporting policies and measures. National Health and Family Planning Commission, together with other 9 departments of Ministry of Tourism, Civil Aviation Administration of China, General Railway Corporation printed and distributed *Guiding Opinions on Accelerating the Construction of Maternal and Child Facilities* to promote the construction of standardized facilities for mothers and infants in public places and the units of employment, and coordinated the efforts of the relevant departments in promoting the establishment of a system and social environment to encourage family planning according to the policy.

**Improving the population development strategy and coordinating the formulation of plans.** We will carry out the research on parallel issues of population development strategy to formulate the Improvement of the *Study Report on Population Development Strategy*, complete the "trends of population development in 2030 and the report on strategic studies", assist in organizing a high-level information conference on population and development, and introducing the effect of the universal two-child policy and population development. We shall formulate the "13th Five-year Plan" for the development of national family planning program and coordinate the compilation of the national population development plan (2016-2030).

**Carrying out the statistical monitoring of family planning and intensifying the analysis on population situation.** We shall print and distribute the *Circular on Strengthening the Management of Birth Population Information* jointly with Department of Development and Reform, Public Security, Civil Affairs and Statistics, and establish a cross-sector sharing mechanism for basic population information. The monitoring and analysis of family planning monitoring sites are organized to guide the local governments to do a good job in routine statistics and population situation analysis, strengthen the monitoring and forecasting of the population at birth, and scientifically determine the situation of the population at birth. We will actively participate in cross-sectoral consultation on the population situation, cooperate with National Development and Reform Commission in the preparation of national population plan and do a good job in the demonstration evaluation and preliminary preparation of national sample survey project on fertility status in 2017.

According to the estimated data from 1‰ of the sampling survey released by National Bureau of Statistics, the total number of births in 2016 reached 17.86 million. According to health and family planning statistics, the annual number of live births in hospitalization is 18.46 million. The birth population increased significantly, and the proportion of two or more children increased significantly too. The effect of the family planning policy adjustment and improvement gradually appeared.

## II. Reform of family planning service management

**Fully implementing the birth registration service system.** *Guiding Opinions of the General Office of National Health and Family Planning Commission on Birth Registration* is printed and distributed to guide the implementation of the spirit of the Central Decision of all places in clarifying the goals and tasks, optimizing the procedures, building a variety of registration platforms, and making solid progress in the registration of births. 27 provinces (autonomous regions, municipalities directly under the Central Government), and Xinjiang Production and Construction Corps have introduced measures for the registration of births. The seminars on the administration of family planning registration services are held to listen to the work in the provinces (autonomous regions, municipalities directly under the Central Government), summarize and promote the experience and practice of "integration of multiple certificates" in various regions.

**Promoting the building of network and teams at the community level for family planning.** We will conscientiously implement the spirit of the decision of the Central Government to guide the local governments in stabilizing and strengthening the family planning network and teams in counties and villages in the reform of primary health and family planning institutions. People's University of China is entrusted to carry out the "Research on the Policy of Old-age Pension Security for Rural Family Planning Professionals". The experience and practice of promoting innovative management mechanisms is summarized, and the experience and practices of the team building in community-level family planning institutions stabilized and strengthened.

**Launching new national excellence creation activities.** *Notice of National Health and Family Planning Commission on Launching a New Round of Activities to Create Advanced Units Providing Quality Family Planning Service across the Country* is printed and distributed to define work objectives, basic principles and evaluation priorities, and develop management methods for the activities. Nankai University is entrusted to carry out "A New Round of Research on the Investigation and Evaluation of the Advanced Units of Quality Family Planning Service across the Country". The seminar and promotion meetings on the new national excellence creation are held to guide all regions to do a good job in the selection of 2016. Twenty-nine provinces (autonomous regions and municipalities directly under the Central Government) and Xinjiang Production and Construction Corps formulated plans and established leading groups. After county level declaration, municipal recommendation and provincial evaluation, 560 counties (county-level cities and districts) are awarded the honorary title of "National Advanced Unit of Quality Family Planning Service in 2014-2016".

**Strengthening the target accountability system and work supervision.** *Opinions on Adhering to and Improving the Family Planning Goal Management Responsibility System* is printed and distributed in the cooperation with the Office of the Central Committee and the General Office of the State Council to coordinate local Party committees and governments to report to the Central Committee on the work of family planning in the region. The supervision and the implementation of the Central Decision is organized and carried out in the 4 provinces of Liaoning, Shandong, Guangdong and Sichuan.

**Population and family planning information construction and application.** We will develop and apply the whole population database, set up a national information platform to connect and communicate family planning information between China and various provinces, establish a national birth population and birth registration information bank, promote the concentration of basic demographic information, social attributes, family relations, whole reproductive history, migration and mobility trajectories, as well as information on reward and assistance, and death. All regions will be urged to strengthen provincial information platform construction to accelerate the development and application of the information system for population and family planning services and promote business collaboration and information sharing. We will organize a survey on the status quo of information construction of family planning at provincial level and hold a national conference on family planning informatization.

**(Ji Chenglian)**

# Chapter XI    Family Development

## 1. Overview of the Work in Family Planning and Family Development in 2016

### I. Family support and guarantee for family-planning households

A system of family planning incentives and assistance should be implemented to encourage local governments to continuously implement various incentive and assistance policies for families with only child and families with two daughters in rural areas before the adjustment of the family planning policy. The implementation of the reward and assistance system for some family planning families in rural areas, the project of "fewer births and quick wealth" in western China and the special assistance system for family planning families should be organized to cooperate with the Ministry of Human Resources and Social Security in the implementation of birth insurance, basic medical insurance, and the related work.

We will provide family planning assistance and care to special families and promote urban-rural integration of special assistance funds. Standards for Information Archives of Special Families of Family Planning, and Notification of the Establishment and Improvement of Contact System for the Special Families of Family Planning are printed and distributed. It is required that all localities establish information files for each family with the only child disabled or dead, and designate one township (street) leader and one village (neighborhood) committee leader as the "dual post" associate to help them fully, accurately and responsibly.

### II. Family development work

The project of "new family planning" will be expanded to increase the number of pilot units nationwide to 84, and the mid-term project evaluation be organized. The "Healthy Families Initiative" shall be launched in the observance of international family day. 2016 China Family Development Report will be issued and the theme essay campaign of "Healthy Family" be carried out. 2016 "China Family Development Tracking Survey" will be organized and implemented and the pilot projects on family scientific parenting, healthy development of adolescents and care for the elderly be carried out continuously.

The first election campaign for "Happy Family" is organized and carried out, and after being elected from different regions and at different levels, 100 "Happy Families across the Country" were born. National promotion activities on the theme of creating happy families have been organized and held to create a happy family, focusing on the story of "Happy Family".

Research on fertility support policies are organized and carried out to guide the local governments to formulate specific policies and measures for extend maternity leave and paternity leave. A special survey on the situation of childcare services for 10,000 mothers of children under the age of three was conducted and the research reports and policy suggestions been submitted to the State Council.

### III. Healthy aging, and a combination of medicine and nutrition

The 2016 China-France seminar on healthy ageing and the 3rd China-France seminar on family development policy were held in France, and Vice Premier Liu Yandong attended and addressed at the meeting. An expert forum on ageing in the Asia-pacific region was convened to launch WHO biennial research project on combination of medicine and nutrition. The "13th Five-year Plan" on Healthy Ageing is compiled. In the health and family planning system, the selection and commendation work of "Model of Respecting for the Aged" is carried out, and 200 commendation units are recommended to National Office for the Aged.

To promote the integration of medicine and nutrition, the *Notice on the License for Institutions with Medical and Nutrition Service* is jointly printed and distributed with Ministry of Civil Affairs. A total of 90 national pilot cities (districts) for the combination of medicine and nutrition are selected, and 6 model cities for the smart and healthy elderly care are identified together with Ministry of Industry and Information Technology. The combined medicine and nutrition in 8 key provinces (autonomous regions and municipalities directly under the Central Government) is jointly supervised and guided, and a special report on the combined medicine and nutrition submitted to the State Council. We will establish a national data monitoring platform for the combined medicine and nutrition, and summarize and analyze the seasonal progress in different regions.

### IV. Comprehensive management of the sex ratio at birth

In Wuling Mountain, we organized and carried out the demonstration activity of "Voluntary Action of Fulfilling Dreams for Girls" in the concentrated areas of extreme poverty, organized and promoted the theme song of "Voluntary Action of Fulfilling Dreams for Girls" — Daisy Flowers.

Six departments jointly launched a nationwide campaign to combat the illegal fetus sex identification and the illegal sex-selective abortion practices, and a total of

7,111 cases were put on records and 6,273 cases were settled in a whole year. And the relevant departments revised and promulgated *Regulations on Prohibiting Fetal Sex Identification and Artificial Termination of Pregnancy by Sex Selection for Non-medical Purposes*. We have completed the final assessment of the "12th Five-year Plan" on the comprehensive control of the sex ratio of the population at birth, and worked out the "13th Five-year Plan".

**(Ji Chenglian)**

# Chapter XII    Publicity of the Work in Health and Family Planning

## 1. China Tobacco Control Mass Communication Activity

The China Tobacco Control Mass Communication Activity was launched in 2008, which was an activity advocated and encouraged by the tobacco control publicity media covering the whole country. To implement the spirit of the "Two Offices" notice, the Kick-off Conference of China Tobacco Control Mass Communication Activity 2017 was held in Beijing on December 29th, 2016. The activity was sponsored by the National Health and Family Planning Commission, organized by China Health Education Center, and supported by the World Health Organization. Wang Hesheng, Deputy Director of the National Health and Family Planning Commission, attended and addressed the meeting.

December 29th, 2016 was the 3rd anniversary of the issuance of *Notice on Relevant Regulations on Leading Cadres to Take the Lead in Banning Smoking in Public Places* by the "Two Offices". The purpose of this meeting was to take the initiative to implement the regulations and requirements of the CPC Central Committee and the State Council on tobacco control, and, on the coming of New Year's Day and the Spring Festival, advocate to continue to create a good social atmosphere of non-smoking, discouraging cigarette smoking and no offering cigarettes.

**(Zhao Yueting)**

## 2. Establishment of China Tobacco Cessation Alliance

The Publicity Department of National Health and Family Planning Commission entrusted the China-Japan Friendship Hospital to take a lead in the establishment of China Tobacco Cessation Alliance and the inaugural conference of China Tobacco Cessation Alliance was held on August 31st, 2016. Academician Wang Chen, also President of China-Japan Friendship Hospital was the newly-elected Chairman of China Tobacco Cessation Alliance. The alliance's counselors are Huang Jiefu and Wang Longde, the former vice ministers of the Ministry of Health, Mao Qun'an, the Director of the Publicity Department of the National Health and Family Planning Commission, academician Zhong Nanshan, academician Sun Yan, academician Chen Junshi, academician Gao Runlin, academician Zhao Jizong, and Wang Ke'an, Director of the ThinkTank Research Center for Health Development. The Alliance has 53 members, consisting of the hospitals directly under or administrated by the National Health and Family Planning Commission and the member units of Tobacco Division of the Respiratory Medicine of Chinese Medical Association. The China Tobacco Cessation Alliance conducted the national smoking cessation clinic survey and made effective evaluation of the overall operation of smoking cessation clinics in China, which was significant to the formulation of national tobacco control policy.

A total of 1,480 institutions participated in the survey and 366 of them were confirmed to provide outpatient services for smoking cessation.

The China Tobacco Cessation Alliance would build China clinical smoking cessation system, promote the establishment of the overall tobacco dependence diagnosis and treatment network in hospitals at the national level, advocate the construction of smoke-free working places, help doctors who smoke to give up smoking, and make use of the hospitals directly under or administrated by the National Health and Family Planning Commission in the treatment of smoking dependence.

**(Zhao Yueting)**

# Chapter XIII    Medical Science, Technology and Education

## 1. Overview of Medical Science, Technology and Education in 2016

### I. The National Conference on Scientific and Technological Innovation in Health was convened

According to the decisions of the Party Group of the National Health and Family Planning Commission and the instructions of Minister Li Bin and in order to comprehensively implement the spirit of the National Conference on Scientific and Technological Innovation and the National Health Conference, the National Health and Family Planning Commission convened the national conference on scientific and technological innovation in health from October 13th to October 14th in 2016. Vice-premier Liu Yandong made important instructions, emphasizing to place scientific and technological innovation in the core position of health work. Li Bin, Minister of National Health and Family Planning Commission, made a systemic deployment of "Six Enhancements" to mobilize the enthusiasm and creativity of medical and health care workers.

### II. System and strategy for scientific and technological innovation

The overall leadership was strengthened and the "Collaboration of Science and Health" system was established with the Ministry of Science and Technology. The *Guiding Opinions on Comprehensively Promoting Scientific and Technological Innovation in Health* and the *Guiding Opinions on Speeding up Transfer and Transformation of Achievements* were jointly issued by five departments, including the National Health and Family Planning Commission and the Ministry of Science and Technology and others. Guiding opinions on scientific and technological innovation projects of the 13th Five-Year Plan, the opening and sharing of scientific and technological resources and other issues were formulated. The strategic counselors of scientific and technological innovation were hired for National Health and Family Planning Commission and a committee of specialists was set up.

### III. Reform of the system for science and technology

The reform of scientific and technological system was accelerated and the tasks such as functional transformation were completed ahead of the schedule. The reconstruction of the specialized management organizations and the research center for the development of medical and health science and technology of the National Health and Family Planning Commission, was basically completed. Seven key research and development projects, including precise medicine, were launched and smoothly implemented. By Coordinating with the Ministry of Finance, the innovation projects of medical and health science and technology of the Chinese Academy of Medical Sciences were launched and implemented. The idea for constructing national laboratory in this field was studied and put forward.

### IV. Development of major science and technology projects

The requirements of the State Council were fully implemented, the focus was laid on the symbolic achievements, and the 13th Five-Year plan for implementing major special projects of science and technology was formulated. The project guidance for the year of 2017 was issued. The National Health and Family Planning Commission completed the third party performance appraisal and participated in the national science and technology innovation achievement exhibition. The technical and administrative management was strengthened and the special work standards for clean government were formulated.

### V. Construction of scientific research base and technical management

In collaboration with the Ministry of Science and Technology, 32 national clinical medical research centers were identified and incorporated into the management of the national scientific research base system. The evaluation of key laboratories at the commission level was completed and the management method and assessment rules were revised. The synergic management mechanism of stem cells clinical research was established and the list of the first batch of institutions filed was released. The *Measures on Ethical Review of Biomedical Research Involving Human Beings* were revised and issued.

### VI. National biosafety work

The National Health and Family Planning Commission took a lead in the establishment of national biosafety coordination mechanism, completed the prevention and control of Zika virus and other infectious diseases and the tasks of ensuring laboratory biosecurity for major events such as the G20 Summit, and strengthened the supervision and control of laboratory biosecurity in accordance with the law.

## VII. The reform of medical education and human resources training

Remarkable results were achieved in the construction of standardized residency training system, and the full coverage of the organizational management system and policy system was achieved. The third-party evaluation was continuously carried out to achieve dynamic management of the bases. The simulation tests consisting of questions from the questions bank for theoretical graduation assessment were carried out in 11 provinces (autonomous regions and municipalities directly under the Central Government), and the construction of quality connotation was significantly strengthened. Seventy-two thousand people were recruited for training, which accounted for 80% of the total of undergraduates in that year, a significant increase compared with 20% before the implementing the training system. More than 190,000 residents were under training. The recruitment of general practitioners, pediatricians and psychiatrists hit a record high, with 8,600 in general practice, an increase of 8% over the year before. Pilot work on a standardized training system for specialized physicians was initiated with three specialties of neurosurgery, respiratory and critical diseases and cardiovascular diseases as the forerunner. The *Opinions on Further Strengthening the Training and Employment of General Practitioners* was researched and formulated, and the training system and employment incentive mechanism were improved. The *Implementation Opinions on Training of Assistant General Practitioners* was jointly issued with other five departments like the Ministry of Education, and 5000 people from township hospitals were recruited to attend the training of "3+2" assistant general medical practitioners. Efforts were made to continue organizing and implementing the free training program for order-oriented medical students. In the Midwest, 5,636 medical students were recruited for township hospitals in 2016, which exceeded the target by 10%, and 32,000 order-oriented medical students were recruited accumulatively. The collaboration between hospitals and medical universities was strengthened, the training of pediatricians was promoted in line with hospital demand, and 8 medical colleges and universities were supported to hold undergraduate programs in pediatrics, with a total enrollment of 870 students. Various forms of further medical education were further advanced and the abilities and qualities of various professionals and technical personnel were continuously improved.

(Zhao Yueting)

# Chapter XIV    International Exchange and Cooperation

## 1. Overview of the International Cooperation and Foreign Exchange in 2016

In 2016, the state leaders attended seven foreign affairs activities sponsored by the National Health and Family Planning Commission or the senior delegations invited by the Commission, and Commission leaders accompanied the state leaders to attend the foreign affairs activities17 times, participated in 42 foreign affairs activities in China and hosted 25 batches of international organizations and foreign ministerial delegations. 18 batches of foreign visits by the Commission leaders and 179 times by the civil servants of the Commission offices were completed, with the total number of 357 person times. The National Health and Family Planning Commission was implementing 162 intergovernmental cooperation agreements.

### I. The arrangements were made for the state leaders to attend important foreign affairs activities in the field of sanitation and health

In July, 2016, President Xi Jinping met with visiting Director-General Margaret Chan of the World Health Organization (WHO), and in November, Prime Minister Li Keqiang met with Margaret Chan and Executive Director of the United Nations Population Fund (UNFPA), Babatunde. The 9th Global Conference on Health Promotion was held in November 2016, with Prime Minister Li Keqiang attending the opening ceremony and making an important speech. A total of 657 delegates from 131 countries were invited to the conference.

The arrangements were completed for Vice Premier Liu Yandong attending the China-US, Sino-British, Sino-French, China-Israel and China-South Africa high-level human exchange mechanism related activities in the health field. The arrangements for series of activities were made coordinately for Professor Peng Liyuan as WHO Goodwill Ambassador for tuberculosis and AIDS prevention and treatment.

### II. We participated in global health affairs in an all-round way to enhance China's influence and voice in global health diplomacy

On behalf of China, we participated in global health management in a more active manner, participated in the discussion of major issues in the global health field as well as the formulation of relevant international standards and norms, and promoted the construction of the destiny community of human health. *China's Global Health*

*Strategy"(2017-2030)* was formulated, which is a strategic, systematic and sustainable planning deployment for our country's participation in the global health management. Li Bin, director of the National Health and Family Planning Commission, led a delegation to attend and chair the opening ceremony of the 69th World Health Conference. The Chinese delegation played a constructive role in the discussion of important topics in the Conference and promoted the adoption of the resolution on safe drug use for children proposed by our country. China International Emergency Medical Team (Shanghai) became the first international emergency medical team.

**III. We participated in the high-level humanity exchange mechanism between China-US, China-Russia, China-Britain, China-France, China-Israel, China-Nepal, as well as the regional cooperation mechanisms between China, Japan and South Korea and China-ASEAN; we also participated in the multilateral cooperative exchange mechanisms of WHO, UNAIDS and UNFPA.**

In line with the national "Belt and Road" initiative, we promoted the construction of "healthy Silk Road" and issued the "Three-Year Implementation Plan" of the "Belt and Road" in the field of health, and promoted the implementing and strengthening cooperation with countries along the line in the field of sanitation and health. The 2nd China-CEE Health Ministers Forum and the 1st China-ASEAN Health Cooperation Forum were held. Cooperating with the construction of "Belt and Road", the three-year plan of the "Belt and Road" health cooperation of the National Health and Family Planning Commission was implemented, and the health cooperation under the multi-bilateral mechanism was promoted comprehensively, systematically and pragmatically.

**IV. The sustainable development agenda 2030 was implemented**

"China-World Health Organization National Cooperation Strategy" (2016-2020)" was signed and issued with WHO; the Ministerial Strategic Dialogue on South-South Cooperation in Population and Development was co-hosted with the United Nations Population Fund. While focusing on deepening the focus of medical reform and learning from international experience, we popularized to the international society the China's successful experience and practice in health development and reform. In 2016, a joint study with the World Bank and WHO on health reform was completed and the research report was published.

## V. We innovated the work of health assistance to foreign countries and implemented new initiatives for health cooperation between China and Africa

We optimized the distribution of medical teams for foreign aid, explored counterpart cooperation among medical institutions, and dispatched medical teams for short-term free consultations. Health assistance to other countries changed from a single medical aid gradually to a three-dimensional approach covering public health, medical care, counterpart cooperation, education and training, etc. The innovation in the mode of dispatching foreign aid medical teams was implemented taking the dispatching mode to aid Trinidad and Tobago as a typical one, and the innovation in foreign aid projects like the "Light Trip" was carried out with positive results. The outcomes of President Xi Jinping's foreign visits were implemented, and the Sino-African public health cooperation plan was launched to support Africa in strengthening the construction in the public health systems and capacity. With the cooperation of the Ministry of Commerce, the "Two 100s" project and the health foreign aid training implementation program were formulated and implemented; a memorandum of understanding was signed with the United States on the cooperation between China and the United States to support the construction of CDC in Africa; the subsidy standards for some foreign aid medical teams in arduous areas were raised and the overall treatment of foreign aid medical teams was improved. Two health diplomats were sent to the African Union mission.

## VI. We deepened the cooperation with Hong Kong, Macao and Taiwan

In November, 2016, Li Bin, director of the National Health and Family Planning Commission, led a delegation to Hong Kong to attend the 3rd Annual Meeting of the Global Emergency Medical Team and the 15th Joint Meeting of Health Administration of the Three Regions. We actively implemented the eight cooperation agreements signed between the National Health and Family Planning Commission and Hong Kong, Macao and Taiwan, and promoted the cooperation with Hong Kong, Macao and Taiwan in the field of medical and health services and scientific research. The social resources in Hong Kong, Macao and Taiwan were explored to support the development of health services in the mainland, and to introduce project funds to support health development in the western and remote poverty-stricken areas. Personnel exchanges with Hong Kong, Macao and Taiwan in medical and health services were strengthen, gradually forming a pattern of great exchanges, great promotion and great development in the field of health in the four areas of the two sides of the Straits.

（ **Chen Ying** ）

# Part V

# Traditional Chinese Medicine

## 1. Overview of the Work in Traditional Chinese Medicine (TCM) in 2016

### I. Coordinating and promoting various tasks

**(1) Implementing the spirit of the National Health and Wellness Conference and *the Outline of the Strategic Plan for the Development of Traditional Chinese Medicine (2016-2030)*.** In 2016, the Party Central Committee and the State Council held the first national health and wellness conference in the new century, which set clear requirements for promoting the revitalization and development of traditional Chinese medicine and giving full play to the unique advantages of traditional Chinese medicine in the construction of healthy China. In February, 2016, the State Council issued *the Outline of the Strategic Plan for the Development of Traditional Chinese Medicine (2016-2030)*, which promotes the development of traditional Chinese medicine and makes it a national strategy, and makes systematic arrangements for promoting the development of traditional Chinese medicine in the new era. The State Administration of Traditional Chinese Medicine compiled and issued five special plans: the 13th Five-Year Plan for the development of Chinese medicine and cultural construction, information construction, talent development, scientific and technological innovation, and "One Belt, One Road". The task requirements for traditional Chinese medicine were put forward in key programs such as the outline of "Healthy China 2030", the outline of health and wellness of the "13th Five-Year Plan", and the outline of deepening medical reform of the "13th Five-Year Plan".

**(2) Promoting the issuance of *Law of the People's Republic of China on Traditional Chinese Medicine*.** At the end of 2015, the Executive Meeting of the State Council passed the *Law of the People's Republic of China on Traditional Chinese Medicine (Draft)"* and submitted it to the Standing Committee of the National People's Congress for deliberation, cooperated with and coordinated relevant parties for the deliberation by the Standing Committee of the National People's Congress. The 25th Meeting of the

Standing Committee of the National People's Congress deliberated and passed the *Law of the People's Republic of China on Traditional Chinese Medicine*. The Law was signed and issued by President Xi Jinping in Order No. 59. It was officially implemented on July 1st, 2017. It is the first time that China has clearly and legally defined the important status, development policy and supporting measures of traditional Chinese medicine. It has made institutional arrangements to solve the problems that have restricted the development of traditional Chinese medicine for many years. It is of epoch-making significance to promote the modernization of governance system and governance capacity of traditional Chinese medicine, guarantee the revitalization and development of traditional Chinese medicine, and safeguard the health and well-being of the people.

(3) **Promoting the publication of the white paper on *Traditional Chinese Medicine in China*.** Information Office of the State Council published the white paper on *Traditional Chinese Medicine in China* for the first time. The white paper system reviews the historical development of traditional Chinese medicine, introduces the policies, measures and achievements of developing traditional Chinese medicine in China, shows the cultural connotation and scientific value of traditional Chinese medicine, and reflects that the state attaches much importance to traditional Chinese medicine.

(4) **Promoting the establishment of an inter-ministerial joint conference system for traditional Chinese medicine work under the State Council.** In August, 2016, the State Council approved the establishment of an inter-ministerial joint conference system for traditional Chinese medicine. Deputy Prime Minister Liu Yandong addressed the conference. The role of the joint conference system was given full play to. Communication and coordination with member entities were strengthened. The division plans of the strategic planning outline departments were implemented. The issuance of a batch of documents was promoted. The mechanism and environment of multi-sector cooperation, up-and-down linkage, and the implementation of the strategic planning outline were formed.

(5) **Promoting the seminar on reform and development of higher education in traditional Chinese medicine.** 2016 was the 60th anniversary of higher education in traditional Chinese medicine in New China. A series of activities were organized to accumulate 60 years of successful experience in higher education of traditional Chinese medicine and promote the reform and development of higher education of traditional Chinese medicine in the new era. 60 distinguished teachers of institutions of higher learning of traditional Chinese medicine were selected and commended together with the National Health and Family Planning Commission and the Ministry of Education. A symposium on reform and development of higher education of

traditional Chinese medicine was held. Liu Yandong presided over the meeting and delivered a speech. He confirmed the achievements in the development of higher education in traditional Chinese medicine, and gave instructions on creating new prospects in higher education in traditional Chinese medicine in the new situation.

**II. Stimulating the potential and vitality of the "five kinds of resources" of traditional Chinese medicine, and promoting the coordinated development of medical care, health care, scientific research, education, industry, culture, and foreign cooperation and exchanges of traditional Chinese medicine**

**(1) Driven by deepening medical reform, the service capacity of traditional Chinese medicine continued to be improved.** The simultaneous arrangements were promoted about the policies of traditional Chinese medicine reform, public hospital reform, family doctor contracting services, etc. reflecting the characteristics of traditional Chinese medicine on the background of overall objectives of deepening medical reform. The leading group of medical reform of the State Council promoted the construction of community-level traditional Chinese medicine clinics nationwide, rational determination of the payment standards for traditional Chinese medicine according to types of diseases, outpatient TCM diagnosis and treatment services included into primary diagnosis, innovative models of TCM diagnosis and treatment, etc. The work mechanism of the bureau's leadership to contact and promote the reform of traditional Chinese medicine of pilot provinces of the national comprehensive medical reform was improved. The monitoring of the medical reform of traditional Chinese medicine was launched. A special fund of 6.9 billion *yuan* was allocated to support the construction of 250 TCM hospitals. The "Innovation Project of Traditional Chinese Medicine Heritage" was included into the "Construction Plan of National Health Security Project" and officially launched. The plans for promoting comprehensive reform of public TCM hospitals and the participation of bureau-owned (bureau-in-charge) hospitals in Beijing medical reform were formulated and implemented. The construction of a hierarchical diagnosis and treatment system was promoted. The experience of the implementation of the 12th Five-Year Plan for the improvement of the basic TCM service capacity was accumulated. The action plan for the "13th Five-Year Plan" was launched to consolidate the basis of hierarchical diagnosis and treatment; TCM technical plans were made in the hierarchical diagnosis and treatment services of trial diseases. The technical requirements of hierarchical diagnosis and treatment were clearly defined. Inspections of large-scale TCM hospitals and special inspections of TCM decoction pieces in the national medical institutions were carried out. Continuous improvement of medical quality and giving full play to the advantages of traditional Chinese medicine were promoted. Handling emergency, infectious disease prevention and control, and treatment of AIDS by using TCM were promoted.

**(2) Focusing on increasing supply, TCM health services had good prospects.**

The reform of "decentralization-control-service" was deepened. Focusing on optimizing service and increasing supply, the development of TCM health services was accelerated. Health projects of preventive treatment with TCM were carried out. Guidelines on promoting the development of TCM health care services were issued. The services provided by TCM practitioners such as health consultation and conditioning in health care institutions were standardized. Social organizations were encouraged to practice traditional Chinese medicine. The selection of demonstration centers (bases, projects) of healthy tourism of traditional Chinese medicine was carried out. The formation of new TCM industries such as TCM health care for the elderly and TCM health tourism was accelerated. Special inspection of the development plan for TCM health service was carried out. 23 provinces (autonomous regions and municipalities directly under the Central Government) issued development plans for the regions. TCM health services became a powerful tool for boosting the development of transformation of dynamism.

**(3) Driven by system construction, TCM technology innovation made remarkable achievements.** Tu Youyou, a researcher, won the top National Science and Technology Award. A group of scientific research projects of traditional Chinese medicine, and the combination of Chinese medicine and Western medicine won the National Science and Technology Progress Award. Two opinions on strengthening the inheritance and innovation of TCM theory and accelerating the construction of TCM science and technology innovation system were issued. The outline of the 13th Five-Year Plan for science and technology development of ethnic minority medicine was issued. The construction of professional organizations of TCM science and technology management was promoted. Preparations for building national TCM laboratories, national key TCM laboratories, 11 additional key TCM research rooms were made. The acceptance of the national TCM clinical research base was completed. 314 items of the 2nd batch of base clinical research projects were launched. The "special research program of TCM modernization " was coordinated and promoted. The protection and utilization of Chinese herbs were strengthened. The pilot program for conducting a general survey on TCM resources was promoted. The construction of a dynamic monitoring system for TCM resources was deepened. The project of TCM standardization was launched.

**(4) Based on strengthening support, the construction of the team of TCM professionals was strengthened.** The State Administration of Traditional Chinese

Medicine established a leading group for talent work, issued opinions on further strengthening TCM talents, and launched the "100 million" talent project for the inheritance and innovation of traditional Chinese medicine. The selection of the 3rd National Master of Traditional Chinese Medicine and national famous TCM practitioners was launched. The 4th advanced training course on professional management of TCM hospitals was held. The expert committee of standardized training for TCM resident physicians was established. Standardized training evaluation was carried out. The connection between degree education and standardized training was promoted. The training of TCM category of assistant general practitioner and the program of special posts as TCM general practitioners were well implemented. The inheritance of academic experience of famous TCM experts continued to be promoted. The 5th batch of 1,435 heirs passed the achievement test after completion of the courses. 500 outstanding TCM clinical talents and 556 TCM nursing backbones were cultivated. 210 inheritance studios of famous and experienced TCM experts and 64 inheritance laboratories of schools of TCM thoughts passed the acceptance test. A total of 122 studios of famous and experienced TCM experts and 102 inheritance studios of famous and experienced TCM experts at the community level were established. 578 TCM nursing talents were selected for training.

(5) **Promoting the construction of TCM culture by expanding channels as a breakthrough.** The implementation plan of "TCM China Trip– TCM Health Culture Promotion Action" was issued TCM health care literacy of Chinese citizens was first released. Inclusion of TCM culture literacy into the "Chinese Citizen Science Quality Benchmark" was promoted. A total of 32 national TCM culture publicity and education bases were added. Base construction supervision was carried out. Publicity activities of TCM health culture were extensively carried out. 12 scientific and educational activities were organized among central state organs. More than 300 cultural science activities of different kinds were carried out in various places. The creation of a batch of TCM cultural masterpieces, especially the broadcast of "Materia Medica China" were supported, which drew much public attention and promoted the development of TCM culture industry.

(6) **Based on cooperation and sharing, the overseas development of traditional Chinese medicine was accelerated.** The "One Belt, One Road" plan for traditional Chinese medicine was jointly issued with the Development and Reform Commission after being deliberated by the National Leading Group for Promoting the Construction of "One Belt, One Road". The 2nd batch of special projects of international cooperation were implemented. Overall arrangements for the overseas development of traditional Chinese medicine were made. Bilateral and multilateral cooperation was deepened. Cooperation and dialogue in traditional Chinese medicine with the countries such

as Russia, South Korea, New Zealand and Italy were strengthened. China had been participating in foreign negotiations. At the 9th global health promotion conference, TCM with its unique charm in health promotion was exhibited. TCM exhibition was unveiled at the 2nd forum of health ministers between China and Central and Eastern European Countries. The sub-forum of TCM internationalization "made its voice heard" once again at the Boao Forum for Asia. The 5th international conference on modernization of traditional Chinese medicine was hosted. Traditional Chinese medicine has attracted much attention on the international stage. The international standardization of traditional Chinese medicine was promoted. The pace of TCM service trade was accelerated. TCM exchanges and cooperation in the four places on both sides of the Taiwan Strait was deepened.

(7) **Taking the main responsibility as the "bovine nose" (starting point), strict administration of the Party was comprehensively implemented.** In cooperation with the inspection team of the CPC Central Committee, special inspections were completed. Inspections and rectifications were seen as major political tasks. Plans were formulated. Division of labor was clarified. Responsibility was compacted. Item lists, rectification lists and lists of duties were made. Efforts were made to rectify each article, implement each item and make sure that every single item was effectively organized, dealt with by taking appropriate measures, and thoroughly rectified. The inspection of the Party groups under the bureau was strengthened and improved to achieve full coverage of the inspections of the entities directly under the bureau. Learning and education about "Two Studies, One Action" were carried out. The spirit of the 6th Plenary Session of the 18th CPC Central Committee was implemented. The construction of TCM ethos was promoted.

(General Office of the State Administration of Traditional Chinese Medicine)

**(Wang Guimin)**

# Part VI
# Data Sheet

## Health Statistical Data

### Number of Medical Health Institutions

| Year | Total | Hospital | | | | Grassroots Medical Health Institution | | | | Professional Public Health Institution | | | |
|------|-------|----------------------|-------------|------------------|--------------------------------------|-----------------|--------------------|-------------------------------|------------------------------------|------------------------------------------------------------------|----------------------------------------------|--------------------------------------------|
| | | Comprehensive Hospital | TCM Hospital | Specialty Hospital | Community Health Service Center (Station) | Township Hospital | Village Health Room | Outpatient Department (Clinic) | Disease Prevention & Control Center | Special Disease Prevention & Treatment Center (Clinic/ Station) | Maternal & Child Care Center (Clinic/Station) | Health Supervision Institution(Center) |
| 1950 | 8915 | 2803 | 2692 | 4 | 85 | | | 3356 | 61 | 30 | 426 | |
| 1955 | 67725 | 3648 | 3351 | 67 | 188 | | | 51600 | 315 | 287 | 3944 | |
| 1960 | 261195 | 6020 | 5173 | 330 | 401 | 24849 | | 213823 | 1866 | 683 | 4213 | |
| 1965 | 224266 | 5330 | 4747 | 131 | 339 | 36965 | | 170430 | 2499 | 822 | 2910 | |
| 1970 | 149823 | 5964 | 5353 | 117 | 385 | 56568 | | 79600 | 1714 | 607 | 1124 | |
| 1975 | 151733 | 7654 | 6817 | 160 | 543 | 54026 | | 80739 | 2912 | 683 | 2128 | |
| 1980 | 180553 | 9902 | 7859 | 678 | 694 | 55413 | | 102474 | 3105 | 1138 | 2745 | |
| 1985 | 978540 | 11955 | 9197 | 1485 | 938 | 47387 | 777674 | 126604 | 3410 | 1566 | 2996 | |
| 1986 | 999102 | 12442 | 9363 | 1646 | 1030 | 46967 | 795963 | 127575 | 3475 | 1635 | 3059 | |
| 1987 | 1012804 | 12962 | 9657 | 1790 | 1097 | 47177 | 807844 | 128459 | 3512 | 1697 | 3082 | |
| 1988 | 1012485 | 13544 | 9916 | 1932 | 1190 | 47529 | 806497 | 128422 | 3532 | 1727 | 3103 | |
| 1989 | 1027522 | 14090 | 10242 | 2046 | 1265 | 47523 | 820798 | 128112 | 3591 | 1747 | 3112 | |
| 1990 | 1012690 | 14377 | 10424 | 2115 | 1362 | 47749 | 803956 | 129332 | 3618 | 1781 | 3148 | |
| 1991 | 1003769 | 14628 | 10562 | 2195 | 1345 | 48140 | 794733 | 128665 | 3652 | 1818 | 3187 | |
| 1992 | 1001310 | 14889 | 10774 | 2269 | 1376 | 46117 | 796523 | 125873 | 3673 | 1845 | 3187 | |
| 1993 | 1000531 | 15436 | 11426 | 2298 | 1438 | 45024 | 806945 | 115161 | 3729 | 1872 | 3115 | |

*Continued*

| Year | Total | Hospital | Comprehensive Hospital | TCM Hospital | Specialty Hospital | | Community Health Service Center (Station) | Township Hospital | Village Health Room | Outpatient Department (Clinic) | | Disease Prevention & Control Center | Special Disease Prevention & Treatment Center (Clinic/ Station) | Maternal & Child Care Center (Clinic/Station) | Health Supervision Institution(Center) |
|---|---|---|---|---|---|---|---|---|---|---|---|---|---|---|---|
| 1994 | 1005271 | 15595 | 11549 | 2336 | 1440 | | | 51929 | 813529 | 105984 | | 3711 | 1905 | 3190 | |
| 1995 | 994409 | 15663 | 11586 | 2361 | 1445 | | | 51797 | 804352 | 104406 | | 3729 | 1895 | 3179 | |
| 1996 | 1078131 | 15833 | 11696 | 2405 | 1473 | | | 51277 | 755565 | 237153 | | 3737 | 1887 | 3172 | |
| 1997 | 1048657 | 15944 | 11771 | 2413 | 1488 | | | 50981 | 733624 | 229474 | | 3747 | 1893 | 3180 | |
| 1998 | 1042885 | 16001 | 11779 | 2443 | 1495 | | | 50071 | 728788 | 229349 | | 3746 | 1889 | 3191 | |
| 1999 | 1017673 | 16678 | 11868 | 2441 | 1533 | | | 49694 | 716677 | 226588 | | 3763 | 1877 | 3180 | |
| 2000 | 1034229 | 16318 | 11872 | 2453 | 1543 | 1000169 | | 49229 | 709458 | 240934 | 11386 | 3741 | 1839 | 3163 | |
| 2001 | 1029314 | 16197 | 11834 | 2478 | 1576 | 995670 | | 48090 | 698966 | 248061 | 11471 | 3813 | 1783 | 3132 | |
| 2002 | 1005004 | 17844 | 12716 | 2492 | 2237 | 973098 | 8211 | 44992 | 698966 | 219907 | 10787 | 3580 | 1839 | 3067 | 571 |
| 2003 | 806243 | 17764 | 12599 | 2518 | 2271 | 774693 | 10101 | 44279 | 514920 | 204468 | 10792 | 3584 | 1749 | 3033 | 838 |
| 2004 | 849140 | 18393 | 12900 | 2611 | 2492 | 817018 | 14153 | 41626 | 551600 | 208794 | 10878 | 3588 | 1583 | 2998 | 1284 |
| 2005 | 882206 | 18703 | 12982 | 2620 | 2682 | 849488 | 17128 | 40907 | 583209 | 207457 | 11177 | 3585 | 1502 | 3021 | 1702 |
| 2006 | 918097 | 19246 | 13120 | 2665 | 3022 | 884818 | 22656 | 39975 | 609128 | 212243 | 11269 | 3548 | 1402 | 3003 | 2097 |
| 2007 | 912263 | 19852 | 13372 | 2720 | 3282 | 878686 | 27069 | 39876 | 613855 | 197083 | 11528 | 3585 | 1365 | 3051 | 2553 |
| 2008 | 891480 | 19712 | 13119 | 2688 | 3437 | 858015 | 24260 | 39080 | 613143 | 180752 | 11485 | 3534 | 1310 | 3011 | 2675 |
| 2009 | 916571 | 20291 | 13364 | 2728 | 3716 | 882153 | 27308 | 38475 | 632770 | 182448 | 11665 | 3536 | 1291 | 3020 | 2809 |
| 2010 | 936927 | 20918 | 13681 | 2778 | 3956 | 901709 | 32739 | 37836 | 648424 | 181781 | 11835 | 3513 | 1274 | 3025 | 2992 |
| 2011 | 954389 | 21979 | 14328 | 2831 | 4283 | 918003 | 32860 | 37295 | 662894 | 184287 | 11926 | 3484 | 1294 | 3036 | 3022 |
| 2012 | 950297 | 23170 | 15021 | 2889 | 4665 | 912620 | 33562 | 37097 | 653419 | 187932 | 12083 | 3490 | 1289 | 3044 | 3088 |
| 2013 | 974398 | 24709 | 15887 | 3015 | 5127 | 915368 | 33965 | 37015 | 648619 | 195176 | 31155 | 3516 | 1271 | 3144 | 2967 |
| 2014 | 981432 | 25860 | 16524 | 3115 | 5478 | 917335 | 34238 | 36902 | 645470 | 200130 | 35029 | 3490 | 1242 | 3098 | 2975 |
| 2015 | 983528 | 27587 | 17430 | 3267 | 6023 | 920770 | 34321 | 36817 | 640536 | 208572 | 31927 | 3478 | 1234 | 3078 | 2986 |
| 2016 | 983394 | 29140 | 18020 | 3462 | 6642 | 926518 | 34327 | 36795 | 638763 | 216187 | 24866 | 3481 | 1213 | 3063 | 2986 |

Notes: The statistical data are from 2017 volume of China Statistical Yearbook of Health and Family Planning. ①Village health room number is included in the number of medical health institution; ②The reason of the fewer community health service centers (stations) in 2008 is that 5,000 rural community health service station in Jiangsu Province is incorporated into village health room;③From 2002, medical colleges and universities, secondary medical colleges, drug test institutions, frontier health quarantines and family planning guidance stations under non-health department is excluded from medical health institution number; ④From 2013, medical health institution number covers family planning technique service institution under former family planning department; ⑤Outpatient clinic before 1996 excludes private clinic.

## Number of All-region Medical

| Region | Total | Hospital | | | | | | | Grassroots Medical Health Institution | | | | | | |
|---|---|---|---|---|---|---|---|---|---|---|---|---|---|---|---|
| | | Subtotal | Comprehensive Hospital | TCM Hospital | Hospital of Traditional Chinese and Western Medicine | National Hospital | Specialty Hospital | Nursing Home | Subtotal | Community Health Service Center | Community Health Service Station | District Health Center | Township Health Center | Village Health Room | Outpatient Clinic |
| Total | 983394 | 29140 | 18020 | 3462 | 510 | 266 | 6642 | 240 | 926518 | 8918 | 25409 | 446 | 36795 | 638763 | 14779 |
| East Region | 357697 | 11221 | 6625 | 1276 | 204 | 8 | 2903 | 205 | 336998 | 4266 | 15767 | 47 | 9352 | 215845 | 9678 |
| Central Region | 314745 | 8500 | 5093 | 1146 | 145 | 14 | 2081 | 21 | 297310 | 2529 | 5222 | 326 | 11538 | 222158 | 2781 |
| West Region | 310952 | 9419 | 6302 | 1040 | 161 | 244 | 1658 | 14 | 292210 | 2123 | 4420 | 73 | 15905 | 200760 | 2320 |
| Beijing | 9773 | 638 | 272 | 154 | 35 | 2 | 169 | 6 | 8908 | 324 | 1591 | | | 2729 | 990 |
| Tianjin | 5443 | 421 | 278 | 53 | 3 | | 87 | | 4844 | 114 | 471 | 5 | 145 | 2528 | 539 |
| Hebei | 78795 | 1618 | 1086 | 201 | 36 | | 295 | | 76003 | 280 | 917 | | 1970 | 60371 | 267 |
| Shanxi | 42204 | 1393 | 693 | 210 | 26 | | 463 | 1 | 40288 | 231 | 698 | 266 | 1353 | 29027 | 356 |
| Inner Mongolia | 24002 | 720 | 402 | 110 | 10 | 61 | 134 | 3 | 22606 | 314 | 881 | | 1321 | 13632 | 285 |
| Liaoning | 36131 | 1190 | 694 | 139 | 10 | 1 | 339 | 7 | 33931 | 378 | 787 | 20 | 1014 | 20120 | 589 |
| Jilin | 20829 | 662 | 375 | 84 | 9 | 3 | 188 | 3 | 19589 | 207 | 188 | 1 | 774 | 10172 | 563 |
| Heilongjiang | 20375 | 1031 | 684 | 138 | 8 | 5 | 195 | 1 | 18256 | 440 | 213 | 11 | 988 | 11384 | 390 |
| Shanghai | 5016 | 349 | 181 | 19 | 8 | | 113 | 28 | 4470 | 307 | 732 | | | 1218 | 683 |
| Jiangsu | 32117 | 1678 | 1032 | 111 | 27 | | 403 | 105 | 29099 | 544 | 2116 | 2 | 1039 | 15475 | 1297 |
| Zhejiang | 31546 | 1130 | 505 | 152 | 31 | | 411 | 31 | 29811 | 467 | 5404 | 7 | 1194 | 11677 | 1389 |
| Anhui | 24385 | 1039 | 678 | 99 | 20 | | 236 | 6 | 22271 | 404 | 1504 | 1 | 1371 | 15276 | 247 |
| Fujian | 27656 | 587 | 356 | 79 | 10 | 1 | 139 | 2 | 26190 | 222 | 333 | | 880 | 18945 | 615 |
| Jiangxi | 38272 | 592 | 382 | 101 | 8 | | 100 | 1 | 36784 | 168 | 423 | 6 | 1585 | 30394 | 167 |
| Shandong | 76997 | 2018 | 1250 | 196 | 21 | 4 | 532 | 15 | 72904 | 518 | 1792 | 4 | 1621 | 53226 | 619 |
| Henan | 71271 | 1596 | 985 | 258 | 28 | | 322 | 3 | 67174 | 424 | 905 | 6 | 2059 | 56774 | 175 |
| Hubei | 36354 | 927 | 551 | 115 | 18 | 3 | 237 | 3 | 34703 | 342 | 889 | 31 | 1139 | 24792 | 484 |
| Hunan | 61055 | 1260 | 745 | 141 | 28 | 3 | 340 | 3 | 58245 | 313 | 402 | 4 | 2269 | 44339 | 399 |
| Guangdong | 49079 | 1381 | 813 | 155 | 17 | | 385 | 11 | 46033 | 1082 | 1484 | 9 | 1192 | 26886 | 2599 |
| Guangxi | 34253 | 543 | 330 | 93 | 17 | 5 | 97 | 1 | 32020 | 150 | 129 | | 1267 | 21011 | 182 |
| Hainan | 5144 | 211 | 158 | 17 | 6 | | 30 | | 4805 | 30 | 140 | | 297 | 2670 | 91 |
| Chongqing | 19933 | 699 | 452 | 76 | 25 | | 142 | 4 | 19044 | 199 | 297 | 13 | 894 | 11240 | 355 |
| Sichuan | 79513 | 2066 | 1362 | 204 | 26 | 36 | 437 | 1 | 76619 | 413 | 538 | 3 | 4490 | 55958 | 383 |
| Guizhou | 28017 | 1220 | 923 | 90 | 20 | 7 | 177 | 3 | 26172 | 167 | 468 | 42 | 1399 | 20652 | 119 |
| Yunnan | 24234 | 1187 | 787 | 131 | 28 | 5 | 236 | | 22395 | 189 | 377 | 4 | 1366 | 13432 | 262 |
| Tibet | 6835 | 145 | 105 | | 1 | 30 | 9 | | 6546 | 8 | 2 | | 678 | 5360 | |
| Shaanxi | 36598 | 1085 | 740 | 157 | 10 | | 176 | 2 | 34017 | 249 | 374 | 9 | 1561 | 25412 | 285 |
| Gansu | 28197 | 446 | 276 | 82 | 12 | 12 | 64 | | 25791 | 201 | 380 | 1 | 1375 | 16748 | 69 |
| Qinghai | 6291 | 199 | 113 | 13 | 2 | 34 | 37 | | 5908 | 30 | 205 | | 405 | 4518 | 5 |
| Ningxia | 4254 | 190 | 123 | 22 | 4 | 2 | 39 | | 3968 | 18 | 124 | | 219 | 2365 | 27 |
| Xinjiang | 18825 | 919 | 689 | 62 | 6 | 52 | 110 | | 17124 | 185 | 645 | 1 | 930 | 10432 | 348 |

## Health Institution in 2016

| Clinic (Infirmary, Nursing Home) | Professional Public Health Institution | | | | | | | | | Other Medical Health Institution | | | | | |
|---|---|---|---|---|---|---|---|---|---|---|---|---|---|---|---|
| | Subtotal | Disease Prevention & Control Center | Special Disease Prevention & Treatment Center (Clinic/Station) | Health Education Center (Station) | Maternal & Child Care Center (Clinic/Station) | First Aid Center | Blood Collecting and Supplying Institution | Health Supervision Institution (Center) | Family Planning Technique Service Center | Subtotal | Sanatorium | Medical Science Research Institution | In-service Medical Training Institution | Statistical Information Center | Others |
| **201408** | **24866** | **3481** | **1213** | **163** | **3063** | **355** | **552** | **2986** | **13053** | **2870** | **171** | **197** | **387** | **75** | **2040** |
| 82043 | 8140 | 1059 | 518 | 59 | 955 | 185 | 190 | 896 | 4278 | 1338 | 104 | 103 | 161 | 40 | 930 |
| 52756 | 7970 | 1082 | 508 | 30 | 984 | 99 | 163 | 944 | 4160 | 965 | 29 | 41 | 139 | 15 | 741 |
| 66609 | 8756 | 1340 | 187 | 74 | 1124 | 71 | 199 | 1146 | 4615 | 567 | 38 | 53 | 87 | 20 | 369 |
| 3274 | 112 | 29 | 25 | | 20 | 12 | 4 | 18 | 4 | 115 | | 28 | 8 | 9 | 70 |
| 1042 | 126 | 24 | 16 | 1 | 21 | 3 | 6 | 19 | 36 | 52 | 3 | 9 | 13 | 1 | 26 |
| 12198 | 1089 | 192 | 11 | 2 | 191 | 5 | 16 | 179 | 493 | 85 | 3 | 2 | | 1 | 79 |
| 8357 | 455 | 136 | 7 | 11 | 134 | 9 | 22 | 131 | 5 | 68 | 8 | 7 | 3 | 2 | 48 |
| 6173 | 600 | 117 | 54 | 23 | 113 | 8 | 18 | 114 | 153 | 76 | 5 | 6 | 4 | 2 | 59 |
| 11023 | 854 | 133 | 85 | 10 | 110 | 13 | 23 | 90 | 390 | 156 | 15 | 6 | 3 | 4 | 128 |
| 7684 | 428 | 68 | 54 | 3 | 71 | 6 | 20 | 39 | 167 | 150 | 9 | 3 | 4 | 1 | 133 |
| 4830 | 1037 | 168 | 109 | | 139 | 14 | 28 | 139 | 440 | 51 | 2 | 6 | 10 | 4 | 29 |
| 1530 | 117 | 20 | 21 | 1 | 21 | 11 | 8 | 18 | 17 | 80 | 4 | 9 | 10 | 3 | 54 |
| 8626 | 1059 | 117 | 42 | 6 | 110 | 43 | 30 | 106 | 605 | 281 | 15 | 9 | 29 | 4 | 224 |
| 9673 | 420 | 101 | 16 | 1 | 87 | 50 | 21 | 101 | 43 | 185 | 16 | 7 | 41 | 5 | 116 |
| 3468 | 983 | 121 | 47 | 4 | 120 | 14 | 22 | 112 | 543 | 92 | 4 | 11 | 19 | 3 | 55 |
| 5195 | 809 | 96 | 24 | | 87 | 7 | 9 | 85 | 501 | 70 | 11 | 8 | 22 | 1 | 28 |
| 4041 | 794 | 147 | 109 | 5 | 112 | 9 | 13 | 110 | 289 | 102 | 3 | 5 | 3 | | 91 |
| 15124 | 1891 | 184 | 125 | 3 | 156 | 17 | 27 | 106 | 1273 | 184 | 17 | 8 | 23 | 5 | 131 |
| 6831 | 2223 | 180 | 21 | 4 | 164 | 32 | 22 | 177 | 1623 | 278 | 2 | 6 | 80 | 1 | 189 |
| 7026 | 557 | 115 | 74 | 1 | 105 | 12 | 21 | 105 | 124 | 167 | | 1 | 19 | 3 | 144 |
| 10519 | 1493 | 147 | 87 | 2 | 139 | 3 | 15 | 131 | 969 | 57 | 1 | 2 | 1 | 1 | 52 |
| 12781 | 1544 | 137 | 135 | 33 | 128 | 21 | 42 | 150 | 898 | 121 | 17 | 17 | 12 | 7 | 68 |
| 9281 | 1650 | 115 | 37 | 1 | 103 | 4 | 28 | 110 | 1252 | 40 | 5 | 14 | 1 | 3 | 17 |
| 1577 | 119 | 26 | 18 | 2 | 24 | 3 | 4 | 24 | 18 | 9 | 3 | | | | 6 |
| 6046 | 156 | 42 | 16 | 4 | 42 | | 11 | 39 | 2 | 34 | 7 | | 6 | 4 | 17 |
| 14834 | 744 | 206 | 25 | 12 | 202 | 17 | 31 | 200 | 51 | 84 | 2 | 6 | 13 | 7 | 56 |
| 3325 | 597 | 100 | 10 | | 101 | 5 | 29 | 95 | 257 | 28 | 1 | 2 | 9 | | 16 |
| 6765 | 593 | 152 | 29 | 8 | 145 | 23 | 16 | 142 | 78 | 59 | 6 | 10 | 7 | 1 | 35 |
| 498 | 142 | 82 | | | 55 | | 4 | 1 | | 2 | 1 | | 1 | | |
| 6127 | 1390 | 119 | 5 | 5 | 116 | 4 | 10 | 115 | 1016 | 106 | 3 | 10 | 36 | 1 | 56 |
| 7017 | 1844 | 103 | 7 | 13 | 100 | 3 | 17 | 93 | 1508 | 116 | 4 | 4 | 10 | 1 | 97 |
| 745 | 180 | 56 | 1 | 4 | 34 | | 9 | 55 | 21 | 4 | | 1 | | | 3 |
| 1215 | 85 | 25 | | 4 | 21 | 2 | 5 | 24 | 4 | 11 | 1 | | | 1 | 9 |
| 4583 | 775 | 223 | 3 | | 92 | 5 | 21 | 158 | 273 | 7 | 3 | | | | 4 |

## Number of All-type Medical

| Institution Type | Total | Urban or Rural Type | | Registration Type | | |
|---|---|---|---|---|---|---|
| | | Urban | Rural | Public | | |
| | | | | State Ownership | Collectivity | |
| Total | 983394 | 172532 | 810862 | 542507 | 139670 | 402837 |
| I. Hospital | 29140 | 15500 | 13640 | 12708 | 11775 | 933 |
| Comprehensive Hospital | 18020 | 8754 | 9266 | 8190 | 7597 | 593 |
| TCM Hospital | 3462 | 1606 | 1856 | 2327 | 2209 | 118 |
| Hospital of Traditional Chinese and Western Medicine | 510 | 300 | 210 | 139 | 125 | 14 |
| National Hospital | 266 | 45 | 221 | 210 | 207 | 3 |
| Specialty Hospital | 6642 | 4608 | 2034 | 1810 | 1612 | 198 |
| Stomatological Hospital | 594 | 452 | 142 | 167 | 142 | 25 |
| Ophthalmic Hospital | 537 | 381 | 156 | 52 | 41 | 11 |
| Otolaryngology Hospital | 95 | 70 | 25 | 10 | 9 | 1 |
| Tumor Hospital | 140 | 118 | 22 | 74 | 72 | 2 |
| Cardiovascular Hospital | 86 | 56 | 30 | 17 | 15 | 2 |
| Thoracopathy Hospital | 20 | 17 | 3 | 15 | 14 | 1 |
| Hematonosis Hospital | 11 | 6 | 5 | 1 | 1 | |
| Obstetrical and Gynecological Hospital | 757 | 556 | 201 | 67 | 60 | 7 |
| Children's Hospital | 117 | 91 | 26 | 68 | 59 | 9 |
| Mental Hospital | 1026 | 513 | 513 | 655 | 606 | 49 |
| Infectious Disease Hospital | 166 | 143 | 23 | 164 | 164 | |
| Dermatology Hospital | 184 | 152 | 32 | 41 | 37 | 4 |
| Tuberculosis Hospital | 34 | 28 | 6 | 33 | 33 | |
| Leprosy Hospital | 28 | 15 | 13 | 28 | 28 | |
| Occupational Disease Hospital | 20 | 18 | 2 | 19 | 18 | 1 |
| Orthopaedic Hospital | 603 | 308 | 295 | 54 | 34 | 20 |
| Rehabilitation Hospital | 495 | 339 | 156 | 163 | 133 | 30 |
| Plastic Surgery Hospital | 62 | 57 | 5 | 3 | 2 | 1 |
| Cosmetic Hospital | 275 | 256 | 19 | 1 | 1 | |
| Other Specialty Hospital | 1392 | 1032 | 360 | 178 | 143 | 35 |
| Nursing Hospital | 240 | 187 | 53 | 32 | 25 | 7 |
| II. Grassroots Medical Health Institution | 926518 | 147745 | 778773 | 502619 | 101293 | 401326 |
| Community Health Service Center (Station) | 34327 | 24889 | 9438 | 26023 | 15645 | 10378 |
| Community Health Service Center | 8918 | 6779 | 2139 | 8281 | 6380 | 1901 |
| Community Health Service Station | 25409 | 18110 | 7299 | 17742 | 9265 | 8477 |
| Health Center | 37241 | 124 | 37117 | 37049 | 28112 | 8937 |
| District Health Center | 446 | 124 | 322 | 440 | 220 | 220 |
| Township Health Hospital | 36795 | | 36795 | 36609 | 27892 | 8717 |
| Central Health Center | 10568 | | 10568 | 10556 | 9216 | 1340 |
| Township Health Center | 26227 | | 26227 | 26053 | 18676 | 7377 |
| Village Health Room | 638763 | | 638763 | 410615 | 40758 | 369857 |
| Outpatient Department | 14779 | 11812 | 2967 | 2516 | 1629 | 887 |
| Comprehensive Outpatient Department | 6806 | 5148 | 1658 | 1832 | 1170 | 662 |
| TCM Outpatient Department | 1539 | 1342 | 197 | 131 | 69 | 62 |
| Outpatient Department of Traditional Chinese and Western Medicine | 355 | 279 | 76 | 38 | 17 | 21 |
| National Medical Outpatient Department | 19 | 5 | 14 | 3 | 1 | 2 |
| Specialty Outpatient Department | 6060 | 5038 | 1022 | 512 | 372 | 140 |
| Clinic, Health Clinic, Infirmary and Nursing Station | 201408 | 110920 | 90488 | 26416 | 15149 | 11267 |
| Clinic | 169367 | 92510 | 76857 | 5390 | 1522 | 3868 |
| Health Clinic and Infirmary | 31964 | 18377 | 13587 | 21023 | 13626 | 7397 |
| Nursing Station | 77 | 33 | 44 | 3 | 1 | 2 |

Note: ①Urban refer to municipalities directly under the central area; Rural refers to county, county-level city, township health center and village

# Health Institutions in 2016

| Registration Type | Non-public | | Host Unit Type | | | |
|---|---|---|---|---|---|---|
| | Joint ownership | Private Ownership | Government Operation | Health and Family Planning department | Social Operation | Private Operation |
| **440887** | **19297** | **366882** | **152179** | **141997** | **480257** | **350957** |
| 16432 | 168 | 12409 | 9605 | 8560 | 6808 | 12727 |
| 9830 | 113 | 7516 | 5488 | 4699 | 4890 | 7642 |
| 1135 | 6 | 881 | 2260 | 2234 | 248 | 954 |
| 371 | 2 | 283 | 123 | 120 | 85 | 302 |
| 56 | 1 | 42 | 198 | 197 | 24 | 44 |
| 4832 | 44 | 3548 | 1519 | 1297 | 1482 | 3641 |
| 427 | 2 | 313 | 147 | 144 | 124 | 323 |
| 485 | 7 | 330 | 45 | 42 | 162 | 330 |
| 85 | 1 | 63 | 8 | 8 | 24 | 63 |
| 66 | 1 | 37 | 68 | 67 | 39 | 33 |
| 69 | | 54 | 12 | 12 | 20 | 54 |
| 5 | | 4 | 12 | 12 | 3 | 5 |
| 10 | | 8 | 1 | 1 | 1 | 9 |
| 690 | 2 | 488 | 62 | 60 | 189 | 506 |
| 49 | | 31 | 59 | 59 | 22 | 36 |
| 371 | 3 | 306 | 600 | 480 | 116 | 310 |
| 2 | | 1 | 161 | 159 | 3 | 2 |
| 143 | | 109 | 35 | 34 | 32 | 117 |
| 1 | | 1 | 30 | 30 | 3 | 1 |
| | | | 26 | 25 | 2 | |
| 1 | | | 14 | 12 | 6 | |
| 549 | 5 | 436 | 33 | 32 | 115 | 455 |
| 332 | 7 | 224 | 93 | 38 | 187 | 215 |
| 59 | | 39 | 2 | 2 | 18 | 42 |
| 274 | 1 | 180 | | | 95 | 180 |
| 1214 | 15 | 924 | 111 | 80 | 321 | 960 |
| 208 | 2 | 139 | 17 | 13 | 79 | 144 |
| 423899 | 19119 | 354305 | 117421 | 114050 | 471008 | 338089 |
| 8304 | 76 | 6732 | 18031 | 16912 | 8797 | 7499 |
| 637 | 5 | 345 | 6229 | 5974 | 2274 | 415 |
| 7667 | 71 | 6387 | 11802 | 10938 | 6523 | 7084 |
| 192 | 4 | 167 | 36764 | 36526 | 301 | 176 |
| 6 | 1 | 5 | 416 | 413 | 23 | 7 |
| 186 | 3 | 162 | 36348 | 36113 | 278 | 169 |
| 12 | | 10 | 10522 | 10458 | 33 | 13 |
| 174 | 3 | 152 | 25826 | 25655 | 245 | 156 |
| 228148 | 18604 | 174448 | 60419 | 60419 | 426180 | 152164 |
| 12263 | 33 | 9811 | 197 | 43 | 4461 | 10121 |
| 4974 | 23 | 4064 | 148 | 38 | 2551 | 4107 |
| 1408 | 2 | 1067 | 2 | | 403 | 1134 |
| 317 | 2 | 281 | 1 | | 68 | 286 |
| 16 | | 15 | | | 3 | 16 |
| 5548 | 6 | 4384 | 46 | 5 | 1436 | 4578 |
| 174992 | 402 | 163147 | 2010 | 150 | 31269 | 168129 |
| 163977 | 277 | 155652 | 211 | 49 | 8717 | 160439 |
| 10941 | 125 | 7434 | 1799 | 101 | 22542 | 7623 |
| 74 | | 61 | | | 10 | 67 |

health room; ②Social Operation includes enterprise, public institution, social group and health institution by other social organizations.

| Institution Type | Total | Urban and Rural Type | | Registration Type | | |
|---|---|---|---|---|---|---|
| | | | | | Public Ownership | |
| | | Urban | Rural | | State Ownership | Collective Ownership |
| III. Professional Public Health Institution | 24866 | 7897 | 16969 | 24568 | 24049 | 519 |
| Disease Prevention and Control Center | 3481 | 1345 | 2136 | 3478 | 3462 | 16 |
| Provincial Ownership | 31 | 31 | | 31 | 31 | |
| Prefecture-level City (Region) Ownership | 416 | 360 | 56 | 416 | 415 | 1 |
| County-level City (District) Ownership | 1209 | 844 | 365 | 1209 | 1207 | 2 |
| County Ownership | 1575 | | 1575 | 1575 | 1573 | 2 |
| Others Ownership | 250 | 110 | 140 | 247 | 236 | 11 |
| Special Disease Prevention and Treatment Center (Institution, Station) | 1213 | 478 | 735 | 1174 | 1125 | 49 |
| Special Disease Prevention and Treatment Center | 189 | 114 | 75 | 180 | 175 | 5 |
| Infectious Disease Prevention and Treatment Center | 12 | 4 | 8 | 12 | 11 | 1 |
| Tuberculosis Prevention and Treatment Center | 20 | 14 | 6 | 20 | 20 | |
| Occupational Disease Prevention and Treatment Center | 37 | 35 | 2 | 35 | 35 | |
| Others | 120 | 61 | 59 | 113 | 109 | 4 |
| Special Disease Prevention and Treatment Institution (Station, Center) | 1024 | 364 | 660 | 994 | 950 | 44 |
| Stomatology Disease Prevention and Treatment Institution (Station, Center) | 97 | 63 | 34 | 83 | 50 | 33 |
| Mental Disease Prevention and Treatment Institution (Station, Center) | 29 | 9 | 20 | 28 | 23 | 5 |
| Dermatosis and Venereal Disease Prevention and Treatment Institution (Station, Center) | 221 | 55 | 166 | 219 | 216 | 3 |
| Tuberculosis Prevention and Treatment Institution (Station, Center) | 344 | 124 | 220 | 343 | 342 | 1 |
| Occupational Disease Prevention and Treatment Institution (Station, Center) | 41 | 33 | 8 | 35 | 35 | |
| Endemic Disease Prevention and Treatment Institution (Station, Center) | 31 | 8 | 23 | 31 | 31 | |
| Schistosomiasis Prevention and Treatment Institution (Station, Center) | 162 | 30 | 132 | 162 | 161 | 1 |
| Drug Rehabilitation Institution (Station, Center) | 12 | 10 | 2 | 11 | 10 | 1 |
| Others | 87 | 32 | 55 | 82 | 82 | |
| Health Education Institution (Station, Center) | 163 | 109 | 54 | 160 | 156 | 4 |
| Maternal and Child Care Center (Institution, Station) | 3063 | 1145 | 1918 | 3050 | 3032 | 18 |
| Provincial Ownership | 25 | 25 | | 25 | 25 | |
| Prefecture-level City (Region) Ownership | 382 | 347 | 35 | 382 | 381 | 1 |
| County-level City (District) Ownership | 1067 | 710 | 357 | 1067 | 1056 | 11 |
| County Ownership | 1486 | | 1486 | 1486 | 1482 | 4 |
| Others | 103 | 63 | 40 | 90 | 88 | 2 |
| Maternal and Child Care Center | 1981 | 688 | 1293 | 1972 | 1961 | 11 |
| Maternal and Child Care Institution | 534 | 280 | 254 | 533 | 530 | 3 |
| Maternal and Child Care Station | 523 | 166 | 357 | 521 | 517 | 4 |
| Reproduction Health Center | 25 | 11 | 14 | 24 | 24 | |
| First Aid Center (Station) | 355 | 238 | 117 | 350 | 344 | 6 |
| Blood Collecting and Supplying Institution | 552 | 348 | 204 | 490 | 485 | 5 |
| Health Supervision Institution (Center) | 2986 | 1133 | 1853 | 2986 | 2974 | 12 |
| Provincial Ownership | 31 | 31 | | 31 | 31 | |
| Prefecture-level City (Region) Ownership | 404 | 358 | 47 | 404 | 403 | 1 |
| County-level City (District) Ownership | 1062 | 740 | 322 | 1062 | 1059 | 3 |
| County Ownership | 1438 | | 1437 | 1438 | 1432 | 6 |
| Others | 51 | 4 | 47 | 51 | 49 | 2 |
| Family Planning Technique Service Institution | 13053 | 3101 | 9952 | 12880 | 12471 | 409 |
| IV. Other Medical Health Institution | 2870 | 1390 | 1480 | 2612 | 2553 | 59 |
| Sanatorium | 171 | 119 | 52 | 155 | 149 | 6 |
| Health Supervision and Testing (Monitoring) Institution | 14 | 8 | 6 | 11 | 11 | |
| Medical Science Research Institution | 197 | 175 | 22 | 197 | 195 | 2 |
| In-service Medical Training Institution | 387 | 118 | 269 | 387 | 383 | 4 |
| Clinical Testing Center (Institution, Station) | 183 | 172 | 11 | 26 | 22 | 4 |
| Statistical Information Center | 75 | 71 | 4 | 74 | 74 | |
| Others | 1843 | 727 | 1116 | 1762 | 1719 | 43 |

Continued

| Registration Type | Non-public | | Host Unit Type | | | |
| --- | --- | --- | --- | --- | --- | --- |
| | Joint Ownership | Private Ownership | Government Operation | Health and Family Planning Department | Social Operation | Private Operation |
| 298 | 5 | 44 | 22859 | 17489 | 1970 | 37 |
| 3 | | | 3374 | 3258 | 107 | |
| | | | 31 | 31 | | |
| | | | 416 | 416 | | |
| | | | 1209 | 1209 | | |
| | | | 1575 | 1575 | | |
| 3 | | | 143 | 27 | 106 | 1 |
| 39 | | 25 | 1106 | 1086 | 83 | 24 |
| 9 | | 6 | 168 | 162 | 18 | 3 |
| | | | 12 | 12 | | |
| | | | 20 | 20 | | |
| 2 | | | 25 | 23 | 12 | |
| 7 | | 6 | 111 | 107 | 6 | 3 |
| 30 | | 19 | 938 | 924 | 65 | 21 |
| 14 | | 10 | 76 | 75 | 9 | 12 |
| 1 | | 1 | 24 | 22 | 4 | 1 |
| 2 | | 1 | 209 | 208 | 10 | 2 |
| 1 | | | 332 | 332 | 12 | |
| 6 | | 4 | 18 | 18 | 20 | 3 |
| | | | 29 | 29 | 2 | |
| | | | 160 | 158 | 2 | |
| 1 | | | 10 | 2 | 2 | |
| 5 | | 3 | 80 | 80 | 4 | 3 |
| 3 | | | 148 | 143 | 15 | |
| 13 | 1 | 5 | 2997 | 2967 | 61 | 5 |
| | | | 25 | 25 | | |
| | | | 382 | 382 | | |
| | | | 1067 | 1067 | | |
| | | | 1486 | 1486 | | |
| 13 | 1 | 5 | 37 | 7 | 61 | 5 |
| 9 | 1 | 4 | 1950 | 1933 | 27 | 4 |
| 1 | | | 521 | 520 | 13 | |
| 2 | | | 505 | 499 | 18 | |
| 1 | | 1 | 21 | 15 | 3 | 1 |
| 5 | | 4 | 313 | 308 | 39 | 3 |
| 62 | 4 | 10 | 474 | 466 | 74 | 4 |
| | | | 2986 | 2936 | | |
| | | | 31 | 31 | | |
| | | | 404 | 404 | | |
| | | | 1062 | 1062 | | |
| | | | 1438 | 1438 | | |
| | | | 51 | 1 | | |
| 173 | | | 11461 | 6325 | 1591 | 1 |
| 258 | 5 | 124 | 2294 | 1898 | 472 | 104 |
| 16 | | 6 | 84 | 39 | 82 | 5 |
| 3 | | 3 | 9 | 8 | 2 | 3 |
| | | | 171 | 166 | 26 | |
| | | | 374 | 370 | 13 | |
| 157 | 2 | 95 | 11 | 10 | 98 | 74 |
| 1 | | | 68 | 66 | 7 | |
| 81 | 3 | 20 | 1577 | 1239 | 244 | 22 |

### Hospital Numbers (Registration Type/Host Unit/Management Type/Class/Institution Type)

| Hospital Type | 2010 | 2012 | 2013 | 2014 | 2015 | 2016 |
|---|---|---|---|---|---|---|
| **Total** | **20918** | **23170** | **24709** | **25860** | **27587** | **29140** |
| Registration Type | | | | | | |
|   Public Hospital | 13850 | 13384 | 13396 | 13314 | 13069 | 12708 |
|   Private Hospital | 7068 | 9786 | 11313 | 12546 | 14518 | 16432 |
| Host Unit | | | | | | |
|   Government Ownership | 9629 | 9637 | 9673 | 9668 | 9651 | 9605 |
|   Society Operation | 5892 | 6029 | 6193 | 6331 | 6570 | 6808 |
|   Private Operation | 5397 | 7504 | 8843 | 9861 | 11366 | 12727 |
| Management Type | | | | | | |
|   Non-profit | 15822 | 16767 | 17269 | 17705 | 18518 | 19065 |
|   Profit | 5096 | 6403 | 7440 | 8155 | 9069 | 10075 |
|   Unknown | | | | | | |
| Hospital Class | | | | | | |
|   Class Three Hospital | 1284 | 1624 | 1787 | 1954 | 2123 | 2232 |
|   Class Two Hospital | 6472 | 6566 | 6709 | 6850 | 7494 | 7944 |
|   Class One Hospital | 5271 | 5962 | 6473 | 7009 | 8759 | 9282 |
| Institution Type | | | | | | |
|   Comprehensive Hospital | 13681 | 15021 | 15887 | 16524 | 17430 | 18020 |
|   TCM Hospital | 2778 | 2889 | 3015 | 3115 | 3267 | 3462 |
|   Hospital of Traditional Chinese and Western Medicine | 256 | 312 | 358 | 384 | 446 | 510 |
|   National Hospital | 198 | 208 | 217 | 233 | 253 | 266 |
|   Specialty Hospital | 3956 | 4665 | 5127 | 5478 | 6023 | 6642 |
|   Nursing Home | 49 | 75 | 105 | 126 | 168 | 240 |

## All-region Public Hospital Numbers in 2016

| Region | All Hospitals | Hospital Class | | | | Institution Type | | | | | | Among Public Hospital: Government-owned Hospital |
|---|---|---|---|---|---|---|---|---|---|---|---|---|
| | | Class Three Hospital | Class Two Hospital | Class One Hospital | Not Evaluated | Comprehensive Hospital | TCM Hospital | Hospital of TCM ★ and Western Medicine | National Hospital | Specialty Hospital | Nursing Home | |
| Total | 12708 | 2060 | 6067 | 2986 | 1595 | 8190 | 2327 | 139 | 210 | 1810 | 32 | 9605 |
| East Region | 4751 | 970 | 2039 | 1190 | 552 | 2999 | 786 | 69 | 4 | 865 | 28 | 3534 |
| Central Region | 4050 | 539 | 1980 | 1064 | 467 | 2654 | 795 | 31 | 5 | 562 | 3 | 2909 |
| West Region | 3907 | 551 | 2048 | 732 | 576 | 2537 | 746 | 39 | 201 | 383 | 1 | 3162 |
| Beijing | 229 | 78 | 67 | 84 | | 136 | 35 | 12 | 1 | 43 | 2 | 144 |
| Tianjin | 151 | 42 | 45 | 64 | | 87 | 22 | 1 | | 41 | | 91 |
| Hebei | 730 | 63 | 391 | 228 | 48 | 486 | 143 | 10 | | 91 | | 517 |
| Shanxi | 670 | 56 | 279 | 146 | 189 | 432 | 127 | 4 | | 107 | | 391 |
| Inner Mongolia | 347 | 60 | 201 | 66 | 20 | 197 | 63 | 2 | 51 | 34 | | 284 |
| Liaoning | 536 | 118 | 217 | 150 | 51 | 336 | 69 | 4 | 1 | 126 | | 380 |
| Jilin | 303 | 45 | 172 | 48 | 38 | 184 | 61 | 5 | 2 | 51 | | 222 |
| Heilongjiang | 665 | 86 | 303 | 245 | 31 | 490 | 90 | 4 | 1 | 79 | 1 | 445 |
| Shanghai | 178 | 47 | 104 | 9 | 18 | 94 | 15 | 7 | | 53 | 9 | 163 |
| Jiangsu | 524 | 137 | 201 | 124 | 62 | 298 | 78 | 12 | | 126 | 10 | 406 |
| Zhejiang | 438 | 129 | 185 | 12 | 112 | 250 | 86 | 8 | | 90 | 4 | 398 |
| Anhui | 367 | 55 | 201 | 78 | 33 | 226 | 80 | 3 | | 57 | 1 | 298 |
| Fujian | 264 | 56 | 145 | 60 | 3 | 151 | 65 | 4 | 1 | 43 | | 235 |
| Jiangxi | 349 | 55 | 184 | 41 | 69 | 224 | 87 | 6 | | 32 | | 264 |
| Shandong | 800 | 134 | 340 | 231 | 95 | 536 | 126 | 4 | 1 | 131 | 2 | 528 |
| Henan | 781 | 80 | 361 | 320 | 20 | 531 | 152 | 3 | | 95 | | 568 |
| Hubei | 416 | 99 | 210 | 76 | 31 | 263 | 84 | 2 | 2 | 64 | 1 | 322 |
| Hunan | 499 | 63 | 270 | 110 | 56 | 304 | 114 | 4 | | 77 | | 399 |
| Guangdong | 747 | 149 | 316 | 166 | 116 | 493 | 132 | 6 | | 115 | 1 | 622 |
| Guangxi | 331 | 61 | 192 | 31 | 47 | 186 | 84 | 11 | 4 | 45 | 1 | 309 |
| Hainan | 154 | 17 | 28 | 62 | 47 | 132 | 15 | 1 | | 6 | | 50 |
| Chongqing | 256 | 33 | 100 | 62 | 61 | 167 | 40 | 7 | | 42 | | 177 |
| Sichuan | 704 | 142 | 374 | 25 | 163 | 409 | 155 | 7 | 36 | 97 | | 593 |
| Guizhou | 298 | 43 | 158 | 56 | 41 | 197 | 59 | 5 | 3 | 34 | | 228 |
| Yunnan | 418 | 58 | 249 | 42 | 69 | 279 | 103 | 1 | 3 | 32 | | 350 |
| Tibet | 107 | 7 | 10 | 78 | 12 | 82 | | | 24 | 1 | | 100 |
| Shaanxi | 511 | 49 | 278 | 127 | 57 | 360 | 111 | 2 | | 38 | | 295 |
| Gansu | 295 | 35 | 166 | 25 | 69 | 191 | 74 | 3 | 9 | 18 | | 233 |
| Qinghai | 108 | 16 | 75 | | 17 | 62 | 13 | | 27 | 6 | | 103 |
| Ningxia | 70 | 13 | 49 | 7 | 1 | 46 | 18 | | | 6 | | 65 |
| Xinjiang | 462 | 34 | 196 | 213 | 19 | 361 | 26 | 1 | 44 | 31 | | 425 |

★ Traditional Chinese Medicine

## All-region Private Hospital Numbers in 2016

| Region | Hospital | Hospital Class | | | | Institution Type | | | | | |
|---|---|---|---|---|---|---|---|---|---|---|---|
| | | Class Three Hospital | Class Two Hospital | Class One Hospital | Not Evaluated | Comprehensive Hospital | TCM Hospital | Hospital of Traditional Chinese and Western Medicine | National Hospital | Specialty Hospital | Nursing Home |
| **Total** | **16432** | **172** | **1877** | **6296** | **8087** | **9830** | **1135** | **371** | **56** | **4832** | **208** |
| East Region | 6470 | 81 | 726 | 2827 | 2836 | 3626 | 490 | 135 | 4 | 2038 | 177 |
| Central Region | 4450 | 57 | 541 | 1670 | 2182 | 2439 | 351 | 114 | 9 | 1519 | 18 |
| West Region | 5512 | 34 | 610 | 1799 | 3069 | 3765 | 294 | 122 | 43 | 1275 | 13 |
| Beijing | 409 | 15 | 59 | 310 | 25 | 136 | 119 | 23 | 1 | 126 | 4 |
| Tianjin | 270 | 0 | 13 | 133 | 124 | 191 | 31 | 2 | | 46 | |
| Hebei | 888 | 6 | 91 | 597 | 194 | 600 | 58 | 26 | | 204 | |
| Shanxi | 723 | 2 | 62 | 185 | 474 | 261 | 83 | 22 | | 356 | 1 |
| Inner Mongolia | 373 | 7 | 71 | 197 | 98 | 205 | 47 | 8 | 10 | 100 | 3 |
| Liaoning | 654 | 6 | 70 | 288 | 290 | 358 | 70 | 6 | | 213 | 7 |
| Jilin | 359 | 1 | 44 | 60 | 254 | 191 | 23 | 4 | 1 | 137 | 3 |
| Heilongjiang | 366 | 6 | 42 | 127 | 191 | 194 | 48 | 4 | 4 | 116 | |
| Shanghai | 171 | 0 | 1 | 2 | 168 | 87 | 4 | 1 | | 60 | 19 |
| Jiangsu | 1154 | 12 | 172 | 565 | 405 | 734 | 33 | 15 | | 277 | 95 |
| Zhejiang | 692 | 3 | 37 | 31 | 621 | 255 | 66 | 23 | | 321 | 27 |
| Anhui | 672 | 11 | 116 | 333 | 212 | 452 | 19 | 17 | | 179 | 5 |
| Fujian | 323 | 8 | 47 | 253 | 15 | 205 | 14 | 6 | | 96 | 2 |
| Jiangxi | 243 | 4 | 29 | 49 | 161 | 158 | 14 | 2 | | 68 | 1 |
| Shandong | 1218 | 16 | 155 | 481 | 566 | 714 | 70 | 17 | 3 | 401 | 13 |
| Henan | 815 | 6 | 95 | 502 | 212 | 454 | 106 | 25 | | 227 | 3 |
| Hubei | 511 | 22 | 91 | 175 | 223 | 288 | 31 | 16 | 1 | 173 | 2 |
| Hunan | 761 | 5 | 62 | 239 | 455 | 441 | 27 | 24 | 3 | 263 | 3 |
| Guangdong | 634 | 13 | 74 | 159 | 388 | 320 | 23 | 11 | | 270 | 10 |
| Guangxi | 212 | 2 | 26 | 111 | 73 | 144 | 9 | 6 | 1 | 52 | |
| Hainan | 57 | 2 | 7 | 8 | 40 | 26 | 2 | 5 | | 24 | |
| Chongqing | 443 | 1 | 27 | 85 | 330 | 285 | 36 | 18 | | 100 | 4 |
| Sichuan | 1362 | 2 | 160 | 241 | 959 | 953 | 49 | 19 | | 340 | 1 |
| Guizhou | 922 | 6 | 88 | 456 | 372 | 726 | 31 | 15 | 4 | 143 | 3 |
| Yunnan | 769 | 9 | 88 | 169 | 503 | 508 | 28 | 27 | 2 | 204 | |
| Tibet | 38 | | 1 | 9 | 28 | 23 | | 1 | 6 | 8 | |
| Shaanxi | 574 | 5 | 55 | 163 | 351 | 380 | 46 | 8 | | 138 | 2 |
| Gansu | 151 | 1 | 18 | 17 | 115 | 85 | 8 | 9 | 3 | 46 | |
| Qinghai | 91 | | 17 | | 74 | 51 | | 2 | 7 | 31 | |
| Ningxia | 120 | | 22 | 37 | 61 | 77 | 4 | 4 | 2 | 33 | |
| Xinjiang | 457 | 1 | 37 | 314 | 105 | 328 | 36 | 5 | 8 | 80 | |

## All-region Hospital Grade in 2016

| Region | Total | Class Three | Grade One | Grade Two | Grade Three | Class Two | Grade One | Grade Two | Grade Three | Class One | Grade One | Grade Two | Grade Three | Not Evaluated |
|---|---|---|---|---|---|---|---|---|---|---|---|---|---|---|
| **Total** | **29140** | **2232** | **1308** | **433** | **36** | **7944** | **4245** | **1537** | **86** | **9282** | **2349** | **631** | **238** | **9682** |
| East Region | 11221 | 1051 | 599 | 188 | 20 | 2765 | 1451 | 432 | 51 | 4017 | 974 | 232 | 177 | 3388 |
| Central Region | 8500 | 596 | 386 | 69 | 11 | 2521 | 1292 | 565 | 25 | 2734 | 835 | 236 | 43 | 2649 |
| West Region | 9419 | 585 | 323 | 176 | 5 | 258 | 1502 | 540 | 10 | 2531 | 540 | 163 | 18 | 3645 |
| Beijing | 638 | 93 | 54 | 1 | 14 | 126 | 39 | 4 | 30 | 394 | 43 | 1 | 148 | 25 |
| Tianjin | 421 | 42 | 31 | 4 | | 58 | 24 | 13 | 9 | 197 | 42 | 7 | 1 | 124 |
| Hebei | 1618 | 69 | 44 | 1 | | 482 | 313 | 50 | 4 | 825 | 171 | 26 | 7 | 242 |
| Shanxi | 1393 | 58 | 41 | 12 | | 341 | 211 | 76 | 1 | 331 | 159 | 52 | 5 | 663 |
| Inner Mongolia | 720 | 67 | 23 | 19 | 4 | 272 | 93 | 93 | 3 | 263 | 41 | 11 | 1 | 118 |
| Liaoning | 1190 | 124 | 64 | 21 | 2 | 287 | 160 | 50 | 1 | 438 | 105 | 18 | 7 | 341 |
| Jilin | 662 | 46 | 29 | 8 | 9 | 216 | 97 | 91 | 10 | 108 | 39 | 20 | 4 | 292 |
| Heilongjiang | 1031 | 92 | 65 | 13 | 2 | 345 | 135 | 150 | 5 | 372 | 144 | 43 | 9 | 222 |
| Shanghai | 349 | 47 | 32 | 5 | | 105 | 58 | 24 | 1 | 11 | 7 | | | 186 |
| Jiangsu | 1678 | 149 | 69 | 46 | | 373 | 122 | 76 | 3 | 689 | 249 | 146 | 7 | 467 |
| Zhejiang | 1130 | 132 | 70 | 62 | | 222 | 123 | 91 | | 43 | 7 | 3 | 2 | 733 |
| Anhui | 1039 | 66 | 41 | 9 | | 317 | 144 | 42 | 1 | 411 | 87 | 45 | 1 | 245 |
| Fujian | 587 | 64 | 34 | 10 | | 192 | 89 | 58 | | 313 | 20 | 2 | 1 | 18 |
| Jiangxi | 592 | 59 | 44 | 9 | | 213 | 168 | 26 | | 90 | 18 | 6 | 2 | 230 |
| Shandong | 2018 | 150 | 83 | 34 | 1 | 495 | 257 | 52 | 3 | 712 | 193 | 21 | 2 | 661 |
| Henan | 1596 | 86 | 51 | 1 | | 456 | 199 | 67 | 4 | 822 | 210 | 34 | 9 | 232 |
| Hubei | 927 | 121 | 72 | 14 | | 301 | 151 | 60 | 2 | 251 | 70 | 15 | 8 | 245 |
| Hunan | 1260 | 68 | 43 | 3 | | 332 | 187 | 53 | 2 | 349 | 108 | 21 | 5 | 511 |
| Guangdong | 1381 | 162 | 108 | 4 | | 390 | 245 | 12 | | 325 | 112 | 6 | 1 | 504 |
| Guangxi | 543 | 63 | 43 | 6 | 1 | 218 | 149 | 16 | | 142 | 33 | 3 | 3 | 120 |
| Hainan | 211 | 19 | 10 | | 3 | 35 | 21 | 2 | | 70 | 25 | 2 | 1 | 87 |
| Chongqing | 699 | 34 | 27 | | | 127 | 60 | 21 | | 147 | 26 | 5 | | 391 |
| Sichuan | 2066 | 144 | 67 | 77 | | 534 | 285 | 185 | | 266 | 111 | 58 | | 1122 |
| Guizhou | 1220 | 49 | 29 | 4 | | 246 | 123 | 22 | 1 | 512 | 19 | 43 | 3 | 413 |
| Yunnan | 1187 | 67 | 34 | 16 | | 337 | 193 | 46 | 1 | 211 | 15 | 11 | 4 | 572 |
| Tibet | 145 | 7 | 2 | 5 | | 11 | 6 | 4 | | 87 | 53 | 2 | 2 | 40 |
| Shaanxi | 1085 | 54 | 34 | 17 | | 333 | 197 | 89 | 3 | 290 | 60 | 14 | | 408 |
| Gansu | 446 | 36 | 17 | 18 | | 184 | 152 | 14 | | 42 | 9 | 3 | | 184 |
| Qinghai | 199 | 16 | 10 | 6 | | 92 | 65 | 18 | 1 | | | | | 91 |
| Ningxia | 190 | 13 | 6 | 7 | | 71 | 36 | 3 | | 44 | 5 | | 1 | 62 |
| Xinjiang | 919 | 35 | 31 | 1 | | 233 | 143 | 29 | 1 | 527 | 168 | 13 | 4 | 124 |

## Grassroots Medical Health Institution Numbers (Registration Type/ Host Unit/Management Type/Class/Institution Type)

| Institution Type | 2010 | 2012 | 2013 | 2014 | 2015 | 2016 |
|---|---|---|---|---|---|---|
| **Total** | **901709** | **912620** | **915368** | **917335** | **920770** | **926518** |
| Registration Type | | | | | | |
|   Public Operation | 460927 | 475544 | 487802 | 491885 | 495986 | 502619 |
|   Private Operation | 440782 | 437076 | 427566 | 425450 | 424784 | 423899 |
| Host Unit | | | | | | |
|   Government Operation | 111290 | 119661 | 117765 | 116948 | 117503 | 117421 |
|   Society Operation | 470858 | 473095 | 476868 | 471722 | 472631 | 471008 |
|   Private Operation | 319561 | 319864 | 320735 | 328665 | 330636 | 338089 |
| Management Type | | | | | | |
|   Non-profit | 675760 | 692158 | 694827 | 695290 | 691375 | 69119 |
|   Profit | 225949 | 220462 | 220541 | 222045 | 229395 | 235392 |
| Institution Class | | | | | | |
|   Community Health Service Center (Station) | 32739 | 33562 | 33965 | 34238 | 34321 | 34327 |
|     Community Health Service Center | 6903 | 8182 | 8488 | 8669 | 8806 | 8918 |
|     Community Health Service Station | 25836 | 25380 | 25477 | 25569 | 25515 | 25409 |
|   Health Center | 38765 | 37707 | 37608 | 37497 | 37341 | 37241 |
|     District Health Center | 929 | 610 | 593 | 595 | 524 | 446 |
|     Township Health Center | 37836 | 37097 | 37015 | 36902 | 36817 | 36795 |
|   Village Health Room | 648424 | 653419 | 648619 | 645470 | 640536 | 638763 |
|   Outpatient Department | 8291 | 10134 | 11126 | 12030 | 13282 | 14779 |
|   Clinic (Infirmary) | 173434 | 177798 | 184050 | 188100 | 195290 | 201408 |

## All-region Community Health Service Center (Station) Numbers Grouped by Number of Beds in 2016

| Region | Community Health Service Center | | | | | | | Community Health Service Station | | | |
|---|---|---|---|---|---|---|---|---|---|---|---|
| | Total | 0 | 1-9 | 10-29 | 30-49 | 50-99 | 100 and above | Total | 0 | 1-9 | 10 and above |
| **Total** | **8918** | **4110** | **492** | **1830** | **1164** | **1051** | **271** | **25409** | **23224** | **1561** | **624** |
| East Region | 4266 | 2231 | 178 | 690 | 513 | 502 | 152 | 15767 | 14883 | 603 | 281 |
| Central Region | 2529 | 920 | 158 | 667 | 380 | 335 | 69 | 5222 | 4569 | 503 | 150 |
| West Region | 2123 | 959 | 156 | 473 | 271 | 214 | 50 | 4420 | 3772 | 455 | 193 |
| Beijing | 324 | 159 | 44 | 72 | 24 | 18 | 7 | 1591 | 1591 | | |
| Tianjin | 114 | 50 | | 17 | 12 | 33 | 2 | 471 | 471 | | |
| Hebei | 280 | 57 | 30 | 102 | 60 | 29 | 2 | 917 | 514 | 230 | 173 |
| Shanxi | 231 | 107 | 17 | 66 | 27 | 13 | 1 | 698 | 592 | 82 | 24 |
| Inner Mongolia | 314 | 145 | 33 | 83 | 33 | 19 | 1 | 881 | 795 | 67 | 19 |
| Liaoning | 378 | 247 | 8 | 54 | 23 | 33 | 13 | 787 | 786 | 1 | |
| Jilin | 207 | 104 | 16 | 43 | 22 | 21 | 1 | 188 | 139 | 41 | 8 |
| Heilongjiang | 440 | 217 | 42 | 92 | 47 | 37 | 5 | 213 | 152 | 33 | 28 |
| Shanghai | 307 | 105 | 2 | 19 | 43 | 84 | 54 | 732 | 732 | | |
| Jiangsu | 544 | 144 | 5 | 116 | 131 | 118 | 30 | 2116 | 2044 | 71 | 1 |
| Zhejiang | 467 | 238 | 41 | 79 | 63 | 38 | 8 | 5404 | 5398 | 5 | 1 |
| Anhui | 404 | 154 | 28 | 123 | 50 | 41 | 8 | 1504 | 1504 | | |
| Fujian | 222 | 105 | 10 | 66 | 23 | 17 | 1 | 333 | 329 | 3 | 1 |
| Jiangxi | 168 | 55 | 17 | 57 | 26 | 11 | 2 | 423 | 273 | 131 | 19 |
| Shandong | 518 | 219 | 16 | 107 | 82 | 73 | 21 | 1792 | 1421 | 270 | 101 |
| Henan | 424 | 148 | 14 | 105 | 86 | 62 | 9 | 905 | 787 | 87 | 31 |
| Hubei | 342 | 80 | 5 | 65 | 61 | 102 | 29 | 889 | 818 | 54 | 17 |
| Hunan | 313 | 55 | 19 | 116 | 61 | 48 | 14 | 402 | 304 | 75 | 23 |
| Guangdong | 1082 | 892 | 22 | 53 | 50 | 52 | 13 | 1484 | 1481 | 2 | 1 |
| Guangxi | 150 | 101 | 6 | 22 | 12 | 8 | 1 | 129 | 126 | 3 | |
| Hainan | 30 | 15 | | 5 | 2 | 7 | 1 | 140 | 116 | 21 | 3 |
| Chongqing | 199 | 63 | | 29 | 37 | 47 | 23 | 297 | 292 | 4 | 1 |
| Sichuan | 413 | 150 | 25 | 111 | 61 | 56 | 10 | 538 | 422 | 60 | 56 |
| Guizhou | 167 | 64 | 18 | 40 | 25 | 19 | 1 | 468 | 468 | | |
| Yunnan | 189 | 77 | 16 | 34 | 31 | 27 | 4 | 377 | 290 | 59 | 28 |
| Tibet | 8 | 1 | 5 | 2 | | | | 2 | 1 | 1 | |
| Shaanxi | 249 | 141 | 19 | 44 | 31 | 13 | 1 | 374 | 338 | 25 | 11 |
| Gansu | 201 | 85 | 27 | 54 | 21 | 13 | 1 | 380 | 255 | 80 | 45 |
| Qinghai | 30 | 13 | 5 | 5 | 3 | 2 | 2 | 205 | 108 | 85 | 12 |
| Ningxia | 18 | 13 | | 4 | | 1 | | 124 | 97 | 22 | 5 |
| Xinjiang | 185 | 106 | 2 | 45 | 17 | 9 | 6 | 645 | 580 | 49 | 16 |

## Village Health Room Numbers

| Year and Region | Village Health Room | | | | | | Administrative Village Number | Percentage of Village Health Point in Administrative Village |
|---|---|---|---|---|---|---|---|---|
| | Total | Village Operation | Township Health Center Point | Joint Operation | Private Operation | Others | | |
| 1990 | 803956 | 266137 | 29963 | 87149 | 381844 | 38863 | 743278 | 86.2 |
| 1995 | 804352 | 297462 | 36388 | 90681 | 354981 | 22876 | 740150 | 88.9 |
| 2000 | 709458 | 300864 | 47101 | 89828 | 255179 | 16486 | 734715 | 89.8 |
| 2005 | 583209 | 313633 | 32396 | 38561 | 180403 | 18216 | 629079 | 85.8 |
| 2010 | 648424 | 365153 | 49678 | 32650 | 177080 | 23863 | 594658 | 92.3 |
| 2012 | 653419 | 370099 | 58317 | 32278 | 167025 | 25700 | 588475 | 93.3 |
| 2013 | 648619 | 371579 | 59896 | 32690 | 158811 | 25643 | 589447 | 93.0 |
| 2014 | 645470 | 349428 | 59396 | 29180 | 160549 | 46917 | 585451 | 93.3 |
| 2015 | 640536 | 353196 | 60231 | 29208 | 153353 | 44548 | 580575 | 93.3 |
| 2016 | 638763 | 351016 | 60419 | 29336 | 152164 | 45828 | 559166 | 92.9 |
| East Region | 215845 | 116014 | 25193 | 8594 | 53268 | 12776 | 222585 | 82.2 |
| Central Region | 222158 | 130912 | 13196 | 12531 | 48919 | 16600 | 173965 | 99.8 |
| West Region | 200760 | 104090 | 22030 | 8211 | 49977 | 16452 | 162616 | 100.0 |
| Beijing | 2729 | 2419 | 7 | 3 | 278 | 22 | 3941 | 69.2 |
| Tianjin | 2528 | 850 | 724 | 122 | 264 | 568 | 3681 | 68.7 |
| Hebei | 60371 | 28727 | 2111 | 1030 | 25138 | 3365 | 48863 | 100.0 |
| Shanxi | 29027 | 19734 | 1024 | 724 | 3652 | 3893 | 28106 | 100.0 |
| Inner Mongolia | 13632 | 5235 | 2132 | 481 | 4867 | 917 | 11078 | 100.0 |
| Liaoning | 20120 | 8692 | 379 | 158 | 10259 | 632 | 11555 | 100.0 |
| Jilin | 10172 | 4063 | 1382 | 1256 | 2982 | 489 | 9327 | 100.0 |
| Heilongjiang | 11384 | 7551 | 1679 | 169 | 1474 | 511 | 9050 | 100.0 |
| Shanghai | 1218 | 913 | 190 | 31 | | 84 | 1590 | 76.6 |
| Jiangsu | 15475 | 8409 | 4062 | 1983 | 23 | 998 | 14477 | 100.0 |
| Zhejiang | 11677 | 7241 | 1319 | 157 | 2010 | 950 | 27568 | 42.4 |
| Anhui | 15276 | 7146 | 2784 | 1923 | 928 | 2495 | 14586 | 100.0 |
| Fujian | 18945 | 11592 | 499 | 231 | 4704 | 1919 | 14407 | 100.0 |
| Jiangxi | 30394 | 13929 | 265 | 1585 | 12935 | 1680 | 17046 | 100.0 |
| Shandong | 53226 | 26732 | 14224 | 4693 | 4202 | 3375 | 74217 | 71.7 |
| Henan | 56774 | 33534 | 814 | 2844 | 16548 | 3034 | 46831 | 100.0 |
| Hubei | 24792 | 15499 | 3603 | 2984 | 1860 | 846 | 25064 | 98.9 |
| Hunan | 44339 | 29456 | 1645 | 1046 | 8540 | 3652 | 23955 | 100.0 |
| Guangdong | 26886 | 19582 | 1533 | 156 | 4917 | 698 | 19734 | 100.0 |
| Guangxi | 21011 | 13638 | 852 | 180 | 5467 | 874 | 14276 | 100.0 |
| Hainan | 2670 | 857 | 145 | 30 | 1473 | 165 | 2552 | 100.0 |
| Chongqing | 11240 | 6763 | 1257 | 357 | 1653 | 1210 | 8064 | 100.0 |
| Sichuan | 55958 | 27024 | 2931 | 2478 | 18950 | 4575 | 45922 | 100.0 |
| Guizhou | 20652 | 9115 | 2170 | 530 | 6868 | 1969 | 14619 | 100.0 |
| Yunnan | 13432 | 10064 | 1319 | 607 | 465 | 977 | 11971 | 100.0 |
| Tibet | 5360 | 1692 | 2478 | 150 | | 1040 | 5259 | 100.0 |
| Shaanxi | 25412 | 19645 | 652 | 455 | 4020 | 640 | 20277 | 100.0 |
| Gansu | 16748 | 6829 | 1637 | 995 | 5316 | 1971 | 16027 | 100.0 |
| Qinghai | 4518 | 1651 | 522 | 538 | 1057 | 750 | 4146 | 100.0 |
| Ningxia | 2365 | 721 | 345 | 207 | 757 | 335 | 2275 | 100.0 |
| Xinjiang | 10432 | 1713 | 5735 | 1233 | 557 | 1194 | 8702 | 100.0 |

Note: Administrative village number is the number of village committee.

## Professional Medical Health Institution Numbers
### (Registration Type/Host Unit/Institution Type)

| Institution Type | 2010 | 2012 | 2013 | 2014 | 2015 | 2016 |
|---|---|---|---|---|---|---|
| **Total** | **11835** | **12083** | **31155** | **35029** | **31927** | **24866** |
| Registration Type | | | | | | |
| Public Operation | 11764 | 12004 | 30824 | 34382 | 31582 | 24568 |
| Private Operation | 71 | 79 | 331 | 401 | 345 | 298 |
| Host Unit | | | | | | |
| Government Operation | 11421 | 11642 | 28269 | 31140 | 29019 | 22859 |
| Society Operation | 396 | 421 | 2858 | 3617 | 2880 | 1969 |
| Private Operation | 18 | 20 | 28 | 26 | 28 | 38 |
| Institution Class | | | | | | |
| Disease Prevention and Control Center | 3513 | 3490 | 3516 | 3490 | 3478 | 3481 |
| Special Disease Prevention and Control Agency | 1274 | 1289 | 1271 | 1242 | 1234 | 1213 |
| Health Education Institution (Station) | 139 | 160 | 169 | 172 | 166 | 163 |
| Maternal and Child Care Center(Institution/Station) | 3025 | 3044 | 3144 | 3098 | 3078 | 3063 |
| First Aid Center (Station) | 245 | 295 | 312 | 325 | 345 | 355 |
| Blood Collecting and Supplying Institution | 530 | 531 | 538 | 541 | 548 | 552 |
| Health Supervision Institution (Center) | 2992 | 3088 | 2967 | 2975 | 2986 | 2986 |
| Family Planning Technique Service Institution | 117 | 186 | 19238 | 23186 | 20092 | 13053 |

Note: In 2013, family planning technique service institutions under former family planning department are included. Because of the villages and towns merge, the family planning and maternity care institutions merge, the family planning technique service institutions declined in the number.

## All-type Personnel in Medical

| Institution Type | Total | Health Technical Worker | | | |
|---|---|---|---|---|---|
| | | Subtotal | Certified (Assistant) | | Registered Nurse |
| | | | Certified Practitioner | Certified Practitioner | |
| **Total** | **11172945** | **8454403** | **3191005** | **2651398** | **3507166** |
| I. Hospital | 6542137 | 5415066 | 1803462 | 1680062 | 2613367 |
| Comprehensive Hospital | 4682477 | 3916565 | 1296844 | 1214397 | 1924425 |
| TCM Hospital | 884394 | 745725 | 265257 | 244641 | 320769 |
| Hospital of Traditional Chinese and Western Medicine | 105358 | 88059 | 31900 | 29835 | 39864 |
| National Hospital | 26167 | 21541 | 8256 | 6970 | 7080 |
| Specialty Hospital | 828863 | 633767 | 199061 | 182386 | 315900 |
| Stomatological Hospital | 48841 | 38796 | 17952 | 16349 | 15370 |
| Ophthalmic Hospital | 49160 | 31550 | 9932 | 9045 | 15431 |
| Otolaryngology Hospital | 7178 | 5461 | 1865 | 1669 | 2606 |
| Tumor Hospital | 82153 | 67418 | 20812 | 20351 | 34226 |
| Cardiovascular Hospital | 19845 | 16233 | 4938 | 4584 | 8307 |
| Thoracopathy Hospital | 10616 | 8905 | 2664 | 2624 | 4933 |
| Hematonosis Hospital | 1735 | 1317 | 284 | 267 | 714 |
| Obstetrical and Gynecological Hospital | 98251 | 73066 | 23271 | 21364 | 37460 |
| Children's Hospital | 61643 | 52225 | 15766 | 15522 | 26938 |
| Mental Hospital | 149039 | 113403 | 29704 | 26747 | 62980 |
| Infectious Disease Hospital | 55452 | 44546 | 13388 | 13045 | 22624 |
| Dermatology Hospital | 10454 | 7519 | 2493 | 2251 | 3254 |
| Tuberculosis Hospital | 11178 | 8897 | 2560 | 2491 | 4742 |
| Leprosy Hospital | 754 | 506 | 213 | 156 | 144 |
| Occupational Disease Hospital | 4791 | 3566 | 1267 | 1221 | 1557 |
| Orthopaedic Hospital | 47984 | 37826 | 12507 | 10316 | 17359 |
| Rehabilitation Hospital | 43807 | 32503 | 9514 | 8231 | 13736 |
| Plastic Surgery Hospital | 5035 | 2960 | 975 | 891 | 1621 |
| Cosmetic Hospital | 19692 | 9842 | 3462 | 3053 | 5102 |
| Other Specialty Hospital | 101255 | 77228 | 25494 | 22209 | 36796 |
| Nursing Hospital | 14878 | 9409 | 2144 | 1833 | 5329 |
| II. Grassroots Medical Health Institution | 3682561 | 2354430 | 1145408 | 764867 | 695781 |
| Community Health Service Center (Station) | 521974 | 446176 | 187699 | 151673 | 162132 |
| Community Health Service Center | 410693 | 347718 | 143217 | 115078 | 122881 |
| Community Health Service Station | 111281 | 98458 | 44482 | 36595 | 39251 |
| Health Center | 1330995 | 1124431 | 458797 | 265301 | 321080 |
| District Health Center | 10154 | 8510 | 3802 | 2399 | 2471 |
| Township Health Hospital | 1320841 | 1115921 | 454995 | 262902 | 318609 |
| Central Health Center | 566880 | 483319 | 194419 | 119596 | 144057 |
| Township Health Center | 753961 | 632602 | 260576 | 143306 | 174552 |
| Village Health Room | 1169224 | 168900 | 147754 | 48483 | 21146 |
| Outpatient Department | 181664 | 149644 | 74473 | 65799 | 53354 |
| Comprehensive Outpatient Department | 95520 | 80314 | 38690 | 34931 | 28355 |
| TCM Outpatient Department | 21015 | 16206 | 9372 | 8785 | 3203 |
| Outpatient Department of Traditional Chinese and Western Medicine | 4125 | 3617 | 1842 | 1671 | 1175 |
| National Medical Outpatient Department | 137 | 104 | 60 | 49 | 25 |
| Specialty Outpatient Department | 60867 | 49403 | 24509 | 20363 | 20596 |
| Clinic, Health Clinic, Infirmary and Nursing Station | 478704 | 465279 | 276685 | 233611 | 138069 |
| Clinic | 395175 | 384686 | 230539 | 196357 | 114097 |
| Health Clinic and Infirmary | 83062 | 80244 | 46051 | 37175 | 23730 |
| Nursing Station | 467 | 349 | 95 | 79 | 242 |

Notes: ①Total number of health workers includes 10,000 civil servants with "Health Supervisor" Certification and 1,000,324 village doctors and health workers; ②The number of health workers in village health room of this Table excludes health workers of township health centers working in village health

## Health Institutions in 2016

| Senior Pharmacist (Assistant Pharmacist) | Technician(Assistant Technician) | Docimaster (Lab Assistant) | Others | Medical Intern | Other Technician | Other Technician | Ground Skilled Staff |
|---|---|---|---|---|---|---|---|
| 439246 | 453185 | 308873 | 863801 | 220964 | 426171 | 483198 | 808849 |
| 278730 | 291553 | 188473 | 427954 | 151488 | 267460 | 320158 | 539453 |
| 184705 | 211095 | 136758 | 299496 | 109410 | 177946 | 217440 | 370526 |
| 56685 | 39556 | 24858 | 63458 | 24396 | 35672 | 36052 | 66945 |
| 5244 | 4433 | 2928 | 6618 | 2010 | 4160 | 5377 | 7762 |
| 2038 | 1077 | 651 | 3090 | 908 | 1474 | 1253 | 1899 |
| 29641 | 35084 | 23093 | 54081 | 14482 | 47563 | 59151 | 88382 |
| 685 | 950 | 362 | 3839 | 1059 | 2342 | 3321 | 4382 |
| 1408 | 1208 | 882 | 3571 | 870 | 4439 | 5668 | 7503 |
| 307 | 292 | 166 | 391 | 132 | 350 | 643 | 724 |
| 2978 | 4060 | 2029 | 5342 | 1270 | 4367 | 4461 | 5907 |
| 606 | 801 | 495 | 1581 | 415 | 898 | 1293 | 1421 |
| 409 | 567 | 361 | 332 | 84 | 650 | 545 | 516 |
| 62 | 117 | 105 | 140 | 50 | 144 | 182 | 92 |
| 3097 | 4918 | 3481 | 4320 | 1246 | 5674 | 7382 | 12129 |
| 2612 | 3154 | 2332 | 3755 | 1228 | 2729 | 3128 | 3561 |
| 5447 | 4636 | 3225 | 10636 | 3144 | 7834 | 9486 | 18316 |
| 2680 | 3342 | 2518 | 2512 | 858 | 3099 | 3587 | 4220 |
| 739 | 507 | 451 | 526 | 118 | 703 | 878 | 1354 |
| 438 | 670 | 482 | 487 | 180 | 604 | 667 | 1010 |
| 53 | 45 | 43 | 51 | 13 | 48 | 74 | 126 |
| 181 | 263 | 214 | 298 | 77 | 486 | 317 | 422 |
| 1796 | 2419 | 1189 | 3745 | 1201 | 2214 | 3125 | 4819 |
| 1570 | 1544 | 958 | 6139 | 777 | 2811 | 3374 | 5119 |
| 103 | 110 | 73 | 151 | 21 | 580 | 463 | 1032 |
| 402 | 435 | 336 | 441 | 158 | 2571 | 2668 | 4611 |
| 4068 | 5046 | 3391 | 5824 | 1581 | 5020 | 7889 | 11118 |
| 417 | 308 | 185 | 1211 | 282 | 645 | 885 | 3939 |
| 138060 | 92884 | 60988 | 282297 | 55136 | 86635 | 73476 | 167696 |
| 34638 | 21074 | 15072 | 40633 | 9253 | 21569 | 21350 | 32879 |
| 28859 | 18982 | 13477 | 33779 | 8175 | 17818 | 16175 | 28982 |
| 5779 | 2092 | 1595 | 6854 | 1078 | 3751 | 5175 | 3897 |
| 76813 | 61844 | 39023 | 205897 | 39817 | 60840 | 43021 | 102703 |
| 593 | 437 | 280 | 1207 | 230 | 469 | 468 | 707 |
| 76220 | 61407 | 38743 | 204690 | 39587 | 60371 | 42553 | 101996 |
| 33081 | 28543 | 17625 | 83219 | 18028 | 23417 | 16570 | 43574 |
| 43139 | 32864 | 21118 | 121471 | 21559 | 36954 | 25983 | 58422 |
|  |  |  |  |  |  |  |  |
| 8110 | 7713 | 5345 | 5994 | 1345 | 4052 | 8673 | 19295 |
| 4722 | 5588 | 3815 | 2959 | 477 | 1882 | 3982 | 9342 |
| 2124 | 559 | 451 | 948 | 269 | 542 | 1153 | 3114 |
| 272 | 212 | 144 | 116 | 21 | 75 | 125 | 308 |
| 10 | 4 | 2 | 5 | 2 | 8 | 5 | 20 |
| 982 | 1350 | 933 | 1966 | 576 | 1545 | 3408 | 6511 |
| 18499 | 2253 | 1548 | 29773 | 4721 | 174 | 432 | 12819 |
| 16235 | 1401 | 882 | 22414 | 3907 | 70 | 274 | 10145 |
| 2262 | 851 | 665 | 7350 | 810 | 75 | 143 | 2600 |
| 2 | 1 | 1 | 9 | 4 | 29 | 15 | 74 |

rooms (They are included into township health centers).

| Institution Type | Total | Health Technical Worker | | | |
|---|---|---|---|---|---|
| | | Subtotal | Certified (Assistant) | | Registered Nurse |
| | | | Practitioner | Certified Practitioner | |
| III. Professional Public Health Institution | 870652 | 646425 | 229484 | 195871 | 189435 |
| Disease Prevention and Control Center | 191627 | 142492 | 70734 | 60322 | 14488 |
| Provincial Ownership | 10852 | 7702 | 3955 | 3867 | 193 |
| Prefecture-level City (Region) Ownership | 43465 | 32784 | 17347 | 16289 | 2275 |
| County-level City (District) Ownership | 59241 | 44091 | 21822 | 18519 | 4990 |
| County Ownership | 70733 | 52570 | 25107 | 19505 | 6414 |
| Others Ownership | 7336 | 5345 | 2503 | 2142 | 616 |
| Special Disease Prevention and Treatment Center (Institution, Station) | 50486 | 38941 | 16186 | 13708 | 12323 |
| Special Disease Prevention and Treatment Center | 19832 | 15457 | 5800 | 5203 | 6098 |
| Infectious Disease Prevention and Treatment Center | 1644 | 1217 | 377 | 344 | 591 |
| Tuberculosis Prevention and Treatment Center | 3455 | 2731 | 841 | 788 | 1327 |
| Occupational Disease Prevention and Treatment Center | 5730 | 4311 | 1695 | 1630 | 1576 |
| Others | 9003 | 7198 | 2887 | 2441 | 2604 |
| Special Disease Prevention and Treatment Institution (Station, Center) | 30654 | 23484 | 10386 | 8505 | 6225 |
| Stomatology Disease Prevention and Treatment Institution (Station, Center) | 2335 | 1913 | 1063 | 889 | 486 |
| Mental Disease Prevention and Treatment Institution (Station, Center) | 1176 | 985 | 347 | 243 | 464 |
| Dermatosis and Venereal Disease Prevention and Treatment Institution (Station, Center) | 6304 | 4748 | 1981 | 1693 | 1332 |
| Tuberculosis Prevention and Treatment Institution (Station, Center) | 8990 | 6747 | 2738 | 2273 | 1686 |
| Occupational Disease Prevention and Treatment Institution (Station, Center) | 2178 | 1682 | 812 | 767 | 313 |
| Endemic Disease Prevention and Treatment Institution (Station, Center) | 837 | 606 | 325 | 284 | 52 |
| Schistosomiasis Prevention and Treatment Institution (Station, Center) | 5412 | 4216 | 1966 | 1499 | 1138 |
| Drug Rehabilitation Institution (Station, Center) | 283 | 148 | 66 | 48 | 43 |
| Others | 3139 | 2439 | 1088 | 809 | 711 |
| Health Education Institution (Station, Center) | 2070 | 915 | 434 | 377 | 118 |
| Maternal and Child Care Center (Institution, Station) | 388238 | 320748 | 116524 | 103360 | 138266 |
| Provincial Ownership | 20481 | 17099 | 5416 | 5404 | 8733 |
| Prefecture-level City (Region) Ownership | 114049 | 94853 | 31563 | 30478 | 45185 |
| County-level City (District) Ownership | 119905 | 98836 | 36927 | 33002 | 41484 |
| County Ownership | 125905 | 103400 | 40283 | 32423 | 39794 |
| Others | 7898 | 6560 | 2335 | 2053 | 3070 |
| Maternal and Child Care Center | 348716 | 289191 | 100505 | 89699 | 129821 |
| Maternal and Child Care Institution | 21678 | 17345 | 9037 | 8041 | 4446 |
| Maternal and Child Care Station | 16979 | 13552 | 6600 | 5311 | 3820 |
| Reproduction Health Center | 865 | 660 | 382 | 309 | 179 |
| First Aid Center (Station) | 15858 | 8301 | 3671 | 3386 | 3362 |
| Blood Collecting and Supplying Institution | 34061 | 24546 | 3712 | 3196 | 11900 |
| Health Supervision Institution (Center) | 81522 | 68165 | | | |
| Provincial Ownership | 2579 | 2133 | | | |
| Prefecture-level City (Region) Ownership | 16023 | 13437 | | | |
| County-level City (District) Ownership | 25360 | 20616 | | | |
| County Ownership | 27091 | 21569 | | | |
| Others | 469 | 410 | | | |
| Family Planning Technique Service Institution | 106790 | 42317 | 18223 | 11522 | 8978 |
| IV. Other Medical Health Institution | 77595 | 38482 | 12651 | 10598 | 8583 |
| Sanatorium | 14329 | 8804 | 3001 | 2698 | 3951 |
| Health Supervision and Testing (Monitoring) Institution | 620 | 247 | 88 | 82 | 5 |
| Medical Science Research Institution | 11127 | 5977 | 1983 | 1916 | 628 |
| In-service Medical Training Institution | 12597 | 5791 | 2096 | 1636 | 1290 |
| Clinical Testing Center (Institution, Station) | 13978 | 6729 | 735 | 668 | 233 |
| Statistical Information Center | 1235 | 71 | 29 | 29 | 6 |
| Others | 23709 | 10863 | 4719 | 3569 | 2470 |

*Continued*

| Senior Pharmacist (Assistant Pharmacist) | Technician(Assistant Technician) | Docimaster (Lab Assistant) | Others | Medical Intern | Other Technician | Managerial Worker | Ground Skilled Staff |
|---|---|---|---|---|---|---|---|
| 20849 | 63428 | 54607 | 143229 | 13725 | 57315 | 77235 | 89677 |
| 2790 | 27346 | 25504 | 27134 | 2654 | 14741 | 13978 | 20416 |
| 100 | 1963 | 1929 | 1491 | 76 | 1317 | 794 | 1039 |
| 474 | 8347 | 8049 | 4341 | 776 | 3388 | 3455 | 3838 |
| 920 | 7807 | 7264 | 8552 | 691 | 4263 | 4483 | 6404 |
| 1226 | 8460 | 7550 | 11363 | 997 | 4846 | 4647 | 8670 |
| 70 | 769 | 712 | 1387 | 114 | 927 | 599 | 465 |
| 2736 | 3700 | 2854 | 3996 | 765 | 3267 | 3337 | 4941 |
| 1004 | 1328 | 1047 | 1227 | 373 | 1321 | 1180 | 1874 |
| 63 | 83 | 73 | 103 | 25 | 108 | 42 | 277 |
| 149 | 246 | 178 | 168 | 79 | 164 | 282 | 278 |
| 254 | 455 | 373 | 331 | 107 | 530 | 400 | 489 |
| 538 | 544 | 423 | 625 | 162 | 519 | 456 | 830 |
| 1732 | 2372 | 1807 | 2769 | 392 | 1946 | 2157 | 3067 |
| 29 | 31 | 13 | 304 | 29 | 129 | 146 | 147 |
| 47 | 26 | 18 | 101 | 13 | 101 | 42 | 48 |
| 597 | 414 | 378 | 424 | 111 | 354 | 423 | 779 |
| 495 | 962 | 647 | 866 | 106 | 674 | 746 | 823 |
| 52 | 251 | 198 | 254 | 21 | 190 | 147 | 159 |
| 25 | 75 | 68 | 129 | 12 | 33 | 70 | 128 |
| 245 | 404 | 323 | 463 | 31 | 284 | 298 | 614 |
| 9 | 17 | 11 | 13 | 3 | 3 | 117 | 15 |
| 233 | 192 | 151 | 215 | 66 | 178 | 168 | 354 |
| 40 | 23 | 19 | 300 | 15 | 616 | 365 | 174 |
| 13468 | 23154 | 17984 | 29336 | 8880 | 18139 | 18290 | 31061 |
| 606 | 1328 | 1136 | 1016 | 468 | 1000 | 829 | 1553 |
| 3809 | 6427 | 5279 | 7869 | 2662 | 5378 | 5722 | 8096 |
| 4319 | 7296 | 5654 | 8810 | 2751 | 5651 | 5603 | 9815 |
| 4496 | 7707 | 5612 | 11120 | 2903 | 5789 | 5689 | 11027 |
| 238 | 396 | 303 | 521 | 96 | 321 | 447 | 570 |
| 12220 | 20333 | 15748 | 26312 | 8298 | 15791 | 15430 | 28304 |
| 711 | 1756 | 1437 | 1395 | 372 | 1298 | 1502 | 1533 |
| 516 | 1008 | 756 | 1608 | 203 | 993 | 1286 | 1148 |
| 21 | 57 | 43 | 21 | 7 | 57 | 72 | 76 |
| 125 | 98 | 70 | 1045 | 520 | 1101 | 1361 | 5095 |
| 304 | 6136 | 6094 | 2494 | 149 | 3042 | 2114 | 4359 |
|  |  |  | 68165 |  | 2056 | 6242 | 5059 |
|  |  |  | 2133 |  | 45 | 248 | 153 |
|  |  |  | 13437 |  | 361 | 1352 | 873 |
|  |  |  | 20616 |  | 835 | 2168 | 1741 |
|  |  |  | 21569 |  | 815 | 2422 | 2285 |
|  |  |  | 410 |  |  | 52 | 7 |
| 1386 | 2971 | 2082 | 10759 | 742 | 14353 | 31548 | 18572 |
| 1607 | 5320 | 4805 | 10321 | 615 | 14761 | 12329 | 12023 |
| 463 | 554 | 382 | 835 | 209 | 932 | 1679 | 2914 |
| 0 | 110 | 108 | 44 | 0 | 54 | 71 | 248 |
| 278 | 465 | 400 | 2623 | 51 | 3022 | 1274 | 854 |
| 383 | 262 | 173 | 1760 | 64 | 3480 | 1624 | 1702 |
| 6 | 3376 | 3354 | 2379 | 73 | 2310 | 1575 | 3364 |
| 8 |  |  | 28 |  | 699 | 389 | 76 |
| 469 | 553 | 388 | 2652 | 218 | 4264 | 5717 | 2865 |

*453*

## Health Worker Numbers

| Year | Health Worker | Health Technical Worker | | | | | | Village Doctor and Health Worker | Other Technician | Managerial Worker | Ground Skilled Staff |
|------|------|------|------|------|------|------|------|------|------|------|------|
| | | | Certified (Assistant) | | Registered Nurse | Senior Pharmacist (Assistant Pharmacist) | Docimaster (Lab Assistant) | | | | |
| | | | Practitioner | Certified Practitioner | | | | | | | |
| 1950 | 611240 | 555040 | 380800 | 327400 | 37800 | 8080 | | | | 21877 | 34323 |
| 1955 | 1052787 | 874063 | 500398 | 402409 | 107344 | 60974 | 15394 | | | 86465 | 92259 |
| 1960 | 1769205 | 1504894 | 596109 | 427498 | 170143 | 119293 | | | | 132034 | 132277 |
| 1965 | 1872300 | 1531600 | 762804 | 510091 | 234546 | 117314 | | | 10996 | 168845 | 160899 |
| 1970 | 6571795 | 1453247 | 702304 | 446251 | 295147 | ... | | 4779280 | 10813 | 156862 | 171593 |
| 1975 | 7435212 | 2057068 | 877716 | 521617 | 379545 | 219904 | 77506 | 4841695 | 14122 | 251420 | 270907 |
| 1980 | 7355483 | 2798241 | 1153234 | 709473 | 465798 | 308438 | 114290 | 3820776 | 27834 | 310805 | 397827 |
| 1985 | 5606105 | 3410910 | 1413281 | 724238 | 636974 | 365145 | 145217 | 1293094 | 46052 | 358812 | 497237 |
| 1986 | 5725854 | 3506517 | 1444150 | 745592 | 680583 | 372760 | 150132 | 1279935 | 50957 | 370056 | 518389 |
| 1987 | 5842621 | 3608618 | 1481754 | 777333 | 717596 | 382121 | 156878 | 1278499 | 57255 | 371167 | 527082 |
| 1988 | 5924557 | 3723756 | 1618174 | 1095926 | 829261 | 394287 | 161615 | 1247045 | 65063 | 368227 | 520466 |
| 1989 | 6028234 | 3809097 | 1718018 | 1257668 | 921687 | 401098 | 166383 | 1241275 | 73530 | 384890 | 519442 |
| 1990 | 6137711 | 3897921 | 1763086 | 1302997 | 974541 | 405978 | 170371 | 1231510 | 85504 | 396694 | 526082 |
| 1991 | 6278458 | 3984974 | 1779545 | 1310933 | 1011943 | 409325 | 176832 | 1253324 | 91265 | 408819 | 540076 |
| 1992 | 6409307 | 4073986 | 1808194 | 1327875 | 1039674 | 413598 | 180754 | 1269061 | 99177 | 417670 | 549413 |
| 1993 | 6540522 | 4117067 | 1831665 | 1372471 | 1056096 | 413025 | 183657 | 1325106 | 113138 | 432903 | 552311 |
| 1994 | 6630710 | 4199217 | 1882180 | 1425375 | 1093544 | 417166 | 186415 | 1323701 | 116921 | 438084 | 552787 |
| 1995 | 6704395 | 4256923 | 1917772 | 1454926 | 1125661 | 418520 | 189488 | 1331017 | 120782 | 450013 | 545660 |
| 1996 | 6735097 | 4311845 | 1941235 | 1475232 | 1162609 | 424952 | 192873 | 1316095 | 125480 | 444571 | 537106 |
| 1997 | 6833962 | 4397805 | 1984867 | 1505342 | 1198228 | 428295 | 198016 | 1317786 | 133369 | 448047 | 536955 |
| 1998 | 6863315 | 4423721 | 1999521 | 1513975 | 1218836 | 423644 | 200846 | 1327633 | 145060 | 435507 | 531394 |
| 1999 | 6894985 | 4458669 | 2044672 | 1561584 | 1244844 | 418574 | 201272 | 1324937 | 150041 | 434997 | 526341 |
| 2000 | 6910383 | 4490803 | 2075843 | 1603266 | 1266838 | 414408 | 200900 | 1319357 | 157533 | 426789 | 515901 |
| 2001 | 6874527 | 4507700 | 2099658 | 1637337 | 1286938 | 404087 | 203378 | 1290595 | 157961 | 412757 | 505514 |
| 2002 | 6528674 | 4269779 | 1843995 | 1463573 | 1246545 | 357659 | 209144 | 1290595 | 179962 | 332628 | 455710 |
| 2003 | 6216971 | 4380878 | 1942364 | 1534045 | 1265959 | 357378 | 209616 | 867778 | 199331 | 318692 | 450292 |
| 2004 | 6332739 | 4485983 | 1999457 | 1582441 | 1308433 | 355451 | 211553 | 883075 | 209422 | 315595 | 438664 |
| 2005 | 6447246 | 4564050 | 2042135 | 1622683 | 1349589 | 349533 | 211495 | 916532 | 225697 | 312826 | 428141 |
| 2006 | 6681184 | 4728350 | 2099064 | 1678030 | 1426339 | 353565 | 218771 | 957459 | 235466 | 323705 | 436204 |
| 2007 | 6964389 | 4913186 | 2122925 | 1715460 | 1558822 | 325212 | 206487 | 931761 | 243460 | 356569 | 519413 |
| 2008 | 7251803 | 5174478 | 2201904 | 1791881 | 1678091 | 330525 | 212618 | 938313 | 255149 | 356854 | 527009 |
| 2009 | 7781448 | 5535124 | 2329206 | 1905436 | 1854818 | 341910 | 220695 | 1050991 | 275006 | 362665 | 557662 |
| 2010 | 8207502 | 5876158 | 2413259 | 1972840 | 2048071 | 353916 | 230572 | 1091863 | 290161 | 370548 | 578772 |
| 2011 | 8616040 | 6202858 | 2466094 | 2020154 | 2244020 | 363993 | 238874 | 1126443 | 305981 | 374885 | 605873 |
| 2012 | 9115705 | 6675549 | 2616064 | 2138836 | 2496599 | 377398 | 249255 | 1094419 | 319117 | 372997 | 653623 |
| 2013 | 9790483 | 7210578 | 2794754 | 2285794 | 2783121 | 395578 | 266607 | 1081063 | 359819 | 420971 | 718052 |
| 2014 | 10234213 | 7589790 | 2892518 | 2374917 | 3004144 | 409595 | 279277 | 1058182 | 379740 | 451250 | 755251 |
| 2015 | 10693881 | 8007537 | 3039135 | 2508408 | 3241469 | 423294 | 293680 | 1031525 | 399712 | 472620 | 782487 |
| 2016 | 11172945 | 8454403 | 3191005 | 2651398 | 3507166 | 439246 | 293680 | 1000324 | 426171 | 483198 | 808849 |

Notes: ①Health workers and health technicians include the 10,000 civil servants with "Health Supervisor" Certification; ②In 2013, health worker number includes the ones serving in family planning service institution directly under the former health and family planning department, but the number before 2013 excludes the ones serving in family planning service institution directly under former population and family planning department; ③Certified (Assistant) practitioner number includes certified (assistant) practitioners in village health room; ④Before 1985, the number of village doctors and health workers refers to the number of barefoot doctors.

## Health Worker Numbers (in accordance with Urban & Rural Region/Registration Type/Host Unit) in 2016

| Type | Total | Health Technical Worker | | | | | | | Village Doctor and Health Worker | Other Technician | Managerial Worker | Ground Skilled Staff |
|---|---|---|---|---|---|---|---|---|---|---|---|---|
| | | Subtotal | Certified (Assistant) | | Registered Nurse | Senior Pharmacist (Assistant Pharmacist) | Docimaster (Lab Assistant) | Others | | | | |
| | | | Practitioner | Certified Practitioner | | | | | | | | |
| **Total** | **11172945** | **8454403** | **3191005** | **2651398** | **2507166** | **439246** | **453185** | **863801** | **1000324** | **426171** | **483198** | **808849** |
| Urban/Rural | | | | | | | | | | | | |
| Cities | 5487317 | 4527708 | 1647676 | 1537354 | 2063019 | 228161 | 241749 | 347103 | | 234224 | 287296 | 438089 |
| Countryside | 5675628 | 3916695 | 1543329 | 1114044 | 1444147 | 211085 | 211436 | 506698 | 1000324 | 191947 | 195902 | 370760 |
| Registration Type | | | | | | | | | | | | |
| Public | 8911762 | 6851079 | 2497032 | 2086876 | 2875221 | 364623 | 384685 | 729518 | 682967 | 360484 | 378219 | 639013 |
| State Ownership | 7630737 | 6272404 | 2199979 | 1914645 | 2714259 | 330623 | 361485 | 666058 | 71948 | 334288 | 357853 | 594244 |
| Collective Ownership | 1281025 | 578675 | 297053 | 172231 | 160962 | 34000 | 23200 | 63469 | 611019 | 26196 | 20366 | 44769 |
| Non-public | 2251183 | 1593324 | 693973 | 564522 | 631945 | 74623 | 68500 | 124283 | 317357 | 65687 | 104979 | 169836 |
| Joint Ownership | 60010 | 21691 | 10694 | 6450 | 7232 | 710 | 925 | 2130 | 34009 | 759 | 1410 | 2141 |
| Private Ownership | 1581837 | 1135647 | 521475 | 420017 | 429691 | 52998 | 44305 | 87178 | 232097 | 41070 | 66161 | 106862 |
| Host Unit | | | | | | | | | | | | |
| Government Ownership | 7599688 | 6218706 | 2191923 | 1873649 | 2646484 | 336385 | 357462 | 686452 | 110362 | 339017 | 340138 | 591465 |
| Health and Family Planning Department | 7317269 | 6009571 | 2116224 | 1807873 | 2557458 | 325414 | 346265 | 66420 | 110362 | 321016 | 312394 | 563926 |
| Society Operation | 1979798 | 1052808 | 463951 | 344137 | 414139 | 48088 | 49909 | 76721 | 701096 | 44041 | 73927 | 107926 |
| Private Ownership | 1583459 | 1172889 | 535131 | 433612 | 446543 | 54773 | 45814 | 90628 | 188866 | 43113 | 96133 | 109458 |

Notes: ①Health workers and health technicians include the 10,000 civil servants with "Health Supervisor" Certification; ②Cities cover municipalities directly under the central area and prefecture jurisdiction; ③Society includes enterprise, public institution, social group and the health institutions run by other social organizations.

## All-region Health Worker Numbers

| Region | Total | Health Technical Worker | | | | | | | | Village Doctor and Health Worker | Other Technician | Managerial Worker | Ground Skilled Staff |
|---|---|---|---|---|---|---|---|---|---|---|---|---|---|
| | | Subtotal | Certified (Assistant) | | Registered Nurse | Senior Pharmacist (Assistant Pharmacist) | Technician (Assistant Technician) | Others | | | | | |
| | | | Practitioner | Certified Practitioner | | | | | | | | | |
| 2015 | 10693881 | 8007537 | 3039135 | 2508408 | 3241469 | 423294 | 428929 | 874710 | 1031525 | 399712 | 472620 | 782487 |
| 2016 | 11172945 | 8454403 | 3191005 | 2651398 | 3507166 | 439246 | 453185 | 863801 | 1000324 | 426171 | 483198 | 808849 |
| East Region | 4793644 | 3711318 | 1440049 | 1228771 | 1546121 | 203523 | 191128 | 330497 | 330296 | 197283 | 194865 | 359882 |
| Central Region | 3322701 | 2452631 | 946830 | 760120 | 1023720 | 123085 | 137664 | 221332 | 368932 | 129137 | 144115 | 227886 |
| West Region | 3046600 | 2280454 | 804126 | 662507 | 937325 | 112638 | 124393 | 301972 | 301096 | 99751 | 144218 | 221081 |
| Beijing | 299460 | 233953 | 89411 | 84276 | 98082 | 13682 | 12150 | 20628 | 3364 | 16179 | 17679 | 28285 |
| Tianjin | 122558 | 94952 | 37804 | 35435 | 36088 | 5579 | 5250 | 10231 | 5140 | 4692 | 9544 | 8230 |
| Hebei | 555115 | 393059 | 177140 | 137687 | 143432 | 16418 | 20006 | 36063 | 82281 | 25601 | 19230 | 34944 |
| Shanxi | 311250 | 225880 | 91699 | 79147 | 92112 | 10385 | 11650 | 20034 | 38593 | 11345 | 13670 | 21762 |
| Inner Mongolia | 221090 | 170406 | 66391 | 56996 | 66445 | 10429 | 8743 | 18398 | 17944 | 9154 | 10230 | 13356 |
| Liaoning | 365729 | 277494 | 109800 | 98985 | 119147 | 13463 | 15383 | 19701 | 25095 | 14697 | 19172 | 29271 |
| Jilin | 223250 | 166605 | 69666 | 61269 | 65749 | 7933 | 8421 | 14836 | 17248 | 8820 | 13906 | 16671 |
| Heilongjiang | 292297 | 221362 | 84422 | 72084 | 85418 | 11550 | 12793 | 27179 | 23464 | 10226 | 16359 | 20886 |
| Shanghai | 217061 | 178196 | 65386 | 61762 | 79373 | 9779 | 10338 | 13320 | 806 | 10702 | 12175 | 15182 |
| Jiangsu | 654117 | 516986 | 204647 | 169889 | 221168 | 27757 | 25685 | 37729 | 32520 | 25219 | 26379 | 53013 |
| Zhejiang | 523598 | 432641 | 168178 | 145017 | 174523 | 26872 | 21979 | 41089 | 8000 | 20383 | 18081 | 44493 |
| Anhui | 388224 | 293732 | 112741 | 90089 | 126350 | 13875 | 17111 | 23655 | 43290 | 14690 | 14312 | 22200 |
| Fujian | 288205 | 219557 | 79685 | 69186 | 95641 | 14336 | 11418 | 18477 | 26502 | 10902 | 8386 | 22858 |
| Jiangxi | 301651 | 220972 | 79187 | 66016 | 95519 | 14246 | 15095 | 16925 | 45079 | 8562 | 8401 | 18637 |
| Shandong | 874110 | 641701 | 244900 | 210806 | 268379 | 33395 | 33137 | 61890 | 118280 | 40184 | 29007 | 44938 |
| Henan | 796480 | 547001 | 206747 | 152056 | 222123 | 25904 | 32713 | 59514 | 113804 | 36512 | 34597 | 64566 |
| Hubei | 494077 | 384532 | 141741 | 117036 | 174918 | 18508 | 19038 | 30327 | 40396 | 20516 | 19870 | 28763 |
| Hunan | 515472 | 392547 | 160627 | 122423 | 161531 | 20684 | 20843 | 28862 | 47058 | 18466 | 23000 | 34401 |
| Guangdong | 819106 | 665257 | 243224 | 199457 | 283793 | 39311 | 32662 | 66267 | 24996 | 26354 | 31176 | 71323 |
| Guangxi | 390601 | 289872 | 96673 | 77826 | 122602 | 16693 | 15740 | 38164 | 34981 | 12326 | 17745 | 35677 |
| Hainan | 74585 | 57522 | 19874 | 16271 | 26495 | 2931 | 3120 | 5102 | 3312 | 2370 | 4036 | 7345 |
| Chongqing | 242826 | 179354 | 64709 | 51474 | 77463 | 8574 | 8748 | 19860 | 21644 | 8385 | 12463 | 20980 |
| Sichuan | 670444 | 495750 | 185414 | 153601 | 207633 | 23998 | 24932 | 53773 | 65450 | 20252 | 31320 | 57672 |
| Guizhou | 277380 | 204621 | 69007 | 55371 | 85993 | 8128 | 11883 | 29610 | 34690 | 10629 | 13874 | 13566 |
| Yunnan | 329760 | 249677 | 85876 | 71460 | 105966 | 10377 | 13625 | 33833 | 36038 | 12770 | 9937 | 21338 |
| Tibet | 29187 | 14829 | 6542 | 4791 | 3833 | 654 | 695 | 3105 | 10905 | 845 | 854 | 1754 |
| Shaanxi | 372646 | 288607 | 85681 | 71585 | 116803 | 14815 | 18539 | 52769 | 32706 | 3388 | 24184 | 23761 |
| Gansu | 186756 | 134641 | 52791 | 42793 | 50530 | 6222 | 7005 | 18093 | 21121 | 7530 | 11809 | 11655 |
| Qinghai | 49653 | 37010 | 13670 | 11757 | 14364 | 1915 | 2104 | 4957 | 6528 | 2119 | 1290 | 2706 |
| Ningxia | 56218 | 44700 | 17070 | 15336 | 18069 | 2722 | 2440 | 4399 | 3559 | 2085 | 2363 | 3511 |
| Xinjiang | 220039 | 170987 | 60302 | 49517 | 57524 | 8111 | 9939 | 25011 | 15530 | 10268 | 8149 | 15105 |

## All-region Health Worker Numbers (Urban) in 2016

| Region | Total | Health Technical Worker | | | | | | | Other Technician | Managerial Worker | Ground Skilled Staff |
|--------|-------|---------|---------------------|----------------------|-------------------|------------------------------------------|----------------------------------|--------|----------|----------|----------|
| | | Subtotal | Certified (Assistant) | | Registered Nurse | Senior Pharmacist (Assistant Pharmacist) | Technician (Assistant Technician ) | Others | | | |
| | | | Practitioner | Certified Practitioner | | | | | | | |
| Total | 5487317 | 4527708 | 1647676 | 1537354 | 2063019 | 228161 | 241749 | 347103 | 234224 | 287296 | 438089 |
| East Region | 2816299 | 2323970 | 863591 | 807455 | 1033450 | 124927 | 123188 | 178814 | 125167 | 136744 | 230418 |
| Central Region | 1387790 | 1151228 | 412709 | 384622 | 548268 | 52302 | 62238 | 75711 | 61533 | 76182 | 98847 |
| West Region | 1283228 | 1052510 | 371376 | 345277 | 481301 | 50932 | 56323 | 92578 | 47524 | 74370 | 108824 |
| Beijing | 295770 | 233627 | 89129 | 84118 | 98038 | 13682 | 12150 | 20628 | 16179 | 17679 | 28285 |
| Tianjin | 109152 | 87682 | 34158 | 32660 | 34179 | 5172 | 4935 | 9238 | 4485 | 9062 | 7923 |
| Hebei | 217819 | 181354 | 73134 | 67069 | 79954 | 7337 | 9606 | 11323 | 11543 | 9609 | 15313 |
| Shanxi | 151566 | 125427 | 47562 | 44533 | 57848 | 5456 | 6473 | 8088 | 6321 | 8436 | 11382 |
| Inner Mongolia | 104620 | 86863 | 31737 | 29848 | 38666 | 5114 | 4475 | 6871 | 4802 | 5730 | 7225 |
| Liaoning | 239128 | 197368 | 75594 | 71965 | 90271 | 9219 | 11057 | 11227 | 9731 | 12929 | 19100 |
| Jilin | 101652 | 82569 | 34295 | 32316 | 35879 | 3568 | 4417 | 4410 | 4705 | 6510 | 7868 |
| Heilongjiang | 155814 | 126899 | 46311 | 43530 | 56522 | 5821 | 6973 | 11272 | 6274 | 10006 | 12635 |
| Shanghai | 210301 | 173076 | 62735 | 60403 | 77729 | 9513 | 10093 | 13006 | 10563 | 11880 | 14782 |
| Jiangsu | 346369 | 286054 | 104107 | 98561 | 132383 | 14959 | 14817 | 19788 | 14359 | 16688 | 29268 |
| Zhejiang | 272166 | 224095 | 83538 | 77745 | 96236 | 13264 | 12376 | 18681 | 11349 | 11506 | 25216 |
| Anhui | 172052 | 144949 | 50999 | 47390 | 70375 | 6332 | 8059 | 9184 | 7881 | 8777 | 10445 |
| Fujian | 135775 | 113533 | 41539 | 39055 | 52049 | 6952 | 5907 | 7086 | 5983 | 4960 | 11299 |
| Jiangxi | 108622 | 91987 | 31050 | 29414 | 44604 | 5099 | 5797 | 5437 | 4241 | 4746 | 7648 |
| Shandong | 373230 | 314660 | 117967 | 109885 | 143337 | 15438 | 15807 | 22111 | 20846 | 15819 | 21905 |
| Henan | 281866 | 231944 | 79779 | 73232 | 111477 | 10369 | 12638 | 17681 | 14191 | 14900 | 20831 |
| Hubei | 227812 | 189786 | 65779 | 61856 | 94382 | 8627 | 9542 | 11456 | 10597 | 11719 | 15710 |
| Hunan | 188406 | 157667 | 56934 | 52351 | 77181 | 7030 | 8339 | 8183 | 7323 | 11088 | 12328 |
| Guangdong | 578021 | 481604 | 171107 | 156260 | 214189 | 27859 | 24667 | 43782 | 18761 | 24329 | 53327 |
| Guangxi | 163596 | 134482 | 46150 | 43383 | 62217 | 7310 | 7070 | 11735 | 5138 | 8430 | 15546 |
| Hainan | 38568 | 30917 | 10583 | 9734 | 15085 | 1532 | 1773 | 1944 | 1368 | 2283 | 4000 |
| Chongqing | 143321 | 114805 | 39928 | 35300 | 53493 | 5567 | 5931 | 9886 | 5661 | 8683 | 14172 |
| Sichuan | 288468 | 233624 | 83251 | 78476 | 109792 | 10812 | 12107 | 17662 | 10425 | 16206 | 28213 |
| Guizhou | 87132 | 72786 | 26570 | 24769 | 33664 | 2804 | 3835 | 5913 | 3958 | 5189 | 5199 |
| Yunnan | 104385 | 87644 | 31351 | 29159 | 40708 | 3910 | 4716 | 6959 | 5138 | 4281 | 7322 |
| Tibet | 9481 | 7250 | 3265 | 2729 | 2495 | 292 | 447 | 751 | 408 | 591 | 1232 |
| Shaanxi | 183402 | 152096 | 47916 | 43736 | 68837 | 7113 | 9079 | 19151 | 1859 | 14981 | 14466 |
| Gansu | 79488 | 64857 | 25229 | 23629 | 28221 | 2994 | 3701 | 4712 | 4167 | 4765 | 5699 |
| Qinghai | 22862 | 19218 | 6601 | 6268 | 8857 | 975 | 986 | 1799 | 1432 | 698 | 1514 |
| Ningxia | 36127 | 30308 | 11276 | 10636 | 13282 | 1730 | 1582 | 2438 | 1412 | 1901 | 2506 |
| Xinjiang | 60346 | 48577 | 18102 | 17344 | 21069 | 2311 | 2394 | 4701 | 3124 | 2915 | 5730 |

Notes: Cities include municipalities directly under the central area and prefecture jurisdiction.

## All-region Health Worker Numbers (Rural) in 2016

| Region | Total | Health Technical Worker | | | | | | | | Village Doctor and Health Worker | Other Technician | Managerial Worker | Ground Skilled Staff |
|---|---|---|---|---|---|---|---|---|---|---|---|---|---|
| | | Subtotal | Certified (Assistant) | | Registered Nurse | Senior Pharmacist (Assistant Pharmacist) | Technician (Assistant Technician) | Others | | | | | |
| | | | Practitioner | Certified Practitioner | | | | | | | | | |
| Total | 5675628 | 3916695 | 1543329 | 1114044 | 1444147 | 211085 | 211436 | 506698 | 1000324 | 191947 | 195902 | 370760 |
| East Region | 1977345 | 1387348 | 576458 | 421316 | 512671 | 78596 | 67940 | 151683 | 330296 | 72116 | 58121 | 129464 |
| Central Region | 1934911 | 1301403 | 534121 | 375498 | 475452 | 70783 | 75426 | 145621 | 368932 | 67604 | 67933 | 129039 |
| West Region | 1763372 | 1227944 | 432750 | 317230 | 456024 | 61706 | 68070 | 209394 | 301096 | 52227 | 69848 | 112257 |
| Beijing | 3690 | 326 | 282 | 158 | 44 | | | | 3364 | | | |
| Tianjin | 13406 | 7270 | 3646 | 2775 | 1909 | 407 | 315 | 993 | 5140 | 207 | 482 | 307 |
| Hebei | 337296 | 211705 | 104006 | 70618 | 63478 | 9081 | 10400 | 24740 | 82281 | 14058 | 9621 | 19631 |
| Shanxi | 159684 | 100453 | 44137 | 34614 | 34264 | 4929 | 5177 | 11946 | 38593 | 5024 | 5234 | 10380 |
| Inner Mongolia | 116470 | 83543 | 34654 | 27148 | 27779 | 5315 | 4268 | 11527 | 17944 | 4352 | 4500 | 6131 |
| Liaoning | 126601 | 80126 | 34206 | 27020 | 28876 | 4244 | 4326 | 8474 | 25095 | 4966 | 6243 | 10171 |
| Jilin | 121598 | 84036 | 35371 | 28953 | 29870 | 4365 | 4004 | 10426 | 17248 | 4115 | 7396 | 8803 |
| Heilongjiang | 136483 | 94463 | 38111 | 28554 | 28896 | 5729 | 5820 | 15907 | 23464 | 3952 | 6353 | 8251 |
| Shanghai | 6760 | 5120 | 2651 | 1359 | 1644 | 266 | 245 | 314 | 806 | 139 | 295 | 400 |
| Jiangsu | 307748 | 230932 | 100540 | 71328 | 88785 | 12798 | 10868 | 17941 | 32520 | 10860 | 9691 | 23745 |
| Zhejiang | 251432 | 208546 | 84640 | 67272 | 78287 | 13608 | 9603 | 22408 | 8000 | 9034 | 6575 | 19277 |
| Anhui | 216172 | 148783 | 61742 | 42699 | 55975 | 7543 | 9052 | 14471 | 43290 | 6809 | 5535 | 11755 |
| Fujian | 152430 | 106024 | 38146 | 30131 | 43592 | 7384 | 5511 | 11391 | 26502 | 4919 | 3426 | 11559 |
| Jiangxi | 193029 | 128985 | 48137 | 36602 | 50915 | 9147 | 9298 | 11488 | 45079 | 4321 | 3655 | 10989 |
| Shandong | 500880 | 327041 | 126933 | 100921 | 125042 | 17957 | 17330 | 39779 | 118280 | 19338 | 13188 | 23033 |
| Henan | 514614 | 315057 | 126968 | 78824 | 110646 | 15535 | 20075 | 41833 | 113804 | 22321 | 19697 | 43735 |
| Hubei | 266265 | 194746 | 75962 | 55180 | 80536 | 9881 | 9496 | 18871 | 40396 | 9919 | 8151 | 13053 |
| Hunan | 327066 | 234880 | 103693 | 70072 | 84350 | 13654 | 12504 | 20679 | 47058 | 11143 | 11912 | 22073 |
| Guangdong | 241085 | 183653 | 72117 | 43197 | 69604 | 11452 | 7995 | 22485 | 24996 | 7593 | 6847 | 17996 |
| Guangxi | 227005 | 155390 | 50523 | 34443 | 60385 | 9383 | 8670 | 26429 | 34981 | 7188 | 9315 | 20131 |
| Hainan | 36017 | 26605 | 9291 | 6537 | 11410 | 1399 | 1347 | 3158 | 3312 | 1002 | 1753 | 3345 |
| Chongqing | 99505 | 64549 | 24781 | 16174 | 23970 | 3007 | 2817 | 9974 | 21644 | 2724 | 3780 | 6808 |
| Sichuan | 381976 | 262126 | 102163 | 75125 | 97841 | 13186 | 12825 | 36111 | 65450 | 9827 | 15114 | 29459 |
| Guizhou | 190248 | 131835 | 42437 | 30602 | 52329 | 5324 | 8048 | 23697 | 34690 | 6671 | 8685 | 8367 |
| Yunnan | 225375 | 162033 | 54525 | 42301 | 65258 | 6467 | 8909 | 26874 | 36038 | 7632 | 5656 | 14016 |
| Tibet | 19706 | 7579 | 3277 | 2062 | 1338 | 362 | 248 | 2354 | 10905 | 437 | 263 | 522 |
| Shaanxi | 189244 | 136511 | 37765 | 27849 | 47966 | 7702 | 9460 | 33618 | 32706 | 1529 | 9203 | 9295 |
| Gansu | 107268 | 69784 | 27562 | 19164 | 22309 | 3228 | 3304 | 13381 | 21121 | 3363 | 7044 | 5956 |
| Qinghai | 26791 | 17792 | 7069 | 5489 | 5507 | 940 | 1118 | 3158 | 6528 | 687 | 592 | 1192 |
| Ningxia | 20091 | 14392 | 5794 | 4700 | 4787 | 992 | 858 | 1961 | 3559 | 673 | 462 | 1005 |
| Xinjiang | 159693 | 122410 | 4200 | 32173 | 46555 | 5800 | 7545 | 20310 | 15530 | 7144 | 5234 | 9375 |

## Number of Health Technical Workers per Thousand People

| Year | Health Technical Worker | | | Certified (Assistant) Practitioner | | | Certified Practitioner | Registered Nurse | | |
|------|-------|-------|-------|-------|-------|-------|------|-------|-------|-------|
| | Total | Urban | Rural | Total | Urban | Rural | | Total | Urban | Rural |
| 1949 | 0.93 | 1.87 | 0.73 | 0.67 | 0.70 | 0.66 | 0.58 | 0.06 | 0.25 | 0.02 |
| 1955 | 1.42 | 3.49 | 1.01 | 0.81 | 1.24 | 0.74 | 0.70 | 0.14 | 0.64 | 0.04 |
| 1960 | 2.37 | 5.67 | 1.85 | 1.04 | 1.97 | 0.90 | 0.79 | 0.23 | 1.04 | 0.07 |
| 1965 | 2.11 | 5.37 | 1.46 | 1.05 | 2.22 | 0.82 | 0.70 | 0.32 | 1.45 | 0.10 |
| 1970 | 1.76 | 4.88 | 1.22 | 0.85 | 1.97 | 0.66 | 0.43 | 0.29 | 1.10 | 0.14 |
| 1975 | 2.24 | 6.92 | 1.41 | 0.95 | 2.66 | 0.65 | 0.57 | 0.41 | 1.74 | 0.18 |
| 1980 | 2.85 | 8.03 | 1.81 | 1.17 | 3.22 | 0.76 | 0.72 | 0.47 | 1.83 | 0.20 |
| 1985 | 3.28 | 7.92 | 2.09 | 1.36 | 3.35 | 0.85 | 0.70 | 0.61 | 1.85 | 0.30 |
| 1990 | 3.45 | 6.59 | 2.15 | 1.56 | 2.95 | 0.98 | 1.15 | 0.86 | 1.91 | 0.43 |
| 1995 | 3.59 | 5.36 | 2.32 | 1.62 | 2.39 | 1.07 | 1.23 | 0.95 | 1.59 | 0.49 |
| 1998 | 3.64 | 5.30 | 2.35 | 1.65 | 2.34 | 1.11 | 1.25 | 1.00 | 1.64 | 0.51 |
| 1999 | 3.64 | 5.24 | 2.38 | 1.67 | 2.33 | 1.14 | 1.27 | 1.02 | 1.64 | 0.52 |
| 2000 | 3.63 | 5.17 | 2.41 | 1.68 | 2.31 | 1.17 | 1.30 | 1.02 | 1.64 | 0.54 |
| 2001 | 3.62 | 5.15 | 2.38 | 1.69 | 2.32 | 1.17 | 1.32 | 1.03 | 1.65 | 0.54 |
| 2002 | 3.41 | ... | ... | 1.47 | ... | ... | 1.17 | 1.00 | ... | ... |
| 2003 | 3.48 | 4.88 | 2.26 | 1.54 | 2.13 | 1.04 | 1.22 | 1.00 | 1.59 | 0.50 |
| 2004 | 3.53 | 4.99 | 2.24 | 1.57 | 2.18 | 1.04 | 1.25 | 1.03 | 1.63 | 0.50 |
| 2005 | 3.50 | 5.82 | 2.69 | 1.56 | 2.46 | 1.26 | 1.24 | 1.03 | 2.10 | 0.65 |
| 2006 | 3.60 | 6.09 | 2.70 | 1.60 | 2.56 | 1.26 | 1.28 | 1.09 | 2.22 | 0.66 |
| 2007 | 3.72 | 6.44 | 2.69 | 1.61 | 2.61 | 1.23 | 1.30 | 1.18 | 2.42 | 0.70 |
| 2008 | 3.90 | 6.68 | 2.80 | 1.66 | 2.68 | 1.26 | 1.35 | 1.27 | 2.54 | 0.76 |
| 2009 | 4.15 | 7.15 | 2.94 | 1.75 | 2.83 | 1.31 | 1.43 | 1.39 | 2.82 | 0.81 |
| 2010 | 4.39 | 7.62 | 3.04 | 1.80 | 2.97 | 1.32 | 1.47 | 1.53 | 3.09 | 0.89 |
| 2011 | 4.58 | 7.90 | 3.19 | 1.82 | 3.00 | 1.33 | 1.49 | 1.66 | 3.29 | 0.98 |
| 2012 | 4.94 | 8.54 | 3.41 | 1.94 | 3.19 | 1.40 | 1.58 | 1.85 | 3.65 | 1.09 |
| 2013 | 5.27 | 9.18 | 3.64 | 2.04 | 3.39 | 1.48 | 1.67 | 2.04 | 4.00 | 1.22 |
| 2014 | 5.56 | 9.70 | 3.77 | 2.12 | 3.54 | 1.51 | 1.74 | 2.20 | 4.30 | 1.31 |
| 2015 | 5.84 | 10.21 | 3.90 | 2.22 | 3.72 | 1.55 | 1.84 | 2.37 | 4.58 | 1.39 |
| 2016 | 6.12 | 10.42 | 4.08 | 2.31 | 3.79 | 1.61 | 1.92 | 2.54 | 4.75 | 1.50 |

Notes: ①Before 2002, the number of certified (assistant) practitioners covers the number of doctors, certified practitioners refer to practitioners and registered nurses are senior nurses and nurses; ②Cities include municipalities directly under the central area and prefecture jurisdiction, and countryside covers counties and county-level cities; ③Denominator refers to the number of resident population.

## All-type Certified (Assistant) Practitioner Numbers

| | Total | | Certified Practitioner | | Certified (Assistant) Practitioner | |
|---|---|---|---|---|---|---|
| | 2015 | 2016 | 2015 | 2016 | 2015 | 2016 |
| **Number (Ten Thousand)** | **303.9** | **319.1** | **250.8** | **265.1** | **53.1** | **54.0** |
| Clinical Type | 232.2 | 243.0 | 191.3 | 201.8 | 40.9 | 41.3 |
| TCM Type | 45.2 | 48.2 | 38.3 | 40.9 | 6.9 | 7.2 |
| Stomatology Type | 15.4 | 16.7 | 12.5 | 13.6 | 2.9 | 3.1 |
| Public Health Type | 11.1 | 11.2 | 8.8 | 8.9 | 2.4 | 2.3 |
| **Constituent (%)** | **100.0** | **100.0** | **100.0** | **100.0** | **100.0** | **100.0** |
| Clinical Type | 76.4 | 76.2 | 76.3 | 76.1 | 77.1 | 76.5 |
| TCM Type | 14.9 | 15.1 | 15.3 | 15.4 | 13.0 | 13.4 |
| Stomatology Type | 5.1 | 5.2 | 5.0 | 5.1 | 5.4 | 5.8 |
| Public Health Type | 3.7 | 3.5 | 3.5 | 3.4 | 4.4 | 4.2 |

## General Medical Practitioner Numbers

| | Total | | | Number of Registered General Medial Practitioner | | | Number of Trained General Practitioner with Certification | | |
|---|---|---|---|---|---|---|---|---|---|
| | 2014 | 2015 | 2016 | 2014 | 2015 | 2016 | 2014 | 2015 | 2016 |
| **Total** | **172597** | **188649** | **209083** | **64156** | **68364** | **77631** | **108441** | **120285** | **131452** |
| Hospital | 30428 | 31382 | 34654 | 9395 | 8936 | 9517 | 21033 | 22446 | 25137 |
| Community Health Service Center (Station) | 68914 | 73288 | 78337 | 31202 | 33169 | 36513 | 37712 | 40119 | 41824 |
| Township Health Center | 70296 | 80975 | 92791 | 22594 | 25434 | 30718 | 47702 | 55541 | 62073 |

Note: General medical practitioner number refers to the total of registered general practitioners and certified (assistant) practitioners with training certification for general practitioner.

## All-region Classified Practitioner of Certification (Assistant Practitioner) Numbers and General Practitioner Numbers in 2016

| Region | Certified (Assistant) Practitioner Number | | | | | General Practitioner Number | | | General Practitioner Number Per Ten Thousand People |
|---|---|---|---|---|---|---|---|---|---|
| | Total | Clinic | TCM | Stomatology | Public Health | Total | Number of Registered General Medicine | Number of Trained General Practitioner with Certification | |
| **Total** | **3191005** | **2430499** | **481590** | **167227** | **111689** | **209083** | **77631** | **131452** | **1.51** |
| East Region | 1440049 | 1093170 | 204743 | 89597 | 52539 | 116537 | 47538 | 68999 | 2.03 |
| Central Region | 946830 | 745942 | 129680 | 40564 | 30644 | 49944 | 17767 | 32177 | 1.16 |
| West Region | 804126 | 591387 | 147167 | 37066 | 28506 | 42602 | 12326 | 30276 | 1.14 |
| Beijing | 89411 | 60897 | 17010 | 8327 | 3177 | 8402 | 4396 | 4006 | 3.87 |
| Tianjin | 37804 | 26895 | 7341 | 2360 | 1208 | 2403 | 1072 | 1331 | 1.54 |
| Hebei | 177140 | 138825 | 26831 | 8102 | 3382 | 9355 | 2288 | 7067 | 1.25 |
| Shanxi | 91699 | 68360 | 14625 | 5572 | 3142 | 4175 | 1629 | 2546 | 1.13 |
| Inner Mongolia | 66391 | 45960 | 13367 | 3879 | 3185 | 3178 | 1126 | 2052 | 1.26 |
| Liaoning | 109800 | 85248 | 12906 | 7568 | 4078 | 4195 | 1582 | 2613 | 0.96 |
| Jilin | 69666 | 52127 | 9671 | 5285 | 2583 | 3384 | 1259 | 2125 | 1.24 |
| Heilongjiang | 84422 | 66053 | 10409 | 5372 | 2588 | 4454 | 1342 | 3112 | 1.17 |
| Shanghai | 65386 | 49370 | 7822 | 4744 | 3450 | 7967 | 5761 | 2206 | 3.29 |
| Jiangsu | 204647 | 161509 | 24122 | 9979 | 9037 | 25162 | 8815 | 16347 | 3.15 |
| Zhejiang | 168178 | 126150 | 24687 | 12073 | 5268 | 22571 | 8111 | 14460 | 4.04 |
| Anhui | 112741 | 92421 | 12479 | 3853 | 3988 | 8625 | 3506 | 5119 | 1.39 |
| Fujian | 79685 | 57344 | 13785 | 5322 | 3234 | 5786 | 1756 | 4030 | 1.49 |
| Jiangxi | 79187 | 62464 | 11466 | 2326 | 2931 | 3641 | 1219 | 2422 | 0.79 |
| Shandong | 244900 | 189639 | 32203 | 14282 | 8776 | 11372 | 3570 | 7802 | 1.14 |
| Henan | 206747 | 161824 | 31685 | 7505 | 5733 | 12129 | 3882 | 8247 | 1.27 |
| Hubei | 141741 | 114104 | 16896 | 6140 | 4601 | 7020 | 2216 | 4804 | 1.19 |
| Hunan | 160627 | 128589 | 22449 | 4511 | 5078 | 6516 | 2714 | 3802 | 0.96 |
| Guangdong | 243224 | 181339 | 36079 | 15726 | 10080 | 18338 | 9721 | 8617 | 1.67 |
| Guangxi | 96673 | 73871 | 14191 | 5036 | 3575 | 5104 | 1268 | 3836 | 1.05 |
| Hainan | 19874 | 15954 | 1957 | 1114 | 849 | 986 | 466 | 520 | 1.08 |
| Chongqing | 64709 | 46404 | 13742 | 2870 | 1693 | 3127 | 868 | 2259 | 1.03 |
| Sichuan | 185414 | 127125 | 46594 | 7316 | 4379 | 10360 | 2296 | 8064 | 1.25 |
| Guizhou | 69007 | 54449 | 9338 | 2472 | 2748 | 3714 | 1610 | 2104 | 1.04 |
| Yunnan | 85876 | 66926 | 11002 | 3943 | 4005 | 4737 | 980 | 3757 | 0.99 |
| Tibet | 6542 | 4445 | 1298 | 160 | 639 | 202 | 130 | 72 | 0.61 |
| Shaanxi | 85681 | 66494 | 12593 | 4381 | 2213 | 2738 | 702 | 2036 | 0.72 |
| Gansu | 52791 | 36474 | 12619 | 2035 | 1663 | 3773 | 1277 | 2496 | 1.45 |
| Qinghai | 13670 | 10329 | 2499 | 416 | 426 | 993 | 382 | 611 | 1.67 |
| Ningxia | 17070 | 12762 | 2176 | 1326 | 806 | 654 | 286 | 368 | 0.97 |
| Xinjiang | 60302 | 46148 | 7748 | 3232 | 3174 | 4022 | 1401 | 2621 | 1.68 |

## Grassroots Medical Health Institution Worker Numbers

| Institution Type | Total | Health Technical Worker | | | | | | | Village Doctor and Health Worker | Other Technician | Managerial Worker | Ground Skilled Staff |
|---|---|---|---|---|---|---|---|---|---|---|---|---|
| | | Subtotal | Certified (Assistant) | | Registered Nurse | Pharmacist (Assistant Pharmacist) | Technician (Assistant Technician) | Others | | | | |
| | | | Practitioner | Certified Practitioner | | | | | | | | |
| 2015 | 3603162 | 2257701 | 1101934 | 731851 | 646607 | 134495 | 88106 | 286559 | 1031525 | 80981 | 69452 | 163503 |
| 2016 | 3682561 | 2354430 | 1145408 | 764867 | 695781 | 138060 | 92884 | 282297 | 1000324 | 86635 | 73476 | 167696 |
| Urban/Rural | | | | | | | | | | | | |
| Cities | 869712 | 772155 | 384857 | 331685 | 271894 | 47101 | 24807 | 43496 | | 20426 | 25636 | 51495 |
| Countryside | 2812849 | 1582275 | 760551 | 433182 | 423887 | 90959 | 68077 | 238801 | 1000324 | 66209 | 47840 | 116201 |
| Registration Type | | | | | | | | | | | | |
| Public | 2657345 | 1698057 | 764021 | 463408 | 492413 | 110780 | 82798 | 248045 | 682967 | 79749 | 60149 | 136423 |
| Non-public | 1025216 | 656373 | 381387 | 301459 | 203368 | 27280 | 10086 | 34252 | 317357 | 6886 | 13327 | 31273 |
| Host Unit | | | | | | | | | | | | |
| Government Ownership | 1793521 | 1424364 | 584749 | 365029 | 424112 | 101939 | 76996 | 236568 | 110362 | 76129 | 55433 | 127233 |
| Society Operation | 1090015 | 359102 | 229557 | 133442 | 94731 | 12523 | 8260 | 14031 | 701096 | 5178 | 7912 | 16727 |
| Private Ownership | 799025 | 570964 | 331102 | 266396 | 176938 | 23598 | 7628 | 31698 | 188866 | 5328 | 10131 | 23736 |
| Management Type | | | | | | | | | | | | |
| Non-profit | 3047709 | 1836044 | 845808 | 514865 | 533980 | 116410 | 85859 | 253987 | 920558 | 83081 | 65513 | 142513 |
| Profit | 634852 | 518386 | 299600 | 250002 | 161801 | 21650 | 7025 | 28310 | 79766 | 3554 | 7963 | 25183 |

## All-region Grassroots Medical Health Institution Worker Numbers

| Institution Type | Total | Health Technical Worker | | | | | | | Village Doctor and Health Worker | Other Technician | Managerial Worker | Ground Skilled Staff |
| | | Subtotal | Certified (Assistant) | | Registered Nurse | Pharmacist (Assistant Pharmacist) | Technician (Assistant Technician) | Others | | | | |
| | | | Practitioner | Certified Practitioner | | | | | | | | |
|---|---|---|---|---|---|---|---|---|---|---|---|---|
| 2015 | 3603162 | 2257701 | 1101934 | 731851 | 646607 | 134495 | 88106 | 286559 | 1031525 | 80981 | 69452 | 163503 |
| 2016 | 3682561 | 2354430 | 1145408 | 764867 | 695781 | 138060 | 92884 | 282297 | 1000324 | 86635 | 73476 | 167696 |
| East Region | 1503701 | 1027010 | 514273 | 361186 | 310384 | 65739 | 38662 | 97952 | 330296 | 38673 | 30050 | 77672 |
| Central Region | 1141886 | 675155 | 343477 | 212826 | 193096 | 36866 | 29287 | 72429 | 368932 | 26932 | 21655 | 49212 |
| West Region | 1036974 | 652265 | 287658 | 190855 | 192301 | 35455 | 24935 | 111916 | 301096 | 21030 | 21771 | 40812 |
| Beijing | 65110 | 50890 | 25139 | 21921 | 15996 | 4351 | 2127 | 3277 | 3364 | 2436 | 2400 | 6020 |
| Tianjin | 28174 | 19357 | 10117 | 8651 | 5084 | 1514 | 915 | 1727 | 5140 | 688 | 1324 | 1665 |
| Hebei | 200306 | 105262 | 65454 | 38562 | 20704 | 4219 | 3062 | 11823 | 82281 | 4433 | 2313 | 6017 |
| Shanxi | 103629 | 57233 | 32138 | 23916 | 15957 | 2505 | 1542 | 5091 | 38593 | 1917 | 1861 | 4025 |
| Inner Mongolia | 68878 | 45787 | 23496 | 17413 | 12017 | 3920 | 1381 | 4973 | 17944 | 1662 | 1389 | 2096 |
| Liaoning | 97227 | 61830 | 31747 | 25429 | 19856 | 2955 | 2205 | 5067 | 25095 | 2226 | 2772 | 5304 |
| Jilin | 70307 | 45564 | 23428 | 18411 | 12645 | 2294 | 1454 | 5743 | 17248 | 1796 | 2220 | 3479 |
| Heilongjiang | 79287 | 48766 | 23725 | 16531 | 12066 | 2814 | 2088 | 8073 | 23464 | 1754 | 2187 | 3116 |
| Shanghai | 54512 | 45016 | 21351 | 18160 | 16120 | 3117 | 2009 | 2419 | 806 | 2093 | 2395 | 4202 |
| Jiangsu | 212776 | 155832 | 81255 | 52400 | 47893 | 9608 | 6442 | 10634 | 32520 | 5876 | 4399 | 14149 |
| Zhejiang | 156816 | 132178 | 67180 | 48627 | 36353 | 9984 | 4727 | 13934 | 8000 | 4081 | 3114 | 9443 |
| Anhui | 133189 | 80686 | 41817 | 24604 | 23618 | 4140 | 4035 | 7076 | 43290 | 2447 | 2362 | 4404 |
| Fujian | 104548 | 67844 | 30076 | 22508 | 22148 | 6030 | 2689 | 6901 | 26502 | 2824 | 1397 | 5981 |
| Jiangxi | 115061 | 62544 | 28525 | 18696 | 18903 | 4952 | 4240 | 5924 | 45079 | 1793 | 1039 | 4606 |
| Shandong | 321582 | 182978 | 85779 | 63005 | 56444 | 10895 | 7768 | 22092 | 118280 | 7578 | 4046 | 8700 |
| Henan | 284804 | 143560 | 73650 | 36664 | 37395 | 6781 | 6936 | 18798 | 113804 | 7810 | 5012 | 14618 |
| Hubei | 175178 | 119321 | 55551 | 36505 | 42008 | 6013 | 4490 | 11259 | 40396 | 5075 | 3734 | 6652 |
| Hunan | 180431 | 117481 | 64643 | 37499 | 30504 | 7367 | 4502 | 10465 | 47058 | 4340 | 3240 | 8312 |
| Guangdong | 239498 | 189076 | 89428 | 57386 | 43056 | 12223 | 6188 | 18181 | 24996 | 5741 | 5208 | 14477 |
| Guangxi | 144195 | 96872 | 38048 | 22713 | 30156 | 6844 | 3932 | 17892 | 34981 | 3525 | 1373 | 7444 |
| Hainan | 23152 | 16747 | 6747 | 4537 | 6730 | 843 | 530 | 1897 | 3312 | 697 | 682 | 1714 |
| Chongqing | 85124 | 55056 | 26759 | 16758 | 16219 | 2800 | 1745 | 7533 | 21644 | 1993 | 2040 | 4391 |
| Sichuan | 242034 | 151985 | 74961 | 50256 | 43219 | 7984 | 4914 | 20907 | 65450 | 4882 | 6939 | 12778 |
| Guizhou | 99401 | 56384 | 22503 | 13345 | 16981 | 2196 | 2821 | 11883 | 34690 | 2626 | 3612 | 2089 |
| Yunnan | 105220 | 62184 | 26899 | 18274 | 19451 | 1909 | 2515 | 11410 | 36038 | 2704 | 1104 | 3190 |
| Tibet | 16046 | 4558 | 2017 | 1346 | 701 | 155 | 33 | 1652 | 10905 | 277 | 64 | 242 |
| Shaanxi | 111383 | 71756 | 26842 | 18484 | 19998 | 4604 | 3936 | 16376 | 32706 | 398 | 3308 | 3215 |
| Gansu | 71033 | 46309 | 19209 | 12330 | 14323 | 2029 | 1386 | 9362 | 21121 | 819 | 717 | 2067 |
| Qinghai | 15669 | 8483 | 4026 | 3135 | 2175 | 461 | 273 | 1548 | 6528 | 239 | 154 | 265 |
| Ningxia | 14097 | 9763 | 4730 | 3735 | 2792 | 749 | 279 | 1213 | 3559 | 246 | 114 | 415 |
| Xinjiang | 63894 | 43128 | 18168 | 13066 | 14269 | 1804 | 1720 | 7167 | 15530 | 1659 | 957 | 2020 |

## All-region Community Health Service Center (Station) Worker Numbers

| Institution Type | Total | Health Technical Worker | | | | | | | Other Technician | Managerial Worker | Ground Skilled Staff |
|---|---|---|---|---|---|---|---|---|---|---|---|
| | | Subtotal | Certified (Assistant) | | Registered Nurse | Pharmacist (Assistant Pharmacist) | Technician (Assistant Technician) | Others | | | |
| | | | Practitioner | Certified Practitioner | | | | | | | |
| 2015 | 504817 | 431158 | 181670 | 146047 | 153393 | 33909 | 20431 | 41755 | 20305 | 20790 | 32564 |
| 2016 | 521974 | 446176 | 187699 | 151673 | 162132 | 34638 | 21074 | 40633 | 21569 | 21350 | 32879 |
| East Region | 294485 | 251628 | 108719 | 88366 | 85891 | 22161 | 11731 | 23126 | 12726 | 10565 | 19566 |
| Central Region | 125471 | 107168 | 45126 | 36183 | 42181 | 6542 | 5235 | 8084 | 5236 | 5823 | 7244 |
| West Region | 102018 | 87380 | 33854 | 27124 | 34060 | 5935 | 4108 | 9423 | 3607 | 4962 | 6069 |
| Beijing | 32801 | 27349 | 12114 | 10146 | 8242 | 3175 | 1286 | 2532 | 1752 | 1360 | 2340 |
| Tianjin | 8516 | 7062 | 3077 | 2740 | 2135 | 704 | 399 | 747 | 381 | 607 | 466 |
| Hebei | 16360 | 14099 | 6859 | 5571 | 5096 | 738 | 667 | 739 | 667 | 781 | 813 |
| Shanxi | 12314 | 10605 | 4763 | 4064 | 4356 | 490 | 346 | 650 | 498 | 575 | 636 |
| Inner Mongolia | 12502 | 10847 | 4578 | 3738 | 4095 | 846 | 408 | 920 | 605 | 525 | 525 |
| Liaoning | 16558 | 13982 | 5834 | 5130 | 5803 | 924 | 688 | 733 | 695 | 971 | 910 |
| Jilin | 8673 | 7001 | 2894 | 2485 | 2697 | 471 | 329 | 610 | 542 | 533 | 597 |
| Heilongjiang | 14994 | 12576 | 4804 | 4036 | 4859 | 874 | 758 | 1281 | 658 | 888 | 872 |
| Shanghai | 35034 | 29159 | 12324 | 10850 | 10720 | 2544 | 1450 | 2121 | 1690 | 1302 | 2883 |
| Jiangsu | 44444 | 37671 | 16149 | 13159 | 12570 | 3326 | 1926 | 3700 | 1952 | 1418 | 3403 |
| Zhejiang | 40060 | 35022 | 15494 | 11613 | 9904 | 3368 | 1680 | 4576 | 1653 | 954 | 2431 |
| Anhui | 18736 | 16609 | 7241 | 5528 | 6573 | 862 | 770 | 1163 | 597 | 774 | 756 |
| Fujian | 12469 | 10631 | 4358 | 3599 | 3845 | 995 | 489 | 944 | 693 | 349 | 796 |
| Jiangxi | 8636 | 7504 | 2894 | 2512 | 3086 | 614 | 540 | 370 | 272 | 380 | 480 |
| Shandong | 34070 | 29421 | 12048 | 9624 | 10323 | 2266 | 1364 | 3420 | 1833 | 1216 | 1600 |
| Henan | 21687 | 18117 | 7856 | 6262 | 6879 | 906 | 947 | 1529 | 1027 | 1092 | 1451 |
| Hubei | 23774 | 20369 | 8228 | 6724 | 8586 | 1231 | 898 | 1426 | 1073 | 995 | 1337 |
| Hunan | 16657 | 14387 | 6446 | 4572 | 5145 | 1094 | 647 | 1055 | 569 | 586 | 1115 |
| Guangdong | 51050 | 44555 | 19533 | 15200 | 15989 | 3946 | 1685 | 3402 | 1330 | 1444 | 3721 |
| Guangxi | 7382 | 6506 | 2571 | 2129 | 2589 | 551 | 281 | 514 | 233 | 200 | 443 |
| Hainan | 3123 | 2677 | 929 | 734 | 1264 | 175 | 97 | 212 | 80 | 163 | 203 |
| Chongqing | 11239 | 9394 | 3587 | 2508 | 3467 | 673 | 476 | 1191 | 405 | 564 | 876 |
| Sichuan | 21597 | 18101 | 7000 | 5712 | 7209 | 1357 | 835 | 1700 | 653 | 1156 | 1687 |
| Guizhou | 8615 | 7162 | 2722 | 2052 | 2952 | 279 | 321 | 888 | 457 | 579 | 417 |
| Yunnan | 7535 | 6508 | 2509 | 1988 | 2571 | 294 | 294 | 840 | 388 | 288 | 351 |
| Tibet | 218 | 170 | 79 | 63 | 31 | 9 | 13 | 38 | 6 | 12 | 30 |
| Shaanxi | 11688 | 9998 | 3406 | 2671 | 3633 | 735 | 631 | 1593 | 67 | 906 | 717 |
| Gansu | 7797 | 7011 | 2874 | 2376 | 2930 | 370 | 268 | 569 | 201 | 229 | 356 |
| Qinghai | 2187 | 1969 | 749 | 640 | 717 | 198 | 74 | 231 | 78 | 65 | 75 |
| Ningxia | 1528 | 1411 | 467 | 383 | 605 | 117 | 44 | 178 | 47 | 30 | 40 |
| Xinjiang | 9730 | 8303 | 3312 | 2864 | 3261 | 506 | 463 | 761 | 467 | 408 | 552 |

## Village Doctor Number and Health Worker Numbers

| Year | Village Doctor and Health Worker | | | Village Doctor and Health Worker Per Village | Village Doctor and Health Worker Per Thousand Agricultural Population |
|---|---|---|---|---|---|
| | Total | Village Doctor | Health Worker | | |
| 1980 | 1463406 | 607879 | 2357370 | 2.10 | 1.79 |
| 1985 | 1293094 | 643022 | 650072 | 1.80 | 1.55 |
| 1990 | 1231510 | 776859 | 454651 | 1.64 | 1.38 |
| 1992 | 1269061 | 816557 | 452504 | 1.73 | 1.41 |
| 1993 | 1325106 | 910664 | 414442 | 1.81 | 1.47 |
| 1994 | 1323701 | 933386 | 390351 | 1.81 | 1.47 |
| 1995 | 1331017 | 955933 | 375084 | 1.81 | 1.48 |
| 1996 | 1316095 | 954630 | 361465 | 1.79 | 1.46 |
| 1997 | 1317786 | 972288 | 345498 | 1.80 | 1.45 |
| 1998 | 1327633 | 990217 | 337416 | 1.81 | 1.46 |
| 1999 | 1324937 | 1009665 | 315272 | 1.82 | 1.45 |
| 2000 | 1319357 | 1019845 | 299512 | 1.81 | 1.44 |
| 2001 | 1290595 | 1021542 | 269053 | 1.82 | 1.41 |
| 2003 | 867778 | 791956 | 75822 | 1.31 | 0.98 |
| 2004 | 883075 | 825672 | 57403 | 1.37 | 1.00 |
| 2005 | 916532 | 864168 | 52364 | 1.46 | 1.05 |
| 2006 | 957459 | 906320 | 51139 | 1.53 | 1.10 |
| 2007 | 931761 | 882218 | 49543 | 1.52 | 1.06 |
| 2008 | 938313 | 893535 | 44778 | 1.55 | 1.06 |
| 2009 | 1050991 | 995449 | 55542 | 1.75 | 1.19 |
| 2010 | 1091863 | 1031828 | 60035 | 1.68 | 1.14 |
| 2011 | 1126443 | 1060548 | 65895 | 1.91 | 1.20 |
| 2012 | 1094419 | 1022869 | 71550 | 1.86 | 1.14 |
| 2013 | 1081063 | 1004502 | 76561 | 1.83 | 1.12 |
| 2014 | 1058182 | 985692 | 72490 | 1.64 | 1.09 |
| 2015 | 1031525 | 962514 | 69011 | 1.78 | 1.07 |
| 2016 | 1000324 | 932936 | 67388 | 1.79 | 1.04 |

Note: ①Before 1985, village doctors refer to barefoot doctors. ②Before 2010, the data are village doctor and health worker per thousand agricultural population

## Village Health Room Worker Numbers

| Host Unit | Total | Certified (Assistant) Practitioner | Registered Nurse | Village Doctor | Health Worker |
|---|---|---|---|---|---|
| 2010 | 1292410 | 173275 | 27272 | 1031828 | 60035 |
| 2011 | 1350222 | 193277 | 30502 | 1060548 | 65895 |
| 2012 | 1371592 | 232826 | 44347 | 1022869 | 71550 |
| 2013 | 1457276 | 291291 | 84922 | 1004502 | 76561 |
| 2014 | 1460389 | 304343 | 97864 | 985692 | 72490 |
| 2015 | 1447712 | 309923 | 106264 | 962514 | 69011 |
| 2016 | 1435766 | 319797 | 115645 | 932936 | 67388 |
| Village Ownership | 678084 | 94844 | 13286 | 534025 | 35929 |
| Township Health Hospital Point | 376904 | 172043 | 94499 | 102303 | 8059 |
| Joint Operation | 72364 | 10907 | 1728 | 55496 | 4233 |
| Private Operation | 223791 | 30713 | 4212 | 175950 | 12916 |
| Others | 84623 | 11290 | 1920 | 65162 | 6251 |

Note: This Table includes certified (assistant) practitioners and registered nurses working in village health rooms under health centers.

## All-region Village Health Room Worker Numbers

| Region | Total | Certified (Assistant) Practitioner | Registered Nurse | Village Doctor and Health Worker | | | Village Doctor and Health Worker Per Village | Village Doctor and Health Worker Per Thousand Agricultural Population |
|--------|-------|------------------------------------|------------------|-------|----------------|----------------|----------------|----------------|
| | | | | Total | Village Doctor | Health Worker | | |
| 2015 | 1447712 | 309923 | 106264 | 1031525 | 962514 | 69011 | 2.26 | 1.50 |
| 2016 | 1435766 | 319797 | 115645 | 1000324 | 932936 | 67388 | 2.25 | 1.49 |
| East Region | 497948 | 125244 | 42408 | 330296 | 315635 | 14661 | 2.31 | 1.57 |
| Central Region | 543598 | 127872 | 46794 | 368932 | 343306 | 25626 | 2.45 | 1.74 |
| West Region | 394220 | 66681 | 26443 | 301096 | 273995 | 27101 | 1.96 | 1.19 |
| Beijing | 4808 | 991 | 453 | 3364 | 3332 | 32 | 1.76 | |
| Tianjin | 6957 | 1392 | 425 | 5140 | 4889 | 251 | 2.75 | 8.06 |
| Hebei | 117602 | 30162 | 5159 | 82281 | 77228 | 5053 | 1.95 | 2.00 |
| Shanxi | 51564 | 9821 | 3150 | 38593 | 35761 | 2832 | 1.78 | 2.04 |
| Inner Mongolia | 27407 | 6717 | 2746 | 17944 | 16697 | 1247 | 2.01 | 1.56 |
| Liaoning | 33395 | 5607 | 2693 | 25095 | 24623 | 472 | 1.66 | 1.45 |
| Jilin | 23277 | 4512 | 1517 | 17248 | 16386 | 862 | 2.29 | 1.30 |
| Heilongjiang | 32372 | 7193 | 1715 | 23464 | 22280 | 1184 | 2.84 | 1.41 |
| Shanghai | 5272 | 3810 | 656 | 806 | 617 | 189 | 4.33 | 7.85 |
| Jiangsu | 67098 | 26684 | 7894 | 32520 | 31175 | 1345 | 4.34 | 1.38 |
| Zhejiang | 25260 | 12680 | 4580 | 8000 | 7590 | 410 | 2.16 | 0.81 |
| Anhui | 67921 | 18602 | 6029 | 43290 | 40470 | 2820 | 4.45 | 1.37 |
| Fujian | 36054 | 7035 | 2517 | 26502 | 25697 | 805 | 1.90 | 1.36 |
| Jiangxi | 61976 | 11847 | 5050 | 45079 | 43496 | 1583 | 2.04 | 1.53 |
| Shandong | 150393 | 21278 | 10835 | 118280 | 113465 | 4815 | 2.83 | 2.17 |
| Henan | 164907 | 37391 | 13712 | 113804 | 103284 | 10520 | 2.90 | 1.78 |
| Hubei | 66668 | 17020 | 9252 | 40396 | 38509 | 1887 | 2.69 | 1.58 |
| Hunan | 74913 | 21486 | 6369 | 47058 | 43120 | 3938 | 1.69 | 1.26 |
| Guangdong | 44550 | 13916 | 5638 | 24996 | 24408 | 588 | 1.66 | 0.88 |
| Guangxi | 41773 | 5753 | 1039 | 34981 | 32038 | 2943 | 1.99 | 1.04 |
| Hainan | 6559 | 1689 | 1558 | 3312 | 2611 | 701 | 2.46 | 0.98 |
| Chongqing | 30372 | 6653 | 2075 | 21644 | 20782 | 862 | 2.70 | 1.72 |
| Sichuan | 83530 | 16649 | 1431 | 65450 | 63530 | 1920 | 1.49 | 1.33 |
| Guizhou | 43841 | 5647 | 3504 | 34690 | 26724 | 7966 | 2.12 | 1.12 |
| Yunnan | 42216 | 3815 | 2363 | 36038 | 33745 | 2293 | 3.14 | 1.04 |
| Tibet | 11412 | 360 | 147 | 10905 | 8489 | 2416 | 2.13 | 4.34 |
| Shaanxi | 42838 | 6933 | 3199 | 32706 | 31080 | 1626 | 1.69 | 1.68 |
| Gansu | 32434 | 6632 | 4681 | 21121 | 18287 | 2834 | 1.94 | 1.67 |
| Qinghai | 9181 | 1971 | 682 | 6528 | 5681 | 847 | 2.03 | 1.90 |
| Ningxia | 5213 | 1090 | 564 | 3559 | 3051 | 508 | 2.20 | 1.40 |
| Xinjiang | 24003 | 4461 | 4012 | 15530 | 13891 | 1639 | 2.30 | 1.23 |

Note: This Table includes certified (assistant) practitioners and registered nurses in village health rooms under township health center.

## All-region Maternal and Child Health Care Center (Institution, Station) Worker Numbers

| Region | Total | Health Technical Worker | | | | | | | Other Technician | Managerial Worker | Ground Skilled Staff |
| | | Subtotal | Certified (Assistant) | | Registered Nurse | Senior Pharmacist (Assistant Pharmacist) | Docimaster (Lab Assistant) | Others | | | |
| | | | Practitioner | Certified Practitioner | | | | | | | |
| 2015 | 351257 | 291361 | 105832 | 93643 | 124414 | 12558 | 21019 | 27538 | 15987 | 15898 | 28011 |
| 2016 | 388238 | 320748 | 116524 | 103360 | 138266 | 13468 | 23154 | 29336 | 18139 | 18290 | 31061 |
| East Region | 153786 | 127240 | 46233 | 42000 | 54246 | 5607 | 8904 | 12250 | 8122 | 6287 | 12137 |
| Central Region | 121830 | 100606 | 37833 | 32790 | 44420 | 3974 | 7316 | 7063 | 5857 | 6068 | 9299 |
| West Region | 112622 | 92902 | 32458 | 28570 | 39600 | 3887 | 6934 | 10023 | 4160 | 5935 | 9625 |
| Beijing | 6597 | 5482 | 2160 | 2109 | 2321 | 254 | 409 | 338 | 256 | 309 | 550 |
| Tianjin | 1453 | 1144 | 551 | 489 | 298 | 48 | 120 | 127 | 71 | 172 | 66 |
| Hebei | 18542 | 14767 | 6670 | 5394 | 5052 | 581 | 1075 | 1389 | 1479 | 759 | 1537 |
| Shanxi | 9274 | 7082 | 3115 | 2704 | 2670 | 272 | 443 | 582 | 607 | 694 | 891 |
| Inner Mongolia | 7773 | 6411 | 2885 | 2576 | 2281 | 285 | 478 | 482 | 434 | 455 | 473 |
| Liaoning | 4838 | 3768 | 1959 | 1766 | 1036 | 143 | 366 | 264 | 244 | 505 | 321 |
| Jilin | 5894 | 4585 | 2258 | 2040 | 1450 | 162 | 347 | 368 | 328 | 629 | 352 |
| Heilongjiang | 7995 | 6428 | 2713 | 2344 | 2244 | 298 | 546 | 627 | 304 | 635 | 628 |
| Shanghai | 3201 | 2705 | 1033 | 1021 | 1313 | 90 | 196 | 73 | 163 | 126 | 207 |
| Jiangsu | 13096 | 10640 | 4412 | 4231 | 4457 | 394 | 693 | 684 | 693 | 624 | 1139 |
| Zhejiang | 18373 | 15590 | 5722 | 5432 | 6652 | 731 | 1025 | 1460 | 921 | 424 | 1438 |
| Anhui | 8633 | 7219 | 2913 | 2646 | 2907 | 281 | 609 | 509 | 400 | 466 | 548 |
| Fujian | 10525 | 8813 | 3146 | 2861 | 3906 | 432 | 782 | 547 | 436 | 271 | 1005 |
| Jiangxi | 15163 | 12952 | 4229 | 3888 | 6228 | 689 | 1086 | 720 | 497 | 459 | 1255 |
| Shandong | 31899 | 26395 | 8984 | 8325 | 11646 | 1080 | 1828 | 2857 | 2049 | 1346 | 2109 |
| Henan | 29597 | 23823 | 8034 | 6447 | 11175 | 896 | 1649 | 2069 | 1642 | 1297 | 2835 |
| Hubei | 21384 | 18436 | 6411 | 5650 | 9108 | 622 | 1152 | 1143 | 1149 | 736 | 1063 |
| Hunan | 23890 | 20081 | 8160 | 7071 | 8638 | 754 | 1484 | 1045 | 930 | 1152 | 1727 |
| Guangdong | 42173 | 35507 | 10868 | 9686 | 16409 | 1746 | 2250 | 4234 | 1550 | 1587 | 3529 |
| Guangxi | 25264 | 20790 | 6060 | 5549 | 9986 | 989 | 1545 | 2210 | 955 | 748 | 2771 |
| Hainan | 3089 | 2429 | 728 | 686 | 1156 | 108 | 160 | 277 | 260 | 164 | 236 |
| Chongqing | 7696 | 6131 | 1926 | 1763 | 2957 | 245 | 479 | 524 | 248 | 533 | 784 |
| Sichuan | 22440 | 18368 | 6055 | 5538 | 8582 | 777 | 1383 | 1571 | 808 | 1166 | 2098 |
| Guizhou | 8839 | 7615 | 3226 | 2738 | 2750 | 255 | 577 | 807 | 303 | 549 | 372 |
| Yunnan | 11745 | 9686 | 3867 | 3261 | 3724 | 286 | 706 | 1103 | 644 | 412 | 1003 |
| Tibet | 511 | 432 | 194 | 120 | 115 | 16 | 28 | 79 | 10 | 25 | 44 |
| Shaanxi | 13560 | 11316 | 3038 | 2532 | 4671 | 547 | 881 | 2179 | 120 | 1102 | 1022 |
| Gansu | 6395 | 5295 | 2399 | 2122 | 2046 | 171 | 292 | 387 | 166 | 369 | 565 |
| Qinghai | 1078 | 865 | 373 | 311 | 297 | 43 | 78 | 74 | 75 | 74 | 64 |
| Ningxia | 2758 | 2272 | 889 | 831 | 847 | 107 | 177 | 252 | 130 | 171 | 185 |
| Xinjiang | 4563 | 3721 | 1546 | 1229 | 1344 | 166 | 310 | 355 | 267 | 331 | 244 |

*467*

## All-region Disease Prevention and Control Center Worker Numbers

| Region | Total | Health Technical Worker | | | | | | | Other Technician | Managerial Worker | Ground Skilled Staff |
|---|---|---|---|---|---|---|---|---|---|---|---|
| | | Subtotal | Certified (Assistant) | | Registered Nurse | Senior Pharmacist (Assistant Pharmacist) | Docimaster (Lab Assistant) | Others | | | |
| | | | Practitioner | Certified Practitioner | | | | | | | |
| 2015 | 190930 | 141698 | 70709 | 59972 | 13798 | 2737 | 26907 | 27547 | 14413 | 14240 | 20579 |
| 2016 | 191627 | 142492 | 70734 | 60322 | 14488 | 2790 | 27346 | 27134 | 14741 | 13978 | 20416 |
| East Region | 67639 | 50873 | 26403 | 23501 | 3840 | 751 | 10554 | 9325 | 5893 | 4607 | 6266 |
| Central Region | 61425 | 42983 | 20263 | 16522 | 5277 | 1062 | 7961 | 8420 | 5448 | 4850 | 8144 |
| West Region | 62563 | 48636 | 24068 | 20299 | 5371 | 977 | 8831 | 9389 | 3400 | 4521 | 6006 |
| Beijing | 3837 | 2958 | 1383 | 1343 | 143 | 11 | 720 | 701 | 449 | 248 | 182 |
| Tianjin | 1795 | 1327 | 750 | 706 | 79 | 12 | 310 | 176 | 190 | 162 | 116 |
| Hebei | 8472 | 5767 | 2577 | 2034 | 366 | 71 | 988 | 1765 | 929 | 538 | 1238 |
| Shanxi | 5033 | 3443 | 1799 | 1509 | 330 | 87 | 725 | 502 | 444 | 527 | 619 |
| Inner Mongolia | 5482 | 4416 | 2374 | 2045 | 355 | 62 | 636 | 989 | 342 | 364 | 360 |
| Liaoning | 7586 | 5650 | 2930 | 2470 | 435 | 84 | 1211 | 990 | 452 | 895 | 589 |
| Jilin | 4934 | 3734 | 1869 | 1593 | 324 | 76 | 640 | 825 | 344 | 477 | 379 |
| Heilongjiang | 6082 | 4405 | 1858 | 1516 | 306 | 83 | 873 | 1285 | 611 | 576 | 490 |
| Shanghai | 3127 | 2272 | 1251 | 1214 | 44 | 3 | 585 | 389 | 341 | 275 | 239 |
| Jiangsu | 7956 | 6135 | 3734 | 3583 | 405 | 102 | 1220 | 674 | 776 | 453 | 592 |
| Zhejiang | 5641 | 4429 | 2459 | 2342 | 214 | 53 | 1242 | 461 | 512 | 269 | 431 |
| Anhui | 4901 | 3838 | 1966 | 1676 | 275 | 68 | 914 | 615 | 357 | 293 | 413 |
| Fujian | 4573 | 3677 | 2081 | 1938 | 247 | 50 | 781 | 518 | 285 | 170 | 441 |
| Jiangxi | 5172 | 4014 | 1836 | 1581 | 722 | 99 | 788 | 569 | 273 | 287 | 598 |
| Shandong | 11743 | 9134 | 4291 | 3772 | 691 | 150 | 1428 | 2574 | 1010 | 787 | 812 |
| Henan | 17255 | 10103 | 4584 | 3396 | 1283 | 243 | 1482 | 2511 | 1832 | 1608 | 3712 |
| Hubei | 8515 | 6701 | 3049 | 2595 | 1243 | 191 | 1210 | 1008 | 777 | 415 | 622 |
| Hunan | 9533 | 6745 | 3302 | 2656 | 794 | 215 | 1329 | 1105 | 810 | 667 | 1311 |
| Guangdong | 11358 | 8432 | 4393 | 3658 | 1049 | 194 | 1837 | 959 | 866 | 676 | 1384 |
| Guangxi | 7781 | 6004 | 2841 | 2487 | 890 | 190 | 1184 | 899 | 562 | 384 | 831 |
| Hainan | 1551 | 1092 | 554 | 441 | 167 | 21 | 232 | 118 | 83 | 134 | 242 |
| Chongqing | 2809 | 2018 | 1015 | 911 | 125 | 21 | 540 | 317 | 237 | 269 | 285 |
| Sichuan | 12307 | 9048 | 4222 | 3646 | 846 | 114 | 1982 | 1884 | 851 | 937 | 1471 |
| Guizhou | 5233 | 4288 | 2347 | 1921 | 378 | 73 | 695 | 795 | 156 | 513 | 276 |
| Yunnan | 8301 | 6767 | 3742 | 3122 | 710 | 88 | 1025 | 1202 | 472 | 342 | 720 |
| Tibet | 1061 | 883 | 545 | 404 | 55 | 8 | 46 | 229 | 26 | 47 | 105 |
| Shaanxi | 6331 | 4875 | 1632 | 1304 | 674 | 168 | 814 | 1587 | 164 | 688 | 604 |
| Gansu | 4671 | 3418 | 1748 | 1504 | 527 | 143 | 568 | 432 | 114 | 477 | 662 |
| Qinghai | 1289 | 997 | 506 | 442 | 160 | 28 | 210 | 93 | 111 | 55 | 126 |
| Ningxia | 1092 | 907 | 535 | 503 | 68 | 9 | 221 | 74 | 50 | 52 | 83 |
| Xinjiang | 6206 | 5015 | 2561 | 2010 | 583 | 73 | 910 | 888 | 315 | 393 | 483 |

## All-region Health Supervision Institution (Center) Worker Numbers

| Region | Total | Health Technical Worker | | | Other Technical Worker | Managerial Worker | Ground Skilled Staff |
|---|---|---|---|---|---|---|---|
| | | Subtotal | Health Supervision Worker | Others | | | |
| 2015 | 80710 | 67942 | 65077 | 2865 | 2029 | 5737 | 5002 |
| 2016 | 81522 | 68165 | 65025 | 3140 | 2056 | 6242 | 5059 |
| East Region | 25406 | 20874 | 19626 | 1248 | 828 | 2064 | 1640 |
| Central Region | 26055 | 20626 | 19211 | 1415 | 879 | 2513 | 2037 |
| West Region | 20061 | 16665 | 16188 | 477 | 349 | 1665 | 1382 |
| Beijing | 1262 | 1185 | 1137 | 48 | 22 | 13 | 42 |
| Tianjin | 770 | 673 | 660 | 13 | 2 | 61 | 34 |
| Hebei | 4487 | 3316 | 2861 | 455 | 261 | 386 | 524 |
| Shanxi | 4341 | 3389 | 3208 | 181 | 115 | 475 | 362 |
| Inner Mongolia | 2681 | 2311 | 2197 | 114 | 58 | 235 | 77 |
| Liaoning | 2577 | 2135 | 2015 | 120 | 71 | 242 | 129 |
| Jilin | 1538 | 1220 | 1085 | 135 | 44 | 194 | 80 |
| Heilongjiang | 2834 | 2410 | 2263 | 147 | 107 | 207 | 110 |
| Shanghai | 1182 | 1027 | 997 | 30 | 27 | 94 | 34 |
| Jiangsu | 3447 | 3064 | 2948 | 116 | 97 | 187 | 99 |
| Zhejiang | 2822 | 2464 | 2414 | 50 | 94 | 134 | 130 |
| Anhui | 2405 | 2040 | 1874 | 166 | 46 | 201 | 118 |
| Fujian | 1711 | 1347 | 1215 | 132 | 48 | 184 | 132 |
| Jiangxi | 1948 | 1548 | 1464 | 84 | 25 | 167 | 208 |
| Shandong | 3362 | 2723 | 2552 | 171 | 103 | 329 | 207 |
| Henan | 6591 | 4767 | 4403 | 364 | 303 | 733 | 788 |
| Hubei | 2987 | 2345 | 2125 | 220 | 152 | 293 | 197 |
| Hunan | 3411 | 2907 | 2789 | 118 | 87 | 243 | 174 |
| Guangdong | 3437 | 2674 | 2574 | 100 | 99 | 384 | 280 |
| Guangxi | 2089 | 1702 | 1603 | 99 | 135 | 149 | 103 |
| Hainan | 349 | 266 | 253 | 13 | 4 | 50 | 29 |
| Chongqing | 1077 | 1027 | 1018 | 9 | 2 | 29 | 19 |
| Sichuan | 2928 | 2497 | 2443 | 54 | 38 | 141 | 252 |
| Guizhou | 1739 | 1460 | 1452 | 8 | 9 | 138 | 132 |
| Yunnan | 1955 | 1577 | 1563 | 14 | 15 | 192 | 171 |
| Tibet | 25 | 21 | 21 | | | 2 | 2 |
| Shaanxi | 2977 | 2261 | 2184 | 77 | 40 | 379 | 297 |
| Gansu | 1832 | 1494 | 1457 | 37 | 20 | 150 | 168 |
| Qinghai | 465 | 348 | 333 | 15 | 16 | 74 | 27 |
| Ningxia | 508 | 462 | 439 | 23 | 9 | 10 | 27 |
| Xinjiang | 1785 | 1505 | 1478 | 27 | 7 | 166 | 107 |

Notes: ①In 2016, there are 1,217 health supervision workers in disease prevention and control center (disease prevention station); ②The total number in This Table includes 10,000 civil servants with health supervision certification.

All-type Medical Health

| Institution Type | Total | Urban and Rural | | Registration Type | | |
|---|---|---|---|---|---|---|
| | | City | Countryside | Public | State Ownership | Collective Ownership |
| Total | 7410453 | 3676235 | 3734218 | 6134450 | 5723768 | 410682 |
| Hospital | 5688875 | 3374900 | 2313975 | 4455238 | 4367239 | 87999 |
| Comprehensive Hospital | 3927857 | 2256239 | 1671618 | 3142788 | 3091342 | 51446 |
| TCM Hospital | 761755 | 361393 | 400362 | 688389 | 674239 | 14150 |
| Hospital of Traditional Chinese and Western Medicine | 89074 | 70077 | 18997 | 60550 | 59050 | 1500 |
| National Hospital | 26484 | 7236 | 19248 | 23640 | 23605 | 35 |
| Specialty Hospital | 844580 | 648021 | 196559 | 533552 | 513944 | 19608 |
| Nursing Hospital | 39125 | 31934 | 7191 | 6319 | 5059 | 1260 |
| Grassroots Medical Health Institution | 1441940 | 155769 | 1286171 | 1403522 | 1083835 | 319687 |
| Community Health Service Center (Station) | 202689 | 148470 | 54219 | 175654 | 123213 | 52441 |
| Community Health Service Center | 182191 | 132719 | 49472 | 166005 | 118140 | 47865 |
| Community Health Service Station | 20498 | 15751 | 4747 | 9649 | 5073 | 4576 |
| Health Center | 1232623 | 3350 | 1229273 | 1225176 | 958607 | 266569 |
| District Health Center | 8732 | 3350 | 5382 | 8589 | 5706 | 2883 |
| Township Health Center | 1223891 | | 1223891 | 1216587 | 952901 | 263686 |
| Outpatient Department | 6474 | 3827 | 2647 | 2566 | 1909 | 657 |
| Nursing Station | 154 | 122 | 32 | 126 | 106 | 20 |
| Special Public Health Institution | 247228 | 122438 | 124790 | 244680 | 242612 | 2068 |
| Special Disease Prevention and Treatment Center (Institution, Station) | 40048 | 23977 | 16071 | 39484 | 37918 | 1566 |
| Special Disease Prevention and Treatment Hospital | 20638 | 15673 | 4965 | 20351 | 19660 | 691 |
| Special Disease Prevention and Treatment Institution (Center) | 19410 | 8304 | 11106 | 19133 | 18258 | 875 |
| Maternal and Child Health Care Hospital (Institution, Station) | 206538 | 98128 | 108410 | 204554 | 204054 | 500 |
| Maternal and Child Health Care Center | 193959 | 96204 | 97755 | 192002 | 191522 | 480 |
| Maternal and Child Health Care Institution (Station) | 12224 | 1768 | 10456 | 12217 | 12197 | 20 |
| First Aid Center (Station) | 642 | 333 | 309 | 642 | 640 | 2 |
| Other Medical Health Institutions | 32410 | 23128 | 9282 | 31010 | 30082 | 928 |
| Sanatorium | 32410 | 23128 | 9282 | 31010 | 30082 | 928 |

Notes: ①Cities cover municipalities directly under the central area and prefecture jurisdiction, while countryside covers county and county-level city;

## Institution Bed Number in 2015

| Registration Type | | | Host Unit | | | | Management | |
|---|---|---|---|---|---|---|---|---|
| Non-public | Joint Ownership | Private Ownership | Government Ownership | Health & Family Planning Department | Social Ownership | Private Ownership | Non-profit | Profit |
| 1276003 | 16323 | 843279 | 5704779 | 5495320 | 828972 | 876702 | 6755237 | 655216 |
| 1233637 | 16031 | 814517 | 4080615 | 3894129 | 763186 | 845074 | 5041777 | 647098 |
| 785069 | 11337 | 508825 | 2818958 | 2702792 | 581648 | 527251 | 3528207 | 399650 |
| 73366 | 365 | 47901 | 682260 | 675204 | 26956 | 52539 | 724900 | 36855 |
| 28524 | 203 | 20588 | 57319 | 56227 | 8966 | 22789 | 74336 | 14738 |
| 2844 | 20 | 2228 | 22507 | 22487 | 1892 | 2085 | 24548 | 1936 |
| 311028 | 3936 | 213533 | 496746 | 435491 | 130023 | 217811 | 657426 | 187154 |
| 32806 | 170 | 21442 | 2825 | 1928 | 13701 | 22599 | 32360 | 6765 |
| 38418 | 292 | 27228 | 1364587 | 1352406 | 47694 | 29659 | 1435220 | 6720 |
| 27035 | 189 | 17090 | 144837 | 140247 | 38455 | 19397 | 199701 | 2988 |
| 16186 | 160 | 8397 | 140982 | 136969 | 31331 | 9878 | 180666 | 1525 |
| 10849 | 29 | 8693 | 3855 | 3278 | 7124 | 9519 | 19035 | 1463 |
| 7447 | 58 | 6683 | 1219234 | 1212149 | 6739 | 6650 | 1232326 | 297 |
| 143 | 30 | 113 | 8292 | 8272 | 282 | 158 | 8729 | 3 |
| 7304 | 28 | 6570 | 1210942 | 1203877 | 6457 | 6492 | 1223597 | 294 |
| 3908 | 45 | 3439 | 516 | 10 | 2362 | 3596 | 3045 | 3429 |
| 28 | | 16 | | | 138 | 16 | 148 | 6 |
| 2548 | | 1174 | 239428 | 236841 | 6241 | 1559 | 246722 | 506 |
| 564 | | 434 | 35015 | 33449 | 4829 | 204 | 39932 | 116 |
| 287 | | 247 | 17432 | 16842 | 3119 | 87 | 20618 | 20 |
| 277 | | 187 | 17583 | 16607 | 1710 | 117 | 19314 | 96 |
| 1984 | | 740 | 203845 | 202832 | 1338 | 1355 | 206148 | 390 |
| 1957 | | 720 | 191445 | 190564 | 1179 | 1335 | 193589 | 370 |
| 7 | | | 12137 | 12112 | 87 | | 12224 | |
| | | | 568 | 560 | 74 | | 642 | |
| 1400 | | 360 | 20149 | 11944 | 11851 | 410 | 31518 | 892 |
| 1400 | | 360 | 20149 | 11944 | 11851 | 410 | 31518 | 892 |

②Society includes enterprise, public institution, social groups and other medical health institutions under other social organizations.

**All-region Medical Health**

| Region | Total | Hospital | | | | | | |
|---|---|---|---|---|---|---|---|---|
| | | Subtotal | Comprehensive Hospital | TCM Hospital | Hospital of Traditional Chinese and Western Medicine | National Hospital | Specialty Hospital | Nursing Hospital |
| **Total** | 7410453 | 5688875 | 3927857 | 761755 | 89074 | 26484 | 844580 | 39125 |
| East Region | 2911065 | 2333615 | 1571346 | 287830 | 44833 | 772 | 392401 | 36433 |
| Central Region | 2359616 | 1755906 | 1229740 | 255195 | 17952 | 985 | 250247 | 1787 |
| West Region | 2139772 | 1599354 | 1126771 | 218730 | 26289 | 24727 | 201932 | 905 |
| Beijing | 117041 | 110073 | 62139 | 14092 | 8482 | 198 | 25012 | 150 |
| Tianjin | 65832 | 57561 | 32780 | 7803 | 1247 | | 15731 | |
| Hebei | 360485 | 270831 | 200148 | 34917 | 6521 | | 29245 | |
| Shanxi | 189689 | 147011 | 101048 | 16201 | 2356 | | 27216 | 190 |
| Inner Mongolia | 139236 | 109676 | 73227 | 13201 | 1017 | 7659 | 14372 | 200 |
| Liaoning | 284384 | 239350 | 162043 | 24740 | 1685 | 300 | 50083 | 499 |
| Jilin | 151195 | 124837 | 84997 | 14721 | 2607 | 137 | 22115 | 260 |
| Heilongjiang | 220054 | 181514 | 127849 | 23056 | 766 | 282 | 29501 | 60 |
| Shanghai | 129166 | 110148 | 63311 | 6047 | 3597 | | 28129 | 9064 |
| Jiangsu | 443060 | 356188 | 224794 | 43781 | 6329 | | 61125 | 20159 |
| Zhejiang | 289870 | 254793 | 160871 | 34003 | 6564 | | 49483 | 3872 |
| Anhui | 281720 | 216281 | 155242 | 29021 | 2250 | | 29160 | 608 |
| Fujian | 174767 | 131892 | 91762 | 17100 | 2831 | 60 | 20059 | 80 |
| Jiangxi | 209097 | 143049 | 100078 | 25461 | 1263 | | 16187 | 60 |
| Shandong | 540994 | 399427 | 283560 | 55779 | 3523 | 214 | 55376 | 975 |
| Henan | 521546 | 387054 | 280443 | 59532 | 2369 | | 44560 | 150 |
| Hubei | 360558 | 256909 | 184034 | 37108 | 3922 | 460 | 31204 | 181 |
| Hunan | 425757 | 299251 | 196049 | 50095 | 2419 | 106 | 50304 | 278 |
| Guangdong | 465142 | 371685 | 266073 | 45889 | 3577 | | 54512 | 1634 |
| Guangxi | 224471 | 148480 | 101035 | 23529 | 5504 | 455 | 17877 | 80 |
| Hainan | 40324 | 31667 | 23865 | 3679 | 477 | | 3646 | |
| Chongqing | 190850 | 136245 | 92583 | 20696 | 3242 | | 19444 | 280 |
| Sichuan | 519205 | 375378 | 251686 | 51905 | 7724 | 1248 | 62765 | 50 |
| Guizhou | 210279 | 159098 | 115509 | 19676 | 2803 | 518 | 20352 | 240 |
| Yunnan | 253555 | 194727 | 142587 | 25222 | 1776 | 383 | 24759 | |
| Tibet | 14456 | 10397 | 8098 | | 50 | 1604 | 645 | |
| Shaanxi | 225400 | 180316 | 133884 | 27668 | 1504 | | 17205 | 55 |
| Gansu | 134346 | 100638 | 71440 | 20674 | 1591 | 798 | 6135 | |
| Qinghai | 34749 | 29156 | 20307 | 2432 | 60 | 3262 | 3095 | |
| Ningxia | 36313 | 32027 | 24921 | 4185 | 256 | 40 | 2625 | |
| Xinjiang | 156912 | 123216 | 91494 | 9542 | 762 | 8760 | 12658 | |

## Institution Bed Numbers in 2016

| | Grassroots Medical Health Institution | | | | | | Professional Public Health Institution | | | | Other Medical Health Institution |
|---|---|---|---|---|---|---|---|---|---|---|---|
| Subtotal | Community Health Service Center | Community Health Service Station | District Health Center | Township Health Center | Outpatient Department | Nursing Station | Subtotal | Special Disease Prevention and Treatment Hospital (Institution, Station) | Maternal and Child Health Care Hospital (Institution, Station) | First Aid Center (Station) | |
| 1441940 | 182191 | 20498 | 8732 | 1223891 | 6474 | 154 | 247228 | 40048 | 206538 | 642 | 32410 |
| 463935 | 86440 | 8039 | 1383 | 365855 | 2082 | 136 | 94159 | 17932 | 75810 | 417 | 19356 |
| 506248 | 56298 | 6064 | 4993 | 436594 | 2293 | 6 | 89639 | 18738 | 70823 | 78 | 7823 |
| 471757 | 39453 | 6395 | 2356 | 421442 | 2099 | 12 | 63430 | 3378 | 59905 | 147 | 5231 |
| 4443 | 4417 | | | | 26 | | 2525 | 554 | 1971 | | |
| 7101 | 2869 | | 110 | 4093 | 29 | | 874 | 744 | 130 | | 296 |
| 76853 | 5893 | 3869 | | 66624 | 467 | | 11796 | 831 | 10910 | 55 | 1005 |
| 37042 | 3087 | 890 | 2742 | 30068 | 249 | 6 | 3786 | 160 | 3616 | 10 | 1850 |
| 24802 | 3974 | 607 | | 20002 | 219 | | 4242 | 394 | 3848 | | 516 |
| 36720 | 5926 | 9 | 269 | 30424 | 92 | | 3334 | 1995 | 1210 | 129 | 4980 |
| 20896 | 2846 | 334 | 50 | 17429 | 237 | | 3164 | 1055 | 2109 | | 2298 |
| 30039 | 6185 | 804 | 174 | 22469 | 407 | | 7551 | 3503 | 4044 | 4 | 950 |
| 16690 | 16690 | | | | | | 1465 | 148 | 1317 | | 863 |
| 77546 | 18175 | 305 | 35 | 58768 | 157 | 106 | 6495 | 1079 | 5411 | 5 | 2831 |
| 24605 | 7150 | 34 | 76 | 17096 | 249 | | 8500 | 448 | 7985 | 67 | 1972 |
| 58613 | 7137 | | | 51305 | 171 | | 6156 | 2339 | 3787 | 30 | 670 |
| 32833 | 3320 | 18 | | 29449 | 46 | | 7502 | 1554 | 5917 | 31 | 2540 |
| 52240 | 2959 | 1325 | 70 | 47672 | 214 | | 11998 | 3004 | 8994 | | 1810 |
| 115017 | 12623 | 3648 | 126 | 97894 | 696 | 30 | 23404 | 4663 | 18611 | 130 | 3146 |
| 111968 | 10089 | 1178 | 288 | 99994 | 419 | | 22379 | 1455 | 20894 | 30 | 145 |
| 87662 | 13981 | 580 | 1489 | 71546 | 66 | | 15987 | 2231 | 13752 | 4 | |
| 107788 | 10014 | 953 | 180 | 96111 | 530 | | 18618 | 4991 | 13627 | | 100 |
| 65634 | 8488 | 24 | 767 | 56075 | 280 | | 26787 | 5822 | 20965 | | 1036 |
| 62207 | 1557 | 12 | | 60565 | 73 | | 12883 | 440 | 12442 | 1 | 901 |
| 6493 | 889 | 132 | | 5432 | 40 | | 1477 | 94 | 1383 | | 687 |
| 50288 | 8716 | 41 | 1120 | 40045 | 366 | | 3612 | 390 | 3222 | | 705 |
| 132023 | 9388 | 1826 | 108 | 120279 | 422 | | 11452 | 274 | 11122 | 56 | 352 |
| 43758 | 2894 | | 959 | 39905 | | | 7323 | 276 | 7047 | | 100 |
| 51206 | 3963 | 719 | 85 | 46225 | 214 | | 6734 | 531 | 6175 | 28 | 888 |
| 3345 | 57 | 3 | | 3285 | | | 674 | | 674 | | 40 |
| 36346 | 2960 | 348 | 80 | 32722 | 236 | | 7970 | 916 | 7054 | | 768 |
| 28631 | 2517 | 1360 | 4 | 24600 | 138 | 12 | 4427 | 32 | 4383 | 12 | 650 |
| 5193 | 517 | 610 | | 4062 | 4 | | 400 | 40 | 360 | | |
| 3218 | 143 | 162 | | 2913 | | | 968 | | 968 | | 100 |
| 30740 | 2767 | 707 | | 26839 | 427 | | 2745 | 85 | 2610 | 50 | 211 |

## Medical Health Institution Bed Numbers (Ten Thousand)

| Year | Total | Hospital | | | | Grassroots Medical Health | | | Professional Public Health | | | Other Medical Health Institution |
|---|---|---|---|---|---|---|---|---|---|---|---|---|
| | | | Comprehensive Hospital | TCM Hospital | Specialty Hospital | Institution | Community Health Service Center (Station) | Township Health Center | Institution | Maternal and Child Health Care Hospital (Institution, Station) | Special Disease Prevention and Treatment Hospital (Institution, Station) | |
| 1950 | 11.91 | 9.71 | 8.46 | 0.01 | 0.74 | | | | | 0.27 | | |
| 1955 | 36.28 | 21.53 | 17.08 | 0.14 | 2.80 | | | | | 0.57 | | |
| 1960 | 97.68 | 59.14 | 44.74 | 1.42 | 7.95 | | | 4.63 | | 0.88 | 1.74 | |
| 1965 | 103.33 | 61.20 | 48.04 | 1.04 | 7.49 | | | 13.25 | | 0.92 | | |
| 1970 | 126.15 | 70.50 | 57.21 | 1.01 | 7.79 | | | 36.80 | | 0.70 | | |
| 1975 | 176.43 | 94.02 | 76.33 | 1.37 | 11.11 | | | 62.03 | | 0.97 | 2.88 | |
| 1980 | 218.44 | 119.58 | 94.11 | 5.00 | 12.87 | | | 77.54 | | 1.64 | 2.73 | |
| 1985 | 248.71 | 150.86 | 112.77 | 11.23 | 16.56 | | | 72.06 | | 3.46 | 2.95 | |
| 1986 | 256.25 | 155.98 | 117.52 | 12.52 | 17.71 | | | 71.12 | | 3.67 | 3.06 | |
| 1987 | 268.50 | 165.34 | 123.71 | 14.21 | 19.03 | | | 72.30 | | 4.00 | 3.07 | |
| 1988 | 279.49 | 174.70 | 129.06 | 15.55 | 20.23 | | | 72.61 | | 4.35 | 3.00 | |
| 1989 | 286.70 | 181.46 | 133.60 | 16.60 | 20.93 | | | 72.30 | | 4.50 | 3.10 | |
| 1990 | 292.54 | 186.89 | 136.90 | 17.57 | 21.95 | | | 72.29 | | 4.66 | 3.10 | |
| 1991 | 299.19 | 192.61 | 140.55 | 18.82 | 22.26 | | | 72.92 | | 4.80 | 3.17 | |
| 1992 | 304.94 | 197.66 | 144.10 | 20.04 | 22.71 | | | 73.28 | | 5.00 | 3.22 | |
| 1993 | 309.90 | 203.64 | 156.63 | 21.35 | 24.37 | | | 73.08 | | 4.50 | 3.03 | |
| 1994 | 313.40 | 207.04 | 158.70 | 22.18 | 24.85 | | | 73.24 | | 4.80 | 2.98 | |
| 1995 | 314.06 | 206.33 | 158.72 | 22.72 | 24.51 | | | 73.31 | | 5.13 | 3.07 | |
| 1996 | 309.96 | 209.65 | 159.73 | 23.75 | 24.86 | | | 73.47 | | 5.60 | 2.83 | |
| 1997 | 313.45 | 211.92 | 161.21 | 24.46 | 24.97 | | | 74.24 | | 6.02 | 3.06 | |
| 1998 | 314.30 | 213.41 | 162.00 | 24.95 | 25.01 | | | 73.77 | | 6.30 | 2.90 | |
| 1999 | 315.90 | 215.07 | 163.25 | 25.33 | 25.03 | | | 73.40 | | 6.63 | 2.93 | |
| 2000 | 317.70 | 216.67 | 164.09 | 25.93 | 25.08 | 76.65 | | 73.48 | 11.86 | 7.12 | 2.84 | 12.52 |
| 2001 | 320.12 | 215.56 | 150.50 | 24.60 | 25.65 | 77.14 | | 74.00 | 12.02 | 7.40 | 2.70 | 15.40 |
| 2002 | 313.61 | 222.18 | 168.38 | 24.67 | 26.21 | 71.05 | 1.20 | 67.13 | 12.37 | 7.98 | 3.18 | 8.01 |
| 2003 | 316.40 | 226.95 | 171.34 | 26.02 | 26.72 | 71.05 | 1.21 | 67.27 | 12.61 | 8.09 | 3.38 | 5.79 |
| 2004 | 326.84 | 236.35 | 177.68 | 27.55 | 28.26 | 71.44 | 1.81 | 66.89 | 12.73 | 8.70 | 3.12 | 6.32 |
| 2005 | 336.75 | 244.50 | 183.47 | 28.77 | 29.21 | 72.58 | 2.50 | 67.82 | 13.58 | 9.41 | 3.34 | 6.09 |
| 2006 | 351.18 | 256.04 | 190.29 | 30.32 | 32.05 | 76.19 | 4.12 | 69.62 | 13.50 | 9.93 | 2.80 | 5.45 |
| 2007 | 370.11 | 267.51 | 197.16 | 32.16 | 34.37 | 85.03 | 7.66 | 74.72 | 13.29 | 10.62 | 2.59 | 4.28 |
| 2008 | 403.87 | 288.29 | 211.28 | 35.03 | 37.77 | 97.10 | 9.80 | 84.69 | 14.66 | 11.73 | 2.64 | 3.82 |
| 2009 | 441.66 | 312.08 | 227.11 | 38.56 | 41.67 | 109.98 | 13.13 | 93.34 | 15.3964 | 12.61 | 2.71 | 4.21 |
| 2010 | 478.68 | 338.74 | 244.95 | 42.42 | 45.95 | 119.22 | 16.88 | 99.43 | 16.45 | 13.44 | 2.93 | 4.26 |
| 2011 | 515.99 | 370.51 | 267.07 | 47.71 | 49.65 | 123.37 | 18.71 | 102.63 | 17.8132 | 14.59 | 3.14 | 4.29 |
| 2012 | 572.48 | 416.15 | 297.99 | 54.80 | 55.74 | 132.43 | 20.32 | 109.93 | 19.8198 | 16.16 | 3.57 | 4.08 |
| 2013 | 618.19 | 457.86 | 325.52 | 60.88 | 62.11 | 134.99 | 19.42 | 113.65 | 21.49 | 17.55 | 3.85 | 3.85 |
| 2014 | 660.12 | 496.12 | 349.99 | 66.50 | 68.58 | 138.12 | 19.59 | 116.72 | 22.30 | 18.48 | 3.76 | 3.58 |
| 2015 | 701.52 | 533.06 | 372.10 | 71.54 | 76.25 | 141.38 | 20.10 | 119.61 | 23.63 | 19.54 | 4.03 | 3.45 |
| 2016 | 741.05 | 568.89 | 392.79 | 76.18 | 84.46 | 144.19 | 20.27 | 122.39 | 24.72 | 20.65 | 4.00 | 3.24 |

## Medical Health Institution Bed Numbers per Thousand People

| Year Region | Medical Health Institution Bed Number | | | Medical Health Institution Bed Number Per Thousand Population | | | Medical Health Institution Bed Number Per Thousand Population |
|---|---|---|---|---|---|---|---|
| | Total | City | Countryside | Total | City | Countryside | |
| 2010 | 4786831 | 2302297 | 2484534 | 3.58 | 5.94 | 2.60 | 1.04 |
| 2012 | 5724775 | 2733403 | 2991372 | 4.24 | 6.88 | 3.11 | 1.14 |
| 2013 | 6181891 | 2948465 | 3233426 | 4.55 | 7.36 | 3.35 | 1.18 |
| 2014 | 6601214 | 3169880 | 3431334 | 4.85 | 7.84 | 3.54 | 1.20 |
| 2015 | 7015214 | 3418194 | 3597020 | 5.11 | 8.27 | 3.71 | 1.24 |
| 2016 | 7410453 | 3654956 | 3755497 | 5.37 | 8.41 | 3.91 | 1.27 |
| | | | | | | | |
| East Region | 2911065 | 1712620 | 1198445 | 5.08 | 8.21 | 3.79 | 1.16 |
| Central Region | 2359616 | 1059178 | 1300438 | 5.46 | 9.12 | 3.71 | 1.24 |
| West Region | 2139772 | 883158 | 1256614 | 5.71 | 8.05 | 4.28 | 1.44 |
| | | | | | | | |
| Beijing | 117041 | 117041 | | 5.39 | 8.64 | | |
| Tianjin | 65832 | 60521 | 5311 | 4.21 | 6.31 | 6.15 | 4.74 |
| Hebei | 360485 | 148711 | 211774 | 4.83 | 8.04 | 3.61 | 1.14 |
| Shanxi | 189689 | 93759 | 95930 | 5.15 | 9.44 | 3.79 | 1.19 |
| Inner Mongolia | 139236 | 70018 | 69218 | 5.53 | 10.22 | 3.94 | 1.14 |
| | | | | | | | |
| Liaoning | 284384 | 190867 | 93517 | 6.50 | 9.95 | 4.07 | 1.33 |
| Jilin | 151195 | 79464 | 71731 | 5.53 | 9.43 | 4.01 | 0.97 |
| Heilongjiang | 220054 | 136868 | 83186 | 5.79 | 10.34 | 3.62 | 0.98 |
| | | | | | | | |
| Shanghai | 129166 | 126010 | 3156 | 5.34 | 9.11 | 4.70 | |
| Jiangsu | 443060 | 244696 | 198364 | 5.54 | 8.41 | 4.07 | 1.20 |
| Zhejiang | 289870 | 158123 | 131747 | 5.19 | 8.58 | 4.25 | 0.55 |
| Anhui | 281720 | 134038 | 147682 | 4.55 | 6.40 | 2.98 | 1.03 |
| Fujian | 174767 | 79658 | 95109 | 4.51 | 6.94 | 3.58 | 1.11 |
| Jiangxi | 209097 | 80351 | 128746 | 4.55 | 8.51 | 3.18 | 1.18 |
| Shandong | 540994 | 245199 | 295795 | 5.44 | 7.95 | 4.28 | 1.42 |
| | | | | | | | |
| Henan | 521546 | 208749 | 312797 | 5.47 | 9.89 | 3.37 | 1.08 |
| Hubei | 360558 | 169620 | 190938 | 6.13 | 8.81 | 4.52 | 1.69 |
| Hunan | 425757 | 156329 | 269428 | 6.24 | 11.41 | 4.53 | 1.61 |
| Guangdong | 465142 | 320355 | 144787 | 4.23 | 7.67 | 2.85 | 1.10 |
| Guangxi | 224471 | 91870 | 132601 | 4.64 | 5.86 | 3.29 | 1.50 |
| Hainan | 40324 | 21439 | 18885 | 4.40 | 9.05 | 2.81 | 0.81 |
| | | | | | | | |
| Chongqing | 190850 | 111387 | 79463 | 6.26 | 6.87 | 4.49 | 2.26 |
| Sichuan | 519205 | 217579 | 301626 | 6.28 | 7.62 | 4.81 | 1.92 |
| Guizhou | 210279 | 65994 | 144285 | 5.92 | 11.88 | 3.69 | 1.02 |
| Yunnan | 253555 | 70046 | 183509 | 5.31 | 10.62 | 4.52 | 1.14 |
| Tibet | 14456 | 6529 | 7927 | 4.37 | 10.65 | 3.01 | 1.25 |
| | | | | | | | |
| Shaanxi | 225400 | 113895 | 111505 | 5.91 | 8.03 | 4.37 | 1.28 |
| Gansu | 134346 | 59962 | 74384 | 5.15 | 7.25 | 3.82 | 1.26 |
| Qinghai | 34749 | 15674 | 19075 | 5.86 | 16.19 | 3.94 | 0.84 |
| Ningxia | 36313 | 23937 | 12376 | 5.38 | 7.88 | 3.33 | 0.78 |
| Xinjiang | 156912 | 36267 | 120645 | 6.54 | 11.27 | 6.18 | 1.38 |

## Total Health Expense

| Year | Total Health Expense (One Hundred Million yuan) | | | | Total Health Expense Constituent (%) | | | Urban & Rural Health Expense(One Hundred Million yuan) | | Total Health Expense Constituent (%) | | | Health Expense in GCP (%) |
|---|---|---|---|---|---|---|---|---|---|---|---|---|---|
| | Total | Government Health Expenditure | Society Health Expenditure | Personal Health Expenditure | Government Health Expenditure | Society Health Expenditure | Personal Health Expenditure | City | Countryside | Total | City | Countryside | |
| 1980 | 143.23 | 51.91 | 60.97 | 30.35 | 36.24 | 42.57 | 21.19 | | | 14.50 | | | 3.15 |
| 1985 | 279.00 | 107.65 | 91.96 | 79.39 | 38.58 | 32.96 | 28.46 | | | 26.40 | | | 3.09 |
| 1986 | 315.90 | 122.23 | 110.35 | 83.32 | 38.69 | 34.93 | 26.38 | | | 29.40 | | | 3.06 |
| 1987 | 379.58 | 127.28 | 137.25 | 115.05 | 33.53 | 36.16 | 30.31 | | | 34.70 | | | 3.14 |
| 1988 | 488.04 | 145.39 | 189.99 | 152.66 | 29.79 | 38.93 | 31.28 | | | 44.00 | | | 3.23 |
| 1989 | 615.50 | 167.83 | 237.84 | 209.83 | 27.27 | 38.64 | 34.09 | | | 54.60 | | | 3.60 |
| 1990 | 747.39 | 187.28 | 293.10 | 267.01 | 25.06 | 39.22 | 35.73 | 396.00 | 351.39 | 65.40 | 158.80 | 38.80 | 3.98 |
| 1991 | 893.49 | 204.05 | 354.41 | 335.03 | 22.84 | 39.67 | 37.50 | 482.60 | 410.89 | 77.10 | 187.60 | 45.10 | 4.08 |
| 1992 | 1096.86 | 228.61 | 431.55 | 436.70 | 20.84 | 39.34 | 39.81 | 597.30 | 499.56 | 93.60 | 222.00 | 54.70 | 4.05 |
| 1993 | 1377.78 | 272.06 | 524.75 | 580.97 | 19.75 | 38.09 | 42.17 | 760.30 | 617.48 | 116.30 | 268.60 | 67.60 | 3.88 |
| 1994 | 1761.24 | 342.28 | 644.91 | 774.05 | 19.43 | 36.62 | 43.95 | 991.50 | 769.74 | 146.90 | 332.60 | 86.30 | 3.63 |
| 1995 | 2155.13 | 387.34 | 767.81 | 999.98 | 17.97 | 35.63 | 46.40 | 1239.50 | 915.63 | 177.90 | 401.30 | 112.90 | 3.53 |
| 1996 | 2709.42 | 461.61 | 875.66 | 1372.15 | 17.04 | 32.32 | 50.64 | 1494.90 | 1214.52 | 221.40 | 467.40 | 150.70 | 3.79 |
| 1997 | 3196.71 | 523.56 | 984.06 | 1689.09 | 16.38 | 30.78 | 52.84 | 1771.40 | 1425.31 | 258.60 | 537.80 | 177.90 | 4.02 |
| 1998 | 3678.72 | 590.06 | 1071.03 | 2017.63 | 16.04 | 29.11 | 54.85 | 1906.92 | 1771.80 | 294.90 | 625.90 | 194.60 | 4.33 |
| 1999 | 4047.50 | 640.96 | 1145.99 | 2260.55 | 15.84 | 28.31 | 55.85 | 2193.12 | 1854.38 | 321.80 | 702.00 | 203.20 | 4.49 |
| 2000 | 4586.63 | 709.52 | 1171.94 | 2705.17 | 15.47 | 25.55 | 58.98 | 2624.24 | 1962.39 | 361.90 | 813.70 | 214.70 | 4.60 |
| 2001 | 5025.93 | 800.61 | 1211.43 | 3013.89 | 15.93 | 24.10 | 59.97 | 2792.95 | 2232.98 | 393.80 | 841.20 | 244.80 | 4.56 |
| 2002 | 5790.03 | 908.51 | 1539.38 | 3342.14 | 15.69 | 26.59 | 57.72 | 3448.24 | 2341.79 | 450.70 | 987.10 | 259.30 | 4.79 |
| 2003 | 6584.10 | 1116.94 | 1788.50 | 3678.66 | 16.96 | 27.16 | 55.87 | 4150.32 | 2433.78 | 509.50 | 1108.90 | 274.70 | 4.82 |
| 2004 | 7590.29 | 1293.58 | 2225.35 | 4071.35 | 17.04 | 29.32 | 53.64 | 4939.21 | 2651.08 | 583.90 | 1261.90 | 301.60 | 4.72 |
| 2005 | 8659.91 | 1552.53 | 2586.41 | 4520.98 | 17.93 | 29.87 | 52.21 | 6305.57 | 2354.34 | 662.30 | 1126.40 | 315.80 | 4.66 |
| 2006 | 9843.34 | 1778.86 | 3210.92 | 4853.56 | 18.07 | 32.62 | 49.31 | 7174.73 | 2668.61 | 748.80 | 1248.30 | 361.90 | 4.52 |
| 2007 | 11573.97 | 2581.58 | 3893.72 | 5098.66 | 22.31 | 33.64 | 44.05 | 8968.70 | 2605.27 | 876.00 | 1516.30 | 358.10 | 4.32 |
| 2008 | 14535.40 | 3593.94 | 5065.60 | 5875.86 | 24.73 | 34.85 | 40.42 | 11251.90 | 3283.50 | 1094.50 | 1861.80 | 455.20 | 4.59 |
| 2009 | 17541.92 | 4816.26 | 6154.49 | 6571.16 | 27.46 | 35.08 | 37.46 | 13535.61 | 4006.31 | 1314.30 | 2176.60 | 562.00 | 5.08 |
| 2010 | 19980.39 | 5732.49 | 7196.61 | 7051.29 | 28.69 | 36.02 | 35.29 | 15508.62 | 4471.77 | 1490.10 | 2315.50 | 666.30 | 4.89 |
| 2011 | 24345.91 | 7464.18 | 8416.45 | 8465.28 | 30.66 | 34.57 | 34.80 | 18571.87 | 5774.04 | 1807.00 | 2697.50 | 879.40 | 5.03 |
| 2012 | 28119.00 | 8431.98 | 10030.70 | 9656.32 | 29.99 | 35.67 | 34.34 | 21280.46 | 6838.54 | 2076.70 | 2999.30 | 1064.80 | 5.26 |
| 2013 | 31668.95 | 9545.81 | 11393.79 | 10729.34 | 30.10 | 36.00 | 33.90 | 23644.95 | 8024.00 | 2327.40 | 3234.10 | 1274.40 | 5.39 |
| 2014 | 35312.40 | 10579.23 | 13437.75 | 11295.41 | 29.96 | 38.05 | 31.99 | 26575.60 | 8736.80 | 2581.70 | 2581.70 | 3558.30 | 5.55 |
| 2015 | 40974.64 | 12475.28 | 16506.71 | 11992.65 | 30.45 | 40.29 | 29.27 | — | — | 2980.80 | — | — | 6.05 |
| 2016 | 46344.88 | 13910.31 | 19096.68 | 13337.90 | 30.01 | 41.21 | 28.78 | — | — | 3351.70 | — | — | 6.22 |

Notes: ① This Table shows accounting numbers, and in 2016, the numbers were calculated initially; ② The data are calculated at the price of that year; ③ From 2001, total health expense excludes expenditures of higher medical education, while from 2006, it includes expenditures for urban and rural medical assistance

## All-region Total Health Expense in 2015

| Year | Total Health Expense (One Hundred Million yuan) | | | | Total Health Expense Constituent (%) | | | Health Expense in GCP (%) | Total Personal Health Expense (yuan) |
|------|-------|----------------------------------|-------------------------------|--------------------------------|----------------------------------|-------------------------------|--------------------------------|------|------|
| | Total | Government Health Expenditure | Society Health Expenditure | Personal Health Expenditure | Government Health Expenditure | Society Health Expenditure | Personal Health Expenditure | | |
| **Whole Country** | **40974.64** | **12475.28** | **16506.71** | **11992.65** | **30.45** | **40.29** | **29.27** | **5.95** | **2980.80** |
| Beijing | 1834.75 | 445.81 | 1069.88 | 319.07 | 24.30 | 58.31 | 17.39 | 7.99 | 8453.14 |
| Tianjin | 752.79 | 202.24 | 317.37 | 233.19 | 26.86 | 42.16 | 30.98 | 4.55 | 4866.32 |
| Hebei | 1861.50 | 552.58 | 622.13 | 686.78 | 29.68 | 33.42 | 36.89 | 6.25 | 2507.10 |
| Shanxi | 922.93 | 298.09 | 319.43 | 305.40 | 32.30 | 34.61 | 33.09 | 7.23 | 2518.82 |
| Inner Mongolia | 829.33 | 271.46 | 255.60 | 302.27 | 32.73 | 30.82 | 36.45 | 4.65 | 3302.78 |
| Liaoning | 1411.95 | 292.79 | 610.70 | 508.46 | 20.74 | 43.25 | 36.01 | 4.92 | 3221.86 |
| Jilin | 833.05 | 252.11 | 274.95 | 305.99 | 30.26 | 33.01 | 36.73 | 5.92 | 3025.98 |
| Heilongjiang | 1043.18 | 284.34 | 383.51 | 375.32 | 27.26 | 36.76 | 35.98 | 6.92 | 2736.56 |
| Shanghai | 1536.60 | 319.94 | 882.39 | 334.27 | 20.82 | 57.43 | 21.75 | 6.12 | 6362.02 |
| Jiangsu | 2974.42 | 674.73 | 1496.00 | 803.69 | 22.68 | 50.30 | 27.02 | 4.24 | 3729.07 |
| Zhejiang | 2250.21 | 500.08 | 1086.54 | 663.60 | 22.22 | 48.29 | 29.49 | 5.25 | 4062.49 |
| Anhui | 1460.42 | 497.29 | 527.68 | 435.46 | 34.05 | 36.13 | 29.82 | 6.64 | 2376.98 |
| Fujian | 1130.61 | 357.42 | 478.01 | 295.19 | 31.61 | 42.28 | 26.11 | 4.35 | 2945.07 |
| Jiangxi | 978.66 | 421.78 | 287.37 | 269.51 | 43.10 | 29.36 | 27.54 | 5.85 | 2143.54 |
| Shandong | 2843.96 | 722.22 | 1212.98 | 908.75 | 25.40 | 42.65 | 31.95 | 4.51 | 2888.09 |
| Henan | 2258.50 | 729.70 | 734.65 | 794.14 | 32.31 | 32.53 | 35.16 | 6.10 | 2382.38 |
| Hubei | 1649.24 | 530.67 | 565.72 | 552.85 | 32.18 | 34.30 | 33.52 | 5.58 | 2818.49 |
| Hunan | 1629.32 | 506.82 | 573.11 | 549.39 | 31.11 | 35.17 | 33.72 | 5.61 | 2402.06 |
| Guangdong | 3301.67 | 956.00 | 1485.88 | 859.78 | 28.96 | 45.00 | 26.04 | 4.53 | 3043.29 |
| Guangxi | 1008.94 | 386.97 | 353.17 | 268.80 | 38.35 | 35.00 | 26.64 | 6.00 | 2103.71 |
| Hainan | 262.61 | 102.70 | 93.61 | 66.31 | 39.11 | 35.64 | 25.25 | 7.09 | 2883.25 |
| Chongqing | 1000.23 | 323.69 | 393.80 | 282.74 | 32.36 | 39.37 | 28.27 | 6.36 | 3315.82 |
| Sichuan | 2164.33 | 696.24 | 825.99 | 642.10 | 32.17 | 38.16 | 29.67 | 7.20 | 2638.14 |
| Guizhou | 754.18 | 371.70 | 206.10 | 176.37 | 49.29 | 27.33 | 23.39 | 7.18 | 2136.78 |
| Yunnan | 1095.19 | 425.76 | 338.20 | 331.22 | 38.88 | 30.88 | 30.24 | 8.04 | 2309.65 |
| Tibet | 103.95 | 72.39 | 25.62 | 5.94 | 69.64 | 24.65 | 5.71 | 10.13 | 3208.66 |
| Shaanxi | 1254.37 | 377.76 | 465.24 | 411.37 | 30.12 | 37.09 | 32.80 | 6.96 | 3307.08 |
| Gansu | 654.07 | 259.10 | 199.60 | 195.37 | 39.61 | 30.52 | 29.87 | 9.63 | 2516.10 |
| Qinghai | 215.82 | 107.08 | 57.17 | 51.58 | 49.61 | 26.49 | 23.90 | 8.93 | 3667.80 |
| Ningxia | 227.86 | 77.14 | 75.90 | 74.82 | 33.85 | 33.31 | 32.83 | 7.83 | 3411.75 |
| Xinjiang | 870.98 | 262.92 | 390.81 | 217.25 | 30.19 | 44.84 | 24.94 | 9.34 | 3691.00 |

## Urban and Rural Resident Medical Health Expenditure

| Year Region | Urban Resident | | | Rural Resident | | |
|---|---|---|---|---|---|---|
| | Annual Cash Consumption Expenditure | | Medical Health Expenditure in Consumption Expenditure (%) | Annual Consumption Expenditure | | Medical Health Expenditure in Consumption Expenditure (%) |
| | Per Person (yuan) | Medical Health Expenditure (yuan) | | Per Person (yuan) | Medical Health Expenditure Per Person (yuan) | |
| 2000 | 4998.0 | 318.1 | 6.4 | 1670.1 | 87.6 | 5.2 |
| 2005 | 7942.9 | 600.9 | 7.6 | 2555.4 | 168.1 | 6.6 |
| 2010 | 13471.5 | 871.8 | 6.5 | 4381.8 | 326.0 | 7.4 |
| 2011 | 15160.9 | 969.0 | 6.4 | 5221.1 | 436.8 | 8.4 |
| 2012 | 16674.3 | 1063.7 | 6.4 | 5908.0 | 513.8 | 8.7 |
| 2013 | 18487.5 | 1136.1 | 6.1 | 7485.1 | 668.2 | 8.9 |
| 2014 | 19968.1 | 1305.6 | 6.5 | 8382.6 | 753.9 | 9.0 |
| 2015 | 21392.4 | 1443.4 | 6.7 | 9222.6 | 846.0 | 9.2 |
| 2016 | 23078.9 | 1630.8 | 7.1 | 10129.8 | 929.2 | 9.2 |
| | | | | | | |
| Beijing | 36642.0 | 2369.5 | 6.5 | 15811.2 | 1336.0 | 8.4 |
| Tianjin | 26229.5 | 1888.1 | 7.2 | 14739.4 | 1159.9 | 7.9 |
| Hebei | 17586.6 | 1500.6 | 8.5 | 9022.8 | 920.5 | 10.2 |
| Shanxi | 15818.6 | 1394.1 | 8.8 | 7421.2 | 794.3 | 10.7 |
| Inner Mongolia | 21876.5 | 1575.7 | 7.2 | 10637.4 | 1117.7 | 10.5 |
| | | | | | | |
| Liaoning | 21556.7 | 1761.9 | 8.2 | 8872.8 | 1064.5 | 12.0 |
| Jilin | 17972.6 | 1924.2 | 10.7 | 8783.3 | 1058.1 | 12.0 |
| Heilongjiang | 17152.1 | 1924.3 | 11.2 | 8391.5 | 1112.8 | 13.3 |
| | | | | | | |
| Shanghai | 36946.1 | 2361.7 | 6.4 | 16152.3 | 1464.3 | 9.1 |
| Jiangsu | 24966.0 | 1594.3 | 6.4 | 12882.5 | 1088.2 | 8.4 |
| Zhejiang | 28661.3 | 1539.0 | 5.4 | 16107.7 | 1246.3 | 7.7 |
| Anhui | 17233.5 | 1073.3 | 6.2 | 8975.2 | 808.2 | 9.0 |
| Fujian | 23520.2 | 1165.3 | 5.0 | 11960.8 | 826.9 | 6.9 |
| Jiangxi | 16731.8 | 841.4 | 5.0 | 8485.6 | 569.7 | 6.7 |
| Shandong | 19853.8 | 1416.1 | 7.1 | 8747.6 | 919.2 | 10.5 |
| | | | | | | |
| Henan | 17154.3 | 1365.5 | 8.0 | 7887.4 | 769.0 | 9.7 |
| Hubei | 18192.3 | 1482.0 | 8.1 | 9803.1 | 985.1 | 10.0 |
| Hunan | 19501.4 | 1174.6 | 6.0 | 9690.6 | 844.1 | 8.7 |
| Guangdong | 25673.1 | 1096.4 | 4.3 | 11103.0 | 723.1 | 6.5 |
| Guangxi | 16321.2 | 866.2 | 5.3 | 7582.0 | 709.7 | 9.4 |
| Hainan | 18448.4 | 1307.1 | 7.1 | 8210.3 | 634.5 | 7.7 |
| | | | | | | |
| Chongqing | 19742.3 | 1394.1 | 7.1 | 8937.7 | 745.9 | 8.3 |
| Sichuan | 19276.8 | 1369.3 | 7.1 | 9250.6 | 839.8 | 9.1 |
| Guizhou | 16914.2 | 872.2 | 5.2 | 6644.9 | 449.5 | 6.8 |
| Yunnan | 17675.0 | 1351.9 | 7.6 | 6830.1 | 577.6 | 8.5 |
| Tibet | 17022.0 | 534.4 | 3.1 | 5579.7 | 136.4 | 2.4 |
| | | | | | | |
| Shaanxi | 18463.9 | 1783.6 | 9.7 | 7900.7 | 958.2 | 12.1 |
| Gansu | 17450.9 | 1390.8 | 8.0 | 6829.8 | 669.8 | 9.8 |
| Qinghai | 19200.6 | 1459.3 | 7.6 | 8566.5 | 1190.9 | 13.9 |
| Ningxia | 18983.9 | 2016.0 | 10.6 | 8414.9 | 926.0 | 11.0 |
| Xinjiang | 19414.7 | 1517.1 | 7.8 | 7697.9 | 731.8 | 9.5 |

## Outpatient Expense for Medical Treatment and Drug per Person/Times

| | Outpatient Expense for Medical Treatment and Drug | | | Percentage of Outpatient Expense for Medical Treatment and Drug (%) | |
|---|---|---|---|---|---|
| | Per Person/Times (yuan) | Drug Fee | Examination Fee | Drug Fee | Examination Fee |
| Hospital Total | | | | | |
| 2010 | 166.8 | 85.6 | 30.0 | 51.3 | 18.0 |
| 2012 | 192.5 | 96.9 | 35.0 | 50.3 | 18.2 |
| 2013 | 206.4 | 101.7 | 37.4 | 49.3 | 18.1 |
| 2014 | 220.0 | 106.3 | 40.3 | 48.3 | 18.3 |
| 2015 | 233.9 | 110.5 | 42.7 | 47.3 | 18.3 |
| 2016 | 245.5 | 111.7 | 45.2 | 45.5 | 18.4 |
| Public Hospital | | | | | |
| 2010 | 167.3 | 87.4 | 30.8 | 52.3 | 18.4 |
| 2012 | 193.4 | 99.3 | 36.2 | 51.3 | 18.7 |
| 2013 | 207.9 | 104.4 | 38.7 | 50.2 | 18.6 |
| 2014 | 221.6 | 109.3 | 41.8 | 49.3 | 18.9 |
| 2015 | 235.2 | 113.7 | 44.3 | 48.4 | 18.8 |
| 2016 | 246.5 | 115.1 | 46.9 | 46.7 | 19.0 |
| Class-three Hospital | | | | | |
| 2010 | 220.2 | 117.6 | 37.9 | 53.4 | 17.2 |
| 2012 | 242.1 | 126.7 | 42.7 | 52.3 | 17.6 |
| 2013 | 256.7 | 132.1 | 45.2 | 51.5 | 17.6 |
| 2014 | 269.8 | 136.0 | 48.4 | 50.4 | 17.9 |
| 2015 | 283.7 | 139.8 | 51.1 | 49.3 | 18.0 |
| 2016 | 294.9 | 139.8 | 53.9 | 47.4 | 18.3 |
| Class-two Hospital | | | | | |
| 2010 | 139.3 | 70.5 | 28.9 | 50.6 | 20.8 |
| 2012 | 157.4 | 77.9 | 33.3 | 49.5 | 21.1 |
| 2013 | 166.2 | 79.6 | 35.2 | 47.9 | 21.2 |
| 2014 | 176.0 | 82.8 | 37.7 | 47.1 | 21.4 |
| 2015 | 184.1 | 85.0 | 39.2 | 46.2 | 21.3 |
| 2016 | 190.6 | 85.5 | 40.6 | 44.9 | 21.3 |
| Class-one Hospital | | | | | |
| 2010 | 93.1 | 51.6 | 11.5 | 55.4 | 12.4 |
| 2012 | 112.0 | 59.9 | 14.7 | 53.5 | 13.1 |
| 2013 | 119.8 | 64.2 | 15.6 | 53.6 | 13.1 |
| 2014 | 125.3 | 66.4 | 17.1 | 53.0 | 13.7 |
| 2015 | 132.9 | 70.6 | 17.6 | 53.1 | 13.3 |
| 2016 | 144.5 | 73.8 | 19.4 | 51.0 | 13.4 |

Note: This Table is calculated at the price of that year.

## Inpatient Expense for Medical Treatment and Drug per Person/Times

| | Inpatient Expense for Medical Treatment and Drug Per Person/Times (yuan) | | | Percentage of Inpatient Expense for Medical Treatment and Drug (%) | |
| --- | --- | --- | --- | --- | --- |
| | | Drug Fee | Examination Fee | Drug Fee | Examination Fee |
| Hospital Total | | | | | |
| 2010 | 6193.9 | 2670.2 | 441.6 | 43.1 | 7.1 |
| 2012 | 6980.4 | 2867.4 | 533.9 | 41.1 | 7.6 |
| 2013 | 7442.3 | 2939.1 | 590.2 | 39.5 | 7.9 |
| 2014 | 7832.3 | 2998.5 | 640.6 | 38.3 | 8.2 |
| 2015 | 8268.1 | 3042.0 | 697.2 | 36.8 | 8.4 |
| 2016 | 8604.7 | 2977.5 | 740.7 | 34.6 | 8.6 |
| Public Hospital | | | | | |
| 2010 | 6415.9 | 2784.3 | 460.8 | 43.4 | 7.2 |
| 2012 | 7325.1 | 3026.7 | 565.4 | 41.3 | 7.7 |
| 2013 | 7858.9 | 3116.3 | 629.8 | 39.7 | 8.0 |
| 2014 | 8290.5 | 3187.1 | 685.2 | 38.4 | 8.3 |
| 2015 | 8833.0 | 3259.6 | 753.4 | 36.9 | 8.5 |
| 2016 | 9229.7 | 3195.6 | 805.2 | 34.6 | 8.7 |
| Class-three Hospital | | | | | |
| 2010 | 10442.4 | 4440.9 | 765.5 | 42.5 | 7.3 |
| 2012 | 11186.8 | 4521.0 | 881.1 | 40.4 | 7.9 |
| 2013 | 11722.4 | 4578.3 | 952.1 | 39.1 | 8.1 |
| 2014 | 12100.2 | 4610.1 | 1007.0 | 38.1 | 8.3 |
| 2015 | 12599.3 | 4641.6 | 1078.1 | 36.8 | 8.6 |
| 2016 | 12847.8 | 4459.0 | 1121.8 | 34.7 | 8.7 |
| Class-two Hospital | | | | | |
| 2010 | 4338.6 | 1944.8 | 303.4 | 44.8 | 7.0 |
| 2012 | 4729.4 | 2033.3 | 352.4 | 43.0 | 7.5 |
| 2013 | 4968.3 | 2028.4 | 389.0 | 40.8 | 7.8 |
| 2014 | 5114.6 | 2003.9 | 417.4 | 39.2 | 8.2 |
| 2015 | 5358.2 | 1981.2 | 456.2 | 37.0 | 8.5 |
| 2016 | 5569.9 | 1913.6 | 487.4 | 34.4 | 8.8 |
| Class-one Hospital | | | | | |
| 2010 | 2844.3 | 1243.7 | 185.9 | 43.7 | 6.5 |
| 2012 | 3285.0 | 1411.3 | 236.1 | 43.0 | 7.2 |
| 2013 | 3561.9 | 1471.2 | 277.7 | 41.3 | 7.8 |
| 2014 | 3737.1 | 1519.8 | 311.5 | 40.7 | 8.3 |
| 2015 | 3844.5 | 1525.3 | 304.4 | 39.7 | 7.9 |
| 2016 | 4312.2 | 1604.3 | 358.2 | 37.2 | 8.3 |

Note: This Table is calculated at the price of that year.

## All-region Medical Health Institution Outpatient Service in 2016

| Region | Diagnosis and Treatment | | Case Number under Observation in Observation Room | Number in Health Examination | Mortality in Emergency (%) | Mortality in Observation Room (%) | Residents' Average Clinic Visits |
|---|---|---|---|---|---|---|---|
| | Per Person/ Times | Outpatient & Emergency | | | | | |
| Total | 7931700496 | 7600341010 | 50770028 | 452901318 | 0.07 | 0.09 | 5.75 |
| East Region | 4048011221 | 3904304707 | 21113813 | 240706251 | 0.06 | 0.10 | 7.06 |
| Central Region | 2029222504 | 1912840340 | 14070188 | 105669256 | 0.10 | 0.08 | 4.69 |
| West Region | 1854466771 | 1783195963 | 15586027 | 106525811 | 0.07 | 0.09 | 4.96 |
| Beijing | 232049739 | 230341187 | 2231032 | 8285398 | 0.09 | 0.14 | 10.68 |
| Tianjin | 120035010 | 115975956 | 1380817 | 4332466 | 0.08 | 0.06 | 7.68 |
| Hebei | 434942997 | 398540236 | 1779112 | 14832028 | 0.16 | 0.09 | 5.82 |
| Shanxi | 129423922 | 119048079 | 490409 | 8032048 | 0.14 | 0.14 | 3.52 |
| Inner Mongolia | 103404189 | 96475841 | 451403 | 5314621 | 0.13 | 0.22 | 4.10 |
| Liaoning | 192941947 | 178598447 | 2528364 | 9330822 | 0.12 | 0.06 | 4.41 |
| Jilin | 107607593 | 95463389 | 505068 | 4476355 | 0.10 | 0.09 | 3.94 |
| Heilongjiang | 118908161 | 109746506 | 521731 | 5755900 | 0.17 | 0.32 | 3.13 |
| Shanghai | 259319129 | 255488722 | 185585 | 8805021 | 0.12 | 2.54 | 10.72 |
| Jiangsu | 551949189 | 536538852 | 1695626 | 27864253 | 0.04 | 0.03 | 6.90 |
| Zhejiang | 555212876 | 544525149 | 1084734 | 84909506 | 0.04 | 0.15 | 9.93 |
| Anhui | 263001944 | 251672653 | 1598351 | 13905370 | 0.08 | 0.02 | 4.25 |
| Fujian | 219266573 | 213139309 | 664021 | 9215055 | 0.02 | 0.04 | 5.66 |
| Jiangxi | 213411742 | 203778881 | 1703886 | 12836018 | 0.03 | 0.02 | 4.65 |
| Shandong | 621629641 | 589695170 | 3743792 | 28545873 | 0.16 | 0.12 | 6.25 |
| Henan | 577769911 | 547689924 | 1612656 | 26358304 | 0.18 | 0.10 | 6.06 |
| Hubei | 354790816 | 339929293 | 3492084 | 17782884 | 0.07 | 0.05 | 6.03 |
| Hunan | 264308415 | 245511615 | 4146003 | 16522377 | 0.07 | 0.10 | 3.87 |
| Guangdong | 812006651 | 793446531 | 5614045 | 42397359 | 0.03 | 0.04 | 7.38 |
| Guangxi | 254233641 | 246765180 | 1745660 | 14028087 | 0.03 | 0.04 | 5.25 |
| Hainan | 48657469 | 48015148 | 206685 | 2188470 | 0.03 | 0.02 | 5.31 |
| Chongqing | 149056718 | 143627905 | 2395851 | 7518300 | 0.08 | 0.02 | 4.89 |
| Sichuan | 464246426 | 446918151 | 2802962 | 28236515 | 0.07 | 0.04 | 5.62 |
| Guizhou | 138444990 | 132360465 | 1401887 | 7840359 | 0.05 | 0.03 | 3.89 |
| Yunnan | 244601498 | 238511658 | 3651970 | 9808110 | 0.03 | 0.06 | 5.13 |
| Tibet | 13941952 | 13269918 | 91398 | 1422031 | 0.04 | 0.02 | 4.22 |
| Shaanxi | 184998227 | 180194257 | 204179 | 8888388 | 0.09 | 0.18 | 4.85 |
| Gansu | 130420565 | 122073254 | 1280303 | 9352515 | 0.10 | 0.56 | 5.00 |
| Qinghai | 23566318 | 21976031 | 416389 | 1476100 | 0.24 | 0.01 | 3.97 |
| Ningxia | 38321962 | 36888941 | 482745 | 1889830 | 0.11 | 0.02 | 5.68 |
| Xinjiang | 109230285 | 104134362 | 661280 | 10750955 | 0.14 | 0.18 | 4.55 |

## All-hospital Diagnosis and Treatment Numbers/Times (Registration Type/Host Unit/Management Type/Class/Institution Type)

Unit: Ten Thousand Person/Times

| Hospital Type | 2010 | 2012 | 2013 | 2014 | 2015 | 2016 |
|---|---|---|---|---|---|---|
| **Total** | **203963.3** | **254161.6** | **274177.7** | **297207.0** | **308364.1** | **326955.9** |
| Registration Type | | | | | | |
| Public Hospital | 187381.1 | 228866.3 | 245510.6 | 264741.6 | 271243.6 | 284771.6 |
| Private Hospital | 16582.2 | 25295.3 | 28667.1 | 32465.4 | 37120.5 | 42184.3 |
| Host Unit | | | | | | |
| Government Ownership | 170421.9 | 211670.3 | 227709.9 | 246725.5 | 253498.0 | 267516.9 |
| Society Operation | 23613.1 | 27439.4 | 28811.2 | 30462.3 | 32173.2 | 34027.1 |
| Private Operation | 9928.3 | 15051.9 | 17656.6 | 20019.1 | 22692.8 | 25411.9 |
| Management Type | | | | | | |
| Non-profit | 194544.1 | 241335.0 | 259373.4 | 280616.3 | 290055.6 | 305891.9 |
| Profit | 9419.2 | 12826.6 | 14804.3 | 16590.7 | 18308.5 | 21064.0 |
| Unknown | | | | | | |
| Hospital Class | | | | | | |
| Class Three Hospital | 76046.3 | 108670.6 | 123821.9 | 139804.4 | 149764.6 | 162784.8 |
| Class Two Hospital | 93120.4 | 105476.7 | 109169.1 | 114708.6 | 117233.1 | 121666.5 |
| Class One Hospital | 14573.6 | 16766.5 | 17617.9 | 18478.1 | 20567.9 | 21790.9 |
| Not Estimated Hospital | 20223.0 | 23247.9 | 23568.8 | 24215.8 | 20798.5 | 20713.7 |
| Institution Type | | | | | | |
| Comprehensive Hospital | 151058.2 | 187353.0 | 201576.5 | 218193.0 | 225675.2 | 238512.9 |
| TCM Hospital | 32770.2 | 40705.2 | 43726.3 | 47164.2 | 48502.6 | 50774.5 |
| Hospital of Traditional Chinese and Western Medicine | 2702.6 | 3769.1 | 4466.1 | 5101.3 | 5401.4 | 5927.3 |
| National Hospital | 553.8 | 645.9 | 760.1 | 792.6 | 966.8 | 968.7 |
| Specialty Hospital | 16821.5 | 21633.7 | 23575.5 | 25867.4 | 27702.5 | 30627.1 |
| Nursing Home | 57.1 | 54.7 | 73.3 | 88.6 | 115.4 | 145.5 |

## All-region Medical Health Institution Inpatient Service in 2016

| Region | Inpatient Number | Discharged Number | Inpatient Surgery Number/ Times | Mortality (%) | Discharged Number Per Bed | Inpatient Number from Outpatient & Emergency Percentage | Residents' Annual Hospitalization Rate |
|---|---|---|---|---|---|---|---|
| Total | 227278325 | 226036388 | 50821967 | 0.4 | 30.5 | 4.4 | 16.5 |
| East Region | 87148862 | 86791381 | 23815996 | 0.4 | 29.9 | 3.1 | 15.2 |
| Central Region | 72061550 | 71613221 | 14057266 | 0.3 | 30.4 | 6.0 | 16.7 |
| West Region | 68067913 | 67631786 | 12948705 | 0.3 | 31.6 | 5.7 | 18.2 |
| Beijing | 3118881 | 3109106 | 1291653 | 1.1 | 26.6 | 1.5 | 14.4 |
| Tianjin | 1620968 | 1623907 | 642346 | 0.6 | 24.7 | 1.6 | 10.4 |
| Hebei | 11177230 | 11071235 | 1942252 | 0.3 | 30.7 | 5.6 | 15.0 |
| Shanxi | 4300809 | 4250371 | 962881 | 0.2 | 22.6 | 5.5 | 11.7 |
| Inner Mongolia | 3294839 | 3279938 | 610639 | 0.6 | 23.6 | 4.8 | 13.1 |
| Liaoning | 6925691 | 6875342 | 1360957 | 0.9 | 24.2 | 5.4 | 15.8 |
| Jilin | 3688295 | 3658655 | 699047 | 1.0 | 24.2 | 5.6 | 13.5 |
| Heilongjiang | 5641399 | 5612284 | 1202127 | 1.0 | 25.5 | 6.8 | 14.8 |
| Shanghai | 3666108 | 3661626 | 1990579 | 1.4 | 28.4 | 1.5 | 15.2 |
| Jiangsu | 13089607 | 13027468 | 3300700 | 0.2 | 29.5 | 3.2 | 16.4 |
| Zhejiang | 8712905 | 8694165 | 2680317 | 0.3 | 30.0 | 1.9 | 15.6 |
| Anhui | 8973150 | 8913610 | 1801024 | 0.3 | 31.7 | 5.4 | 14.5 |
| Fujian | 5350435 | 5338778 | 1323388 | 0.1 | 30.6 | 3.6 | 13.8 |
| Jiangxi | 7454683 | 7420483 | 1304691 | 0.2 | 35.5 | 6.8 | 16.2 |
| Shandong | 16917849 | 16842011 | 3518739 | 0.4 | 31.2 | 5.2 | 17.0 |
| Henan | 16018202 | 15938947 | 3147635 | 0.2 | 30.7 | 5.0 | 16.8 |
| Hubei | 11975693 | 11908419 | 2717043 | 0.4 | 33.0 | 5.5 | 20.3 |
| Hunan | 14009319 | 13910452 | 2222818 | 0.1 | 32.7 | 9.1 | 20.5 |
| Guangdong | 15468824 | 15448632 | 5564568 | 0.5 | 33.3 | 2.6 | 14.1 |
| Guangxi | 8603641 | 8584441 | 1431667 | 0.4 | 38.2 | 5.1 | 17.8 |
| Hainan | 1100364 | 1099111 | 200497 | 0.3 | 27.3 | 3.2 | 12.0 |
| Chongqing | 6313679 | 6280342 | 1131716 | 0.3 | 32.9 | 6.6 | 20.7 |
| Sichuan | 16559605 | 16472683 | 3234578 | 0.4 | 31.7 | 5.6 | 20.0 |
| Guizhou | 6619276 | 6546079 | 1260351 | 0.2 | 31.2 | 7.4 | 18.6 |
| Yunnan | 8194449 | 8168550 | 1880660 | 0.3 | 32.3 | 5.1 | 17.2 |
| Tibet | 343803 | 287103 | 49821 | 0.2 | 19.9 | 3.4 | 10.4 |
| Shaanxi | 5806543 | 6755281 | 1430247 | 0.3 | 30.0 | 6.1 | 17.9 |
| Gansu | 4001955 | 3968855 | 609333 | 0.2 | 29.6 | 5.7 | 15.3 |
| Qinghai | 911845 | 907275 | 155391 | 0.2 | 26.1 | 5.6 | 15.4 |
| Ningxia | 1067163 | 1055863 | 245153 | 0.2 | 29.1 | 3.8 | 15.8 |
| Xinjiang | 5351115 | 5325376 | 909149 | 0.4 | 34.0 | 6.4 | 22.3 |

## All-hospital Inpatient Numbers (Registration Type/Host Unit/Management Type/Class/Institution Type)

| Hospital Type | 2010 | 2012 | 2013 | 2014 | 2015 | 2016 |
|---|---|---|---|---|---|---|
| **Total** | **9523.8** | **12727.4** | **14007.4** | **15375.1** | **16086.8** | **17527.7** |
| Registration Type | | | | | | |
| Public Hospital | 8724.2 | 11331.2 | 12315.2 | 13414.8 | 13721.4 | 14750.5 |
| Private Hospital | 799.5 | 1396.3 | 1692.3 | 1960.3 | 2365.4 | 2777.2 |
| Host Unit | | | | | | |
| Government Ownership | 8065.1 | 10590.4 | 11534.9 | 12586.5 | 12905.2 | 13937.8 |
| Society Operation | 939.8 | 1220.4 | 1309.8 | 1450.2 | 1595.5 | 1765.2 |
| Private Operation | 518.9 | 916.7 | 1162.8 | 1338.4 | 1586.1 | 1824.7 |
| Management Type | | | | | | |
| Non-profit | 9082.4 | 11997.1 | 13095.6 | 14332.5 | 14894.9 | 16144.7 |
| Profit | 441.4 | 730.3 | 911.8 | 1042.7 | 1192 | 1383.0 |
| Hospital Class | | | | | | |
| Class Three Hospital | 3096.8 | 4726.4 | 5450.1 | 6291.0 | 6828.9 | 7686.2 |
| Class Two Hospital | 5115.7 | 6241.6 | 6620.9 | 7005.7 | 7121.2 | 7570.3 |
| Class One Hospital | 463.7 | 648.9 | 729.2 | 798.0 | 965.2 | 1039.3 |
| Not Estimated Hospital | 847.5 | 1110.6 | 1207.2 | 1280.3 | 1171.7 | 1231.9 |
| Institution Type | | | | | | |
| Comprehensive Hospital | 7505.5 | 9914.9 | 10848.0 | 11844.1 | 12335.4 | 13402.3 |
| TCM Hospital | 1167.7 | 1641.7 | 1826.7 | 2010.6 | 2101.8 | 2278.6 |
| Hospital of Traditional Chinese and Western Medicine | 91.3 | 129.7 | 155.6 | 177.9 | 203.3 | 229.0 |
| National Hospital | 24.3 | 34.1 | 40.7 | 49.3 | 56.2 | 59.6 |
| Specialty Hospital | 732.8 | 1004.1 | 1132.4 | 1286.8 | 1380.5 | 1545.6 |
| Nursing Home | 2.1 | 3.0 | 4.1 | 6.5 | 9.6 | 12.6 |

## Medical Health Institution Bed Utilization in 2016

| Institution Type | Actual Available Bed Days (Day) | Average Available Bed | Actual Using Bed Days (Day) | Discharge Total Bed Days (Day) | Hospital Bed Turnover Times | Hospital Bed Working Days (Day) | Hospital Bed Utilization Rate (%) | Average Hospitalization Days |
|---|---|---|---|---|---|---|---|---|
| Total | 2579030278 | 7065836 | 2057968370 | 1978739734 | 32.0 | 291.3 | 79.8 | 8.8 |
| I. Hospital | 1986184210 | 5441601 | 1694087028 | 1639944609 | 32.0 | 311.3 | 85.3 | 9.4 |
| Comprehensive Hospital | 1380484814 | 3782150 | 1190039853 | 1163611986 | 35.2 | 314.6 | 86.2 | 8.7 |
| TCM Hospital | 267556110 | 733030 | 227287787 | 222496721 | 31.0 | 310.1 | 84.9 | 9.8 |
| Hospital of Traditional Chinese and Western Medicine | 30480546 | 83508 | 24545866 | 23843058 | 27.2 | 293.9 | 80.5 | 10.5 |
| National Hospital | 8746252 | 23962 | 6181197 | 6098159 | 24.6 | 258.0 | 70.7 | 10.4 |
| Specialty Hospital | 287269233 | 787039 | 237146540 | 217778572 | 19.5 | 301.3 | 82.6 | 14.2 |
| Stomatological Hospital | 3429713 | 9396 | 1209922 | 1199855 | 14.9 | 128.8 | 35.3 | 8.6 |
| Ophthalmic Hospital | 10870902 | 29783 | 6344390 | 6155338 | 49.8 | 213.0 | 58.4 | 4.2 |
| Otolaryngology Hospital | 1941659 | 5320 | 1076594 | 994146 | 33.7 | 202.4 | 55.4 | 5.5 |
| Tumor Hospital | 26057009 | 71389 | 27091493 | 27304338 | 34.1 | 379.5 | 104.0 | 11.2 |
| Cardiovascular Hospital | 5062072 | 13869 | 3973281 | 3808593 | 28.5 | 286.5 | 78.5 | 9.6 |
| Thoracopathy Hospital | 3042297 | 8335 | 2804066 | 2793696 | 27.8 | 336.4 | 92.2 | 12.1 |
| Hematonosis Hospital | 494298 | 1354 | 360961 | 346446 | 19.9 | 266.5 | 73.0 | 12.8 |
| Obstetrical and Gynecological Hospital | 18720077 | 51288 | 11050925 | 10823675 | 35.9 | 215.5 | 59.0 | 5.9 |
| Children's Hospital | 13400141 | 36713 | 12980339 | 12749178 | 48.5 | 353.6 | 96.9 | 7.2 |
| Mental Hospital | 108637357 | 297637 | 103730723 | 89159327 | 5.8 | 348.5 | 95.5 | 51.7 |
| Infectious Disease Hospital | 18339108 | 50244 | 16157270 | 15942120 | 19.6 | 321.6 | 88.1 | 16.2 |
| Dermatology Hospital | 2319639 | 6355 | 1063524 | 954033 | 13.7 | 167.3 | 45.8 | 10.9 |
| Tuberculosis Hospital | 4707218 | 12896 | 4313777 | 4247014 | 22.1 | 334.5 | 91.6 | 14.9 |
| Leprosy Hospital | 501753 | 1375 | 114437 | 29274 | 1.3 | 83.2 | 22.8 | 16.5 |
| Occupational Disease Hospital | 1372580 | 3760 | 1142402 | 1101856 | 15.3 | 303.8 | 83.2 | 19.2 |
| Orthopaedic Hospital | 17423504 | 47736 | 11961598 | 11362651 | 22.6 | 250.6 | 68.7 | 10.5 |
| Rehabilitation Hospital | 18866108 | 51688 | 12838786 | 10901819 | 11.8 | 248.4 | 68.1 | 17.9 |
| Plastic Surgery Hospital | 616496 | 1689 | 242207 | 232053 | 21.1 | 143.4 | 39.3 | 6.5 |
| Cosmetic Hospital | 1634180 | 4477 | 387842 | 321106 | 17.6 | 86.6 | 23.7 | 4.1 |
| Other Specialty Hospital | 29833122 | 81735 | 18302003 | 17352054 | 22.9 | 223.9 | 61.3 | 9.3 |
| Nursing Hospital | 11647255 | 31910 | 8885785 | 6116113 | 3.7 | 278.5 | 76.3 | 51.3 |
| II. Grassroots Medical Health Institution | 497325644 | 1362536 | 296981687 | 275925799 | 30.4 | 218.0 | 59.7 | 6.7 |
| Community Health Service Center (Station) | 66221637 | 181429 | 35817787 | 31196052 | 17.9 | 197.4 | 54.1 | 9.6 |
| Community Health Service Center | 61215866 | 167715 | 33437208 | 30098904 | 18.5 | 199.4 | 54.6 | 9.7 |
| Community Health Service Station | 5005771 | 13714 | 2380579 | 1097148 | 10.9 | 173.6 | 47.6 | 7.4 |
| Health Center | 431056461 | 1180977 | 261121184 | 244722761 | 32.2 | 221.1 | 60.6 | 6.4 |
| District Health Center | 3002169 | 8225 | 1526897 | 1363457 | 23.2 | 185.6 | 50.9 | 7.2 |
| Township Health Hospital | 428054292 | 1172751 | 259594287 | 243359304 | 32.2 | 221.4 | 60.6 | 6.4 |
| Central Health Center | 189202341 | 518363 | 120513495 | 113998590 | 34.2 | 232.5 | 63.7 | 6.4 |
| Township Health Center | 238851951 | 654389 | 139080792 | 129360714 | 30.7 | 212.5 | 58.2 | 6.4 |
| Outpatient Department | | | | | | | | 0.0 |
| Nursing Station | 47546 | 130 | 42716 | 6986 | 18.0 | 327.9 | 89.8 | 3.0 |
| III. Professional Public Health Institution | 85491157 | 234222 | 61768114 | 59112878 | 42.0 | 263.7 | 72.3 | 6.0 |
| Special Disease Prevention and Control Center (Institution, Station) | 13753170 | 37680 | 9751332 | 8700562 | 14.1 | 258.8 | 70.9 | 16.4 |
| Maternal and Child Care Center (Institution, Station) | 71737987 | 196542 | 52016782 | 50412316 | 47.4 | 264.7 | 72.5 | 5.4 |
| Maternal and Child Care Center | 67579260 | 185149 | 50360939 | 48880865 | 48.7 | 272.0 | 74.5 | 5.4 |
| IV. Other Medical Health Institution | 10029267 | 27477 | 5131541 | 3756448 | 16.2 | 186.8 | 51.2 | 8.4 |
| Sanatorium | 10029267 | 27477 | 5131541 | 3756448 | 16.2 | 186.8 | 51.2 | 8.4 |
| Clinical Examination Center | | | | | | | | |

## All-region Hospital Bed Utilization in 2016

| Region | Hospital Bed Working Days | | | Hospital Bed Utilization Rate (%) | | | Average Hospitalization Days | | |
|---|---|---|---|---|---|---|---|---|---|
| | Total | Public | Private | Total | Public | Private | Total | Public | Private |
| **Total** | **311.3** | **332.2** | **229.2** | **85.3** | **91** | **62.8** | **9.4** | **9.6** | **8.6** |
| East Region | 313.0 | 334.1 | 227.5 | 85.7 | 91.5 | 62.3 | 9.4 | 9.5 | 9.1 |
| Central Region | 312.8 | 329.2 | 240.3 | 85.7 | 90.2 | 65.8 | 9.6 | 9.9 | 8.3 |
| West Region | 307.4 | 332.9 | 221.6 | 84.2 | 91.2 | 60.7 | 9.2 | 9.4 | 8.3 |
| Beijing | 300.1 | 328.0 | 196.1 | 82.2 | 89.8 | 53.7 | 10.5 | 10.5 | 10.5 |
| Tianjin | 299.6 | 323.3 | 190.4 | 82.1 | 88.6 | 52.2 | 10.3 | 10.4 | 9.1 |
| Hebei | 315.0 | 333.8 | 228.2 | 86.3 | 91.4 | 62.5 | 8.8 | 9.0 | 7.4 |
| Shanxi | 277.1 | 293.8 | 202.3 | 75.9 | 80.5 | 55.4 | 10.5 | 10.7 | 9.3 |
| Inner Mongolia | 272.7 | 293.2 | 156.1 | 74.7 | 80.3 | 42.8 | 9.9 | 10.0 | 9.0 |
| Liaoning | 305.9 | 329.8 | 200.7 | 83.8 | 90.4 | 55.0 | 10.8 | 11.1 | 9.4 |
| Jilin | 285.9 | 304.9 | 202.2 | 78.3 | 83.5 | 55.4 | 9.6 | 9.9 | 7.9 |
| Heilongjiang | 301.9 | 317.0 | 201.6 | 82.7 | 86.9 | 55.2 | 10.7 | 10.9 | 9.5 |
| Shanghai | 349.6 | 362.1 | 273.6 | 95.8 | 99.2 | 75.0 | 10.1 | 9.7 | 16.5 |
| Jiangsu | 318.7 | 345.6 | 252.9 | 87.3 | 94.7 | 69.3 | 9.6 | 9.7 | 9.3 |
| Zhejiang | 326.3 | 350.4 | 238.9 | 89.4 | 96.0 | 65.5 | 9.9 | 9.6 | 12.7 |
| Anhui | 309.7 | 331.0 | 243.0 | 84.8 | 90.7 | 66.6 | 8.8 | 9.1 | 7.9 |
| Fujian | 299.1 | 315.1 | 213.6 | 81.9 | 86.3 | 58.5 | 8.7 | 9.0 | 7.2 |
| Jiangxi | 326.3 | 335.3 | 275.0 | 89.4 | 91.9 | 75.3 | 9.1 | 9.3 | 7.9 |
| Shandong | 310.4 | 330.9 | 222.4 | 85.0 | 90.7 | 60.9 | 8.9 | 9.1 | 8.2 |
| Henan | 320.7 | 332.6 | 274.4 | 87.9 | 91.1 | 75.2 | 9.7 | 10.0 | 8.5 |
| Hubei | 335.7 | 353.1 | 237.8 | 92.0 | 96.7 | 65.2 | 9.7 | 9.9 | 8.4 |
| Hunan | 313.9 | 335.4 | 228.9 | 86.0 | 91.9 | 62.7 | 9.5 | 9.9 | 7.8 |
| Guangdong | 306.5 | 325.8 | 212.6 | 84.0 | 89.3 | 58.2 | 8.8 | 8.8 | 8.5 |
| Guangxi | 321.1 | 329.6 | 241.2 | 88.0 | 90.3 | 66.1 | 8.6 | 8.6 | 9.1 |
| Hainan | 285.4 | 294.3 | 199.2 | 78.2 | 80.6 | 54.6 | 9.0 | 9.1 | 7.6 |
| Chongqing | 308.0 | 336.8 | 240.0 | 84.4 | 92.3 | 65.8 | 9.2 | 9.6 | 7.9 |
| Sichuan | 329.1 | 360.7 | 252.0 | 90.2 | 98.8 | 69.0 | 10.1 | 10.4 | 9.1 |
| Guizhou | 285.4 | 329.0 | 205.1 | 78.2 | 90.1 | 56.2 | 8.5 | 8.7 | 8.1 |
| Yunnan | 303.0 | 341.6 | 201.6 | 83.0 | 93.6 | 55.2 | 8.6 | 8.8 | 7.6 |
| Tibet | 271.8 | 285.7 | 217.3 | 74.5 | 78.3 | 59.5 | 9.2 | 10.5 | 5.2 |
| Shaanxi | 300.1 | 324.8 | 208.2 | 82.2 | 89.0 | 57.0 | 9.2 | 9.3 | 8.2 |
| Gansu | 301.6 | 309.9 | 217.3 | 82.6 | 84.9 | 59.5 | 9.1 | 9.2 | 7.3 |
| Qinghai | 271.5 | 287.1 | 171.9 | 74.4 | 78.7 | 47.1 | 9.3 | 9.5 | 7.9 |
| Ningxia | 308.1 | 328.2 | 216.2 | 84.4 | 89.9 | 59.2 | 9.3 | 9.5 | 8.2 |
| Xinjiang | 315.8 | 335.7 | 192.2 | 86.5 | 92.0 | 52.7 | 8.7 | 8.9 | 6.6 |

## Grassroots Medical Health Institution Service Volume

| Institution Type | Diagnosis &Treatment Persons/Times (Ten Thousand Persons/Times) | | | | Inpatient Number (Ten Thousand Persons) | | | |
|---|---|---|---|---|---|---|---|---|
| | 2013 | 2014 | 2015 | 2016 | 2013 | 2014 | 2015 | 2016 |
| **Total** | **432431.0** | **436394.9** | **434192.7** | **436663.3** | **4300.7** | **4094.2** | **4036.6** | **4164.8** |
| Host Unit | | | | | | | | |
|   Government Operation | 171467.8 | 173616.9 | 176140.4 | 179037.5 | 4171.4 | 3966.1 | 3910.7 | 4047.3 |
|   Non-government Operation | 260963.2 | 262777.9 | 258052.3 | 257625.8 | 129.3 | 128.0 | 125.9 | 117.5 |
| Institution Type | | | | | | | | |
|   Community Health Service Center | 50788.6 | 53618.8 | 55902.6 | 56327 | 292.1 | 298.1 | 305.5 | 313.7 |
|     Government Operation | 42221.5 | 44252.3 | 46441.8 | 46703.4 | 233.4 | 237.0 | 242.0 | 251.5 |
|   Community Health Service Station | 14921.2 | 14912.0 | 14742.5 | 15561.9 | 30.1 | 23.0 | 16.5 | 15 |
|     Government Operation | 3997.8 | 3524.6 | 3265.9 | 3795.7 | 5.5 | 4.5 | 4.1 | 4 |
|   District Health Center | 999.7 | 892.7 | 792.1 | 881.4 | 20.9 | 19.5 | 17.8 | 19.2 |
|   Township Health Center | 100712.7 | 102865.9 | 105464.3 | 108233.0 | 3937.2 | 3732.6 | 3676.1 | 3799.9 |
|     Government Operation | 99985.7 | 102099.0 | 104610.6 | 107467.5 | 3911.6 | 3705.3 | 3647.0 | 3772.7 |
|   Village Health Room | 201218.4 | 198628.7 | 189406.9 | 185263.6 | | | | |
|   Outpatient Department | 8378.6 | 8786.1 | 9394.2 | 10288.7 | 20.3 | 20.8 | 20.4 | 16.7 |
|   Clinic (Infirmary) | 55411.8 | 56690.8 | 58490.1 | 60107.6 | 0.2 | 0.2 | 0.3 | 0.3 |
| **Constituent (%)** | **100.0** | **100.0** | **100.0** | **100.0** | **100.0** | **100.0** | **100.0** | **100.0** |
| Host Unit | | | | | | | | |
|   Government Operation | 39.7 | 39.8 | 40.6 | 41.0 | 97.0 | 96.9 | 96.9 | 97.2 |
|   Non-government Operation | 60.3 | 60.2 | 59.4 | 59.0 | 3.0 | 3.1 | 3.1 | 2.8 |
| Institution Type | | | | | | | | |
|   Community Health Service Center | 11.7 | 12.3 | 12.9 | 12.9 | 6.8 | 7.3 | 7.6 | 7.5 |
|   Community Health Service Station | 3.5 | 3.4 | 3.4 | 3.6 | 0.7 | 0.6 | 0.4 | 0.4 |
|   District Health Center | 0.2 | 0.2 | 0.2 | 0.2 | 0.5 | 0.5 | 0.4 | 0.5 |
|   Township Health Center | 23.3 | 23.6 | 24.3 | 24.8 | 91.5 | 91.2 | 91.1 | 91.2 |
|   Village Health Room | 46.5 | 45.5 | 43.6 | 42.4 | | | | |
|   Outpatient Department | 1.9 | 2.0 | 2.2 | 2.4 | 0.5 | 0.5 | 0.5 | 0.4 |
|   Clinic (Infirmary) | 12.8 | 13.0 | 13.5 | 13.8 | | | | |

## Community Health Service Institutions, Beds, Personnel Numbers

| | 2010 | 2012 | 2013 | 2014 | 2015 | 2016 |
|---|---|---|---|---|---|---|
| **Total Institution** | **32739** | **33562** | **33965** | **34238** | **34321** | **34327** |
| Community Health Service Center | 6903 | 8182 | 8488 | 8669 | 8806 | 8918 |
| Community Health Service Station | 25836 | 25380 | 25477 | 25569 | 25515 | 25409 |
| Host Unit | | | | | | |
| Government Operation | 18390 | 19579 | 18638 | 18306 | 18246 | 18031 |
| Non-government Operation | 14349 | 13983 | 15327 | 8835 | 16075 | 16296 |
| Hospital Bed | | | | | | |
| No Bed | 25285 | 25805 | 26628 | 26973 | 27357 | 27334 |
| 1-9 | 3211 | 2769 | 2438 | 2301 | 2053 | 2053 |
| 10-49 | 3210 | 3764 | 3656 | 3701 | 3573 | 3575 |
| 50-99 | 797 | 959 | 973 | 998 | 1057 | 1086 |
| 100 and above | 236 | 265 | 270 | 265 | 281 | 279 |
| **Total Bed** | **168814** | **203210** | **194241** | **195913** | **200979** | **202689** |
| Community Health Service Center | 137628 | 163556 | 167998 | 171754 | 178410 | 182191 |
| Community Health Service Station | 31186 | 39654 | 26243 | 24159 | 22569 | 20498 |
| **Personnel Number** | **389516** | **454160** | **476073** | **488771** | **504817** | **521974** |
| Health Technician | 331322 | 386952 | 406218 | 417503 | 431158 | 446176 |
| #Certified (Assistant) Practitioner | 144225 | 167414 | 173838 | 176998 | 181670 | 187699 |
| Registered Nurse | 106528 | 128652 | 139104 | 145672 | 153393 | 162132 |
| Other Technician | 14879 | 17589 | 18929 | 18963 | 20305 | 21569 |
| Managerial Worker | 18652 | 19802 | 20020 | 20380 | 20790 | 21350 |
| Ground Skilled Staff | 24663 | 29817 | 30906 | 31925 | 32564 | 32879 |

## Department Beds, Outpatients and Emergency Person/Times, Discharged Numbers and Constituent in Community Health Service Centers in 2016

| Department Type | Hospital Bed | | Outpatient & Emergency | | Hospital Discharge | |
|---|---|---|---|---|---|---|
| | Number | Constituent (%) | Person/Times | Constituent (%) | Number | Constituent (%) |
| **Total** | **182191** | **100.0** | **53790.9** | **100.0** | **310.2** | **100.0** |
| Prevention and Health Department | 1796 | 1.0 | 3176.4 | 5.9 | 1.7 | 0.6 |
| General Medical Department | 58067 | 31.9 | 26881.4 | 50.0 | 83.4 | 26.9 |
| Internal Medicine | 57898 | 31.8 | 9003.1 | 16.7 | 123.6 | 39.9 |
| Surgical Department | 18489 | 10.1 | 1964.9 | 3.7 | 30.9 | 10.0 |
| Pediatrics Department | 4843 | 2.7 | 1377.0 | 2.6 | 9.1 | 2.9 |
| Gynaecology and Obstetrics Department | 10957 | 6.0 | 1657.2 | 3.1 | 20.3 | 6.5 |
| TCM Department | 7346 | 4.0 | 5174.8 | 9.6 | 11.8 | 3.8 |
| Total | 22795 | 12.5 | 4556.1 | 8.5 | 29.3 | 9.4 |

## All-region Medical Service in Community Health Service Centers (Station)

| Region | Community Health Service Center | | | | | | Community Health Service Station | |
|---|---|---|---|---|---|---|---|---|
| | Diagnosis & Treatment Number | Inpatient Number | Bed Utilization Rate (%) | Average Hospitalization Days | Average-day Diagnosis & Treatment by a Doctor | Average-day Hospitalization Bed in the charge of a Doctor | Diagnosis &Treatment Number | Doctor's Average-day Diagnosis & Treatment |
| 2010 | 347404131 | 2180577 | 56.1 | 10.4 | 13.6 | 0.7 | 137111392 | 13.6 |
| 2012 | 454751077 | 2686554 | 55.5 | 10.1 | 14.8 | 0.7 | 143935953 | 14.0 |
| 2013 | 507885866 | 2920630 | 57.0 | 9.8 | 15.7 | 0.7 | 149211933 | 14.3 |
| 2014 | 536187933 | 2980571 | 55.6 | 9.9 | 16.1 | 0.7 | 149119766 | 14.4 |
| 2015 | 559025520 | 3055499 | 54.7 | 9.8 | 16.3 | 0.7 | 147424820 | 14.1 |
| 2016 | 563270221 | 3137143 | 54.6 | 9.7 | 15.9 | 0.6 | 155618949 | 14.5 |
| East Region | 442167544 | 1131554 | 54.2 | 12.9 | 20.0 | 0.5 | 84470083 | 17.8 |
| Central Region | 63273926 | 1088955 | 52.2 | 8.2 | 8.2 | 0.9 | 41323118 | 12.5 |
| West Region | 57828751 | 916634 | 58.9 | 7.6 | 10.4 | 1.0 | 29825748 | 11.0 |
| Beijing | 46681738 | 25480 | 31.7 | 18.1 | 17.1 | 0.1 | 5993398 | 21.2 |
| Tianjin | 15441163 | 12977 | 21.7 | 12.1 | 22.9 | 0.2 | 2685347 | 31.1 |
| Hebei | 6895241 | 60561 | 44.2 | 9.2 | 8.7 | 0.6 | 9975584 | 10.9 |
| Shanxi | 3793301 | 40363 | 41.9 | 10.9 | 6.7 | 0.5 | 4052933 | 6.9 |
| Inner Mongolia | 4155017 | 55386 | 50.5 | 9.1 | 6.6 | 0.7 | 3684881 | 7.7 |
| Liaoning | 9966429 | 64929 | 37.1 | 9.9 | 9.9 | 0.5 | 5567997 | 12.6 |
| Jilin | 3817026 | 23690 | 30.0 | 9.9 | 6.1 | 0.3 | 708477 | 9.2 |
| Heilongjiang | 6335315 | 73599 | 39.2 | 9.9 | 6.1 | 0.5 | 1113469 | 7.2 |
| Shanghai | 85802333 | 74638 | 88.6 | 62.9 | 27.8 | 1.2 | | |
| Jiangsu | 63735422 | 345414 | 51.7 | 9.0 | 19.1 | 0.7 | 14204424 | 21.0 |
| Zhejiang | 88243821 | 62032 | 40.1 | 15.3 | 24.2 | 0.2 | 3858577 | 24.1 |
| Anhui | 10604947 | 127432 | 43.8 | 7.6 | 11.0 | 0.8 | 10773076 | 13.4 |
| Fujian | 13613062 | 59750 | 35.8 | 6.5 | 16.1 | 0.3 | 3317343 | 13.8 |
| Jiangxi | 3523832 | 44610 | 50.9 | 7.8 | 8.5 | 0.8 | 3525512 | 12.5 |
| Shandong | 18195310 | 240313 | 51.8 | 8.5 | 9.8 | 0.8 | 14917388 | 13.9 |
| Henan | 11818678 | 155168 | 48.0 | 9.3 | 9.3 | 0.9 | 9392157 | 14.6 |
| Hubei | 14978080 | 331316 | 62.0 | 8.0 | 9.3 | 1.2 | 9343703 | 21.9 |
| Hunan | 8402747 | 292777 | 66.7 | 7.2 | 6.6 | 1.2 | 2413791 | 7.2 |
| Guangdong | 92630944 | 162040 | 50.8 | 8.7 | 22.7 | 0.3 | 21895331 | 29.2 |
| Guangxi | 7195669 | 31586 | 50.8 | 7.2 | 14.2 | 0.3 | 1772739 | 13.5 |
| Hainan | 962081 | 23420 | 60.4 | 5.7 | 10.5 | 1.2 | 2054694 | 15.1 |
| Chongqing | 6851133 | 281928 | 73.5 | 7.7 | 8.5 | 1.9 | 1162443 | 12.5 |
| Sichuan | 18982791 | 230501 | 62.7 | 8.0 | 13.8 | 1.0 | 4608993 | 12.7 |
| Guizhou | 2458598 | 79761 | 50.1 | 5.3 | 7.3 | 1.0 | 2869103 | 9.1 |
| Yunnan | 4527000 | 92036 | 55.7 | 7.0 | 11.8 | 1.4 | 2632256 | 11.3 |
| Tibet | 66510 | | 14.3 | | 3.8 | | 14100 | 6.3 |
| Shaanxi | 4481252 | 50162 | 41.6 | 8.7 | 8.3 | 0.6 | 2939811 | 11.5 |
| Gansu | 3272253 | 40554 | 57.1 | 5.8 | 8.1 | 0.7 | 3252177 | 10.9 |
| Qinghai | 689455 | 8975 | 47.8 | 7.8 | 7.4 | 0.5 | 1767696 | 18.8 |
| Ningxia | 377544 | 1029 | 60.0 | 10.3 | 14.0 | 0.7 | 1660520 | 19.9 |
| Xinjiang | 4771529 | 44716 | 50.6 | 8.8 | 10.7 | 0.7 | 3461029 | 9.7 |

## Township Health Service Institution, Beds, Personnel Numbers

| | 2010 | 2012 | 2013 | 2014 | 2015 | 2016 |
|---|---|---|---|---|---|---|
| **Total Institution** | **37836** | **37097** | **37015** | **36902** | **36817** | **36795** |
| Community Health Service Center | 10373 | 10590 | 10538 | 10540 | 10579 | 10568 |
| Community Health Service Station | 27463 | 26507 | 26477 | 26362 | 26238 | 26227 |
| Host Unit | | | | | | |
| Government Operation | 37217 | 36667 | 36593 | 36445 | 36344 | 36348 |
| Non-government Operation | 619 | 430 | 422 | 457 | 473 | 447 |
| Hospital Bed | | | | | | |
| No Bed | 1482 | 1474 | 1463 | 1427 | 1519 | 1592 |
| 1-9 | 7075 | 5965 | 5848 | 5515 | 5358 | 5240 |
| 10-49 | 23701 | 22805 | 22261 | 22162 | 21785 | 21453 |
| 50-99 | 4637 | 5530 | 5990 | 6214 | 6486 | 6780 |
| 100 and above | 941 | 1323 | 1453 | 1584 | 1669 | 1730 |
| **Total Bed** | **994329** | **1099262** | **1136492** | **1167245** | **1196122** | **1223891** |
| Central Health Center | 421441 | 477898 | 497944 | 511732 | 528268 | 539026 |
| Township Health Hospital | 572888 | 621364 | 638548 | 655513 | 667854 | 684865 |
| **Personnel Number** | **1151349** | **1204996** | **1233858** | **1247299** | **1277697** | **1320841** |
| Health Technician | 973059 | 1017096 | 1043441 | 1053348 | 1078532 | 1115921 |
| #Certified (Assistant) Practitioner | 422648 | 423350 | 434025 | 432831 | 440889 | 454995 |
| Registered Nurse | 217693 | 247355 | 270210 | 281864 | 298881 | 318609 |
| Other Technician | 53508 | 52520 | 54401 | 55774 | 57654 | 60371 |
| Managerial Worker | 43983 | 42669 | 41709 | 41677 | 42202 | 42553 |
| Ground Skilled Staff | 80799 | 92711 | 94307 | 96500 | 99309 | 101996 |

## Departmental Beds, Outpatient & Emergency Persons/Times, Discharged Numbers and the Constituent in Township Health Institutions in 2016

| Department Type | Bed | | Outpatient & Emergency | | Hospital Discharge | |
|---|---|---|---|---|---|---|
| | Piece | Constituent (%) | Persons/Times | Constituent (%) | Person | Constituent (%) |
| **Total** | **1223891** | **100.0** | **105259.1** | **100.0** | **3780.7** | **100.0** |
| Prevention and Health Department | 7611 | 0.6 | 2327.2 | 2.2 | 10.8 | 0.3 |
| General Medical Department | 260107 | 21.3 | 25105.5 | 23.9 | 796.7 | 21.1 |
| Internal Medicine | 443153 | 36.2 | 42076.4 | 40.0 | 1679.9 | 44.4 |
| Surgery Department | 190360 | 15.6 | 9701.6 | 9.2 | 479.0 | 12.7 |
| Pediatrics Department | 92015 | 7.5 | 8194.9 | 7.8 | 296.4 | 7.8 |
| Gynaecology and Obstetrics Department | 118731 | 9.7 | 5979.0 | 5.7 | 268.2 | 7.1 |
| TCM Department | 48775 | 4.0 | 6148.5 | 5.8 | 136.0 | 3.6 |
| Others | 63139 | 5.2 | 5726.0 | 5.4 | 113.5 | 3.0 |

## Medical Service in Township Health Hospital

| Year | Diagnosis & Treatment Number (One Thousand Million Times) | Inpatient Number (Ten Thousand Persons) | Hospital Bed Turnover Times (Times) | Hospital Bed Utilization Rate (%) | Average Hospitalization Days (Day) |
|---|---|---|---|---|---|
| 1984 | 12.65 | 1893 | 27.9 | 49.1 | 6.0 |
| 1985 | 11.00 | 1771 | 26.4 | 46.0 | 5.9 |
| 1986 | 11.18 | 1782 | 26.9 | 46.0 | 5.9 |
| 1987 | 11.30 | 1959 | 28.5 | 47.4 | 5.6 |
| 1988 | 11.36 | 2031 | 29.2 | 47.3 | 5.6 |
| 1989 | 10.60 | 1935 | 28.3 | 44.6 | 5.4 |
| 1990 | 10.65 | 1958 | 28.6 | 43.4 | 5.2 |
| 1991 | 10.82 | 2016 | 29.1 | 43.5 | 5.1 |
| 1992 | 10.34 | 1960 | 28.7 | 42.9 | 5.1 |
| 1993 | 8.98 | 1855 | 27.9 | 38.4 | 4.6 |
| 1994 | 9.73 | 1913 | 29.4 | 40.5 | 4.6 |
| 1995 | 9.38 | 1960 | 29.9 | 40.2 | 4.6 |
| 1996 | 9.44 | 1916 | 28.6 | 37.0 | 4.4 |
| 1997 | 9.16 | 1918 | 26.0 | 34.5 | 4.5 |
| 1998 | 8.74 | 1751 | 24.4 | 33.3 | 4.6 |
| 1999 | 8.38 | 1688 | 24.2 | 32.8 | 4.6 |
| 2000 | 8.24 | 1708 | 24.8 | 33.2 | 4.6 |
| 2001 | 8.24 | 1700 | 23.7 | 31.3 | 4.5 |
| 2002 | 7.10 | 1625 | 28.0 | 34.7 | 4.0 |
| 2003 | 6.91 | 1608 | 28.1 | 36.2 | 4.2 |
| 2004 | 6.81 | 1599 | 27.0 | 37.1 | 4.4 |
| 2005 | 6.79 | 1622 | 25.8 | 37.7 | 4.6 |
| 2006 | 7.01 | 1836 | 28.8 | 39.4 | 4.6 |
| 2007 | 7.59 | 2662 | 36.7 | 48.4 | 4.8 |
| 2008 | 8.27 | 3313 | 42.0 | 55.8 | 4.4 |
| 2009 | 8.77 | 3808 | 42.9 | 60.7 | 4.8 |
| 2010 | 8.74 | 3630 | 38.4 | 59.0 | 5.2 |
| 2011 | 8.66 | 3449 | 35.2 | 58.1 | 5.6 |
| 2012 | 9.68 | 3908 | 37.4 | 62.1 | 5.7 |
| 2013 | 10.07 | 3937 | 36.1 | 62.8 | 5.9 |
| 2014 | 10.29 | 3733 | 33.2 | 60.5 | 6.3 |
| 2015 | 10.55 | 3676 | 32.0 | 59.9 | 6.4 |
| 2016 | 10.82 | 3800 | 32.2 | 60.6 | 6.4 |
| Central Health Center | 4.51 | 1781 | 34.2 | 63.7 | 6.4 |
| Township Health Center | 6.32 | 2019 | 30.7 | 58.2 | 6.4 |

Note: Diagnosis & treatment number/times and inpatient number before 1993 is estimated.

## TCM Institution Diagnosis & Treatment Persons/Times

| Institution | 2010 | 2012 | 2013 | 2014 | 2015 | 2016 |
|---|---|---|---|---|---|---|
| **Diagnosis and Treatment with TCM(Ten Thousand Persons)** | **61264.1** | **74695.2** | **81409.4** | **87430.9** | **90912.4** | **96225.1** |
| **TCM Hospital** | **36026.5** | **45120.2** | **48952.5** | **53058.1** | **54870.9** | **57670.4** |
| TCM Hospital | 32770.2 | 40705.2 | 43726.3 | 47164.2 | 48502.6 | 50774.5 |
| Hospital of Traditional Chinese and Western Medicine | 2702.6 | 3769.1 | 4466.1 | 5101.3 | 5401.4 | 5927.3 |
| National Hospital | 553.8 | 645.9 | 760.1 | 792.6 | 966.8 | 968.7 |
| **TCM Outpatient** | **975.9** | **1290.8** | **1433.6** | **1525.5** | **1761.9** | **1978.3** |
| TCM Outpatient | 808.9 | 1069.5 | 1221.6 | 1304.8 | 1567.4 | 1757.4 |
| Outpatient of Traditional Chinese and Western Medicine | 164.6 | 217.8 | 207.9 | 218.5 | 192.1 | 217.9 |
| Outpatient of National Medicine | 2.4 | 3.5 | 4.1 | 2.2 | 2.4 | 3.0 |
| **TCM Clinic** | **9178.3** | **10250.2** | **11059.3** | **11342.0** | **11781.4** | **12517.9** |
| TCM Clinic | 6796.1 | 7857.7 | 8616.7 | 8870.1 | 9215.8 | 9886.0 |
| Clinic of Traditional Chinese and Western Medicine | 2283.8 | 2291.0 | 2341.5 | 2362.0 | 2446.7 | 2517.9 |
| Clinic of National Medicine | 98.3 | 101.5 | 101.1 | 110.0 | 118.8 | 114.1 |
| **Other TCM Clinical Departments in Institutions** | **15083.4** | **18033.9** | **19964.0** | **21505.3** | **22498.3** | **24058.5** |
| **Total Diagnosis & Treatment in TCM Diagnosis & Treatment (%)** | **14.7** | **15.1** | **15.4** | **15.6** | **15.7** | **15.8** |

## TCM Clinical Department Diagnosis & Treatment Persons/Times in Other Institutions

| Institution | 2010 | 2012 | 2013 | 2014 | 2015 | 2016 |
|---|---|---|---|---|---|---|
| **Outpatient & Emergency Number (Ten Thousand Persons/Times)** | **15083.4** | **18033.9** | **19574.1** | **21505.3** | **22498.3** | **24058.5** |
| Comprehensive Hospital | 8089.2 | 8826.9 | 9429.7 | 10114.9 | 10069.2 | 10286.8 |
| Specialty Hospital | 390.2 | 496.5 | 527.8 | 570.6 | 563.5 | 635.7 |
| Community Health Service Center (Station) | 2512.9 | 3846.0 | 4503.5 | 5094.5 | 5571.7 | 6178.5 |
| Township Health Hospital | 3419.5 | 4185.6 | 4756.8 | 5195.4 | 5662.9 | 6148.5 |
| Other Institution | 671.6 | 679.0 | 746.2 | 534.0 | 631.1 | 809.0 |
| **Diagnosis & Treatment Percentage in the Same Institution** | | | | | | |
| Comprehensive Hospital | 5.4 | 4.7 | 4.7 | 4.6 | 4.5 | 4.3 |
| Specialty Hospital | 2.3 | 2.3 | 2.2 | 2.2 | 2.0 | 2.1 |
| Community Health Service Center (Station) | 5.2 | 6.4 | 6.9 | 7.4 | 7.9 | 8.6 |
| Township Health Hospital | 3.9 | 4.3 | 4.7 | 5.1 | 5.4 | 5.7 |
| Other Institution | 1.0 | 0.3 | 0.4 | 0.6 | 0.7 | 0.8 |

## TCM Village Room Diagnosis & Treatment Persons/Times

| | 2010 | 2012 | 2013 | 2014 | 2015 | 2016 |
|---|---|---|---|---|---|---|
| **TCM Diagnosis & Treatment Number (Ten Thousand Persons)** | **50468.3** | **62152.4** | **66848.1** | **66716.5** | **76569.4** | **74455.3** |
| TCM Priority | 4550.2 | 5170.7 | 5648.9 | 5648.5 | 6187.8 | 5919.9 |
| Traditional Chinese and Western Medicine Priority | 45918.1 | 56981.7 | 61199.1 | 61068.1 | 70381.6 | 68535.3 |
| **TCM Percentage in Village Room Diagnosis & Treatment (%)** | **30.5** | **32.3** | **33.2** | **33.6** | **40.4** | **40.2** |

## All-region Diagnosis & Treatment in TCM Institution (Ten Thousand Persons/Times) in 2016

| Region | Total | TCM Hospital | | | | TCM Outpatient | TCM Clinic | TCM Clinical Department in Other Institution |
|---|---|---|---|---|---|---|---|---|
| | | TCM Hospital | Hospital of Traditional Chinese and Western Medicine | National Hospital | | | | |
| Total | 96225.1 | 57670.4 | 50774.5 | 5927.3 | 968.7 | 1978.3 | 12517.9 | 24058.5 |
| East Region | 52972.4 | 31650.8 | 27605.9 | 3990.3 | 54.5 | 1650.0 | 4928.6 | 14743.0 |
| Central Region | 18788.2 | 12539.1 | 11720.7 | 788.0 | 30.5 | 145.5 | 2336.8 | 3766.8 |
| West Region | 24464.5 | 13480.5 | 11447.9 | 1149.0 | 883.7 | 182.8 | 5252.5 | 5548.7 |
| Beijing | 6134.9 | 4008.6 | 3243.2 | 751.7 | 13.8 | 167.6 | 104.0 | 1854.7 |
| Tianjin | 2395.5 | 1461.6 | 1351.8 | 109.8 | | 98.5 | 30.6 | 804.7 |
| Hebei | 3453.7 | 2102.2 | 1800.8 | 301.4 | | 17.5 | 619.0 | 715.0 |
| Shanxi | 1459.0 | 732.2 | 677.2 | 55.0 | | 15.0 | 353.3 | 358.5 |
| Inner Mongolia | 1865.7 | 1017.2 | 627.1 | 17.5 | 372.7 | 16.1 | 474.4 | 358.1 |
| Liaoning | 1717.0 | 1075.0 | 1007.8 | 46.9 | 20.4 | 21.1 | 278.8 | 342.0 |
| Jilin | 1305.6 | 894.1 | 762.3 | 126.5 | 5.2 | 20.4 | 228.7 | 162.4 |
| Heilongjiang | 1443.5 | 1037.1 | 1001.7 | 28.6 | 6.8 | 19.6 | 151.7 | 235.1 |
| Shanghai | 4447.2 | 2314.2 | 1573.4 | 740.7 | | 130.7 | 39.4 | 1963.0 |
| Jiangsu | 6763.3 | 4667.6 | 4141.0 | 526.6 | | 113.4 | 361.4 | 1621.0 |
| Zhejiang | 8858.8 | 5248.3 | 4582.5 | 665.8 | | 721.1 | 747.5 | 2142.0 |
| Anhui | 2152.7 | 1557.8 | 1475.5 | 82.3 | | 20.3 | 181.4 | 393.2 |
| Fujian | 3069.7 | 1784.7 | 1557.8 | 220.5 | 6.5 | 115.1 | 467.4 | 702.5 |
| Jiangxi | 1912.0 | 1321.7 | 1234.7 | 87.1 | | 10.9 | 278.4 | 300.9 |
| Shandong | 4987.3 | 3000.5 | 2825.2 | 161.3 | 13.9 | 18.4 | 688.6 | 1279.9 |
| Henan | 4785.4 | 3263.6 | 3193.1 | 70.5 | | 9.7 | 386.0 | 1126.1 |
| Hubei | 3219.2 | 2050.0 | 1752.3 | 280.4 | 17.2 | 37.4 | 353.0 | 778.7 |
| Hunan | 2510.8 | 1682.6 | 1623.8 | 57.6 | 1.2 | 12.0 | 404.2 | 412.0 |
| Guangdong | 10750.8 | 5714.8 | 5280.9 | 433.8 | | 243.3 | 1521.9 | 3270.9 |
| Guangxi | 2937.1 | 1900.2 | 1594.5 | 278.5 | 27.3 | 8.8 | 449.2 | 578.9 |
| Hainan | 394.1 | 273.3 | 241.5 | 31.8 | | 3.4 | 70.0 | 47.4 |
| Chongqing | 2280.0 | 1201.4 | 1123.2 | 78.2 | | 16.9 | 592.9 | 468.9 |
| Sichuan | 7242.1 | 3365.1 | 2858.5 | 447.4 | 59.3 | 54.1 | 1844.0 | 1978.9 |
| Guizhou | 1300.9 | 811.2 | 696.1 | 101.7 | 13.4 | 12.2 | 249.0 | 228.4 |
| Yunnan | 2501.3 | 1567.3 | 1480.4 | 72.7 | 14.1 | 37.7 | 367.4 | 528.9 |
| Tibet | 217.7 | 148.4 | 0.0 | 3.1 | 145.3 | | 40.6 | 28.7 |
| Shaanxi | 2170.8 | 1266.5 | 1205.2 | 61.2 | | 23.1 | 428.0 | 453.3 |
| Gansu | 1949.6 | 989.1 | 904.7 | 55.4 | 29.0 | 3.0 | 430.4 | 527.2 |
| Qinghai | 304.4 | 216.9 | 146.8 | 2.5 | 67.6 | | 46.1 | 41.4 |
| Ningxia | 539.0 | 334.8 | 325.4 | 6.9 | 2.6 | 6.0 | 85.5 | 112.6 |
| Xinjiang | 1155.8 | 662.3 | 485.9 | 23.8 | 152.6 | 4.9 | 245.2 | 243.4 |

## Mortality of Children under 5 and Pregnant & Parturient Women in Monitored Region

| Year | Newborn Mortality (‰) | | | Infant Mortality(‰) | | | Children under 5 Mortality(‰) | | | Pregnant & Parturient Women Mortality (Hundred Thousandth) | | |
|------|-------|------|-------------|-------|------|-------------|-------|------|-------------|-------|------|-------------|
| | Total | City | Countryside | Total | City | Countryside | Total | City | Countryside | Total | City | Countryside |
| 2000 | 22.8 | 9.5 | 25.8 | 32.2 | 11.8 | 37.0 | 39.7 | 13.8 | 45.7 | 53.0 | 29.3 | 69.6 |
| 2001 | 21.4 | 10.6 | 23.9 | 30.0 | 13.6 | 33.8 | 35.9 | 16.3 | 40.4 | 50.2 | 33.1 | 61.9 |
| 2002 | 20.7 | 9.7 | 23.2 | 29.2 | 12.2 | 33.1 | 34.9 | 14.6 | 39.6 | 43.2 | 22.3 | 58.2 |
| 2003 | 18.0 | 8.9 | 20.1 | 25.5 | 11.3 | 28.7 | 29.9 | 14.8 | 33.4 | 51.3 | 27.6 | 65.4 |
| 2004 | 15.4 | 8.4 | 17.3 | 21.5 | 10.1 | 24.5 | 25.0 | 12.0 | 28.5 | 48.3 | 26.1 | 63.0 |
| 2005 | 13.2 | 7.5 | 14.7 | 19.0 | 9.1 | 21.6 | 22.5 | 10.7 | 25.7 | 47.7 | 25.0 | 53.8 |
| 2006 | 12.0 | 6.8 | 13.4 | 17.2 | 8.0 | 19.7 | 20.6 | 9.6 | 23.6 | 41.1 | 24.8 | 45.5 |
| 2007 | 10.7 | 5.5 | 12.8 | 15.3 | 7.7 | 18.6 | 18.1 | 9.0 | 21.8 | 36.6 | 25.2 | 41.3 |
| 2008 | 10.2 | 5.0 | 12.3 | 14.9 | 6.5 | 18.4 | 18.5 | 7.9 | 22.7 | 34.2 | 29.2 | 36.1 |
| 2009 | 9.0 | 4.5 | 10.8 | 13.8 | 6.2 | 17.0 | 17.2 | 7.6 | 21.1 | 31.9 | 26.6 | 34.0 |
| 2010 | 8.3 | 4.1 | 10.0 | 13.1 | 5.8 | 16.1 | 16.4 | 7.3 | 20.1 | 30.0 | 29.7 | 30.1 |
| 2011 | 7.8 | 4.0 | 9.4 | 12.1 | 5.8 | 14.7 | 15.6 | 7.1 | 19.1 | 26.1 | 25.2 | 26.5 |
| 2012 | 6.9 | 3.9 | 8.1 | 10.3 | 5.2 | 12.4 | 13.2 | 5.9 | 16.2 | 24.5 | 22.2 | 25.6 |
| 2013 | 6.3 | 3.7 | 7.3 | 9.5 | 5.2 | 11.3 | 12.0 | 6.0 | 14.5 | 23.2 | 22.4 | 23.6 |
| 2014 | 5.9 | 3.5 | 6.9 | 8.9 | 4.8 | 10.7 | 11.7 | 5.9 | 14.2 | 21.7 | 20.5 | 22.2 |
| 2015 | 5.4 | 3.3 | 6.4 | 8.1 | 4.7 | 9.6 | 10.7 | 5.8 | 12.9 | 20.1 | 19.8 | 20.2 |
| 2016 | 4.9 | 2.9 | 5.7 | 7.5 | 4.2 | 9.0 | 10.2 | 5.2 | 12.4 | 19.9 | 19.5 | 20.0 |

## Mortality of Major Disease and Death Constituent of Pregnant and Parturient Monitored Region

| | Mortality of Major Disease (Hundred Thousandth) | | | | | | Mortality Percentage (%) | | | | | |
|---|---|---|---|---|---|---|---|---|---|---|---|---|
| | Obstetric Hemorrhage | Pregnancy Hypertension | Heart Disease | Amniotic Fluid Embolism | Puerperal Infection | Hepatopathy | Obstetric Hemorrhage | Pregnancy Hypertension | Heart Disease | Amniotic Fluid Embolism | Puerperal Infection | Hepatopathy |
| **Total** | | | | | | | | | | | | |
| 2010 | 8.3 | 3.7 | 3.3 | 2.8 | 0.4 | 0.9 | 27.8 | 12.3 | 10.9 | 9.2 | 1.2 | 3.1 |
| 2012 | 6.6 | 2.0 | 2.7 | 3.2 | 0.4 | 0.8 | 27.0 | 8.0 | 10.9 | 12.9 | 1.4 | 3.2 |
| 2013 | 6.6 | 2.6 | 1.8 | 3.1 | 0.2 | 0.6 | 28.2 | 11.4 | 7.8 | 13.3 | 0.6 | 2.6 |
| 2014 | 5.7 | 2.0 | 2.5 | 3.2 | 0.2 | 1.0 | 26.3 | 9.1 | 11.4 | 14.9 | 1.1 | 4.6 |
| 2015 | 4.2 | 2.3 | 3.3 | 1.9 | 0.1 | 1.0 | 21.1 | 11.6 | 16.4 | 9.5 | 0.7 | 4.7 |
| 2016 | 4.7 | 1.6 | 2.0 | 2.2 | 0.2 | 0.7 | 23.5 | 7.8 | 10.2 | 10.9 | 1.0 | 3.8 |
| **City** | | | | | | | | | | | | |
| 2010 | 8.0 | 1.9 | 2.8 | 2.5 | 0.3 | 0.9 | 27.1 | 6.3 | 9.4 | 8.3 | 1.0 | 3.1 |
| 2012 | 5.7 | 1.5 | 1.5 | 3.9 | 0.3 | 0.8 | 25.6 | 7.0 | 7.0 | 17.4 | 1.2 | 3.5 |
| 2013 | 5.6 | 2.1 | 2.1 | 2.7 | 0.0 | 0.9 | 25.0 | 9.2 | 9.2 | 11.8 | 0.0 | 3.9 |
| 2014 | 4.3 | 1.4 | 2.3 | 2.7 | 0.2 | 0.8 | 21.2 | 7.1 | 11.1 | 13.1 | 1.0 | 4.0 |
| 2015 | 3.5 | 0.9 | 5.2 | 0.7 | 0.2 | 0.7 | 17.9 | 4.8 | 26.2 | 3.6 | 1.2 | 3.6 |
| 2016 | 4.0 | 0.5 | 2.4 | 1.6 | 0.3 | 0.3 | 20.3 | 2.7 | 12.2 | 8.1 | 1.4 | 1.4 |
| **Countryside** | | | | | | | | | | | | |
| 2010 | 8.4 | 4.3 | 3.4 | 2.8 | 0.4 | 0.9 | 28.0 | 14.2 | 11.3 | 9.4 | 1.3 | 3.1 |
| 2012 | 7.0 | 2.1 | 3.1 | 2.9 | 0.4 | 0.8 | 27.5 | 8.4 | 12.2 | 11.5 | 1.5 | 3.1 |
| 2013 | 6.9 | 2.8 | 1.7 | 3.3 | 0.2 | 0.5 | 29.3 | 12.1 | 7.3 | 13.8 | 0.9 | 2.2 |
| 2014 | 6.3 | 2.2 | 2.6 | 3.4 | 0.3 | 1.1 | 28.3 | 10.0 | 11.6 | 15.5 | 1.2 | 4.8 |
| 2015 | 4.5 | 3.0 | 2.4 | 2.4 | 0.1 | 1.1 | 22.5 | 14.7 | 12.0 | 12.0 | 0.5 | 5.2 |
| 2016 | 4.9 | 1.9 | 1.9 | 2.4 | 0.2 | 0.9 | 24.7 | 9.6 | 9.6 | 11.9 | 0.9 | 4.6 |

## Pregnant and Parturient Women Health

| Year | Live Birth Number | High-risk Parturient Women Proportion (%) | Card Opening Rate (%) | System Management Rate (%) | Prenatal Examination Rate (%) | Postpartum Visit Rate (%) | Institutional Delivery Rate (%) | | | New-method Delivery Rate (%) | | |
|---|---|---|---|---|---|---|---|---|---|---|---|---|
| | | | | | | | Total | City | Countryside | Total | City | Countryside |
| 1980 | ... | ... | ... | ... | ... | ... | ... | ... | ... | 91.4 | 98.7 | 90.3 |
| 1985 | ... | ... | ... | ... | ... | ... | 43.7 | 73.6 | 36.4 | 94.5 | 98.7 | 93.5 |
| 1990 | 14517207 | ... | ... | ... | ... | ... | 50.6 | 74.2 | 45.1 | 94.0 | 98.6 | 93.9 |
| 1991 | 15293237 | ... | ... | ... | ... | ... | 50.6 | 72.8 | 45.5 | 93.7 | 98.1 | 93.2 |
| 1992 | 11746275 | ... | 76.6 | ... | 69.7 | 69.7 | 52.7 | 71.7 | 41.2 | 84.1 | 91.2 | 82.0 |
| 1993 | 10170690 | ... | 75.7 | ... | 72.2 | 71.0 | 56.5 | 68.3 | 51.0 | 83.6 | 81.1 | 84.7 |
| 1994 | 11044607 | ... | 79.1 | ... | 76.3 | 74.5 | 65.6 | 76.4 | 50.4 | ... | ... | 87.4 |
| 1995 | 11539613 | ... | 81.4 | ... | 78.7 | 78.8 | 58.0 | 70.7 | 50.2 | ... | ... | 87.6 |
| 1996 | 11412028 | 7.3 | 82.4 | 65.5 | 83.7 | 80.1 | 60.7 | 76.5 | 51.7 | ... | ... | 95.5 |
| 1997 | 11286021 | 8.1 | 84.5 | 68.3 | 85.9 | 82.3 | 61.7 | 76.4 | 53.0 | ... | ... | 91.8 |
| 1998 | 10961516 | 8.6 | 86.2 | 72.3 | 87.1 | 83.9 | 66.2 | 79.0 | 58.1 | ... | ... | 92.6 |
| 1999 | 10698467 | 9.2 | 87.9 | 75.4 | 89.3 | 85.9 | 70.0 | 83.3 | 61.5 | 96.8 | 98.9 | 95.4 |
| 2000 | 10987691 | 10.0 | 88.6 | 77.2 | 89.4 | 86.2 | 72.9 | 84.9 | 65.2 | 96.6 | 98.8 | 95.2 |
| 2001 | 10690630 | 11.1 | 89.4 | 78.6 | 90.3 | 87.2 | 76.0 | 87.0 | 69.0 | 97.3 | 99.0 | 96.1 |
| 2002 | 10591949 | 11.9 | 89.2 | 78.2 | 90.1 | 86.7 | 78.7 | 89.4 | 71.6 | 96.7 | 98.6 | 95.4 |
| 2003 | 10188005 | 11.8 | 87.6 | 75.5 | 88.9 | 85.4 | 79.4 | 89.9 | 72.6 | 95.9 | 98.5 | 94.1 |
| 2004 | 10892614 | 12.4 | 88.3 | 76.4 | 89.7 | 85.9 | 82.8 | 91.4 | 77.1 | 97.3 | 98.9 | 96.2 |
| 2005 | 11415809 | 12.8 | 88.5 | 76.7 | 89.8 | 86.0 | 85.9 | 93.2 | 81.0 | 97.5 | 98.7 | 96.7 |
| 2006 | 11770056 | 13.0 | 88.2 | 76.5 | 89.7 | 85.7 | 88.4 | 94.1 | 84.6 | 97.8 | 98.7 | 97.2 |
| 2007 | 12506498 | 13.7 | 89.3 | 77.3 | 90.9 | 86.7 | 91.7 | 95.8 | 88.8 | 98.4 | 99.1 | 97.9 |
| 2008 | 13307045 | 15.7 | 89.3 | 78.1 | 91.0 | 87.0 | 94.5 | 97.5 | 92.3 | 99.1 | 99.6 | 98.7 |
| 2009 | 13825431 | 16.4 | 90.9 | 80.9 | 92.2 | 88.7 | 96.3 | 98.5 | 94.7 | 99.3 | 99.8 | 99.0 |
| 2010 | 14218657 | 17.1 | 92.9 | 84.1 | 94.1 | 90.8 | 97.8 | 99.2 | 96.7 | 99.6 | 99.9 | 99.4 |
| 2011 | 14507141 | 17.7 | 93.8 | 85.2 | 93.7 | 91.0 | 98.7 | 99.6 | 98.1 | 99.7 | 99.9 | 99.6 |
| 2012 | 15442995 | 18.5 | 94.8 | 87.6 | 95.0 | 92.6 | 99.2 | 99.7 | 98.8 | 99.8 | 99.9 | 99.7 |
| 2013 | 15108153 | 19.4 | 95.7 | 89.5 | 95.6 | 93.5 | 99.5 | 99.9 | 99.2 | 99.9 | 100.0 | 99.7 |
| 2014 | 15178881 | 20.7 | 95.8 | 90.0 | 96.2 | 93.9 | 99.6 | 99.9 | 99.4 | 99.9 | 100.0 | 99.8 |
| 2015 | 14544524 | 22.6 | 96.4 | 91.5 | 96.5 | 94.5 | 99.7 | 99.9 | 99.5 | 99.9 | 100.0 | 99.9 |
| 2016 | 18466561 | 24.7 | 96.6 | 91.6 | 96.6 | 94.6 | 99.8 | 100.0 | 99.6 | 99.9 | 100.0 | 99.9 |

Note: The live birth number in 2016 is from the monthly report of the national hospital delivery, including the household and non-household live birth number; the live birth numbers in 2015 and before, are from the annual report on maternal and child health, including the household live birth number only.

### All-region Pregnant and

| Region | Live Birth Number | High-risk Parturient Women Proportion (%) | Card Opening Rate (%) | System Management Rate (%) | Prenatal Examination Rate (%) | Postpartum Visit Rate (%) | Institutional Delivery Rate (%) | | |
|---|---|---|---|---|---|---|---|---|---|
| | | | | | | | Total | City | County |
| **Total** | **18466561** | **24.7** | **96.6** | **91.6** | **96.6** | **94.6** | **99.8** | **100.0** | **99.6** |
| Beijing | 279434 | 62.8 | 100.0 | 96.3 | 98.7 | 96.5 | 100.0 | 100.0 | 100.0 |
| Tianjin | 133703 | 54.0 | 98.1 | 95.2 | 97.2 | 96.4 | 100.0 | 100.0 | 100.0 |
| Hebei | 1084347 | 14.9 | 96.1 | 88.9 | 96.0 | 92.3 | 100.0 | 100.0 | 100.0 |
| Shanxi | 439105 | 17.8 | 96.7 | 87.4 | 96.0 | 92.6 | 99.9 | 100.0 | 99.9 |
| Inner Mongolia | 252151 | 30.2 | 97.6 | 93.8 | 97.2 | 95.4 | 100.0 | 100.0 | 100.0 |
| Liaoning | 358553 | 25.7 | 98.3 | 91.8 | 97.7 | 94.0 | 100.0 | 100.0 | 100.0 |
| Jilin | 198344 | 37.7 | 98.5 | 92.0 | 97.3 | 96.0 | 100.0 | 100.0 | 100.0 |
| Heilongjiang | 209949 | 18.1 | 98.6 | 94.4 | 97.9 | 96.4 | 100.0 | 100.0 | 100.0 |
| Shanghai | 230185 | 48.8 | 100.0 | 95.9 | 98.4 | 98.1 | 100.0 | 100.0 | 100.0 |
| Jiangsu | 881545 | 34.8 | 99.7 | 100.0 | 100.0 | 100.0 | 100.0 | 100.0 | 100.0 |
| Zhejiang | 729313 | 56.1 | 99.8 | 96.3 | 98.8 | 98.1 | 100.0 | 100.0 | 100.0 |
| Anhui | 809344 | 27.4 | 94.8 | 87.2 | 94.1 | 92.0 | 100.0 | 100.0 | 100.0 |
| Fujian | 625495 | 38.9 | 97.1 | 91.7 | 97.2 | 94.2 | 100.0 | 100.0 | 100.0 |
| Jiangxi | 633049 | 17.5 | 96.4 | 89.6 | 96.1 | 94.9 | 100.0 | 100.0 | 100.0 |
| Shandong | 1642236 | 14.4 | 95.5 | 91.8 | 95.3 | 93.2 | 100.0 | 100.0 | 100.0 |
| Henan | 1612803 | 17.6 | 90.7 | 86.0 | 94.4 | 90.2 | 100.0 | 100.0 | 100.0 |
| Hubei | 673005 | 22.5 | 98.2 | 92.8 | 97.2 | 95.3 | 100.0 | 100.0 | 100.0 |
| Hunan | 845126 | 31.6 | 97.1 | 92.9 | 96.8 | 95.2 | 100.0 | 100.0 | 100.0 |
| Guangdong | 1906484 | 24.5 | 96.8 | 92.1 | 97.2 | 95.2 | 99.9 | 100.0 | 99.7 |
| Guangxi | 842870 | 25.5 | 99.9 | 97.4 | 99.4 | 98.7 | 100.0 | 100.0 | 100.0 |
| Hainan | 131526 | 16.2 | 96.3 | 87.2 | 96.4 | 89.9 | 99.8 | 99.8 | 99.8 |
| Chongqing | 337287 | 18.9 | 97.7 | 90.9 | 97.0 | 93.4 | 99.6 | 100.0 | 99.0 |
| Sichuan | 911007 | 19.2 | 96.0 | 93.8 | 96.1 | 95.2 | 98.7 | 99.9 | 98.0 |
| Guizhou | 541625 | 11.6 | 95.2 | 89.5 | 94.8 | 93.4 | 99.0 | 98.9 | 99.0 |
| Yunnan | 668898 | 33.1 | 99.0 | 91.2 | 98.5 | 97.8 | 99.6 | 99.8 | 99.5 |
| Tibet | 41030 | 7.2 | 87.9 | 74.4 | 90.2 | 87.4 | 91.7 | 99.5 | 90.5 |
| Shaanxi | 510900 | 22.4 | 98.5 | 95.1 | 98.2 | 97.4 | 100.0 | 99.9 | 100.0 |
| Gansu | 372701 | 13.3 | 97.3 | 93.6 | 97.2 | 96.2 | 99.5 | 99.7 | 99.5 |
| Qinghai | 63242 | 13.6 | 93.4 | 90.6 | 94.7 | 93.5 | 97.3 | 99.8 | 96.8 |
| Ningxia | 115053 | 30.4 | 99.7 | 97.2 | 99.2 | 98.5 | 99.9 | 100.0 | 99.9 |
| Xinjiang | 386251 | 29.4 | 95.2 | 84.7 | 94.5 | 92.5 | 98.8 | 99.6 | 98.4 |

## Parturient Women Health in 2016

| New-method Delivery Rate (%) | | | Pregnant & Parturient Women Mortality (Hundred Thousandth) | | | Death Constituent of Pregnant and Parturient Women (%) | | | | |
|---|---|---|---|---|---|---|---|---|---|---|
| Total | City | County | Total | City | County | Obstetric Hemorrhage | Pregnancy Hypertension | Internal Medical Complication | Amniotic Fluid Embolism | Others |
| **99.9** | **100.0** | **99.9** | | | | | | | | |
| 100.0 | 100.0 | 100.0 | 10.5 | 11.1 | 9.5 | 12.5 | | 31.3 | 18.8 | 37.5 |
| 100.0 | 100.0 | 100.0 | 9.4 | 10.3 | 5.9 | 12.5 | 0.0 | 62.5 | 12.5 | 12.5 |
| 100.0 | 100.0 | 100.0 | 11.1 | 9.5 | 12.2 | 19.6 | 7.2 | 27.8 | 20.6 | 24.7 |
| 100.0 | 100.0 | 100.0 | 12.1 | 12.3 | 12.0 | 12.8 | 10.3 | 28.2 | 15.4 | 33.3 |
| 100.0 | 100.0 | 100.0 | 15.6 | 14.6 | 16.4 | 16.1 | 12.9 | 25.8 | 22.6 | 22.6 |
| 100.0 | 100.0 | 100.0 | 9.2 | 10.5 | 4.7 | 14.8 | 7.4 | 33.3 | 11.1 | 33.3 |
| 100.0 | 100.0 | 100.0 | 14.6 | 9.4 | 29.9 | 16.0 | 4.0 | 16.0 | 8.0 | 56.0 |
| 100.0 | 100.0 | 100.0 | 14.8 | 16.2 | 12.2 | 22.2 | 14.8 | 22.2 | 18.5 | 22.2 |
| 100.0 | 100.0 | 100.0 | 3.4 | 3.4 | | | 33.3 | 66.7 | 0.0 | 0.0 |
| 100.0 | 100.0 | 100.0 | 2.2 | 2.0 | 2.7 | 18.8 | | 43.8 | 25.0 | 12.5 |
| 100.0 | 100.0 | 100.0 | 5.7 | 4.6 | 8.3 | 12.0 | 4.0 | 56.0 | 4.0 | 24.0 |
| 100.0 | 100.0 | 100.0 | 13.0 | 10.7 | 14.3 | 21.2 | 8.1 | 39.4 | 15.2 | 16.2 |
| 100.0 | 100.0 | 100.0 | 8.5 | 8.9 | 8.1 | 11.1 | 8.9 | 26.7 | 24.4 | 28.9 |
| 100.0 | 100.0 | 100.0 | 9.9 | 12.3 | 8.7 | 11.5 | 4.9 | 29.5 | 21.3 | 32.8 |
| 100.0 | 100.0 | 100.0 | 9.6 | 8.8 | 10.4 | 13.0 | 6.5 | 32.4 | 21.3 | 26.9 |
| 100.0 | 100.0 | 100.0 | 9.4 | 11.1 | 8.6 | 14.9 | 10.5 | 26.9 | 29.1 | 18.7 |
| 100.0 | 100.0 | 100.0 | 8.6 | 7.3 | 10.6 | 10.7 | 1.8 | 32.1 | 14.3 | 41.1 |
| 100.0 | 100.0 | 100.0 | 13.8 | 15.0 | 13.2 | 11.8 | 9.1 | 30.0 | 22.7 | 26.4 |
| 100.0 | 100.0 | 99.9 | 7.5 | 6.8 | 10.3 | 18.0 | 2.0 | 32.0 | 31.0 | 17.0 |
| 100.0 | 100.0 | 100.0 | 12.7 | 13.7 | 12.1 | 11.7 | 10.6 | 33.0 | 29.8 | 14.9 |
| 99.8 | 99.8 | 99.9 | 17.7 | 20.7 | 11.5 | 5.3 | 5.3 | 42.1 | 21.1 | 26.3 |
| 99.9 | 100.0 | 99.7 | 13.1 | 11.1 | 16.2 | 24.4 | 7.3 | 31.7 | 17.1 | 19.5 |
| 99.7 | 100.0 | 99.5 | 17.5 | 12.3 | 20.6 | 27.4 | 10.4 | 29.6 | 8.9 | 23.7 |
| 99.9 | 99.9 | 99.9 | 22.4 | 24.5 | 21.5 | 31.0 | 6.0 | 26.0 | 13.0 | 24.0 |
| 99.9 | 100.0 | 99.9 | 23.3 | 13.8 | 26.8 | 32.0 | 6.4 | 24.8 | 14.4 | 22.4 |
| 98.0 | 100.0 | 97.6 | 109.9 | 13.4 | 124.9 | 42.6 | 4.9 | 23.0 | 8.2 | 21.3 |
| 100.0 | 100.0 | 100.0 | 9.5 | 9.3 | 9.6 | 11.1 | 11.1 | 16.7 | 38.9 | 22.2 |
| 100.0 | 100.0 | 99.9 | 17.1 | 14.9 | 18.2 | 39.2 | 2.0 | 9.8 | 21.6 | 27.5 |
| 99.7 | 100.0 | 99.7 | 31.5 | 10.2 | 35.5 | 15.0 | 15.0 | 35.0 | 10.0 | 25.0 |
| 100.0 | 100.0 | 100.0 | 20.0 | 12.3 | 27.9 | 25.0 | 12.5 | 25.0 | 18.8 | 18.8 |
| 99.1 | 99.7 | 98.9 | 31.9 | 21.3 | 37.1 | 24.5 | 12.3 | 30.2 | 12.3 | 20.8 |

## All-region Married Women of Childbearing Age Birth Control Rate (%)

| Region | 2010 | 2011 | 2012 | 2013 | 2014 | 2015 | 2016 |
|---|---|---|---|---|---|---|---|
| **Total** | **89.1** | **88.6** | **87.9** | **87.3** | 86.6 | 86.1 | 83.0 |
| Beijing | 84.6 | 83.6 | 82.7 | 79.0 | 78.3 | 76.6 | 73.0 |
| Tianjin | 90.7 | 91.0 | 91.2 | 91.3 | 90.5 | 90.2 | 88.0 |
| Hebei | 90.8 | 91.2 | 90.9 | 90.9 | 90.8 | 90.8 | 89.5 |
| Shanxi | 90.1 | 91.3 | 91.4 | 92.8 | 91.2 | 91.0 | 88.4 |
| Inner Mongolia | 91.5 | 90.7 | 90.6 | 90.1 | 89.8 | 90.0 | 90.0 |
| Liaoning | 88.2 | 88.2 | 85.9 | 87.1 | 86.0 | 85.0 | 79.4 |
| Jilin | 89.9 | 89.6 | 89.8 | 89.8 | 89.5 | 89.4 | 87.0 |
| Heilongjiang | 92.6 | 92.1 | 91.7 | 91.3 | 91.2 | 90.8 | 90.5 |
| Shanghai | 82.8 | 80.5 | 81.6 | 83.1 | 81.0 | 78.8 | 75.6 |
| Jiangsu | 90.0 | 89.4 | 88.2 | 88.2 | 88.4 | 88.5 | 87.3 |
| Zhejiang | 88.6 | 88.0 | 87.4 | 87.1 | 86.1 | 86.2 | 82.3 |
| Anhui | 90.4 | 89.8 | 89.3 | 88.6 | 89.7 | 90.1 | 89.2 |
| Fujian | 81.6 | 82.8 | 82.3 | 81.4 | 80.3 | 79.3 | 77.8 |
| Jiangxi | 93.9 | 94.6 | 94.6 | 90.4 | 82.2 | 83.6 | 83.9 |
| Shandong | 89.6 | 87.9 | 90.3 | 88.7 | 84.9 | 81.7 | 83.7 |
| Henan | 89.6 | 89.8 | 90.0 | 89.8 | 89.8 | 89.7 | 83.3 |
| Hubei | 86.1 | 86.9 | 85.3 | 82.6 | 84.4 | 84.2 | 80.4 |
| Hunan | 92.2 | 86.1 | 87.8 | 88.4 | 89.8 | 89.7 | 85.6 |
| Guangdong | 89.9 | 87.2 | 80.9 | 80.4 | 81.4 | 81.5 | 81.9 |
| Guangxi | 87.1 | 87.2 | 87.6 | 87.1 | 86.8 | 86.5 | 85.0 |
| Hainan | 79.2 | 81.6 | 81.0 | 80.8 | 80.7 | 81.3 | 81.5 |
| Chongqing | 90.8 | 89.4 | 79.7 | 80.3 | 82.0 | 78.7 | 64.4 |
| Sichuan | 88.3 | 90.6 | 89.3 | 88.2 | 85.7 | 84.8 | 79.0 |
| Guizhou | 88.2 | 88.1 | 89.0 | 89.0 | 89.1 | 88.7 | 85.4 |
| Yunnan | 86.2 | 87.9 | 87.2 | 86.4 | 86.0 | 86.8 | 78.2 |
| Tibet | 78.0 | 75.3 | 81.3 | 75.2 | | | 61.4 |
| Shaanxi | 91.3 | 91.4 | 91.7 | 91.3 | 91.1 | 91.2 | 77.9 |
| Gansu | 87.9 | 88.1 | 85.0 | 88.3 | 82.3 | 81.2 | 67.6 |
| Qinghai | 84.9 | 85.1 | 85.9 | 86.3 | 87.7 | 88.1 | 87.1 |
| Ningxia | 90.5 | 91.5 | 93.2 | 91.7 | 92.3 | 93.0 | 92.4 |
| Xinjiang | 82.7 | 83.2 | 82.0 | 81.5 | 73.0 | 83.5 | 83.3 |

## Birth Insurance

| Year Region | Year-end Birth Insurance Number (Ten Thousand Persons) | Preferential Treatment Enjoyment (Ten Thousand Persons) | Fund Revenue (One Hundred Million yuan) | | |
|---|---|---|---|---|---|
| | | | Fund Revenue | Fund Expenditure | Accumulative Balance |
| 2010 | 12335.9 | 210.7 | 159.6 | 109.9 | 261.4 |
| 2012 | 15428.7 | 352.7 | 304.2 | 219.3 | 427.6 |
| 2013 | 16392.0 | 522.0 | 368.4 | 282.8 | 514.7 |
| 2014 | 17038.7 | 613.4 | 446.1 | 368.1 | 592.7 |
| 2015 | 17771.0 | 641.9 | 501.7 | 411.5 | 684.4 |
| 2016 | 18443.0 | ... | ... | ... | ... |
| | | | | | |
| East Region | 11124.4 | 423.3 | 343.8 | 288.1 | 395.3 |
| Central Region | 11124.4 | 423.3 | 343.8 | 288.1 | 395.3 |
| West Region | 11124.4 | 423.3 | 343.8 | 288.1 | 395.3 |
| | | | | | |
| Beijing | 941.6 | 52.8 | 51.0 | 52.7 | 32.8 |
| Tianjin | 269.7 | 19.4 | 11.1 | 10.4 | 20.0 |
| Hebei | 713.0 | 18.5 | 14.5 | 10.0 | 24.2 |
| Shanxi | 456.5 | 8.0 | 8.6 | 6.2 | 19.6 |
| Inner Mongolia | 302.6 | 7.8 | 8.0 | 5.2 | 14.1 |
| | | | | | |
| Liaoning | 789.3 | 29.6 | 18.9 | 18.5 | 14.3 |
| Jilin | 367.5 | 14.0 | 6.5 | 4.8 | 12.2 |
| Heilongjiang | 357.1 | 6.4 | 7.1 | 4.5 | 15.5 |
| | | | | | |
| Shanghai | 735.4 | 22.9 | 48.7 | 38.2 | 17.2 |
| Jiangsu | 1471.7 | 95.3 | 34.8 | 43.0 | 66.8 |
| Zhejiang | 1285.2 | 51.0 | 38.7 | 29.8 | 40.3 |
| Anhui | 499.3 | 15.9 | 10.8 | 8.9 | 14.9 |
| Fujian | 598.3 | 14.0 | 16.5 | 13.8 | 25.4 |
| Jiangxi | 251.3 | 4.7 | 5.0 | 2.7 | 10.2 |
| Shandong | 1111.3 | 48.1 | 36.0 | 30.1 | 43.8 |
| | | | | | |
| Henan | 609.5 | 16.5 | 15.6 | 12.2 | 29.3 |
| Hubei | 500.2 | 22.3 | 11.7 | 8.0 | 23.9 |
| Hunan | 544.0 | 20.5 | 11.8 | 8.7 | 23.8 |
| Guangdong | 3081.8 | 67.0 | 71.1 | 39.6 | 105.3 |
| Guangxi | 307.9 | 9.6 | 9.0 | 5.5 | 17.6 |
| Hainan | 127.1 | 4.7 | 2.5 | 2.0 | 5.2 |
| | | | | | |
| Chongqing | 354.3 | 18.3 | 7.6 | 10.0 | 7.3 |
| Sichuan | 670.3 | 24.8 | 17.5 | 16.7 | 25.6 |
| Guizhou | 263.6 | 7.5 | 4.6 | 3.4 | 8.6 |
| Yunnan | 289.8 | 12.0 | 9.2 | 8.7 | 13.0 |
| Tibet | 23.8 | 0.7 | 0.8 | 0.7 | 1.3 |
| | | | | | |
| Shaanxi | 265.3 | 6.4 | 5.1 | 3.7 | 15.2 |
| Gansu | 154.1 | 3.5 | 4.3 | 2.7 | 8.3 |
| Qinghai | 48.0 | 5.0 | 2.3 | 1.0 | 4.3 |
| Ningxia | 73.7 | 2.6 | 2.3 | 1.7 | 2.9 |
| Xinjiang | 307.9 | 12.4 | 10.0 | 8.2 | 21.6 |

Notes: ①The data in This Table come from Ministry of Human Resources and Social Security; ②All-region figures are from 2015.

## Morbidity and Mortality Orders of Mandatory Reported Class A and B Infectious Diseases in 2016

| Order | Morbidity | | Mortality | |
|---|---|---|---|---|
| | Disease Name | Infected Number | Disease Name | Death Toll |
| 1 | Viral Hepatitis | 1221479 | AIDS | 14091 |
| 2 | Tuberculosis | 836236 | Tuberculosis | 2465 |
| 3 | Syphilis | 438199 | Rabies | 592 |
| 4 | Bacillary and Amebic Dysentery | 123283 | Viral Hepatitis | 537 |
| 5 | Gonorrhoea | 115024 | Human Avian Influenza H7N9 | 73 |
| 6 | Scarlet Fever | 59282 | Epidemic Hemorrhagic Fever | 53 |
| 7 | Brucellosis | 54360 | Syphilis | 48 |
| 8 | AIDS | 47139 | Measles | 47 |
| 9 | Measles | 24820 | Malaria | 18 |
| 10 | Schistosomiasis | 10899 | Epidemic Encephalitis B | 16 |
| 11 | Typhoid and Paratyphoid Fever | 8853 | Neonatal Tetanus | 10 |
| 12 | Epidemic Hemorrhagic Fever | 5584 | Epidemic Cerebrospinal Meningitis | 4 |
| 13 | Whooping Cough | 3189 | Bacillary and Amebic Dysentery | 3 |
| 14 | Dengue | 2924 | Human Avian Influenza | 3 |
| 15 | Malaria | 2050 | Whooping Cough | 2 |
| 16 | Rabies | 1237 | Gonorrhoea | 2 |
| 17 | Epidemic Encephalitis B | 644 | Scarlet Fever | 1 |
| 18 | Leptospirosis | 374 | Brucellosis | 1 |
| 19 | Neonatal Tetanus | 354 | Typhoid and Paratyphoid Fever | 1 |
| 20 | Anthrax | 264 | Leptospirosis | 1 |
| 21 | Human Avian Influenza H7N9 | 177 | Anthrax | — |
| 22 | Epidemic Cerebrospinal Meningitis | 101 | Plague | — |
| 23 | Cholera | 27 | SARS | — |
| 24 | Human Avian Influenza | 1 | Polio | — |
| 25 | Plague | — | Diphtheria | — |
| 26 | SARS | — | Schistosomiasis | — |
| 27 | Polio | — | Dengue | — |
| 28 | Diphtheria | — | Cholera | — |

**Morbidity and Mortality Orders of Mandatory Reported Class A and B Infectious Diseases in 2016**

| Order | Morbidity | | Mortality | |
|---|---|---|---|---|
| | Disease Name | Morbidity (Hundred Thousandth) | Disease Name | Mortality (Hundred Thousandth) |
| 1 | Viral Hepatitis | 89.11 | AIDS | 1.03 |
| 2 | Tuberculosis | 61.00 | Tuberculosis | 0.18 |
| 3 | Syphilis | 31.97 | Rabies | 0.04 |
| 4 | Bacillary and Amebic Dysentery | 8.99 | Viral Hepatitis | 0.04 |
| 5 | Gonorrhoea | 8.39 | Human Avian Influenza H7N9 | 0.01 |
| 6 | Scarlet Fever | 4.32 | Epidemic Hemorrhagic Fever | 0.00 |
| 7 | Brucellosis | 3.97 | Syphilis | 0.00 |
| 8 | AIDS | 3.44 | Measles | 0.00 |
| 9 | Measles | 1.81 | Malaria | 0.00 |
| 10 | Schistosomiasis | 0.80 | Epidemic Encephalitis B | 0.00 |
| 11 | Typhoid and Paratyphoid Fever | 0.65 | Neonatal Tetanus | 0.00 |
| 12 | Epidemic Hemorrhagic Fever | 0.41 | Epidemic Cerebrospinal Meningitis | 0.00 |
| 13 | Whooping Cough | 0.23 | Bacillary and Amebic Dysentery | 0.00 |
| 14 | Dengue | 0.21 | Human Avian Influenza | 0.00 |
| 15 | Malaria | 0.15 | Gonorrhoea | 0.00 |
| 16 | Rabies | 0.09 | Scarlet Fever | 0.00 |
| 17 | Epidemic Encephalitis B | 0.05 | Brucellosis | 0.00 |
| 18 | Leptospirosis | 0.03 | Typhoid and Paratyphoid Fever | 0.00 |
| 19 | Anthrax | 0.03 | Whooping Cough | 0.00 |
| 20 | Neonatal Tetanus | 0.02 | Leptospirosis | — |
| 21 | Human Avian Influenza H7N9 | 0.01 | Anthrax | — |
| 22 | Epidemic Cerebrospinal Meningitis | 0.01 | Plague | — |
| 23 | Cholera | 0.00 | SARS | — |
| 24 | Human Avian Influenza | 0.00 | Polio | — |
| 25 | Plague | — | Diphtheria | — |
| 26 | SARS | — | Schistosomiasis | — |
| 27 | Polio | — | Dengue | — |
| 28 | Diphtheria | — | Cholera | — |

Note: The morbidity and mortality unit of Neonatal Tetanus is ‰.

## All-region Morbidity and Mortality of Mandatory Reported Class A and B Infectious Diseases in 2016

| Region | Total | | Plague | | Cholera | | Viral Hepatitis | |
|---|---|---|---|---|---|---|---|---|
| | Morbidity (Hundred Thousandth) | Mortality (Hundred Thousandth) | Morbidity (Hundred Thousandth) | Mortality (Hundred Thousandth) | Morbidity (Hundred Thousandth) | Mortality (Hundred Thousandth) | Morbidity (Hundred Thousandth) | Mortality (Hundred Thousandth) |
| Total | 215.68 | 1.31 | 0.00 | | 0.00 | | 89.11 | 0.04 |
| Beijing | 137.99 | 0.80 | | | 0.01 | | 13.29 | 0.48 |
| Tianjin | 129.66 | 0.32 | | | | | 16.88 | 0.01 |
| Hebei | 178.97 | 0.28 | | | | | 92.00 | 0.02 |
| Shanxi | 243.87 | 0.44 | | | | | 143.78 | 0.03 |
| Inner Mongolia | 250.37 | 0.33 | | | | | 112.07 | 0.07 |
| Liaoning | 200.70 | 0.57 | | | | | 75.85 | 0.03 |
| Jilin | 145.87 | 0.61 | | | | | 52.43 | 0.04 |
| Heilongjiang | 181.02 | 0.69 | | | | | 39.23 | 0.05 |
| Shanghai | 184.00 | 0.60 | | | 0.01 | | 55.70 | 0.15 |
| Jiangsu | 114.56 | 0.51 | | | 0.01 | | 28.46 | 0.01 |
| Zhejiang | 195.31 | 0.71 | | | 0.01 | | 36.66 | 0.01 |
| Anhui | 205.99 | 0.70 | | | | | 87.45 | 0.01 |
| Fujian | 258.79 | 0.47 | | | 0.00 | | 130.22 | 0.03 |
| Jiangxi | 224.09 | 1.10 | | | 0.00 | | 100.17 | 0.02 |
| Shandong | 137.19 | 0.31 | | | | | 62.99 | 0.04 |
| Henan | 192.25 | 1.53 | | | 0.00 | | 89.67 | 0.04 |
| Hubei | 249.93 | 0.84 | | | 0.01 | | 133.79 | 0.04 |
| Hunan | 238.24 | 1.44 | | | | | 105.95 | 0.01 |
| Guangdong | 320.16 | 1.01 | | | 0.00 | | 166.40 | 0.03 |
| Guangxi | 254.26 | 6.04 | | | | | 118.23 | 0.06 |
| Hainan | 321.47 | 0.90 | | | | | 158.40 | 0.04 |
| Chongqing | 263.60 | 2.63 | | | | | 89.01 | 0.05 |
| Sichuan | 184.90 | 2.73 | | | | | 64.27 | 0.03 |
| Guizhou | 254.21 | 2.19 | | | 0.00 | | 66.54 | 0.01 |
| Yunnan | 187.90 | 4.30 | 0.00 | | | | 55.06 | 0.04 |
| Tibet | 287.09 | 0.46 | | | | | 63.99 | 0.03 |
| Shaanxi | 194.26 | 0.51 | | | | | 77.33 | 0.02 |
| Gansu | 200.18 | 0.45 | | | | | 69.51 | |
| Qinghai | 426.63 | 0.93 | | | | | 209.83 | 0.10 |
| Ningxia | 225.97 | 0.39 | | | | | 54.26 | 0.02 |
| Xinjiang | 606.70 | 4.27 | | | | | 232.75 | 0.04 |

*Continued*

| Region | Hepatitis A | | Hepatitis B | | Hepatitis C | | Hepatitis D | | Hepatitis E | |
|---|---|---|---|---|---|---|---|---|---|---|
| | Morbidity (Hundred Thousandth) | Mortality (Hundred Thousandth) | Morbidity (Hundred Thousandth) | Mortality (Hundred Thousandth) | Morbidity (Hundred Thousandth) | Mortality (Hundred Thousandth) | Morbidity (Hundred Thousandth) | Mortality (Hundred Thousandth) | Morbidity (Hundred Thousandth) | Mortality (Hundred Thousandth) |
| **Total** | **1.55** | **0.00** | **68.74** | **0.03** | **15.09** | **0.01** | **0.03** | | **2.04** | **0.00** |
| Beijing | 0.65 | | 7.81 | 0.39 | 3.59 | 0.09 | | | 1.12 | |
| Tianjin | 0.39 | | 11.98 | | 3.57 | | | | 0.64 | 0.01 |
| Hebei | 0.54 | 0.00 | 77.89 | 0.02 | 11.69 | 0.00 | 0.05 | | 1.01 | |
| Shanxi | 2.60 | | 115.59 | 0.02 | 22.00 | 0.01 | 0.05 | | 1.81 | |
| Inner Mongolia | 0.83 | | 82.32 | 0.06 | 28.00 | 0.01 | 0.04 | | 0.57 | |
| Liaoning | 6.77 | | 44.20 | 0.01 | 18.36 | 0.01 | 0.02 | | 3.36 | 0.01 |
| Jilin | 0.86 | | 30.64 | 0.03 | 19.41 | 0.02 | | | 0.79 | |
| Heilongjiang | 0.76 | 0.00 | 24.49 | 0.02 | 11.17 | 0.02 | 0.03 | | 0.96 | 0.00 |
| Shanghai | 0.97 | | 41.63 | 0.14 | 9.57 | | 0.02 | | 2.95 | 0.01 |
| Jiangsu | 0.75 | | 17.73 | 0.00 | 4.05 | 0.00 | 0.00 | | 3.45 | 0.00 |
| Zhejiang | 0.86 | | 25.04 | 0.01 | 4.88 | 0.00 | 0.04 | | 3.42 | 0.00 |
| Anhui | 0.82 | | 69.55 | 0.01 | 10.76 | 0.00 | 0.03 | | 2.34 | |
| Fujian | 1.17 | | 114.63 | 0.02 | 6.91 | 0.00 | 0.05 | | 2.17 | 0.00 |
| Jiangxi | 0.60 | | 89.35 | 0.02 | 6.81 | | 0.05 | | 1.55 | |
| Shandong | 0.38 | | 55.58 | 0.04 | 4.87 | 0.00 | 0.02 | | 1.08 | 0.00 |
| Henan | 0.24 | | 64.46 | 0.03 | 23.89 | 0.01 | 0.02 | | 0.67 | |
| Hubei | 1.42 | | 108.60 | 0.04 | 16.38 | 0.00 | 0.04 | | 4.66 | 0.00 |
| Hunan | 0.84 | 0.00 | 81.83 | 0.01 | 19.72 | 0.00 | 0.05 | | 1.73 | |
| Guangdong | 1.48 | | 139.42 | 0.02 | 21.10 | 0.01 | 0.04 | | 2.87 | 0.00 |
| Guangxi | 1.17 | 0.00 | 91.07 | 0.05 | 19.49 | 0.01 | 0.04 | | 3.31 | |
| Hainan | 0.68 | | 115.23 | | 35.32 | 0.04 | 0.08 | | 4.57 | |
| Hubei | 2.94 | | 67.54 | 0.04 | 14.23 | 0.00 | 0.02 | | 2.48 | |
| Hunan | 2.41 | 0.00 | 47.16 | 0.02 | 12.13 | 0.00 | 0.02 | | 1.44 | |
| Guangdong | 0.78 | | 49.85 | 0.01 | 13.70 | 0.00 | 0.05 | | 1.57 | |
| Guangxi | 2.09 | | 29.04 | 0.01 | 20.74 | 0.03 | 0.01 | | 3.01 | 0.00 |
| Hainan | 2.38 | | 59.48 | 0.03 | 1.64 | | 0.03 | | 0.09 | |
| Hubei | 0.78 | | 55.30 | 0.01 | 20.00 | 0.01 | 0.02 | | 0.72 | |
| Hunan | 2.62 | | 38.07 | | 27.28 | | 0.03 | | 0.64 | |
| Guangdong | 5.57 | | 162.42 | 0.09 | 38.92 | 0.02 | 0.12 | | 1.97 | |
| Guangxi | 2.55 | | 38.76 | 0.02 | 12.40 | | 0.02 | | 0.27 | |
| Hainan | 15.15 | | 167.33 | 0.03 | 46.01 | 0.02 | 0.06 | | 1.85 | |

Continued

| Region | Among Which Unclassified Hepatitis | | Dysentery | | Typhoid and Paratyphoid Fever | | AIDS | |
|---|---|---|---|---|---|---|---|---|
| | Morbidity (Hundred Thousandth) | Mortality (Hundred Thousandth) | Morbidity (Hundred Thousandth) | Mortality (Hundred Thousandth) | Morbidity (Hundred Thousandth) | Mortality (Hundred Thousandth) | Morbidity (Hundred Thousandth) | Mortality (Hundred Thousandth) |
| Total | 1.66 | 0.00 | 8.99 | 0.00 | 0.80 | 0.00 | 3.97 | 1.03 |
| Beijing | 0.12 | | 41.07 | | 0.06 | | 3.62 | 0.15 |
| Tianjin | 0.29 | | 52.68 | | 0.14 | | 1.79 | 0.20 |
| Hebei | 0.83 | 0.00 | 11.50 | | 0.44 | | 0.79 | 0.16 |
| Shanxi | 1.73 | | 8.91 | | 0.87 | | 1.45 | 0.27 |
| Inner Mongolia | 0.31 | | 5.71 | 0.00 | 0.20 | | 1.14 | 0.15 |
| Liaoning | 3.14 | | 9.43 | | 0.33 | | 2.31 | 0.29 |
| Jilin | 0.73 | | 3.00 | | 0.05 | | 1.99 | 0.46 |
| Heilongjiang | 1.82 | | 6.75 | | 0.06 | | 1.48 | 0.23 |
| Shanghai | 0.57 | | 0.54 | | 0.08 | | 2.27 | 0.21 |
| Jiangsu | 2.48 | | 4.05 | | 0.40 | | 2.02 | 0.28 |
| Zhejiang | 2.43 | 0.00 | 3.92 | | 0.86 | | 3.37 | 0.44 |
| Anhui | 3.95 | | 12.29 | | 0.62 | | 2.17 | 0.39 |
| Fujian | 5.29 | | 1.27 | | 1.84 | | 2.43 | 0.29 |
| Jiangxi | 1.82 | 0.00 | 8.91 | | 0.67 | | 3.01 | 0.86 |
| Shandong | 1.06 | 0.00 | 4.40 | | 0.11 | | 0.74 | 0.12 |
| Henan | 0.39 | | 12.63 | 0.00 | 0.20 | | 3.17 | 1.28 |
| Hubei | 2.70 | | 7.08 | | 0.49 | | 2.18 | 0.60 |
| Hunan | 1.77 | | 5.62 | | 1.50 | | 4.15 | 1.17 |
| Guangdong | 1.50 | | 2.57 | | 1.40 | | 3.80 | 0.82 |
| Guangxi | 3.15 | | 6.66 | | 2.34 | | 12.48 | 5.57 |
| Hainan | 2.53 | | 3.40 | | 0.36 | | 1.92 | 0.64 |
| Chongqing | 1.80 | | 23.66 | | 0.38 | | 10.20 | 2.08 |
| Sichuan | 1.11 | | 6.93 | 0.00 | 0.43 | | 11.16 | 2.47 |
| Guizhou | 0.60 | | 8.00 | | 1.49 | | 7.42 | 1.73 |
| Yunnan | 0.17 | | 8.85 | | 4.81 | | 12.04 | 3.99 |
| Tibet | 0.37 | | 20.56 | | 0.03 | | 1.57 | 0.12 |
| Shaanxi | 0.51 | | 11.67 | | 0.11 | | 2.13 | 0.35 |
| Gansu | 0.88 | | 24.34 | | 0.13 | | 1.55 | 0.24 |
| Qinghai | 0.83 | | 15.45 | | 0.12 | | 2.97 | 0.49 |
| Ningxia | 0.27 | | 20.63 | | 0.31 | | 1.26 | 0.18 |
| Xinjiang | 2.35 | | 15.68 | 0.00 | 0.56 | 0.00 | 8.14 | 2.83 |

*Continued*

| Region | Gonorrhoea | | Syphilis | | Polio | | Measles | |
|---|---|---|---|---|---|---|---|---|
| | Morbidity (Hundred Thousandth) | Mortality (Hundred Thousandth) | Morbidity (Hundred Thousandth) | Mortality (Hundred Thousandth) | Morbidity (Hundred Thousandth) | Mortality (Hundred Thousandth) | Morbidity (Hundred Thousandth) | Mortality (Hundred Thousandth) |
| **Total** | **8.39** | **0.00** | **31.97** | **0.00** | | | **1.81** | **0.00** |
| Beijing | 6.58 | | 22.92 | 0.01 | | | 5.75 | |
| Tianjin | 2.06 | | 16.60 | | | | 3.63 | 0.01 |
| Hebei | 1.91 | 0.00 | 12.88 | 0.00 | | | 2.46 | 0.00 |
| Shanxi | 3.57 | | 25.30 | 0.01 | | | 0.41 | |
| Inner Mongolia | 8.91 | | 38.12 | 0.01 | | | 1.12 | |
| Liaoning | 5.85 | | 37.41 | 0.00 | | | 0.26 | |
| Jilin | 4.97 | | 18.36 | | | | 0.31 | |
| Heilongjiang | 4.01 | | 24.30 | 0.01 | | | 0.29 | |
| Shanghai | 28.03 | | 57.07 | 0.01 | | | 0.69 | |
| Jiangsu | 9.03 | | 29.70 | 0.00 | | | 0.94 | |
| Zhejiang | 32.75 | | 62.16 | | | | 0.59 | |
| Anhui | 6.05 | | 37.14 | 0.01 | | | 1.17 | 0.00 |
| Fujian | 15.42 | | 58.51 | 0.01 | | | 0.63 | |
| Jiangxi | 8.00 | | 28.70 | | | | 0.50 | 0.00 |
| Shandong | 4.15 | | 15.54 | 0.00 | | | 4.47 | 0.01 |
| Henan | 3.13 | | 15.44 | 0.01 | | | 1.19 | 0.00 |
| Hubei | 4.74 | | 21.67 | 0.00 | | | 1.21 | |
| Hunan | 4.82 | | 33.43 | 0.00 | | | 1.16 | 0.00 |
| Guangdong | 19.80 | | 48.73 | 0.01 | | | 1.17 | |
| Guangxi | 10.23 | | 15.41 | 0.01 | | | 0.08 | |
| Hainan | 20.36 | | 50.69 | | | | 1.76 | |
| Chongqing | 6.79 | | 54.86 | 0.01 | | | 1.13 | |
| Sichuan | 3.56 | | 28.35 | 0.00 | | | 0.99 | |
| Guizhou | 6.41 | | 30.37 | 0.01 | | | 0.09 | |
| Yunnan | 8.64 | | 35.96 | | | | 0.34 | |
| Tibet | 1.39 | | 35.25 | | | | 6.82 | |
| Shaanxi | 4.53 | | 26.09 | | | | 0.89 | |
| Gansu | 3.24 | | 18.61 | | | | 11.14 | |
| Qinghai | 2.52 | | 48.47 | | | | 10.55 | 0.03 |
| Ningxia | 4.72 | | 56.70 | 0.03 | | | 0.76 | |
| Xinjiang | 7.29 | | 89.05 | 0.01 | | | 17.14 | 0.02 |

*Continued*

| Region | Whooping Cough | | Diphtheria | | Epidemic Cerebrospinal Meningitis | | Scarlet Fever | |
|---|---|---|---|---|---|---|---|---|
| | Morbidity (Hundred Thousandth) | Mortality (Hundred Thousandth) | Morbidity (Hundred Thousandth) | Mortality (Hundred Thousandth) | Morbidity (Hundred Thousandth) | Mortality (Hundred Thousandth) | Morbidity (Hundred Thousandth) | Mortality (Hundred Thousandth) |
| **Total** | 041 | 0.00 | | | 0.01 | 0.00 | 4.32 | |
| Beijing | 0.42 | 0.01 | | | | | 12.08 | |
| Tianjin | 2.02 | | | | | | 11.21 | |
| Hebei | 0.49 | | | | 0.01 | | 5.21 | |
| Shanxi | 0.30 | | | | 0.01 | 0.00 | 7.69 | |
| Inner Mongolia | 0.04 | | | | | | 10.35 | |
| Liaoning | 0.00 | | | | 0.00 | | 10.36 | |
| Jilin | 0.01 | | | | | | 7.68 | |
| Heilongjiang | 0.07 | | | | 0.00 | | 7.43 | |
| Shanghai | 0.02 | | | | 0.00 | | 12.10 | |
| Jiangsu | 0.02 | | | | 0.01 | | 2.80 | |
| Zhejiang | 0.26 | | | | 0.01 | | 4.46 | |
| Anhui | 0.04 | | | | 0.00 | | 1.33 | |
| Fujian | 0.01 | | | | 0.00 | | 1.59 | |
| Jiangxi | 0.12 | | | | 0.00 | | 0.10 | |
| Shandong | 1.42 | | | | 0.00 | | 7.22 | |
| Henan | 0.12 | | | | 0.01 | | 1.56 | |
| Hubei | 0.09 | | | | 0.00 | | 1.73 | |
| Hunan | 0.12 | | | | 0.00 | | 1.15 | |
| Guangdong | 0.54 | | | | 0.00 | 0.00 | 2.40 | |
| Guangxi | 0.01 | | | | 0.00 | | 1.09 | |
| Hainan | | | | | | | 0.07 | |
| Chongqing | 2.03 | | | | 0.00 | | 1.60 | |
| Sichuan | 0.43 | | | | 0.00 | | 2.10 | |
| Guizhou | 0.18 | | | | 0.00 | | 2.05 | |
| Yunnan | 0.09 | | | | 0.00 | | 3.59 | |
| Tibet | 0.03 | | | | | | 2.44 | |
| Shaanxi | 1.57 | | | | 0.01 | | 8.07 | |
| Gansu | 0.46 | | | | | | 5.50 | |
| Qinghai | 0.05 | | | | | | 6.49 | |
| Ningxia | 0.04 | | | | | | 14.52 | |
| Xinjiang | 1.66 | | | | 0.19 | 0.03 | 12.69 | |

*Continued*

| Region | Epidemic Hemorrhagic Fever | | Rabies | | Leptospirosis | | Brucellosis | |
|---|---|---|---|---|---|---|---|---|
| | Morbidity (Hundred Thousandth) | Mortality (Hundred Thousandth) | Morbidity (Hundred Thousandth) | Mortality (Hundred Thousandth) | Morbidity (Hundred Thousandth) | Mortality (Hundred Thousandth) | Morbidity (Hundred Thousandth) | Mortality (Hundred Thousandth) |
| Total | 065 | 0.00 | 0.05 | 0.04 | 0.03 | 0.00 | 3.44 | 0.00 |
| Beijing | 0.04 | | 0.01 | 0.01 | | | 0.88 | |
| Tianjin | 0.20 | | 0.03 | 0.03 | | | 1.18 | |
| Hebei | 0.58 | 0.00 | 0.04 | 0.03 | 0.00 | | 5.08 | |
| Shanxi | 0.02 | | 0.07 | 0.03 | | | 12.52 | |
| Inner Mongolia | 0.42 | 0.00 | 0.02 | 0.01 | | | 23.78 | |
| Liaoning | 1.97 | 0.01 | | | | | 5.34 | |
| Jilin | 1.87 | 0.01 | | | | | 5.38 | |
| Heilongjiang | 3.15 | 0.02 | | | | | 14.01 | |
| Shanghai | 0.02 | | 0.00 | 0.00 | | | 0.05 | |
| Jiangsu | 0.41 | 0.01 | 0.06 | 0.06 | | | 0.18 | |
| Zhejiang | 0.62 | | 0.03 | 0.04 | 0.02 | | 0.17 | |
| Anhui | 0.34 | | 0.04 | 0.04 | 0.08 | | 0.13 | |
| Fujian | 0.95 | | 0.00 | 0.00 | 0.07 | | 0.20 | |
| Jiangxi | 1.48 | 0.01 | 0.02 | 0.02 | 0.04 | 0.00 | 0.14 | |
| Shandong | 1.00 | 0.01 | 0.03 | 0.03 | 0.00 | | 3.95 | |
| Henan | 0.19 | 0.00 | 0.09 | 0.07 | | | 4.21 | |
| Hubei | 0.40 | 0.01 | 0.05 | 0.05 | 0.00 | | 0.45 | |
| Hunan | 0.87 | 0.00 | 0.09 | 0.09 | 0.03 | | 0.24 | |
| Guangdong | 0.38 | 0.00 | 0.04 | 0.04 | 0.04 | | 0.35 | |
| Guangxi | 0.01 | | 0.12 | 0.12 | 0.03 | | 0.60 | |
| Hainan | 0.03 | | 0.04 | 0.04 | 0.04 | | 0.05 | |
| Chongqing | 0.04 | | 0.07 | 0.07 | 0.02 | | 0.14 | |
| Sichuan | 0.13 | 0.00 | 0.02 | 0.02 | 0.06 | | 0.14 | |
| Guizhou | 0.17 | | 0.14 | 0.14 | 0.01 | | 0.32 | 0.00 |
| Yunnan | 0.46 | | 0.10 | 0.10 | 0.22 | | 0.59 | |
| Tibet | 0.03 | | 0.03 | 0.03 | | | 0.31 | |
| Shaanxi | 2.46 | 0.00 | 0.04 | 0.03 | | | 2.50 | |
| Gansu | 0.07 | | 0.03 | 0.03 | | | 6.71 | |
| Qinghai | | | 0.02 | | | | 0.25 | |
| Ningxia | 0.06 | | 0.03 | 0.04 | | | 32.34 | 0.02 |
| Xinjiang | 0.00 | | 0.00 | 0.00 | | | 35.60 | |

*Continued*

| Region | Anthrax | | Epidemic Encephalitis B | | Tuberculosis | | Malaria | | Dengue | |
|---|---|---|---|---|---|---|---|---|---|---|
| | Morbidity (Hundred Thousandth) | Mortality (Hundred Thousandth) | Morbidity (Hundred Thousandth) | Mortality (Hundred Thousandth) | Morbidity (Hundred Thousandth) | Mortality (Hundred Thousandth) | Morbidity (Hundred Thousandth) | Mortality (Hundred Thousandth) | Morbidity (Hundred Thousandth) | Mortality (Hundred Thousandth) |
| **Total** | **0.03** | **0.00** | **0.09** | **0.00** | **61.00** | **0.18** | **0.23** | **0.00** | **0.15** | |
| Beijing | 0.05 | | 0.00 | | 31.01 | 0.13 | 0.15 | 0.01 | 0.04 | |
| Tianjin | | | | | 21.14 | 0.06 | 0.07 | | 0.02 | |
| Hebei | 0.01 | | 0.01 | | 45.34 | 0.06 | 0.12 | 0.00 | 0.01 | |
| Shanxi | | | 0.28 | 0.02 | 38.65 | 0.08 | 0.04 | | | |
| Inner Mongolia | 0.15 | 0.00 | 0.00 | | 48.30 | 0.08 | 0.02 | 0.00 | | |
| Liaoning | 0.05 | | | | 51.40 | 0.24 | 0.12 | | 0.02 | |
| Jilin | | | | | 49.76 | 0.10 | 0.06 | | 0.00 | |
| Heilongjiang | 0.05 | | | | 80.16 | 0.40 | 0.02 | | | |
| Shanghai | | | 0.00 | | 27.28 | 0.22 | 0.10 | | 0.02 | |
| Jiangsu | | | 0.02 | | 35.93 | 0.12 | 0.38 | | 0.02 | |
| Zhejiang | | | 0.03 | | 48.78 | 0.20 | 0.38 | 0.00 | 0.10 | |
| Anhui | | | 0.05 | 0.01 | 56.77 | 0.22 | 0.24 | 0.00 | 0.00 | |
| Fujian | | | | | 42.74 | 0.14 | 0.30 | | 2.54 | |
| Jiangxi | | | 0.01 | | 71.99 | 0.18 | 0.11 | | 0.01 | |
| Shandong | | | 0.12 | 0.00 | 30.78 | 0.10 | 0.25 | 0.00 | 0.01 | |
| Henan | | | 0.26 | 0.02 | 60.13 | 0.10 | 0.22 | 0.00 | 0.01 | |
| Hubei | | | 0.01 | | 74.70 | 0.14 | 0.25 | | 0.02 | |
| Hunan | | | 0.07 | 0.00 | 75.50 | 0.16 | 0.22 | | 0.03 | |
| Guangdong | | | 0.03 | 0.00 | 71.82 | 0.09 | 0.13 | 0.00 | 0.50 | |
| Guangxi | 0.00 | | 0.02 | | 86.27 | 0.29 | 0.63 | | 0.01 | |
| Hainan | | | 0.02 | | 84.18 | 0.18 | 0.09 | | 0.02 | |
| Chongqing | | | 0.15 | | 73.34 | 0.44 | 0.13 | | 0.04 | |
| Sichuan | 0.07 | | 0.14 | 0.00 | 65.66 | 0.19 | 0.41 | 0.00 | 0.02 | |
| Guizhou | 0.01 | | 0.18 | 0.01 | 130.66 | 0.29 | 0.10 | | 0.01 | |
| Yunnan | 0.03 | | 0.22 | 0.01 | 55.47 | 0.16 | 0.70 | | 0.69 | |
| Tibet | 0.28 | | | | 154.37 | 0.28 | | | | |
| Shaanxi | 0.02 | | 0.32 | | 56.30 | 0.11 | 0.22 | 0.00 | 0.02 | |
| Gansu | 0.32 | 0.00 | 0.32 | 0.01 | 58.13 | 0.16 | 0.06 | | | |
| Qinghai | 1.19 | | | | 128.70 | 0.31 | 0.02 | | | |
| Ningxia | 0.10 | | | | 40.04 | 0.10 | 0.12 | | | |
| Xinjiang | 0.06 | | 0.00 | | 185.66 | 1.32 | 0.03 | | | |

*Continued*

| Region | Schistosomiasis | | Neonatal Tetanus | | Human Avian Influenza | | Human Avian Influenza H7N9 | |
|---|---|---|---|---|---|---|---|---|
| | Morbidity (Hundred Thousandth) | Mortality (Hundred Thousandth) | Morbidity (Hundred Thousandth) | Mortality (Hundred Thousandth) | Morbidity (Hundred Thousandth) | Mortality (Hundred Thousandth) | Morbidity (Hundred Thousandth) | Morbidity (Hundred Thousandth) |
| **Total** | **0.21** | | **0.01** | **0.00** | | **0.00** | **0.02** | **0.01** |
| Beijing | 0.00 | | | | | | 0.00 | 0.00 |
| Tianjin | | | | | | | 0.01 | 0.01 |
| Hebei | | | | | | | 0.01 | 0.00 |
| Shanxi | | | 0.00 | | | | | |
| Inner Mongolia | | | | | | | | |
| Liaoning | | | 0.00 | | | | 0.00 | 0.00 |
| Jilin | | | 0.01 | | | | | |
| Heilongjiang | | | | | | | | |
| Shanghai | 0.00 | | 0.01 | | | | 0.02 | 0.00 |
| Jiangsu | 0.00 | | 0.00 | | | | 0.13 | 0.03 |
| Zhejiang | 0.01 | | 0.02 | | | | 0.10 | 0.02 |
| Anhui | 0.05 | | 0.00 | | | | 0.04 | 0.02 |
| Fujian | | | 0.02 | | | | 0.04 | 0.01 |
| Jiangxi | 0.09 | | 0.01 | | | | 0.01 | |
| Shandong | | | 0.00 | | | | 0.00 | 0.00 |
| Henan | 0.00 | | 0.01 | 0.00 | | | 0.00 | |
| Hubei | 1.03 | | 0.01 | | | | 0.00 | |
| Hunan | 3.28 | | 0.00 | | | | 0.02 | 0.01 |
| Guangdong | 0.00 | | 0.03 | | | | 0.03 | 0.01 |
| Guangxi | | | 0.02 | | | | | |
| Hainan | | | 0.02 | | | | | |
| Chongqing | 0.00 | | | | | | | |
| Sichuan | 0.00 | | 0.01 | | | 0.00 | | |
| Guizhou | | | 0.03 | 0.00 | | | 0.00 | |
| Yunnan | 0.01 | | 0.01 | | | | | |
| Tibet | | | | | | | | |
| Shaanxi | | | 0.00 | | | | | |
| Gansu | | | 0.03 | | | | | |
| Qinghai | | | | | | | | |
| Ningxia | | | 0.05 | | | | | |
| Xinjiang | 0.00 | | 0.09 | | | | | |

## Top Ten Malignant Tumor Mortality (Total)

| Order | 2004—2005 | | 1990—1992 | | 1973—1975 | |
| --- | --- | --- | --- | --- | --- | --- |
| | Disease Name | Mortality (Hundred Thousandth) | Disease Name | Mortality (Hundred Thousandth) | Disease Name | Mortality (Hundred Thousandth) |
| 1 | Lung Cancer | 30.83 | Gastric Cancer | 25.16 | Gastric Cancer | 19.54 |
| 2 | Liver Cancer | 26.26 | Liver Cancer | 20.37 | Esophagus Cancer | 18.83 |
| 3 | Gastric Cancer | 24.71 | Lung Cancer | 17.54 | Liver Cancer | 12.54 |
| 4 | Esophagus Cancer | 15.21 | Esophagus Cancer | 17.38 | Lung Cancer | 7.09 |
| 5 | Colorectal Cancer | 7.25 | Colorectal Cancer | 5.30 | Cervical Cancer | 5.23 |
| 6 | Leukemia | 3.84 | Leukemia | 3.64 | Colorectal Cancer | 4.60 |
| 7 | Brain Tumor | 3.13 | Cervical Cancer | 1.89 | Leukemia | 2.72 |
| 8 | Female Breast Cancer | 2.90 | Nasopharynx Cancer | 1.74 | Nasopharynx Cancer | 2.32 |
| 9 | Pancreatic Cancer | 2.62 | Female Breast Cancer | 1.72 | Female Breast Cancer | 1.65 |
| 10 | Osteocarcinoma | 1.70 | | | | |
| | Malignant Tumor Total | 134.80 | Malignant Tumor Total | 108.26 | Malignant Tumor Total | 83.65 |

Source: Retrospective Sampling Survey on Malignant Tumor in China (1973—1975、1990—1992、2004—2005).

## Top Ten Malignant Tumor Mortality (Male)

| Order | 2004—2005 | | 1990—1992 | | 1973—1975 | |
| --- | --- | --- | --- | --- | --- | --- |
| | Disease Name | Mortality (Hundred Thousandth) | Disease Name | Mortality (Hundred Thousandth) | Disease Name | Mortality (Hundred Thousandth) |
| 1 | Lung Cancer | 41.34 | Gastric Cancer | 32.84 | Gastric Cancer | 25.12 |
| 2 | Liver Cancer | 37.54 | Liver Cancer | 29.01 | Esophagus Cancer | 23.34 |
| 3 | Gastric Cancer | 32.46 | Lung Cancer | 24.03 | Liver Cancer | 17.60 |
| 4 | Esophagus Cancer | 20.65 | Esophagus Cancer | 22.14 | Lung Cancer | 9.28 |
| 5 | Colorectal Cancer | 8.19 | Colorectal Cancer | 5.76 | Colorectal Cancer | 4.85 |
| 6 | Leukemia | 4.27 | Leukemia | 3.96 | Leukemia | 3.00 |
| 7 | Brain Tumor | 3.50 | Nasopharynx Cancer | 2.34 | Nasopharynx Cancer | 2.94 |
| 8 | Pancreatic Cancer | 2.94 | | | | |
| 9 | Bladder Cancer | 2.13 | | | | |
| 10 | Nasopharynx Cancer | 2.05 | | | | |
| | Malignant Tumor Total | 169.19 | Malignant Tumor Total | 134.91 | Malignant Tumor Total | 96.31 |

## Top Ten Malignant Tumor Mortality (Female)

| Order | 2004—2005 | | 1990—1992 | | 1973—1975 | |
| --- | --- | --- | --- | --- | --- | --- |
| | Disease Name | Mortality (Hundred Thousandth) | Disease Name | Mortality (Hundred Thousandth) | Disease Name | Mortality (Hundred Thousandth) |
| 1 | Lung Cancer | 19.84 | Gastric Cancer | 17.02 | Esophagus Cancer | 14.11 |
| 2 | Gastric Cancer | 16.59 | Esophagus Cancer | 12.34 | Gastric Cancer | 13.72 |
| 3 | Liver Cancer | 14.44 | Liver Cancer | 11.21 | Cervical Cancer | 10.70 |
| 4 | Esophagus Cancer | 9.51 | Lung Cancer | 10.66 | Liver Cancer | 7.26 |
| 5 | Colorectal Cancer | 6.26 | Colorectal Cancer | 4.82 | Lung Cancer | 4.79 |
| 6 | Female Breast Cancer | 5.90 | Female Breast Cancer | 3.89 | Female Breast Cancer | 4.33 |
| 7 | Leukemia | 3.41 | Female Breast Cancer | 3.53 | Female Breast Cancer | 3.37 |
| 8 | Cervical Cancer | 2.86 | Leukemia | 3.30 | Leukemia | 2.42 |
| 9 | Brain Cancer | 2.74 | Nasopharynx Cancer | 1.10 | Nasopharynx Cancer | 1.67 |
| 10 | Cervical Cancer | 2.71 | | | | |
| | Malignant Tumor Total | 98.97 | Malignant Tumor Total | 80.04 | Malignant Tumor Total | 70.43 |

## Urban Resident Major Disease Mortality and Constituent in 2016

| Disease Name | Total | | | Male | | | Female | | |
|---|---|---|---|---|---|---|---|---|---|
| | Mortality (Hundred Thousandth) | Constituent (%) | Order | Mortality (Hundred Thousandth) | Constituent (%) | Order | Mortality (Hundred Thousandth) | Constituent (%) | Order |
| Infectious Disease (including Respiratory TB) | 6.46 | 1.05 | 10 | 9.01 | 1.29 | 8 | 3.85 | 0.73 | 10 |
| Parasitic Disease | 0.05 | 0.01 | 17 | 0.05 | 0.01 | 16 | 0.06 | 0.01 | 17 |
| Malignant Tumor | 160.07 | 26.06 | 1 | 200.97 | 28.73 | 1 | 118.05 | 22.42 | 2 |
| Diseases of Blood, Hematopoietic Organ and Immune Disease | 1.37 | 0.22 | 15 | 1.40 | 0.20 | 15 | 1.33 | 0.25 | 15 |
| Endocrine, Nutritional and Metabolic Disease | 20.43 | 3.33 | 6 | 19.42 | 2.60 | 6 | 21.47 | 4.08 | 6 |
| Mental Disorder | 2.72 | 0.44 | 11 | 2.60 | 0.37 | 11 | 2.83 | 0.54 | 11 |
| Nervous System Disease | 7.50 | 1.22 | 8 | 7.63 | 1.09 | 9 | 7.37 | 1.40 | 8 |
| Heart Disease | 138.70 | 22.58 | 3 | 142.30 | 20.34 | 2 | 135.00 | 25.64 | 1 |
| Cerebrovascular Disease | 126.41 | 20.58 | 3 | 139.50 | 19.94 | 3 | 112.95 | 21.46 | 3 |
| Respiratory System Disease | 69.03 | 11.24 | 4 | 79.65 | 11.39 | 4 | 58.12 | 11.04 | 4 |
| Digestive System Disease | 14.05 | 2.29 | 7 | 17.38 | 2.48 | 7 | 10.62 | 2.02 | 7 |
| Musculoskeletal and Connective Tissue Disease | 2.25 | 0.37 | 12 | 1.78 | 0.25 | 13 | 2.73 | 0.52 | 12 |
| Genitourinary System Disease | 6.58 | 1.07 | 9 | 7.44 | 1.06 | 10 | 5.69 | 1.08 | 9 |
| Pregnancy, Puerperal Childbirth Complication | 0.09 | 0.02 | 16 | | | | 0.19 | 0.04 | 16 |
| Perinatal Disease | 1.87 | 0.30 | 13 | 2.24 | 0.32 | 12 | 1.49 | 0.28 | 13 |
| Congenital Malformation, Deformation and Chromosomal Abnormality | 1.55 | 0.25 | 14 | 1.74 | 0.25 | 14 | 1.37 | 0.26 | 14 |
| Injury and External Cause Poisoning | 37.34 | 6.08 | 5 | 48.12 | 6.88 | 5 | 26.25 | 4.99 | 5 |
| Acatalepsy | 2.18 | 0.36 | | 2.92 | 0.42 | | 1.43 | 0.27 | |
| Other Disease | 6.06 | 0.99 | | 5.03 | 0.72 | | 7.11 | 1.35 | |

## Rural Resident Major Disease Mortality and Constituent in 2016

| Disease Name | Total | | | Male | | | Female | | |
|---|---|---|---|---|---|---|---|---|---|
| | Mortality (Hundred Thousandth) | Constituent (%) | Order | Mortality (Hundred Thousandth) | Constituent (%) | Order | Mortality (Hundred Thousandth) | Constituent (%) | Order |
| Infectious Disease (including Respiratory TB) | 7.76 | 1.14 | 8 | 10.57 | 1.36 | 8 | 4.84 | 0.83 | 10 |
| Parasitic Disease | 0.07 | 0.01 | 17 | 0.09 | 0.01 | 16 | 0.05 | 0.01 | 17 |
| Malignant Tumor | 155.83 | 22.92 | 2 | 199.41 | 25.73 | 1 | 110.45 | 19.02 | 3 |
| Diseases of Blood, Hematopoietic Organ and Immune Disease | 1.15 | 0.17 | 15 | 1.21 | 0.16 | 15 | 1.10 | 0.19 | 15 |
| Endocrine, Nutritional and Metabolic Disease | 15.72 | 2.31 | 6 | 13.90 | 1.79 | 7 | 17.61 | 3.03 | 6 |
| Mental Disorder | 2.85 | 0.42 | 11 | 2.78 | 0.36 | 11 | 2.92 | 0.50 | 11 |
| Nervous System Disease | 7.54 | 1.11 | 9 | 7.43 | 0.96 | 10 | 7.65 | 1.32 | 8 |
| Heart Disease | 151.18 | 22.24 | 3 | 154.07 | 19.88 | 3 | 148.17 | 25.52 | 1 |
| Cerebrovascular Disease | 158.15 | 23.26 | 1 | 173.81 | 22.42 | 2 | 141.84 | 24.43 | 2 |
| Respiratory System Disease | 81.72 | 12.02 | 4 | 90.54 | 11.68 | 4 | 72.54 | 12.49 | 4 |
| Digestive System Disease | 14.31 | 2.11 | 7 | 18.40 | 2.37 | 6 | 10.06 | 1.73 | 7 |
| Musculoskeletal and Connective Tissue Disease | 1.68 | 0.25 | 14 | 1.38 | 0.18 | 14 | 1.99 | 0.34 | 12 |
| Genitourinary System Disease | 7.38 | 1.09 | 10 | 8.61 | 1.11 | 9 | 6.10 | 1.05 | 9 |
| Pregnancy, Puerperal Childbirth Complication | 0.12 | 0.02 | 16 | | | | 0.24 | 0.04 | 16 |
| Perinatal Disease | 2.12 | 0.31 | 12 | 2.59 | 0.33 | 12 | 1.63 | 0.28 | 13 |
| Congenital Malformation, Deformation and Chromosomal Abnormality | 1.74 | 0.26 | 13 | 1.91 | 0.25 | 13 | 1.56 | 0.27 | 14 |
| Injury and External Cause Poisoning | 54.48 | 8.01 | 5 | 72.54 | 9.36 | 5 | 35.68 | 6.15 | 5 |
| Acatalepsy | 2.11 | 0.31 | | 2.44 | 0.31 | | 1.76 | 0.30 | |
| Other Diseases | 6.17 | 0.91 | | 4.99 | 0.64 | | 7.40 | 1.27 | |

## New Rural Co-operative Medical System

| Year | NCMS Participator (Hundred Million) | NCMS Participating Rate (%) | Per Capita Financing (yuan) | Current-Year Fund Expenditure (Hundred Million yuan) | Compensation Beneficiary (Hundred Million Persons/Times) |
|---|---|---|---|---|---|
| 2010 | 8.36 | 96.00 | 156.57 | 1187.84 | 10.87 |
| 2012 | 8.05 | 98.26 | 308.50 | 2408.00 | 17.45 |
| 2013 | 8.02 | 98.70 | 370.59 | 2909.20 | 19.42 |
| 2014 | 7.36 | 98.90 | 410.89 | 2890.40 | 16.52 |
| 2015 | 6.70 | 98.80 | 490.30 | 2933.41 | 16.53 |
| 2016 | 2.75 | 99.36 | 559.00 | 1363.64 | 6.57 |

## All Region New Rural Co-operative Medical Service in 2016

| Region | NCMS Participator (Ten Thousand) | Per Capita Financing (yuan) | Current-year Financing Total (Hundred Million yuan) | Compensation Beneficiary (Ten Thousand Persons/Times) | Fund Utilization Rate (%) |
|---|---|---|---|---|---|
| Total | 27516 | 559 | 1538.15 | 65657.62 | 88.65 |
| Liaoning | 1847 | 585 | 108.05 | 3230.76 | 87.84 |
| Jilin | 1281 | 577 | 73.93 | 820.57 | 85.08 |
| Heilongjiang | 1404 | 598 | 83.99 | 3184.96 | 90.65 |
| Jiangsu | 3395 | 601 | 204.11 | 14589.55 | 92.94 |
| Anhui | 5121 | 557 | 285.45 | 9531.56 | 84.66 |
| Jiangxi | 3226 | 531 | 171.33 | 6064.90 | 88.36 |
| Hainan | 475 | 544 | 25.87 | 1113.85 | 85.66 |
| Guizhou | 3025 | 507 | 153.50 | 5567.93 | 80.60 |
| Yunnan | 3266 | 548 | 179.00 | 10425.01 | 91.42 |
| Shaanxi | 2578 | 565 | 145.72 | 6415.76 | 95.76 |
| Gansu | 1898 | 565 | 107.20 | 4712.77 | 91.33 |

Note: The data of Tianjin, Zhejiang, Shandong, Guangdong, Chongqing, Qinghai and Ningxia are not included.

## Urban Resident and Employee Basic Medical Insurance

| Year and Region | Participator (Ten Thousand Persons) | | | | | Urban Employee Basic Medical Insurance Revenue and Expenditure | | |
|---|---|---|---|---|---|---|---|---|
| | Total | Urban Resident Basic Medical Insurance | Urban Employee Basic Medical Insurance | On-post Staff | Retiree | Fund Revenue | Fund Expenditure | Accumulative Balance |
| 2010 | 43263 | 19528 | 23735 | 17791 | 5944 | 3955.4 | 3271.6 | 4741.2 |
| 2012 | 53641 | 27156 | 26486 | 19861 | 6624 | 6061.9 | 4868.5 | 6884.2 |
| 2013 | 57073 | 29629 | 27443 | 20501 | 6942 | 7061.6 | 5829.9 | 8129.3 |
| 2014 | 59747 | 31451 | 28296 | 21041 | 7255 | 8037.9 | 6696.6 | 9449.8 |
| 2015 | 66582 | 37689 | 28893 | 21362 | 7531 | 9083.5 | 7531.5 | 10997.1 |
| 2016 | 74839 | 45315 | 29524 | ... | ... | ... | ... | ... |
| | | | | | | | | |
| East Region | 38531 | 21485 | 17046 | 13176 | 3870 | 5626.7 | 4585.0 | 6951.6 |
| Central Region | 14337 | 7919 | 6417 | 4386 | 2032 | 1628.7 | 1404.5 | 1892.9 |
| West Region | 13714 | 8284 | 5430 | 3800 | 1629 | 1828.3 | 1542.0 | 2152.6 |
| | | | | | | | | |
| Beijing | 1657 | 181 | 1476 | 1206 | 270 | 786.3 | 719.4 | 294.0 |
| Tianjin | 1054 | 532 | 522 | 332 | 190 | 235.2 | 203.9 | 111.6 |
| Hebei | 1664 | 707 | 957 | 657 | 300 | 304.7 | 237.0 | 441.2 |
| Shanxi | 1114 | 463 | 651 | 471 | 179 | 178.5 | 154.0 | 243.5 |
| Inner Mongolia | 1008 | 531 | 477 | 336 | 141 | 154.1 | 129.2 | 169.3 |
| | | | | | | | | |
| Liaoning | 2396 | 745 | 1651 | 1054 | 598 | 383.6 | 369.6 | 358.2 |
| Jilin | 1381 | 805 | 576 | 376 | 200 | 135.5 | 117.1 | 179.2 |
| Heilongjiang | 1595 | 721 | 874 | 544 | 330 | 229.8 | 213.0 | 273.5 |
| | | | | | | | | |
| Shanghai | 1719 | 273 | 1446 | 981 | 466 | 733.1 | 501.9 | 1107.3 |
| Jiangsu | 4014 | 1585 | 2429 | 1818 | 611 | 781.9 | 665.7 | 979.6 |
| Zhejiang | 4964 | 2971 | 1993 | 1639 | 354 | 687.0 | 503.5 | 1059.6 |
| Anhui | 1738 | 974 | 763 | 542 | 221 | 193.7 | 168.8 | 226.1 |
| Fujian | 1301 | 542 | 759 | 613 | 147 | 243.5 | 183.8 | 411.9 |
| Jiangxi | 1530 | 946 | 585 | 384 | 201 | 126.7 | 100.7 | 155.2 |
| Shandong | 9236 | 7331 | 1904 | 1465 | 440 | 563.2 | 507.1 | 582.0 |
| | | | | | | | | |
| Henan | 2345 | 1144 | 1201 | 864 | 337 | 268.0 | 227.5 | 337.8 |
| Hubei | 1972 | 1023 | 949 | 653 | 296 | 265.8 | 236.4 | 222.1 |
| Hunan | 2662 | 1844 | 819 | 552 | 267 | 230.7 | 187.0 | 255.5 |
| Guangdong | 10136 | 6424 | 3712 | 3272 | 440 | 859.3 | 653.3 | 1542.9 |
| Guangxi | 1078 | 572 | 506 | 357 | 149 | 147.9 | 127.2 | 195.8 |
| Hainan | 390 | 193 | 196 | 141 | 56 | 48.9 | 39.8 | 63.3 |
| | | | | | | | | |
| Chongqing | 3266 | 2678 | 589 | 415 | 174 | 204.1 | 185.4 | 187.4 |
| Sichuan | 2651 | 1272 | 1379 | 960 | 419 | 434.8 | 356.1 | 583.2 |
| Guizhou | 956 | 583 | 373 | 268 | 105 | 112.0 | 97.2 | 88.0 |
| Yunnan | 1141 | 673 | 468 | 328 | 141 | 179.2 | 156.8 | 204.3 |
| Tibet | 62 | 28 | 34 | 26 | 8 | 20.3 | 14.3 | 36.0 |
| | | | | | | | | |
| Shaanxi | 1247 | 667 | 580 | 393 | 187 | 184.2 | 149.6 | 238.6 |
| Gansu | 635 | 327 | 308 | 208 | 100 | 91.0 | 80.6 | 82.1 |
| Qinghai | 195 | 100 | 96 | 65 | 30 | 46.7 | 38.9 | 61.6 |
| Ningxia | 585 | 470 | 115 | 83 | 32 | 40.4 | 35.6 | 50.5 |
| Xinjiang | 891 | 385 | 506 | 363 | 143 | 213.6 | 171.1 | 255.8 |

Notes: ①The data of this table come from Ministry of Human Resources and Social Security; ②All regions are the figures of 2015.

## Ministry of Civil Affairs Medical Assistance

| Year and Region | Assisting Medical Insurance Participator (Persons/Times) | Direct Medical Assistance (Persons/Times) | Assisting Expenditure for Medical Insurance Participator (Ten Thousand yuan) | Direct Medical Assistance Expenditure (Ten Thousand yuan) |
|---|---|---|---|---|
| 2010 | 60766645 | 14793185 | 215670 | 1042328 |
| 2012 | 58775602 | 21736398 | 374766 | 1663140 |
| 2013 | 63588271 | 21263657 | 444488 | 1804597 |
| 2014 | 67237218 | 23953340 | 484468 | 2041295 |
| 2015 | 62130148 | 25158725 | 544835 | 2145715 |
| 2016 | 55604175 | 26961185 | 633541 | 2327458 |
| | | | | |
| East Region | 10274079 | 11452733 | 192839 | 713408 |
| Central Region | 19554051 | 6929407 | 224245 | 766582 |
| West Region | 25776045 | 8579045 | 216457 | 847468 |
| | | | | |
| Beijing | 66909 | 94607 | 6847 | 16550 |
| Tianjin | 236536 | 226537 | 9445 | 28416 |
| Hebei | 1984983 | 333674 | 26832 | 60815 |
| Shanxi | 1509982 | 236796 | 16060 | 56293 |
| Inner Mongolia | 1559631 | 320896 | 12869 | 67000 |
| | | | | |
| Liaoning | 948462 | 637412 | 16886 | 40744 |
| Jilin | 630705 | 485938 | 10179 | 51296 |
| Heilongjiang | 2393574 | 650948 | 31380 | 102208 |
| | | | | |
| Shanghai | 97632 | 183475 | 5038 | 33334 |
| Jiangsu | 1364106 | 3498117 | 27671 | 107520 |
| Zhejiang | 161378 | 2799561 | 7842 | 100834 |
| Anhui | 3461357 | 874851 | 49682 | 103017 |
| Fujian | 634669 | 1544235 | 12229 | 50497 |
| Jiangxi | 2091712 | 1816576 | 25554 | 132621 |
| Shandong | 2200170 | 828131 | 33457 | 96885 |
| | | | | |
| Henan | 3539301 | 656877 | 30252 | 83778 |
| Hubei | 2426720 | 982385 | 27905 | 127925 |
| Hunan | 3500700 | 1225036 | 33233 | 109445 |
| Guangdong | 2346902 | 1191976 | 41746 | 162532 |
| Guangxi | 1727855 | 595218 | 16451 | 66797 |
| Hainan | 232332 | 115008 | 4845 | 15281 |
| | | | | |
| Chongqing | 1555873 | 3615445 | 19110 | 82689 |
| Sichuan | 5366451 | 1561706 | 56798 | 160025 |
| Guizhou | 2814051 | 375514 | 12797 | 76502 |
| Yunnan | 5481548 | 736094 | 38778 | 66609 |
| Tibet | 48760 | 56853 | 1868 | 19400 |
| | | | | |
| Shaanxi | 739900 | 383176 | 9156 | 111147 |
| Gansu | 4104566 | 291316 | 18350 | 72944 |
| Qinghai | 725426 | 163582 | 9058 | 28282 |
| Ningxia | 328571 | 114927 | 3624 | 26741 |
| Xinjiang | 1323413 | 364318 | 17596 | 69333 |

Note: The data of This Table are from Ministry of Civil Affairs.

**(Wang Ruisi)**

# Demographic Data

## Population and Composition

Unit: Ten Thousand Persons

| Year | Total Population (Year End) | Grouped by Gender | | | | Grouped by Urban and Rural | | | |
|---|---|---|---|---|---|---|---|---|---|
| | | Male | | Female | | Urban | | Rural | |
| | | Population Number | Proportion (%) | Population Number | Proportion (%) | Population Number | Proportion (%) | Population Number | Proportion (%) |
| 1949 | 54167 | 28145 | 51.96 | 26022 | 48.04 | 5765 | 10.64 | 48402 | 89.36 |
| 1950 | 55196 | 28669 | 51.94 | 26527 | 48.06 | 6169 | 11.18 | 49027 | 88.82 |
| 1951 | 56300 | 29231 | 51.92 | 27069 | 48.08 | 6632 | 11.78 | 49668 | 88.22 |
| 1955 | 61465 | 31809 | 51.75 | 29656 | 48.25 | 8285 | 13.48 | 53180 | 86.52 |
| 1960 | 66207 | 34283 | 51.78 | 31924 | 48.22 | 13073 | 19.75 | 53134 | 80.25 |
| 1965 | 72538 | 37128 | 51.18 | 35410 | 48.82 | 13045 | 17.98 | 59493 | 82.02 |
| 1970 | 82992 | 42686 | 51.43 | 40306 | 48.57 | 14424 | 17.38 | 68568 | 82.62 |
| 1971 | 85229 | 43819 | 51.41 | 41410 | 48.59 | 14711 | 17.26 | 70518 | 82.74 |
| 1972 | 87177 | 44813 | 51.40 | 42364 | 48.60 | 14935 | 17.13 | 72242 | 82.87 |
| 1973 | 89211 | 45876 | 51.42 | 43335 | 48.58 | 15345 | 17.20 | 73866 | 82.80 |
| 1974 | 90859 | 46727 | 51.43 | 44132 | 48.57 | 15595 | 17.16 | 75264 | 82.84 |
| 1975 | 92420 | 47564 | 51.47 | 44856 | 48.53 | 16030 | 17.34 | 76390 | 82.66 |
| 1976 | 93717 | 48257 | 51.49 | 45460 | 48.51 | 16341 | 17.44 | 77376 | 82.56 |
| 1977 | 94974 | 48908 | 51.50 | 46066 | 48.50 | 16669 | 17.55 | 78305 | 82.45 |
| 1978 | 96259 | 49567 | 51.49 | 46692 | 48.51 | 17245 | 17.92 | 79014 | 82.08 |
| 1979 | 97542 | 50192 | 51.46 | 47350 | 48.54 | 18495 | 18.96 | 79047 | 81.04 |
| 1980 | 98705 | 50785 | 51.45 | 47920 | 48.55 | 19140 | 19.39 | 79565 | 80.61 |
| 1981 | 100072 | 51519 | 51.48 | 48553 | 48.52 | 20171 | 20.16 | 79901 | 79.84 |
| 1982 | 101654 | 52352 | 51.50 | 49302 | 48.50 | 21480 | 21.13 | 80174 | 78.87 |
| 1983 | 103008 | 53152 | 51.60 | 49856 | 48.40 | 22274 | 21.62 | 80734 | 78.38 |
| 1984 | 104357 | 53848 | 51.60 | 50509 | 48.40 | 24017 | 23.01 | 80340 | 76.99 |
| 1985 | 105851 | 54725 | 51.70 | 51126 | 48.30 | 25094 | 23.71 | 80757 | 76.29 |
| 1986 | 107507 | 55581 | 51.70 | 51926 | 48.30 | 26366 | 24.52 | 81141 | 75.48 |
| 1987 | 109300 | 56290 | 51.50 | 53010 | 48.50 | 27674 | 25.32 | 81626 | 74.68 |
| 1988 | 111026 | 57201 | 51.52 | 53825 | 48.48 | 28661 | 25.81 | 82365 | 74.19 |
| 1989 | 112704 | 58099 | 51.55 | 54605 | 48.45 | 29540 | 26.21 | 83164 | 73.79 |
| 1990 | 114333 | 58904 | 51.52 | 55429 | 48.48 | 30195 | 26.41 | 84138 | 73.59 |
| 1991 | 115823 | 59466 | 51.34 | 56357 | 48.66 | 31203 | 26.94 | 84620 | 73.06 |
| 1992 | 117171 | 59811 | 51.05 | 57360 | 48.95 | 32175 | 27.46 | 84996 | 72.54 |
| 1993 | 118517 | 60472 | 51.02 | 58045 | 48.98 | 33173 | 27.99 | 85344 | 72.01 |
| 1994 | 119850 | 61246 | 51.10 | 58604 | 48.90 | 34169 | 28.51 | 85681 | 71.49 |
| 1995 | 121121 | 61808 | 51.03 | 59313 | 48.97 | 35174 | 29.04 | 85947 | 70.96 |
| 1996 | 122389 | 62200 | 50.82 | 60189 | 49.18 | 37304 | 30.48 | 85085 | 69.52 |
| 1997 | 123626 | 63131 | 51.07 | 60495 | 48.93 | 39449 | 31.91 | 84177 | 68.09 |
| 1998 | 124761 | 63940 | 51.25 | 60821 | 48.75 | 41608 | 33.35 | 83153 | 66.65 |
| 1999 | 125786 | 64692 | 51.43 | 61094 | 48.57 | 43748 | 34.78 | 82038 | 65.22 |
| 2000 | 126743 | 65437 | 51.63 | 61306 | 48.37 | 45906 | 36.22 | 80837 | 63.78 |

*Continued*

| Year | Total Population (Year End) | Grouped by Gender | | | | Grouped by Urban and Rural | | | |
|------|------|------|------|------|------|------|------|------|------|
| | | Male | | Female | | Urban | | Rural | |
| | | Population Number | Proportion (%) | Population Number | Proportion (%) | Population Number | Proportion (%) | Population Number | Proportion (%) |
| 2001 | 127627 | 65672 | 51.46 | 61955 | 48.54 | 48064 | 37.66 | 79563 | 62.34 |
| 2002 | 128453 | 66115 | 51.47 | 62338 | 48.53 | 50212 | 39.09 | 78241 | 60.91 |
| 2003 | 129227 | 66556 | 51.50 | 62671 | 48.50 | 52376 | 40.53 | 76851 | 59.47 |
| 2004 | 129988 | 66976 | 51.52 | 63012 | 48.48 | 54283 | 41.76 | 75705 | 58.24 |
| 2005 | 130756 | 67375 | 51.53 | 63381 | 48.47 | 56212 | 42.99 | 74544 | 57.01 |
| 2006 | 131448 | 67728 | 51.52 | 63720 | 48.48 | 58288 | 44.34 | 73160 | 55.66 |
| 2007 | 132129 | 68048 | 51.50 | 64081 | 48.50 | 60633 | 45.89 | 71496 | 54.11 |
| 2008 | 132802 | 68357 | 51.47 | 64445 | 48.53 | 62403 | 46.99 | 70399 | 53.01 |
| 2009 | 133450 | 68647 | 51.44 | 64803 | 48.56 | 64512 | 48.34 | 68938 | 51.66 |
| 2010 | 134091 | 68748 | 51.27 | 65343 | 48.73 | 66978 | 49.95 | 67113 | 50.05 |
| 2011 | 134735 | 69068 | 51.26 | 65667 | 48.74 | 69079 | 51.27 | 65656 | 48.73 |
| 2012 | 135404 | 69395 | 51.25 | 66009 | 48.75 | 71182 | 52.57 | 64222 | 47.43 |
| 2013 | 136072 | 69728 | 51.24 | 66344 | 48.76 | 73111 | 53.73 | 62961 | 46.27 |
| 2014 | 136782 | 70079 | 51.23 | 66703 | 48.77 | 74916 | 54.77 | 61866 | 45.23 |
| 2015 | 137462 | 70414 | 51.22 | 67048 | 48.78 | 77116 | 56.10 | 60346 | 43.90 |
| 2016 | 138271 | 70815 | 51.31 | 67456 | 48.79 | 79298 | 57.35 | 58973 | 42.65 |

Notes: The collective data in This Column are selected from Volume 2017 China Statistical Yearbook.

①The data of 1981 and before are from household registration; The data of 1982, 1990, 2000 and 2010 are estimated by current-year population census; The data of other years are current-year sample population estimation (the same as in the following tables). ②Total population and population by gender include on-service military men, who are included into urban population by urban and rural.

## Birth Rate, Mortality and Natural Growth Rate

Unit: (‰)

| Year | Birth Rate | Mortality | Natural Growth Rate | Year | Birth Rate | Mortality | Natural Growth Rate |
|------|------|------|------|------|------|------|------|
| 1978 | 18.25 | 6.25 | 12.00 | 1998 | 15.64 | 6.50 | 9.14 |
| 1980 | 18.21 | 6.34 | 11.87 | 1999 | 14.64 | 6.46 | 8.18 |
| 1981 | 20.91 | 6.36 | 14.55 | 2000 | 14.03 | 6.45 | 7.58 |
| 1982 | 22.28 | 6.60 | 15.68 | 2001 | 13.38 | 6.43 | 6.95 |
| 1983 | 20.19 | 6.90 | 13.29 | 2002 | 12.86 | 6.41 | 6.45 |
| 1984 | 19.90 | 6.82 | 13.08 | 2003 | 12.41 | 6.40 | 6.01 |
| 1985 | 21.04 | 6.78 | 14.26 | 2004 | 12.29 | 6.42 | 5.87 |
| 1986 | 22.43 | 6.86 | 15.57 | 2005 | 12.40 | 6.51 | 5.89 |
| 1987 | 23.33 | 6.72 | 16.61 | 2006 | 12.09 | 6.81 | 5.28 |
| 1988 | 22.37 | 6.64 | 15.73 | 2007 | 12.10 | 6.93 | 5.17 |
| 1989 | 21.58 | 6.54 | 15.04 | 2008 | 12.14 | 7.06 | 5.08 |
| 1990 | 21.06 | 6.67 | 14.39 | 2009 | 11.95 | 7.08 | 4.87 |
| 1991 | 19.68 | 6.70 | 12.98 | 2010 | 11.90 | 7.11 | 4.79 |
| 1992 | 18.24 | 6.64 | 11.60 | 2011 | 11.93 | 7.14 | 4.79 |
| 1993 | 18.09 | 6.64 | 11.45 | 2012 | 12.10 | 7.15 | 4.95 |
| 1994 | 17.70 | 6.49 | 11.21 | 2013 | 12.08 | 7.16 | 4.92 |
| 1995 | 17.12 | 6.57 | 10.55 | 2014 | 12.37 | 7.16 | 5.21 |
| 1996 | 16.98 | 6.56 | 10.42 | 2015 | 12.07 | 7.11 | 4.96 |
| 1997 | 16.57 | 6.51 | 10.06 | 2016 | 12.95 | 7.09 | 5.86 |

## Mobile Population

Unit: Hundred Million Persons

| Year | Population of Registered and Actual Residence Separation | Mobile Population |
|------|----------------------------------------------------------|-------------------|
| 2000 | 1.44 | 1.21 |
| 2005 | | 1.47 |
| 2010 | 2.61 | 2.21 |
| 2011 | 2.71 | 2.30 |
| 2012 | 2.79 | 2.36 |
| 2013 | 2.89 | 2.45 |
| 2014 | 2.98 | 2.53 |
| 2015 | 2.94 | 2.47 |
| 2016 | 2.92 | 2.45 |

Note: The data of 2000 and 2010 are from current-year population census, the data of other years are sample population estimation.

## Average Life Expectancy

Unit: year (of age)

| Year | Total | Male | Female |
|------|-------|------|--------|
| 1981 | 67.77 | 66.28 | 69.27 |
| 1990 | 68.55 | 66.84 | 70.47 |
| 1996 | 70.80 | | |
| 2000 | 71.40 | 69.63 | 73.33 |
| 2005 | 72.95 | 70.83 | 75.25 |
| 2010 | 74.83 | 72.38 | 77.37 |
| 2015 | 76.34 | 73.64 | 79.43 |

## Population Age Structure and Dependency Ratio

Unit: Ten Thousand Persons

| Year | Total Population (Year End) | Grouped by Age | | | | | | Total Dependency Ratio (%) | Children's Dependency Ratio (%) | Old-age Dependency Ratio (%) |
|------|------|------|------|------|------|------|------|------|------|------|
| | | 0-14 | | 15-64 | | 65 and above | | | | |
| | | Population | Proportion (%) | Population | Proportion (%) | Population | Proportion (%) | | | |
| 1982 | 101654 | 34146 | 33.6 | 62517 | 61.5 | 4991 | 4.9 | 62.6 | 54.6 | 8.0 |
| 1987 | 109300 | 31347 | 28.7 | 71985 | 65.9 | 5968 | 5.4 | 51.8 | 43.5 | 8.3 |
| 1990 | 114333 | 31659 | 27.7 | 76306 | 66.7 | 6368 | 5.6 | 49.8 | 41.5 | 8.3 |
| 1991 | 115823 | 32095 | 27.7 | 76791 | 66.3 | 6938 | 6.0 | 50.8 | 41.8 | 9.0 |
| 1992 | 117171 | 32339 | 27.6 | 77614 | 66.2 | 7218 | 6.2 | 51.0 | 41.7 | 9.3 |
| 1993 | 118517 | 32177 | 27.2 | 79051 | 66.7 | 7289 | 6.2 | 49.9 | 40.7 | 9.2 |
| 1994 | 119850 | 32360 | 27.0 | 79868 | 66.6 | 7622 | 6.4 | 50.1 | 40.5 | 9.5 |
| 1995 | 121121 | 32218 | 26.6 | 81393 | 67.2 | 7510 | 6.2 | 48.8 | 39.6 | 9.2 |
| 1996 | 122389 | 32311 | 26.4 | 82245 | 67.2 | 7833 | 6.4 | 48.8 | 39.3 | 9.5 |
| 1997 | 123626 | 32093 | 26.0 | 83448 | 67.5 | 8085 | 6.5 | 48.1 | 38.5 | 9.7 |
| 1998 | 124761 | 32064 | 25.7 | 84338 | 67.6 | 8359 | 6.7 | 47.9 | 38.0 | 9.9 |
| 1999 | 125786 | 31950 | 25.4 | 85157 | 67.7 | 8679 | 6.9 | 47.7 | 37.5 | 10.2 |
| 2000 | 126743 | 29012 | 22.9 | 88910 | 70.1 | 8821 | 7.0 | 42.6 | 32.6 | 9.9 |
| 2001 | 127627 | 28716 | 22.5 | 89849 | 70.4 | 9062 | 7.1 | 42.0 | 32.0 | 10.1 |

*Continued*

| Year | Total Population (Year End) | Grouped by Age | | | | | | Total Dependency Ratio (%) | Children's Dependency Ratio (%) | Old-age Dependency Ratio (%) |
|---|---|---|---|---|---|---|---|---|---|---|
| | | 0-14 | | 15-64 | | 65 and above | | | | |
| | | Population | Proportion (%) | Population | Proportion (%) | Population | Proportion (%) | | | |
| 2002 | 128453 | 28774 | 22.4 | 90302 | 70.3 | 9377 | 7.3 | 42.2 | 31.9 | 10.4 |
| 2003 | 129227 | 28559 | 22.1 | 90976 | 70.4 | 9692 | 7.5 | 42.0 | 31.4 | 10.7 |
| 2004 | 129988 | 27947 | 21.5 | 92184 | 70.9 | 9857 | 7.6 | 41.0 | 30.3 | 10.7 |
| 2005 | 130756 | 26504 | 20.3 | 94197 | 72.0 | 10055 | 7.7 | 38.8 | 28.1 | 10.7 |
| 2006 | 131448 | 25961 | 19.8 | 95068 | 72.3 | 10419 | 7.9 | 38.3 | 27.3 | 11.0 |
| 2007 | 132129 | 25660 | 19.4 | 95833 | 72.5 | 10636 | 8.1 | 37.9 | 26.8 | 11.1 |
| 2008 | 132802 | 25166 | 19.0 | 96680 | 72.7 | 10956 | 8.3 | 37.4 | 26.0 | 11.3 |
| 2009 | 133450 | 24659 | 18.5 | 97484 | 73.0 | 11307 | 8.5 | 36.9 | 25.3 | 11.6 |
| 2010 | 134091 | 22259 | 16.6 | 99938 | 74.5 | 11894 | 8.9 | 34.2 | 22.3 | 11.9 |
| 2011 | 134735 | 22164 | 16.5 | 100283 | 74.4 | 12288 | 9.1 | 34.4 | 22.1 | 12.3 |
| 2012 | 135404 | 22287 | 16.5 | 100403 | 74.1 | 12714 | 9.4 | 34.9 | 22.2 | 12.7 |
| 2013 | 136072 | 22329 | 16.4 | 100582 | 73.9 | 13161 | 9.7 | 35.3 | 22.2 | 13.1 |
| 2014 | 136782 | 22558 | 16.5 | 100469 | 73.4 | 13755 | 10.1 | 36.2 | 22.5 | 13.7 |
| 2015 | 137462 | 22715 | 16.5 | 100361 | 73.0 | 14386 | 10.5 | 37.0 | 22.6 | 14.3 |
| 2016 | 138271 | 23008 | 16.7 | 100260 | 72.5 | 15003 | 10.8 | 37.9 | 22.9 | 15.0 |

## Year-end Sub-region Population

Unit: Ten Thousand Persons

| Region | 2005 | 2006 | 2007 | 2008 | 2009 | 2010 | 2011 | 2012 | 2013 | 2014 | 2015 | 2016 |
|---|---|---|---|---|---|---|---|---|---|---|---|---|
| **Whole Country** | **130756** | **131448** | **132129** | **132802** | **133450** | **134091** | **134735** | **135404** | **136072** | **136782** | **137462** | **138271** |
| Beijing | 1538 | 1601 | 1676 | 1771 | 1860 | 1962 | 2019 | 2069 | 2115 | 2152 | 2171 | 2173 |
| Tianjin | 1043 | 1075 | 1115 | 1176 | 1228 | 1299 | 1355 | 1413 | 1472 | 1517 | 1547 | 1562 |
| Hebei | 6851 | 6898 | 6943 | 6989 | 7034 | 7194 | 7241 | 7288 | 7333 | 7384 | 7425 | 7470 |
| Shanxi | 3355 | 3375 | 3393 | 3411 | 3427 | 3574 | 3593 | 3611 | 3630 | 3648 | 3664 | 3682 |
| Inner Mongolia | 2403 | 2415 | 2429 | 2444 | 2458 | 2472 | 2482 | 2490 | 2498 | 2505 | 2511 | 2520 |
| Liaoning | 4221 | 4271 | 4298 | 4315 | 4341 | 4375 | 4383 | 4389 | 4390 | 4391 | 4382 | 4378 |
| Jilin | 2716 | 2723 | 2730 | 2734 | 2740 | 2747 | 2749 | 2750 | 2751 | 2752 | 2753 | 2733 |
| Heilongjiang | 3820 | 3823 | 3824 | 3825 | 3826 | 3833 | 3834 | 3834 | 3835 | 3833 | 3812 | 3799 |
| Shanghai | 1890 | 1964 | 2064 | 2141 | 2210 | 2303 | 2347 | 2380 | 2415 | 2426 | 2415 | 2420 |
| Jiangsu | 7588 | 7656 | 7723 | 7762 | 7810 | 7869 | 7899 | 7920 | 7939 | 7960 | 7976 | 7999 |
| Zhejiang | 4991 | 5072 | 5155 | 5212 | 5276 | 5447 | 5463 | 5477 | 5498 | 5508 | 5539 | 5590 |
| Anhui | 6120 | 6110 | 6118 | 6135 | 6131 | 5957 | 5968 | 5988 | 6030 | 6083 | 6144 | 6196 |
| Fujian | 3557 | 3585 | 3612 | 3639 | 3666 | 3693 | 3720 | 3748 | 3774 | 3806 | 3839 | 3874 |
| Jiangxi | 4311 | 4339 | 4368 | 4400 | 4432 | 4462 | 4488 | 4504 | 4522 | 4542 | 4566 | 4592 |
| Shandong | 9248 | 9309 | 9367 | 9417 | 9470 | 9588 | 9637 | 9685 | 9733 | 9789 | 9847 | 9947 |
| Henan | 9380 | 9392 | 9360 | 9429 | 9487 | 9405 | 9388 | 9406 | 9413 | 9436 | 9480 | 9532 |
| Hubei | 5710 | 5693 | 5699 | 5711 | 5720 | 5728 | 5758 | 5779 | 5799 | 5816 | 5852 | 5885 |
| Hunan | 6326 | 6342 | 6355 | 6380 | 6406 | 6570 | 6596 | 6639 | 6691 | 6737 | 6783 | 6822 |

*Continued*

| Region | 2005 | 2006 | 2007 | 2008 | 2009 | 2010 | 2011 | 2012 | 2013 | 2014 | 2015 | 2016 |
|---|---|---|---|---|---|---|---|---|---|---|---|---|
| Guangdong | 9194 | 9442 | 9660 | 9893 | 10130 | 10441 | 10505 | 10594 | 10644 | 10724 | 10849 | 10999 |
| Guangxi | 4660 | 4719 | 4768 | 4816 | 4856 | 4610 | 4645 | 4682 | 4719 | 4754 | 4796 | 4838 |
| Hainan | 828 | 836 | 845 | 854 | 864 | 869 | 877 | 887 | 895 | 903 | 911 | 917 |
| Chongqing | 2798 | 2808 | 2816 | 2839 | 2859 | 2885 | 2919 | 2945 | 2970 | 2991 | 3017 | 3048 |
| Sichuan | 8212 | 8169 | 8127 | 8138 | 8185 | 8045 | 8050 | 8076 | 8107 | 8140 | 8204 | 8262 |
| Guizhou | 3730 | 3690 | 3632 | 3596 | 3537 | 3479 | 3469 | 3484 | 3502 | 3508 | 3530 | 3555 |
| Yunnan | 4450 | 4483 | 4514 | 4543 | 4571 | 4602 | 4631 | 4659 | 4687 | 4714 | 4742 | 4771 |
| Tibet | 280 | 285 | 289 | 292 | 296 | 300 | 303 | 308 | 312 | 318 | 324 | 331 |
| Shaanxi | 3690 | 3699 | 3708 | 3718 | 3727 | 3735 | 3743 | 3753 | 3764 | 3775 | 3793 | 3813 |
| Gansu | 2545 | 2547 | 2548 | 2551 | 2555 | 2560 | 2564 | 2578 | 2582 | 2591 | 2600 | 2610 |
| Qinghai | 543 | 548 | 552 | 554 | 557 | 563 | 568 | 573 | 578 | 583 | 588 | 593 |
| Ningxia | 596 | 604 | 610 | 618 | 625 | 633 | 639 | 647 | 654 | 662 | 668 | 675 |
| Xinjiang | 2010 | 2050 | 2095 | 2131 | 2159 | 2185 | 2209 | 2233 | 2264 | 2298 | 2360 | 2398 |

Note: The data of 2010 are from current-year population census estimation; the data of other years are sample population estimation. The data of different regions are of permanent population.

## Year-end Sub-region Urban Population Proportion

Unit: (%)

| Region | 2008 | 2009 | 2010 | 2011 | 2012 | 2013 | 2014 | 2015 | 2016 |
|---|---|---|---|---|---|---|---|---|---|
| **Whole Country** | **46.99** | **48.34** | **49.95** | **51.27** | **52.57** | **53.73** | **54.77** | **56.10** | **57.35** |
| Beijing | 84.90 | 85.00 | 85.96 | 86.20 | 86.20 | 86.30 | 86.35 | 86.50 | 86.5 |
| Tianjin | 77.23 | 78.01 | 79.55 | 80.50 | 81.55 | 82.01 | 82.27 | 82.64 | 82.93 |
| Hebei | 41.90 | 43.74 | 44.50 | 45.60 | 46.80 | 48.12 | 49.33 | 51.33 | 53.32 |
| Shanxi | 45.11 | 45.99 | 48.05 | 49.68 | 51.26 | 52.56 | 53.79 | 55.03 | 56.21 |
| Inner Mongolia | 51.71 | 53.40 | 55.50 | 56.62 | 57.74 | 58.71 | 59.51 | 60.30 | 61.19 |
| Liaoning | 60.05 | 60.35 | 62.10 | 64.05 | 65.65 | 66.45 | 67.05 | 67.35 | 67.37 |
| Jilin | 53.21 | 53.32 | 53.35 | 53.40 | 53.70 | 54.20 | 54.81 | 55.31 | 55.97 |
| Heilongjiang | 55.40 | 55.50 | 55.66 | 56.50 | 56.90 | 57.40 | 58.01 | 58.80 | 59.2 |
| Shanghai | 88.60 | 88.60 | 89.30 | 89.30 | 89.30 | 89.60 | 89.60 | 87.60 | 87.9 |
| Jiangsu | 54.30 | 55.60 | 60.58 | 61.90 | 63.00 | 64.11 | 65.21 | 66.52 | 67.72 |
| Zhejiang | 57.60 | 57.90 | 61.62 | 62.30 | 63.20 | 64.00 | 64.87 | 65.80 | 67 |
| Anhui | 40.50 | 42.10 | 43.01 | 44.80 | 46.50 | 47.86 | 49.15 | 50.50 | 51.99 |
| Fujian | 53.00 | 55.10 | 57.10 | 58.10 | 59.60 | 60.77 | 61.80 | 62.60 | 63.6 |
| Jiangxi | 41.36 | 43.18 | 44.06 | 45.70 | 47.51 | 48.87 | 50.22 | 51.62 | 53.1 |
| Shandong | 47.60 | 48.32 | 49.70 | 50.95 | 52.43 | 53.75 | 55.01 | 57.01 | 59.02 |
| Henan | 36.03 | 37.70 | 38.50 | 40.57 | 42.43 | 43.80 | 45.20 | 46.85 | 48.5 |
| Hubei | 45.20 | 46.00 | 49.70 | 51.83 | 53.50 | 54.51 | 55.67 | 56.85 | 58.1 |
| Hunan | 42.15 | 43.20 | 43.30 | 45.10 | 46.65 | 47.96 | 49.28 | 50.89 | 52.75 |
| Guangdong | 63.37 | 63.40 | 66.18 | 66.50 | 67.40 | 67.76 | 68.00 | 68.71 | 69.2 |
| Guangxi | 38.16 | 39.20 | 40.00 | 41.80 | 43.53 | 44.81 | 46.01 | 47.06 | 48.08 |
| Hainan | 48.00 | 49.13 | 49.80 | 50.50 | 51.60 | 52.74 | 53.76 | 55.12 | 56.78 |

*Continued*

| Region | 2008 | 2009 | 2010 | 2011 | 2012 | 2013 | 2014 | 2015 | 2016 |
|--------|------|------|------|------|------|------|------|------|------|
| Chongqing | 49.99 | 51.59 | 53.02 | 55.02 | 56.98 | 58.34 | 59.60 | 60.94 | 62.6 |
| Sichuan | 37.40 | 38.70 | 40.18 | 41.83 | 43.53 | 44.90 | 46.30 | 47.69 | 49.21 |
| Guizhou | 29.11 | 29.89 | 33.81 | 34.96 | 36.41 | 37.83 | 40.01 | 42.01 | 44.15 |
| Yunnan | 33.00 | 34.00 | 34.70 | 36.80 | 39.31 | 40.48 | 41.73 | 43.33 | 45.03 |
| Tibet | 21.90 | 22.30 | 22.67 | 22.71 | 22.75 | 23.71 | 25.75 | 27.74 | 29.56 |
| Shaanxi | 42.10 | 43.50 | 45.76 | 47.30 | 50.02 | 51.31 | 52.57 | 53.92 | 55.34 |
| Gansu | 33.56 | 34.89 | 36.12 | 37.15 | 38.75 | 40.13 | 41.68 | 43.19 | 44.69 |
| Qinghai | 40.86 | 41.90 | 44.72 | 46.22 | 47.44 | 48.51 | 49.78 | 50.30 | 51.63 |
| Ningxia | 44.98 | 46.10 | 47.90 | 49.82 | 50.67 | 52.01 | 53.61 | 55.23 | 56.29 |
| Xinjiang | 39.64 | 39.85 | 43.01 | 43.54 | 43.98 | 44.47 | 46.07 | 47.23 | 48.35 |

Note: The data of 2010 are from current-year population census estimation; the data of other years are sample population estimation. Some provincial data of 2008-2009 are revised by 2010 population census.

## Sub-region Urban and Rural Population Composition, Birth Rate, Mortality and Natural Growth Rate in 2016

| Region | Total Population (Year End) | | | | | Birth Rate (‰) | Mortality (‰) | Natural Growth Rate (‰) |
|--------|----------------------------|--|--|--|--|----------------|---------------|-------------------------|
| | (Ten Thousand Persons) | Urban | | Rural | | | | |
| | | Population | Proportion (%) | Population | Proportion (%) | | | |
| **Whole Country** | 138271 | 79298 | 57.35 | 58973 | 42.65 | 12.95 | 7.09 | 5.86 |
| Beijing | 2173 | 1880 | 86.50 | 293 | 13.50 | 9.32 | 5.20 | 4.12 |
| Tianjin | 1562 | 1295 | 82.93 | 267 | 17.07 | 7.37 | 5.54 | 1.83 |
| Hebei | 7470 | 3983 | 53.32 | 3487 | 46.68 | 12.42 | 6.36 | 6.06 |
| Shanxi | 3682 | 2070 | 56.21 | 1612 | 43.79 | 10.29 | 5.52 | 4.77 |
| Inner Mongolia | 2520 | 1542 | 61.19 | 978 | 38.81 | 9.03 | 5.69 | 3.34 |
| Liaoning | 4378 | 2949 | 67.37 | 1429 | 32.63 | 6.60 | 6.78 | -0.18 |
| Jilin | 2733 | 1530 | 55.97 | 1203 | 44.03 | 5.55 | 5.60 | -0.05 |
| Heilongjiang | 3799 | 2249 | 59.20 | 1550 | 40.80 | 6.12 | 6.61 | -0.49 |
| Shanghai | 2420 | 2127 | 87.90 | 293 | 12.10 | 9.00 | 5.00 | 4.00 |
| Jiangsu | 7999 | 5417 | 67.72 | 2582 | 32.28 | 9.76 | 7.03 | 2.73 |
| Zhejiang | 5590 | 3745 | 67.00 | 1845 | 33.00 | 11.22 | 5.52 | 5.70 |
| Anhui | 6196 | 3221 | 51.99 | 2975 | 48.01 | 13.02 | 5.96 | 7.06 |
| Fujian | 3874 | 2464 | 63.60 | 1410 | 36.40 | 14.50 | 6.20 | 8.30 |
| Jiangxi | 4592 | 2438 | 53.10 | 2154 | 46.90 | 13.45 | 6.16 | 7.29 |
| Shandong | 9947 | 5871 | 59.02 | 4076 | 40.98 | 17.89 | 7.05 | 10.84 |
| Henan | 9532 | 4623 | 48.50 | 4909 | 51.50 | 13.26 | 7.11 | 6.15 |
| Hubei | 5885 | 3419 | 58.10 | 2466 | 41.90 | 12.04 | 6.97 | 5.07 |
| Hunan | 6822 | 3599 | 52.75 | 3223 | 47.25 | 13.57 | 7.01 | 6.56 |
| Guangdong | 10999 | 7611 | 69.20 | 3388 | 30.80 | 11.85 | 4.41 | 7.44 |
| Guangxi | 4838 | 2326 | 48.08 | 2512 | 51.92 | 13.82 | 5.95 | 7.87 |
| Hainan | 917 | 521 | 56.78 | 396 | 43.22 | 14.57 | 6.00 | 8.57 |

*Continued*

| Region | Total Population (Year End) | | | | | Birth Rate (‰) | Mortality (‰) | Natural Growth Rate (‰) |
|---|---|---|---|---|---|---|---|---|
| | (Ten Thousand Persons) | Urban | | Rural | | | | |
| | | Population | Proportion (%) | Population | Proportion (%) | | | |
| Chongqing | 3048 | 1908 | 62.60 | 1140 | 37.40 | 11.77 | 7.24 | 4.53 |
| Sichuan | 8262 | 4066 | 49.21 | 4196 | 50.79 | 10.48 | 6.99 | 3.49 |
| Guizhou | 3555 | 1570 | 44.15 | 1985 | 55.85 | 13.43 | 6.93 | 6.50 |
| Yunnan | 4771 | 2148 | 45.03 | 2623 | 54.97 | 13.16 | 6.55 | 6.61 |
| Tibet | 331 | 98 | 29.56 | 233 | 70.44 | 15.79 | 5.11 | 10.68 |
| Shaanxi | 3813 | 2110 | 55.34 | 1703 | 44.66 | 10.64 | 6.23 | 4.41 |
| Gansu | 2610 | 1166 | 44.69 | 1444 | 55.31 | 12.18 | 6.18 | 6.00 |
| Qinghai | 593 | 306 | 51.63 | 287 | 48.37 | 14.70 | 6.18 | 8.52 |
| Ningxia | 675 | 380 | 56.29 | 295 | 43.71 | 13.69 | 4.72 | 8.97 |
| Xinjiang | 2398 | 1159 | 48.35 | 1239 | 51.65 | 15.34 | 4.26 | 11.08 |

Notes: ①The data of this table are the estimation from sample check data in 2016 and the population data of the whole nation are revised according to sample error and check error, while the sub-region population data are not revised; ②Total population of the whole nation includes on-service military men, who are not included into sub-region data.

## Population Numbers by Age and Gender in 2016

| Age | Population Number | | | Proportion in Total Population | | | Sex Ratio (Female=100) |
|---|---|---|---|---|---|---|---|
| | (Person) | Male | Female | (%) | Male | Female | |
| **Total** | **1158019** | **593087** | **564932** | **100** | **51.22** | **48.78** | **104.98** |
| 0-4 | 68447 | 36703 | 31744 | 5.91 | 3.17 | 2.74 | 115.62 |
| 5-9 | 63831 | 34666 | 29165 | 5.51 | 2.99 | 2.52 | 118.86 |
| 10-14 | 60420 | 32773 | 27647 | 5.22 | 2.83 | 2.39 | 118.54 |
| 15-19 | 61562 | 33199 | 28363 | 5.32 | 2.87 | 2.45 | 117.05 |
| 20-24 | 79102 | 41366 | 37736 | 6.83 | 3.57 | 3.26 | 109.62 |
| 25-29 | 106663 | 54225 | 52439 | 9.21 | 4.68 | 4.53 | 103.41 |
| 30-34 | 87573 | 44070 | 43503 | 7.56 | 3.81 | 3.76 | 101.3 |
| 35-39 | 80485 | 40992 | 39492 | 6.95 | 3.54 | 3.41 | 103.8 |
| 40-44 | 94730 | 48342 | 46388 | 8.18 | 4.17 | 4.01 | 104.21 |
| 45-49 | 104623 | 53194 | 51429 | 9.03 | 4.59 | 4.44 | 103.43 |
| 50-54 | 97608 | 49491 | 48116 | 8.43 | 4.27 | 4.16 | 102.86 |
| 55-59 | 59638 | 30264 | 29374 | 5.15 | 2.61 | 2.54 | 103.03 |
| 60-64 | 67696 | 33810 | 33887 | 5.85 | 2.92 | 2.93 | 99.77 |
| 65-69 | 48454 | 23878 | 24576 | 4.18 | 2.06 | 2.12 | 97.16 |
| 70-74 | 31677 | 15545 | 16132 | 2.74 | 1.34 | 1.39 | 96.36 |
| 75-79 | 22449 | 10744 | 11705 | 1.94 | 0.93 | 1.01 | 91.79 |
| 80-84 | 14331 | 6446 | 7884 | 1.24 | 0.56 | 0.68 | 81.76 |
| 85-89 | 6416 | 2613 | 3803 | 0.55 | 0.23 | 0.33 | 68.73 |
| 90-94 | 1902 | 630 | 1271 | 0.16 | 0.05 | 0.11 | 49.58 |
| 95+ | 413 | 134 | 279 | 0.04 | 0.01 | 0.02 | 48.25 |

Notes: ①This table is the sample check data of population changes in 2016and the sampling ratio is 0.837‰; ②There is an error in totaling and item adding because of the sub-region weighting totaling (the same in the following tables).

## Sub-region Population Age Composition and Dependency Ratio in 2016

| Region | Population Number (Person) | | | | Total Dependency Ratio (%) | | |
|---|---|---|---|---|---|---|---|
| | | 0-14 | 15-64 | 65 and above | | Children & Juvenile Dependency Ratio | Aging Population Dependency Ratio |
| **Whole Country** | **1158019** | **192698** | **839679** | **125642** | **37.91** | **22.95** | **14.96** |
| Beijing | 18132 | 1973 | 14031 | 2129 | 29.23 | 14.06 | 15.17 |
| Tianjin | 13046 | 1421 | 10142 | 1482 | 28.63 | 14.01 | 14.62 |
| Hebei | 62750 | 11584 | 44321 | 6845 | 41.58 | 26.14 | 15.44 |
| Shanxi | 30910 | 4747 | 23475 | 2688 | 31.67 | 20.22 | 11.45 |
| Inner Mongolia | 21136 | 2705 | 16436 | 1995 | 28.60 | 16.46 | 12.14 |
| Liaoning | 36668 | 3900 | 27919 | 4849 | 31.34 | 13.97 | 17.37 |
| Jilin | 22945 | 2903 | 17552 | 2490 | 30.72 | 16.54 | 14.19 |
| Heilongjiang | 31874 | 3204 | 24865 | 3805 | 28.19 | 12.89 | 15.30 |
| Shanghai | 20188 | 1953 | 15618 | 2617 | 29.26 | 12.50 | 16.76 |
| Jiangsu | 66998 | 9199 | 48750 | 9048 | 37.43 | 18.87 | 18.56 |
| Zhejiang | 46831 | 6063 | 35319 | 5449 | 32.59 | 17.17 | 15.43 |
| Anhui | 52056 | 9128 | 36958 | 5969 | 40.85 | 24.70 | 16.15 |
| Fujian | 32474 | 5940 | 23303 | 3231 | 39.36 | 25.49 | 13.87 |
| Jiangxi | 38576 | 8187 | 26687 | 3702 | 44.55 | 30.68 | 13.87 |
| Shandong | 83464 | 14140 | 59599 | 9725 | 40.04 | 23.72 | 16.32 |
| Henan | 80140 | 16659 | 55405 | 8075 | 44.64 | 30.07 | 14.57 |
| Hubei | 49384 | 7645 | 36023 | 5716 | 37.09 | 21.22 | 15.87 |
| Hunan | 57310 | 10431 | 40065 | 6814 | 43.04 | 26.03 | 17.01 |
| Guangdong | 92107 | 15417 | 69603 | 7086 | 32.33 | 22.15 | 10.18 |
| Guangxi | 40677 | 8686 | 28048 | 3943 | 45.03 | 30.97 | 14.06 |
| Hainan | 7698 | 1520 | 5543 | 635 | 38.88 | 27.43 | 11.45 |
| Chongqing | 25560 | 3949 | 18041 | 3570 | 41.68 | 21.89 | 19.79 |
| Sichuan | 69457 | 11086 | 48858 | 9513 | 42.16 | 22.69 | 19.47 |
| Guizhou | 29915 | 6663 | 20373 | 2879 | 46.83 | 32.70 | 14.13 |
| Yunnan | 40141 | 7839 | 28939 | 3362 | 38.71 | 27.09 | 11.62 |
| Tibet | 2789 | 671 | 1980 | 139 | 40.88 | 33.87 | 7.01 |
| Shaanxi | 32014 | 4750 | 23826 | 3439 | 34.37 | 19.93 | 14.43 |
| Gansu | 21960 | 3725 | 16049 | 2186 | 36.83 | 23.21 | 13.62 |
| Qinghai | 4987 | 983 | 3643 | 360 | 36.87 | 26.98 | 9.89 |
| Ningxia | 5666 | 1085 | 4140 | 441 | 36.85 | 26.20 | 10.65 |
| Xinjiang | 20165 | 4541 | 14165 | 1458 | 42.35 | 32.06 | 10.30 |

Notes: This table is the sample check data of population changes in 2016 and the sampling ratio is 0.837‰

## Sub-region Households, Population, Sex Ratio and Household in 2016

| Region | Households(Family) | | | Population Number(Person) | | | Sex Ratio (Female=100) |
|---|---|---|---|---|---|---|---|
| | | Family Household | Collective Household | | Male | Female | |
| **Whole Country** | **371070** | **364431** | **6638** | **1158019** | **593087** | **564932** | **104.98** |
| Beijing | 6793 | 6372 | 421 | 18132 | 9324 | 8808 | 105.85 |
| Tianjin | 4497 | 4145 | 352 | 13046 | 6961 | 6085 | 114.39 |
| Hebei | 19210 | 19130 | 80 | 62750 | 32082 | 30668 | 104.61 |
| Shanxi | 9835 | 9768 | 67 | 30910 | 15909 | 15002 | 106.04 |
| Inner Mongolia | 7654 | 7467 | 187 | 21136 | 10675 | 10461 | 102.05 |
| Liaoning | 13389 | 13344 | 45 | 36668 | 18503 | 18165 | 101.86 |
| Jilin | 8038 | 8016 | 22 | 22945 | 11665 | 11280 | 103.41 |
| Heilongjiang | 11521 | 11460 | 61 | 31874 | 16104 | 15770 | 102.11 |
| Shanghai | 8127 | 7801 | 325 | 20188 | 10382 | 9806 | 105.87 |
| Jiangsu | 20935 | 20355 | 580 | 66998 | 33738 | 33260 | 101.44 |
| Zhejiang | 17378 | 16889 | 489 | 46831 | 24377 | 22454 | 108.56 |
| Anhui | 15687 | 15635 | 52 | 52056 | 26727 | 25329 | 105.52 |
| Fujian | 10591 | 10310 | 281 | 32474 | 16540 | 15934 | 103.80 |
| Jiangxi | 10585 | 10482 | 102 | 38576 | 20069 | 18506 | 108.45 |
| Shandong | 28939 | 28783 | 156 | 83464 | 42579 | 40886 | 104.14 |
| Henan | 22955 | 22834 | 120 | 80140 | 40834 | 39306 | 103.89 |
| Hubei | 15757 | 15304 | 453 | 49384 | 25352 | 24032 | 105.49 |
| Hunan | 17503 | 17414 | 89 | 57310 | 29286 | 28024 | 104.51 |
| Guangdong | 29620 | 27857 | 1763 | 92107 | 48869 | 43238 | 113.02 |
| Guangxi | 11484 | 11410 | 74 | 40677 | 21161 | 19516 | 108.43 |
| Hainan | 2037 | 2020 | 17 | 7698 | 4058 | 3641 | 111.46 |
| Chongqing | 9209 | 9132 | 77 | 25560 | 12992 | 12568 | 103.37 |
| Sichuan | 22929 | 22751 | 178 | 69457 | 34682 | 34775 | 99.73 |
| Guizhou | 8986 | 8940 | 46 | 29915 | 15438 | 14476 | 106.65 |
| Yunnan | 11282 | 11002 | 279 | 40141 | 20285 | 19855 | 102.16 |
| Tibet | 686 | 675 | 10 | 2789 | 1410 | 1380 | 102.18 |
| Shaanxi | 9758 | 9510 | 248 | 32014 | 16160 | 15854 | 101.93 |
| Gansu | 6374 | 6253 | 21 | 21960 | 11134 | 10826 | 102.85 |
| Qinghai | 1482 | 1471 | 11 | 4987 | 2564 | 2423 | 105.80 |
| Ningxia | 1783 | 1776 | 8 | 5666 | 2925 | 2741 | 106.70 |
| Xinjiang | 6046 | 6025 | 22 | 20165 | 10303 | 9861 | 104.48 |

Notes: This table is the sample check data of population changes in 2016 and the sampling ratio is 0.837‰

*Continued*

| Region | Family Household (Person) | | | Collective Household (Person) | | | Average Household Scale (Person/Household) |
|---|---|---|---|---|---|---|---|
| | | Male | Female | | Male | Female | |
| **Whole Country** | **1132138** | **578632** | **553506** | **25881** | **14455** | **11426** | **3.11** |
| Beijing | 16695 | 8334 | 8361 | 1437 | 990 | 447 | 2.62 |
| Tianjin | 11472 | 5759 | 5714 | 1574 | 1202 | 371 | 2.77 |
| Hebei | 62372 | 31900 | 30472 | 378 | 182 | 196 | 3.26 |
| Shanxi | 30383 | 15674 | 14709 | 528 | 235 | 293 | 3.11 |
| Inner Mongolia | 20376 | 10431 | 9945 | 760 | 244 | 516 | 2.73 |
| Liaoning | 36513 | 18415 | 18099 | 155 | 88 | 66 | 2.74 |
| Jilin | 22881 | 11632 | 11249 | 64 | 33 | 31 | 2.85 |
| Heilongjiang | 31496 | 16026 | 15470 | 378 | 78 | 300 | 2.75 |
| Shanghai | 19303 | 9799 | 9505 | 885 | 583 | 302 | 2.47 |
| Jiangsu | 64769 | 32742 | 32027 | 2229 | 997 | 1233 | 3.18 |
| Zhejiang | 45228 | 23147 | 22081 | 1603 | 1230 | 373 | 2.68 |
| Anhui | 51868 | 26628 | 25240 | 188 | 99 | 88 | 3.32 |
| Fujian | 31399 | 15935 | 15464 | 1075 | 605 | 470 | 3.05 |
| Jiangxi | 38169 | 19714 | 18455 | 406 | 355 | 51 | 3.64 |
| Shandong | 82708 | 42383 | 40325 | 757 | 196 | 561 | 2.87 |
| Henan | 79392 | 40566 | 38826 | 748 | 268 | 480 | 3.48 |
| Hubei | 47625 | 24326 | 23299 | 1759 | 1026 | 733 | 3.11 |
| Hunan | 56440 | 28711 | 27729 | 870 | 575 | 295 | 3.24 |
| Guangdong | 86392 | 45364 | 41028 | 5715 | 3504 | 2210 | 3.10 |
| Guangxi | 40474 | 21028 | 19446 | 203 | 133 | 70 | 3.55 |
| Hainan | 7626 | 4021 | 3605 | 72 | 37 | 35 | 3.78 |
| Chongqing | 25129 | 12700 | 12430 | 430 | 292 | 138 | 2.75 |
| Sichuan | 68636 | 34421 | 34215 | 821 | 261 | 560 | 3.02 |
| Guizhou | 29753 | 15332 | 14421 | 161 | 106 | 55 | 3.33 |
| Yunnan | 39058 | 19907 | 19152 | 1082 | 378 | 704 | 3.55 |
| Tibet | 2721 | 1363 | 1357 | 69 | 46 | 22 | 4.03 |
| Shaanxi | 30710 | 15580 | 15130 | 1304 | 580 | 725 | 3.23 |
| Gansu | 21887 | 11097 | 10791 | 73 | 38 | 35 | 3.45 |
| Qinghai | 4945 | 2534 | 2411 | 42 | 30 | 12 | 3.36 |
| Ningxia | 5634 | 2907 | 2727 | 32 | 17 | 14 | 3.17 |
| Xinjiang | 20082 | 10257 | 9824 | 83 | 46 | 37 | 3.33 |

## Sub-region Population by Gender, Household Registration in 2016

Unit : Person

| Region | Population Number | | | Living in This Town, County, District with Household in This Town, County, District | | |
|---|---|---|---|---|---|---|
| | Total | Male | Female | Total | Male | Female |
| **Whole Country** | **1158019** | **593087** | **564932** | **942716** | **482318** | **460399** |
| Beijing | 18132 | 9324 | 8808 | 9455 | 4880 | 4575 |
| Tianjin | 13046 | 6961 | 6085 | 8877 | 4475 | 4402 |
| Hebei | 62750 | 32082 | 30668 | 55837 | 28693 | 27144 |
| Shanxi | 30910 | 15909 | 15002 | 25804 | 13372 | 12431 |
| Inner Mongolia | 21136 | 10675 | 10461 | 14779 | 7614 | 7165 |
| Liaoning | 36668 | 18503 | 18165 | 31115 | 15742 | 15373 |
| Jilin | 22945 | 11665 | 11280 | 18604 | 9559 | 9045 |
| Heilongjiang | 31874 | 16104 | 15770 | 28037 | 14289 | 13748 |
| Shanghai | 20188 | 10382 | 9806 | 8873 | 4487 | 4386 |
| Jiangsu | 66998 | 33738 | 33260 | 53868 | 27174 | 26694 |
| Zhejiang | 46831 | 24377 | 22454 | 32066 | 16216 | 15849 |
| Anhui | 52056 | 26727 | 25329 | 46350 | 23932 | 22418 |
| Fujian | 32474 | 16540 | 15934 | 22138 | 11099 | 11038 |
| Jiangxi | 38576 | 20069 | 18506 | 34634 | 17957 | 16678 |
| Shandong | 83464 | 42579 | 40886 | 72028 | 36978 | 35050 |
| Henan | 80140 | 40834 | 39306 | 71781 | 36669 | 35112 |
| Hubei | 49384 | 25352 | 24032 | 40121 | 20499 | 19622 |
| Hunan | 57310 | 29286 | 28024 | 50311 | 25654 | 24657 |
| Guangdong | 92107 | 48869 | 43238 | 59496 | 30832 | 28664 |
| Guangxi | 40677 | 21161 | 19516 | 36161 | 18866 | 17294 |
| Hainan | 7698 | 4058 | 3641 | 6493 | 3463 | 3030 |
| Chongqing | 25560 | 12992 | 12568 | 19522 | 9901 | 9621 |
| Sichuan | 69457 | 34682 | 34775 | 59453 | 29921 | 29532 |
| Guizhou | 29915 | 15438 | 14476 | 26176 | 13579 | 12597 |
| Yunnan | 40141 | 20285 | 19855 | 35181 | 17976 | 17205 |
| Tibet | 2789 | 1410 | 1380 | 2636 | 1329 | 1307 |
| Shaanxi | 32014 | 16160 | 15854 | 27306 | 13877 | 13429 |
| Gansu | 21960 | 11134 | 10826 | 20165 | 10257 | 9908 |
| Qinghai | 4987 | 2564 | 2423 | 4277 | 2185 | 2092 |
| Ningxia | 5666 | 2925 | 2741 | 4432 | 2280 | 2153 |
| Xinjiang | 20165 | 10303 | 9861 | 16743 | 8565 | 8178 |

Notes: This table is the sample check data of population changes in 2016 and the sampling ratio is 0.837‰

*Continued*

Unit : Person

| Region | Living in This Town, County, District, Leaving Household Place for More Than Half a Year | | | Living in This Town, County, District with Undetermined Household | | | Living in Hong Kong, Macao, Taiwan with Household in This Town, County, District | | |
|---|---|---|---|---|---|---|---|---|---|
| | Subtotal | Male | Female | Subtotal | Male | Female | Subtotal | Male | Female |
| **Whole Country** | **209164** | **107641** | **101524** | **4781** | **2408** | **2373** | **1357** | **721** | **636** |
| Beijing | 8541 | 4373 | 4168 | 46 | 31 | 15 | 90 | 40 | 50 |
| Tianjin | 4149 | 2477 | 1671 | 12 | 6 | 6 | 8 | 3 | 6 |
| Hebei | 6352 | 3102 | 3250 | 544 | 276 | 268 | 17 | 12 | 6 |
| Shanxi | 4993 | 2479 | 2514 | 112 | 56 | 55 | 2 | 1 | 1 |
| Inner Mongolia | 6286 | 3025 | 3261 | 66 | 33 | 34 | 5 | 3 | 2 |
| Liaoning | 5447 | 2701 | 2746 | 53 | 29 | 23 | 53 | 31 | 22 |
| Jilin | 4173 | 2021 | 2152 | 30 | 13 | 18 | 138 | 72 | 66 |
| Heilongjiang | 3749 | 1767 | 1983 | 63 | 33 | 29 | 25 | 15 | 10 |
| Shanghai | 11110 | 5799 | 5310 | 45 | 21 | 24 | 161 | 74 | 87 |
| Jiangsu | 12858 | 6405 | 6452 | 184 | 99 | 85 | 88 | 61 | 27 |
| Zhejiang | 14502 | 8032 | 6470 | 157 | 81 | 76 | 106 | 48 | 58 |
| Anhui | 5466 | 2688 | 2777 | 225 | 96 | 128 | 16 | 10 | 6 |
| Fujian | 9707 | 5090 | 4617 | 300 | 163 | 137 | 330 | 187 | 142 |
| Jiangxi | 3812 | 2049 | 1764 | 127 | 64 | 63 | 2 | | 2 |
| Shandong | 11192 | 5467 | 5725 | 189 | 103 | 86 | 55 | 30 | 25 |
| Henan | 8144 | 4069 | 4074 | 200 | 87 | 113 | 16 | 9 | 7 |
| Hubei | 8984 | 4722 | 4262 | 227 | 105 | 122 | 53 | 28 | 25 |
| Hunan | 6682 | 3459 | 3223 | 305 | 167 | 138 | 13 | 7 | 6 |
| Guangdong | 32027 | 17746 | 14281 | 543 | 279 | 264 | 41 | 12 | 29 |
| Guangxi | 4266 | 2185 | 2082 | 235 | 100 | 135 | 15 | 10 | 5 |
| Hainan | 1146 | 568 | 578 | 47 | 21 | 26 | 12 | 6 | 6 |
| Chongqing | 5857 | 2992 | 2865 | 176 | 98 | 78 | 5 | 1 | 4 |
| Sichuan | 9775 | 4637 | 5138 | 195 | 99 | 95 | 35 | 25 | 10 |
| Guizhou | 3569 | 1771 | 1798 | 160 | 83 | 77 | 10 | 6 | 4 |
| Yunnan | 4750 | 2208 | 2541 | 190 | 93 | 97 | 19 | 7 | 12 |
| Tibet | 142 | 74 | 68 | 11 | 7 | 5 | | | |
| Shaanxi | 4608 | 2237 | 2371 | 82 | 34 | 48 | 19 | 13 | 6 |
| Gansu | 1711 | 839 | 872 | 73 | 33 | 40 | 12 | 5 | 7 |
| Qinghai | 679 | 363 | 316 | 29 | 15 | 14 | 1 | 1 | |
| Ningxia | 1219 | 637 | 582 | 13 | 7 | 6 | 2 | 1 | |
| Xinjiang | 3271 | 1659 | 1612 | 143 | 75 | 68 | 7 | 5 | 3 |

## All-region Population by Gender and Marriage in 2016

Unit : Person

| Region | Total | | | Unmarried | | | Married | | |
|---|---|---|---|---|---|---|---|---|---|
| | | Male | Female | | Male | Female | | Male | Female |
| **Whole Country** | 965321 | 488944 | 476376 | 182568 | 107984 | 74584 | 710768 | 354610 | 356158 |
| Beijing | 16160 | 8275 | 7885 | 3434 | 2038 | 1396 | 11730 | 5933 | 5798 |
| Tianjin | 11624 | 6217 | 5407 | 2224 | 1281 | 943 | 8625 | 4679 | 3947 |
| Hebei | 51166 | 25832 | 25334 | 7397 | 4459 | 2938 | 40290 | 19972 | 20317 |
| Shanxi | 26163 | 13383 | 12780 | 5328 | 3095 | 2233 | 19253 | 9684 | 9569 |
| Inner Mongolia | 18431 | 9303 | 9128 | 3415 | 1799 | 1615 | 13801 | 7055 | 6746 |
| Liaoning | 32768 | 16513 | 16254 | 5355 | 3132 | 2223 | 24269 | 12147 | 12123 |
| Jilin | 20043 | 10116 | 9927 | 2940 | 1712 | 1228 | 15254 | 7668 | 7586 |
| Heilongjiang | 28670 | 14444 | 14226 | 4791 | 2688 | 2104 | 21042 | 10579 | 10463 |
| Shanghai | 18236 | 9347 | 8889 | 3103 | 1761 | 1343 | 14057 | 7260 | 6796 |
| Jiangsu | 57799 | 28713 | 29085 | 9063 | 5070 | 3993 | 44561 | 22214 | 22347 |
| Zhejiang | 40768 | 21118 | 19650 | 6981 | 4361 | 2620 | 30912 | 15820 | 15092 |
| Anhui | 42927 | 21710 | 21218 | 7570 | 4603 | 2966 | 32254 | 15933 | 16321 |
| Fujian | 26534 | 13292 | 13241 | 4207 | 2537 | 1670 | 20412 | 10164 | 10248 |
| Jiangxi | 30389 | 15452 | 14937 | 5829 | 3626 | 2203 | 22395 | 11104 | 11290 |
| Shandong | 69325 | 34752 | 34573 | 10634 | 6207 | 4426 | 53971 | 26796 | 27175 |
| Henan | 63480 | 31520 | 31960 | 12159 | 6931 | 5228 | 47045 | 22823 | 24221 |
| Hubei | 41739 | 21236 | 20503 | 7885 | 4886 | 2999 | 30667 | 15152 | 15516 |
| Hunan | 46880 | 23678 | 23201 | 8152 | 5002 | 3150 | 34753 | 17226 | 17527 |
| Guangdong | 76689 | 40344 | 36345 | 21475 | 12922 | 8553 | 51226 | 26207 | 25019 |
| Guangxi | 31991 | 16441 | 15550 | 7430 | 4632 | 2798 | 22134 | 11003 | 11131 |
| Hainan | 6178 | 3228 | 2950 | 1645 | 1042 | 602 | 4159 | 2063 | 2096 |
| Chongqing | 21611 | 10852 | 10759 | 3699 | 2205 | 1494 | 15938 | 7880 | 8059 |
| Sichuan | 58371 | 28868 | 29503 | 10583 | 6132 | 4451 | 42053 | 20548 | 21505 |
| Guizhou | 23252 | 11848 | 11404 | 5120 | 3084 | 2036 | 16077 | 7938 | 8138 |
| Yunnan | 32301 | 16265 | 16036 | 7063 | 4071 | 2992 | 22774 | 11309 | 11465 |
| Tibet | 2119 | 1076 | 1043 | 649 | 344 | 304 | 1306 | 679 | 628 |
| Shaanxi | 27265 | 13659 | 13606 | 5849 | 3278 | 2572 | 19383 | 9618 | 9765 |
| Gansu | 18235 | 9127 | 9109 | 3801 | 2202 | 1599 | 13025 | 6411 | 6614 |
| Qinghai | 4004 | 2065 | 1938 | 856 | 523 | 344 | 2772 | 1403 | 1369 |
| Ningxia | 4581 | 2345 | 2236 | 889 | 534 | 355 | 3402 | 1710 | 1692 |
| Xinjiang | 15624 | 7925 | 7699 | 3044 | 1828 | 1216 | 11229 | 5633 | 5595 |

Note: This table is the sample check data of population changes in 2016 and the sampling ratio is 0.837‰

Continued
Unit: Person

| Region | Divorced | | | Widowed | | |
|---|---|---|---|---|---|---|
| | | Male | Female | | Male | Female |
| **Whole Country** | **18408** | **10415** | **7993** | **53577** | **15935** | **37641** |
| Beijing | 341 | 151 | 191 | 654 | 153 | 501 |
| Tianjin | 228 | 109 | 119 | 547 | 148 | 399 |
| Hebei | 732 | 470 | 262 | 2748 | 931 | 1817 |
| Shanxi | 375 | 239 | 136 | 1208 | 366 | 842 |
| Inner Mongolia | 351 | 202 | 149 | 865 | 247 | 618 |
| Liaoning | 1221 | 660 | 561 | 1923 | 576 | 1347 |
| Jilin | 735 | 410 | 325 | 1114 | 326 | 788 |
| Heilongjiang | 1181 | 660 | 520 | 1656 | 517 | 1140 |
| Shanghai | 366 | 164 | 202 | 709 | 162 | 548 |
| Jiangsu | 890 | 493 | 397 | 3285 | 937 | 2348 |
| Zhejiang | 732 | 429 | 303 | 2143 | 508 | 1634 |
| Anhui | 692 | 439 | 253 | 2412 | 734 | 1677 |
| Fujian | 409 | 227 | 183 | 1506 | 366 | 1140 |
| Jiangxi | 427 | 245 | 182 | 1739 | 476 | 1263 |
| Shandong | 769 | 489 | 281 | 3950 | 1260 | 2691 |
| Henan | 769 | 497 | 272 | 3507 | 1268 | 2239 |
| Hubei | 785 | 456 | 329 | 2402 | 742 | 1659 |
| Hunan | 965 | 574 | 391 | 3009 | 876 | 2133 |
| Guangdong | 888 | 438 | 450 | 3100 | 777 | 2324 |
| Guangxi | 499 | 278 | 221 | 1928 | 528 | 1400 |
| Hainan | 73 | 46 | 27 | 301 | 76 | 225 |
| Chongqing | 620 | 312 | 309 | 1352 | 455 | 897 |
| Sichuan | 1589 | 890 | 699 | 4145 | 1298 | 2847 |
| Guizhou | 567 | 339 | 228 | 1489 | 487 | 1002 |
| Yunnan | 629 | 369 | 260 | 1835 | 515 | 1320 |
| Tibet | 46 | 15 | 32 | 117 | 38 | 79 |
| Shaanxi | 404 | 247 | 158 | 1628 | 516 | 1112 |
| Gansu | 277 | 165 | 112 | 1132 | 349 | 783 |
| Qinghai | 149 | 76 | 73 | 226 | 64 | 163 |
| Ningxia | 93 | 50 | 43 | 197 | 51 | 146 |
| Xinjiang | 604 | 277 | 327 | 747 | 186 | 561 |

## Sub-region Population of 6 and above by Gender and Education in 2016

Unit : Person

| Region | 6 and above | | | No Schooling | | | Elementary School | | |
|---|---|---|---|---|---|---|---|---|---|
| | Subtotal | Male | Female | Subtotal | Male | Female | Subtotal | Male | Female |
| **Whole Country** | 1077322 | 549723 | 527599 | 61448 | 18267 | 43181 | 275939 | 131541 | 144398 |
| Beijing | 17001 | 8721 | 8279 | 313 | 74 | 238 | 1631 | 741 | 890 |
| Tianjin | 12401 | 6619 | 5781 | 333 | 96 | 239 | 1902 | 962 | 941 |
| Hebei | 57884 | 29438 | 28446 | 2752 | 783 | 1968 | 14776 | 6989 | 7787 |
| Shanxi | 29052 | 14883 | 14169 | 909 | 300 | 609 | 5620 | 2607 | 3014 |
| Inner Mongolia | 19913 | 10053 | 9860 | 1013 | 332 | 681 | 4312 | 2011 | 2301 |
| Liaoning | 35135 | 17741 | 17395 | 782 | 244 | 537 | 6838 | 3131 | 3708 |
| Jilin | 21860 | 11076 | 10784 | 675 | 234 | 441 | 5106 | 2436 | 2670 |
| Heilongjiang | 30868 | 15574 | 15294 | 1295 | 482 | 813 | 6952 | 3302 | 3649 |
| Shanghai | 19274 | 9910 | 9364 | 651 | 152 | 500 | 2528 | 1165 | 1363 |
| Jiangsu | 62953 | 31572 | 31381 | 3908 | 1055 | 2853 | 14012 | 6325 | 7687 |
| Zhejiang | 44145 | 22940 | 21204 | 2916 | 764 | 2153 | 12079 | 5864 | 6215 |
| Anhui | 48183 | 24636 | 23547 | 3549 | 1059 | 2491 | 13091 | 6056 | 7035 |
| Fujian | 29688 | 14977 | 14710 | 1953 | 453 | 1500 | 9407 | 4307 | 5100 |
| Jiangxi | 35394 | 18318 | 17076 | 1830 | 524 | 1306 | 10875 | 5118 | 5756 |
| Shandong | 77354 | 39172 | 38183 | 5230 | 1404 | 3824 | 18766 | 8764 | 10002 |
| Henan | 73743 | 37393 | 36351 | 4323 | 1455 | 2868 | 17933 | 8781 | 9151 |
| Hubei | 46004 | 23522 | 22482 | 2690 | 704 | 1986 | 10885 | 5115 | 5770 |
| Hunan | 53099 | 27041 | 26057 | 1984 | 618 | 1366 | 13315 | 6310 | 7004 |
| Guangdong | 85168 | 45148 | 40020 | 3194 | 908 | 2286 | 18686 | 8842 | 9844 |
| Guangxi | 36994 | 19136 | 17857 | 1697 | 468 | 1228 | 10350 | 4895 | 5455 |
| Hainan | 7037 | 3708 | 3329 | 332 | 106 | 227 | 1570 | 751 | 820 |
| Chongqing | 24087 | 12182 | 11906 | 1070 | 287 | 783 | 7581 | 3667 | 3914 |
| Sichuan | 65259 | 32466 | 32793 | 5508 | 1674 | 3835 | 21287 | 10482 | 10805 |
| Guizhou | 27172 | 13928 | 13244 | 3117 | 924 | 2192 | 9233 | 4698 | 4535 |
| Yunnan | 36930 | 18655 | 18276 | 3219 | 1032 | 2186 | 14306 | 7186 | 7120 |
| Tibet | 2512 | 1272 | 1240 | 982 | 410 | 571 | 786 | 448 | 338 |
| Shaanxi | 29889 | 15052 | 14837 | 1685 | 542 | 1143 | 6847 | 3172 | 3674 |
| Gansu | 20445 | 10322 | 10122 | 1793 | 550 | 1244 | 6813 | 3264 | 3549 |
| Qinghai | 4581 | 2359 | 2223 | 605 | 219 | 386 | 1602 | 790 | 812 |
| Ningxia | 5210 | 2681 | 2529 | 350 | 99 | 251 | 1394 | 672 | 722 |
| Xinjiang | 18087 | 9230 | 8857 | 790 | 315 | 475 | 5455 | 2692 | 2763 |

Note: This table is the sample check data of population changes in 2016 and the sampling ratio is 0.837‰.

*Continued*
Unit : Person

| Region | Junior High School | | | High School | | | Secondary School | | |
|---|---|---|---|---|---|---|---|---|---|
| | Subtotal | Male | Female | Subtotal | Male | Female | Subtotal | Male | Female |
| **Whole Country** | **418395** | **225166** | **193229** | **137409** | **77412** | **59997** | **44762** | **23914** | **20848** |
| Beijing | 4070 | 2156 | 1914 | 2228 | 1120 | 1108 | 1030 | 530 | 500 |
| Tianjin | 4169 | 2393 | 1776 | 1560 | 851 | 708 | 1261 | 713 | 548 |
| Hebei | 25765 | 13774 | 11991 | 6712 | 3731 | 2981 | 1913 | 1062 | 851 |
| Shanxi | 12675 | 6648 | 6027 | 4588 | 2559 | 2029 | 1319 | 692 | 628 |
| Inner Mongolia | 7552 | 4194 | 3359 | 2701 | 1332 | 1369 | 694 | 383 | 312 |
| Liaoning | 15399 | 8081 | 7318 | 4161 | 2183 | 1977 | 1626 | 857 | 768 |
| Jilin | 9333 | 4861 | 4472 | 3020 | 1632 | 1389 | 633 | 317 | 316 |
| Heilongjiang | 13491 | 7074 | 6417 | 4089 | 2229 | 1860 | 883 | 452 | 431 |
| Shanghai | 6199 | 3304 | 2895 | 2840 | 1570 | 1269 | 1264 | 690 | 574 |
| Jiangsu | 22540 | 11931 | 10609 | 8530 | 5018 | 3512 | 3506 | 1735 | 1770 |
| Zhejiang | 15554 | 8711 | 6843 | 5296 | 3035 | 2261 | 1594 | 875 | 720 |
| Anhui | 20802 | 11277 | 9526 | 4940 | 2953 | 1987 | 1286 | 686 | 600 |
| Fujian | 10337 | 5799 | 4538 | 3121 | 1823 | 1298 | 1449 | 750 | 699 |
| Jiangxi | 13502 | 7243 | 6259 | 4831 | 2845 | 1986 | 1180 | 610 | 570 |
| Shandong | 30835 | 16546 | 14289 | 9083 | 5233 | 3850 | 3942 | 2161 | 1781 |
| Henan | 32979 | 17355 | 15624 | 10694 | 5911 | 4783 | 1944 | 1003 | 940 |
| Hubei | 17461 | 9295 | 8166 | 6345 | 3685 | 2660 | 2218 | 1205 | 1013 |
| Hunan | 20403 | 10477 | 9926 | 9071 | 5055 | 4016 | 2142 | 1144 | 997 |
| Guangdong | 33330 | 18439 | 14890 | 13313 | 7791 | 5522 | 4866 | 2693 | 2172 |
| Guangxi | 16376 | 9019 | 7357 | 3932 | 2240 | 1692 | 1684 | 915 | 770 |
| Hainan | 3197 | 1715 | 1482 | 841 | 516 | 325 | 412 | 225 | 187 |
| Chongqing | 8112 | 4272 | 3839 | 3380 | 1882 | 1498 | 907 | 478 | 429 |
| Sichuan | 23637 | 12591 | 11046 | 6827 | 3756 | 3071 | 2131 | 1110 | 1022 |
| Guizhou | 9951 | 5670 | 4281 | 2201 | 1221 | 980 | 766 | 391 | 374 |
| Yunnan | 12135 | 6834 | 5301 | 2850 | 1511 | 1339 | 1210 | 636 | 574 |
| Tibet | 466 | 273 | 193 | 128 | 71 | 58 | 18 | 11 | 6 |
| Shaanxi | 11835 | 6364 | 5471 | 4485 | 2521 | 1964 | 1216 | 697 | 518 |
| Gansu | 6337 | 3461 | 2876 | 2700 | 1546 | 1154 | 610 | 317 | 293 |
| Qinghai | 1390 | 804 | 585 | 428 | 246 | 183 | 112 | 59 | 52 |
| Ningxia | 1821 | 1013 | 807 | 655 | 364 | 291 | 189 | 104 | 84 |
| Xinjiang | 6743 | 3591 | 3151 | 1860 | 981 | 878 | 758 | 410 | 348 |

*531*

*Continued*

Unit : Person

| Region | Junior College | | | College | | | Graduate College | | |
|---|---|---|---|---|---|---|---|---|---|
| | Subtotal | Male | Female | Subtotal | Male | Female | Subtotal | Male | Female |
| **Whole Country** | **74338** | **38819** | **35519** | **59235** | **31341** | **27894** | **5797** | **3263** | **2533** |
| Beijing | 2320 | 1130 | 1190 | 4152 | 2170 | 1982 | 1257 | 799 | 458 |
| Tianjin | 1501 | 738 | 762 | 1517 | 780 | 737 | 158 | 86 | 72 |
| Hebei | 3596 | 1858 | 1737 | 2220 | 1163 | 1057 | 150 | 77 | 73 |
| Shanxi | 2269 | 1198 | 1071 | 1490 | 788 | 702 | 182 | 91 | 91 |
| Inner Mongolia | 1966 | 1043 | 923 | 1609 | 729 | 881 | 65 | 29 | 35 |
| Liaoning | 2974 | 1512 | 1461 | 3005 | 1552 | 1453 | 352 | 180 | 173 |
| Jilin | 1444 | 727 | 717 | 1517 | 803 | 715 | 132 | 67 | 65 |
| Heilongjiang | 2060 | 1055 | 1005 | 1971 | 914 | 1057 | 128 | 65 | 62 |
| Shanghai | 2323 | 1214 | 1109 | 2915 | 1499 | 1416 | 553 | 315 | 238 |
| Jiangsu | 5797 | 2924 | 2873 | 4190 | 2313 | 1877 | 471 | 271 | 200 |
| Zhejiang | 3296 | 1705 | 1591 | 3186 | 1871 | 1315 | 223 | 116 | 107 |
| Anhui | 2634 | 1517 | 1117 | 1771 | 1030 | 741 | 110 | 59 | 51 |
| Fujian | 1815 | 979 | 836 | 1504 | 809 | 695 | 102 | 57 | 45 |
| Jiangxi | 1856 | 1050 | 806 | 1251 | 887 | 364 | 70 | 40 | 30 |
| Shandong | 5409 | 2757 | 2652 | 3742 | 2115 | 1628 | 348 | 192 | 156 |
| Henan | 3904 | 1842 | 2061 | 1850 | 977 | 873 | 116 | 67 | 49 |
| Hubei | 3236 | 1822 | 1414 | 2904 | 1549 | 1355 | 266 | 147 | 119 |
| Hunan | 3800 | 2089 | 1711 | 2201 | 1244 | 957 | 183 | 105 | 79 |
| Guangdong | 6197 | 3448 | 2749 | 5296 | 2869 | 2427 | 286 | 157 | 128 |
| Guangxi | 1879 | 1014 | 865 | 983 | 529 | 454 | 92 | 57 | 36 |
| Hainan | 404 | 237 | 167 | 275 | 155 | 119 | 6 | 3 | 2 |
| Chongqing | 1836 | 971 | 865 | 1135 | 585 | 550 | 67 | 40 | 27 |
| Sichuan | 3511 | 1798 | 1713 | 2243 | 996 | 1247 | 115 | 60 | 55 |
| Guizhou | 1060 | 552 | 509 | 824 | 465 | 359 | 21 | 8 | 13 |
| Yunnan | 1566 | 795 | 772 | 1580 | 629 | 951 | 64 | 32 | 32 |
| Tibet | 60 | 29 | 31 | 71 | 30 | 41 | 1 | | 1 |
| Shaanxi | 2319 | 1067 | 1252 | 1382 | 628 | 754 | 121 | 60 | 61 |
| Gansu | 1185 | 643 | 541 | 938 | 507 | 431 | 68 | 34 | 34 |
| Qinghai | 244 | 132 | 112 | 192 | 104 | 88 | 8 | 5 | 4 |
| Ningxia | 448 | 240 | 208 | 333 | 176 | 157 | 20 | 12 | 9 |
| Xinjiang | 1432 | 732 | 699 | 989 | 477 | 512 | 62 | 31 | 30 |

## Sub-region Illiteracy of 15 and above by Age in 2016

| Region | 15 and above (Person) | | | Illiteracy (Person) | | | Illiteracy Proportion in Population of 15 and above (%) | | |
|---|---|---|---|---|---|---|---|---|---|
| | | Male | Female | | Male | Female | | Male | Female |
| **Whole Country** | 965321 | 488944 | 476376 | 50980 | 13402 | 37578 | 5.28 | 2.74 | 7.89 |
| Beijing | 16160 | 8275 | 7885 | 252 | 52 | 201 | 1.56 | 0.62 | 2.54 |
| Tianjin | 11624 | 6217 | 5407 | 262 | 66 | 196 | 2.26 | 1.07 | 3.62 |
| Hebei | 51166 | 25832 | 25334 | 2097 | 473 | 1623 | 4.10 | 1.83 | 6.41 |
| Shanxi | 26163 | 13383 | 12780 | 660 | 198 | 462 | 2.52 | 1.48 | 3.61 |
| Inner Mongolia | 18431 | 9303 | 9128 | 859 | 252 | 607 | 4.66 | 2.71 | 6.65 |
| Liaoning | 32768 | 16513 | 16254 | 553 | 144 | 409 | 1.69 | 0.87 | 2.52 |
| Jilin | 20043 | 10116 | 9927 | 496 | 151 | 345 | 2.47 | 1.49 | 3.48 |
| Heilongjiang | 28670 | 14444 | 14226 | 1031 | 356 | 675 | 3.60 | 2.47 | 4.74 |
| Shanghai | 18236 | 9347 | 8889 | 567 | 114 | 454 | 3.11 | 1.22 | 5.10 |
| Jiangsu | 57799 | 28713 | 29085 | 3361 | 790 | 2571 | 5.81 | 2.75 | 8.84 |
| Zhejiang | 40768 | 21118 | 19650 | 2443 | 568 | 1875 | 5.99 | 2.69 | 9.54 |
| Anhui | 42927 | 21710 | 21218 | 2923 | 810 | 2114 | 6.81 | 3.73 | 9.96 |
| Fujian | 26534 | 13292 | 13241 | 1628 | 314 | 1314 | 6.14 | 2.37 | 9.92 |
| Jiangxi | 30389 | 15452 | 14937 | 1469 | 358 | 1111 | 4.83 | 2.32 | 7.44 |
| Shandong | 69325 | 34752 | 34573 | 4547 | 1089 | 3458 | 6.56 | 3.13 | 10.00 |
| Henan | 63480 | 31520 | 31960 | 3586 | 1076 | 2510 | 5.65 | 3.41 | 7.85 |
| Hubei | 41739 | 21236 | 20503 | 2352 | 552 | 1800 | 5.64 | 2.60 | 8.78 |
| Hunan | 46880 | 23678 | 23201 | 1588 | 430 | 1158 | 3.39 | 1.82 | 4.99 |
| Guangdong | 76689 | 40344 | 36345 | 2204 | 429 | 1775 | 2.87 | 1.06 | 4.88 |
| Guangxi | 31991 | 16441 | 15550 | 1212 | 241 | 971 | 3.79 | 1.47 | 6.25 |
| Hainan | 6178 | 3228 | 2950 | 286 | 77 | 209 | 4.63 | 2.38 | 7.10 |
| Chongqing | 21611 | 10852 | 10759 | 869 | 203 | 666 | 4.02 | 1.87 | 6.19 |
| Sichuan | 58371 | 28868 | 29503 | 4799 | 1336 | 3463 | 8.22 | 4.63 | 11.74 |
| Guizhou | 23252 | 11848 | 11404 | 2758 | 742 | 2017 | 11.86 | 6.26 | 17.68 |
| Yunnan | 32301 | 16265 | 16036 | 2853 | 842 | 2010 | 8.83 | 5.18 | 12.54 |
| Tibet | 2119 | 1076 | 1043 | 871 | 360 | 511 | 41.12 | 33.47 | 49.02 |
| Shaanxi | 27265 | 13659 | 13606 | 1423 | 427 | 996 | 5.22 | 3.13 | 7.32 |
| Gansu | 18235 | 9127 | 9109 | 1587 | 460 | 1127 | 8.70 | 5.04 | 12.38 |
| Qinghai | 4004 | 2065 | 1938 | 538 | 192 | 347 | 13.45 | 9.27 | 17.90 |
| Ningxia | 4581 | 2345 | 2236 | 312 | 82 | 230 | 6.82 | 3.50 | 10.30 |
| Xinjiang | 15624 | 7925 | 7699 | 591 | 219 | 373 | 3.79 | 2.76 | 4.84 |

Note: ①This table is the sample check data of population changes in 2016 and the sampling ratio is 0.837‰; ②Illiteracy population in this table refers to the illiterate people and people lack of literacy.

## Sub-region Household by Family Scale in 2016

Unit: Household

| Region | | Family Household (Number) | | | | | | | | | |
|---|---|---|---|---|---|---|---|---|---|---|---|
| | | One Family Member | Two Family Members | Three Family Members | Four Family Members | Five Family Members | Six Family Members | Seven Family Members | Eight Family Members | Nine Family Members | Ten Family Members and More |
| **Whole Country** | 364431 | 51347 | 93925 | 95094 | 64894 | 35430 | 15813 | 4744 | 1777 | 743 | 664 |
| Beijing | 6372 | 1327 | 1969 | 1872 | 631 | 414 | 104 | 32 | 18 | 4 | 1 |
| Tianjin | 4145 | 584 | 1258 | 1386 | 571 | 253 | 76 | 11 | 4 | | 1 |
| Hebei | 19130 | 1967 | 4991 | 4779 | 3851 | 1965 | 1169 | 287 | 76 | 29 | 17 |
| Shanxi | 9768 | 953 | 2481 | 2902 | 2222 | 821 | 296 | 59 | 24 | 5 | 4 |
| Inner Mongolia | 7467 | 898 | 2484 | 2568 | 1010 | 374 | 108 | 19 | 6 | 2 | |
| Liaoning | 13344 | 1817 | 4450 | 4469 | 1487 | 851 | 207 | 49 | 10 | 2 | 2 |
| Jilin | 8016 | 1036 | 2556 | 2509 | 972 | 663 | 215 | 41 | 19 | 4 | 1 |
| Heilongjiang | 11460 | 1467 | 3861 | 3895 | 1223 | 762 | 181 | 50 | 18 | 3 | 1 |
| Shanghai | 7801 | 1758 | 2694 | 2044 | 718 | 477 | 84 | 22 | 4 | 1 | 1 |
| Jiangsu | 20355 | 2446 | 5302 | 5493 | 3224 | 2576 | 943 | 238 | 89 | 23 | 22 |
| Zhejiang | 16889 | 3657 | 5150 | 4076 | 2272 | 1130 | 453 | 97 | 35 | 17 | 2 |
| Anhui | 15635 | 1563 | 3746 | 4200 | 3196 | 1627 | 887 | 266 | 91 | 44 | 16 |
| Fujian | 10310 | 1788 | 2685 | 2322 | 1746 | 1024 | 514 | 132 | 54 | 20 | 25 |
| Jiangxi | 10482 | 819 | 2081 | 2444 | 2465 | 1459 | 751 | 272 | 92 | 57 | 42 |
| Shandong | 28783 | 3798 | 8302 | 8594 | 5300 | 1957 | 668 | 111 | 29 | 20 | 5 |
| Henan | 22834 | 2072 | 4979 | 5475 | 5243 | 2809 | 1614 | 429 | 118 | 51 | 44 |
| Hubei | 15304 | 1934 | 3910 | 4344 | 2684 | 1576 | 617 | 134 | 65 | 27 | 14 |
| Hunan | 17414 | 2247 | 4004 | 4551 | 3487 | 1831 | 864 | 256 | 94 | 43 | 37 |
| Guangdong | 27857 | 6693 | 6051 | 5169 | 4502 | 2758 | 1376 | 688 | 304 | 146 | 170 |
| Guangxi | 11410 | 1548 | 2075 | 2623 | 2407 | 1401 | 710 | 314 | 148 | 80 | 103 |
| Hainan | 2020 | 206 | 327 | 412 | 511 | 295 | 148 | 62 | 28 | 12 | 20 |
| Chongqing | 9132 | 1975 | 2562 | 2164 | 1379 | 701 | 245 | 70 | 30 | 3 | 5 |
| Sichuan | 22751 | 3609 | 6011 | 5634 | 4043 | 2250 | 846 | 240 | 83 | 25 | 11 |
| Guizhou | 8940 | 1166 | 2033 | 1999 | 1835 | 1058 | 548 | 192 | 69 | 27 | 14 |
| Yunnan | 11002 | 1092 | 2077 | 2568 | 2578 | 1481 | 825 | 235 | 90 | 29 | 28 |
| Tibet | 675 | 94 | 115 | 121 | 126 | 75 | 52 | 32 | 24 | 16 | 21 |
| Shaanxi | 9510 | 1136 | 2295 | 2415 | 2002 | 1078 | 421 | 97 | 43 | 10 | 13 |
| Gansu | 6353 | 630 | 1387 | 1684 | 1234 | 746 | 436 | 150 | 50 | 19 | 16 |
| Qinghai | 1471 | 212 | 303 | 350 | 285 | 168 | 94 | 33 | 14 | 4 | 7 |
| Ningxia | 1776 | 168 | 449 | 523 | 371 | 157 | 75 | 23 | 8 | 2 | 1 |
| Xinjiang | 6025 | 687 | 1339 | 1511 | 1321 | 694 | 286 | 105 | 43 | 17 | 21 |

Note: This table is the sample check data of population changes in 2016 and the sampling ratio is 0.837‰.

**(Wang Ruisi)**

# Statistical Data of Family Planning

## Policy Coincidence Rate of Child/Times Birth in Statistical Year of 2016

| Region | Policy Coincidence Rate | Policy Coincidence Rate of One Child | Policy Coincidence Rate of Two Children | Policy Coincidence Rate of More Children |
|---|---|---|---|---|
| **Whole Country** | **96.47** | **98.28** | **99.02** | **48.27** |
| Beijing | 98.82 | 99.78 | 96.81 | 78.81 |
| Tianjin | 99.73 | 100.00 | 100.00 | 73.70 |
| Hebei | 96.24 | 99.79 | 99.88 | 30.66 |
| Shanxi | 99.05 | 99.89 | 99.89 | 57.83 |
| Inner Mongolia | 98.35 | 98.65 | 99.57 | 75.65 |
| Liaoning | 98.82 | 99.73 | 97.43 | 80.18 |
| Jilin | 98.76 | 99.82 | 99.29 | 64.00 |
| Heilongjiang | 99.04 | 99.36 | 99.62 | 61.88 |
| Shanghai | 99.57 | 99.60 | 99.68 | 91.76 |
| Jiangsu | 99.24 | 99.91 | 99.98 | 57.53 |
| Zhejiang | 98.71 | 99.73 | 99.46 | 51.56 |
| Anhui | 90.11 | 85.79 | 95.76 | 67.39 |
| Fujian | 95.63 | 99.85 | 99.90 | 32.00 |
| Jiangxi | 91.50 | 100.00 | 100.00 | 20.80 |
| Shandong | 96.95 | 96.87 | 99.60 | 28.86 |
| Henan | 99.06 | 100.00 | 100.00 | 38.47 |
| Hubei | 98.19 | 99.84 | 99.63 | 61.48 |
| Hunan | 95.28 | 99.85 | 99.77 | 38.98 |
| Guangdong | 97.05 | 99.52 | 98.12 | 52.68 |
| Guangxi | 95.76 | 98.38 | 99.02 | 36.78 |
| Hainan | 95.57 | 99.93 | 99.91 | 39.46 |
| Chongqing | 95.97 | 100.00 | 96.64 | 54.90 |
| Sichuan | 96.23 | 99.65 | 95.55 | 50.75 |
| Guizhou | 93.74 | 93.46 | 98.72 | 47.82 |
| Yunnan | 89.59 | 89.62 | 97.48 | 29.34 |
| Tibet | 100.00 | 100.00 | 100.00 | 100.00 |
| Shaanxi | 99.60 | 99.96 | 99.83 | 66.48 |
| Gansu | 98.36 | 99.94 | 99.91 | 60.93 |
| Qinghai | 98.90 | 99.79 | 99.98 | 83.36 |
| Ningxia | 96.41 | 98.10 | 99.77 | 71.06 |
| Xinjiang | 99.18 | 99.86 | 99.82 | 96.65 |

Note: The source of this column statistical data is from Grassroots Guidance Department of National Health and Family Planning Committee.

## People with All Contraception at the End of Statistical Year of 2016

Unit: Person

| Region | Total | Male Sterilization | Female Sterilization | Intrauterine Device | Subcutaneous Implant | Oral And Injected Contraceptives | Condom | Externally Applied Drug | Others |
|---|---|---|---|---|---|---|---|---|---|
| **Whole Country** | **221236313** | **7639978** | **57138116** | **117321009** | **519443** | **1771327** | **35751619** | **340721** | **754100** |
| Beijing | 1532935 | 250 | 7840 | 284066 | 959 | 22581 | 1209316 | 1583 | 6340 |
| Tianjin | 1472380 | 1713 | 61161 | 659491 | 1348 | 16816 | 708036 | 4133 | 19682 |
| Hebei | 12771467 | 348209 | 2527476 | 8470891 | 11227 | 59148 | 1176201 | 4007 | 174308 |
| Shanxi | 5802977 | 18713 | 1617706 | 3976235 | 3315 | 17236 | 150542 | 85 | 19145 |
| Inner Mongolia | 4097207 | 2333 | 495188 | 2717436 | 7694 | 24098 | 845000 | 448 | 5010 |
| Liaoning | 6031049 | 287 | 124579 | 4823338 | 6324 | 59534 | 996108 | 12522 | 8357 |
| Jilin | 4171655 | 888 | 168616 | 3298333 | 81297 | 16008 | 603731 | 1990 | 792 |
| Heilongjiang | 6306280 | 691 | 401352 | 5117654 | 15804 | 79726 | 665439 | 5504 | 20110 |
| Shanghai | 3200268 | 6740 | 86841 | 1313177 | 4356 | 82802 | 1633606 | 17885 | 54861 |
| Jiangsu | 12970322 | 101168 | 1065271 | 8586550 | 7694 | 98372 | 3034874 | 34478 | 41915 |
| Zhejiang | 7748608 | 16767 | 1519761 | 3653989 | 7998 | 39067 | 2477853 | 10431 | 22742 |
| Anhui | 12404011 | 153227 | 4629746 | 5962490 | 23577 | 103007 | 1513694 | 1599 | 16671 |
| Fujian | 5966564 | 285254 | 2397174 | 2461175 | 8790 | 12197 | 797426 | 920 | 3628 |
| Jiangxi | 8302331 | 8990 | 3876258 | 2963476 | 4169 | 24073 | 1396643 | 11674 | 17048 |
| Shandong | 15617577 | 957281 | 2793176 | 8747615 | 22064 | 4572 | 3088445 | 1633 | 2791 |
| Henan | 18769289 | 1978661 | 7625997 | 8048367 | 51321 | 68313 | 954439 | 12641 | 29550 |
| Hubei | 11150076 | 276468 | 3082923 | 5960134 | 36643 | 131339 | 1638520 | 3283 | 20766 |
| Hunan | 12255080 | 140367 | 4632616 | 5505412 | 21691 | 12858 | 1872173 | 30839 | 39124 |
| Guangdong | 18722919 | 1177588 | 6874180 | 4611382 | 6821 | 71899 | 5949115 | 14935 | 16999 |
| Guangxi | 8781712 | 687310 | 2668791 | 4681085 | 970 | 89007 | 590699 | 57357 | 6493 |
| Hainan | 1300130 | 6334 | 511265 | 628670 | 274 | 2031 | 149311 | 1124 | 1121 |
| Chongqing | 3194944 | 151461 | 43954 | 2374298 | 5694 | 99472 | 503649 | 11974 | 4442 |
| Sichuan | 9499459 | 349345 | 236378 | 7251263 | 65202 | 193477 | 1242796 | 7819 | 153179 |
| Guizhou | 5794712 | 670889 | 3062513 | 1824581 | 3401 | 6902 | 217003 | 1119 | 8304 |
| Yunnan | 7376406 | 186740 | 1789424 | 4770404 | 18902 | 133629 | 440638 | 16832 | 19837 |
| Tibet | 494529 | 52 | 37421 | 71104 | 46875 | 93834 | 215712 | 26434 | 3097 |
| Shaanxi | 5601959 | 100402 | 2089332 | 2833469 | 36298 | 82366 | 444256 | 13146 | 2690 |
| Gansu | 3566639 | 2704 | 1870276 | 1415902 | 5589 | 33193 | 232504 | 1071 | 5400 |
| Qinghai | 1023387 | 687 | 345948 | 554968 | 5758 | 37664 | 64836 | 10174 | 3352 |
| Ningxia | 1224065 | 196 | 328469 | 602495 | 1963 | 27068 | 251053 | 3133 | 9688 |
| Xinjiang | 4085376 | 8263 | 166484 | 3151559 | 5425 | 29038 | 688001 | 19948 | 16658 |

Note: The statistical time is September 30, 2016 (the same in the following tables).

## Comparison of All Contraception People at the End of Statistical Year of 2016 with the Same Period of Last Year

Unit: Person

| Region | Total | Male Sterilization | Female Sterilization | Intrauterine Device | Subcutaneous Implant | Oral And Injected Contraceptives | Condom | Externally Applied Drug | Others |
|---|---|---|---|---|---|---|---|---|---|
| **Whole Country** | **–396360629** | **–9851662** | **–64626434** | **–160940407** | **–791007** | **–2858254** | **–32485671** | **–333427** | **–744129** |
| Beijing | –3069855 | –3061 | –41348 | –1512723 | –2788 | –31425 | –1190370 | –1693 | –5860 |
| Tianjin | –2823846 | –10930 | –107515 | –1352689 | –9653 | –30971 | –618034 | –7842 | –11049 |
| Hebei | –22773624 | –414790 | –3091110 | –9633862 | –16330 | –228362 | –1036078 | –4343 | –164124 |
| Shanxi | –10256241 | –25189 | –1801092 | –4214980 | –3892 | –30851 | –128824 | –96 | –13941 |
| Inner Mongolia | –7806578 | –11654 | –598524 | –3598200 | –8892 | –30373 | –805317 | –557 | –3363 |
| Liaoning | –12593524 | –18976 | –229686 | –6172431 | –18631 | –68765 | –996875 | –10941 | –4427 |
| Jilin | –8485706 | –17748 | –204588 | –4131685 | –17372 | –9202 | –630047 | –1903 | 0 |
| Heilongjiang | –12371434 | –13778 | –555898 | –5900879 | –12799 | –98185 | –604123 | –5720 | –17616 |
| Shanghai | –6902902 | –31314 | –250828 | –3310380 | –23852 | –153597 | –1838791 | –18941 | –61975 |
| Jiangsu | –24840079 | –169659 | –1624950 | –11522735 | –42238 | –443881 | –2787748 | –34009 | –28690 |
| Zhejiang | –14526895 | –39829 | –1747338 | –6369864 | –21015 | –66621 | –2375306 | –12012 | –19975 |
| Anhui | –20711058 | –216910 | –5228352 | –7632898 | –29315 | –106548 | –993911 | –850 | –11427 |
| Fujian | –9818049 | –324019 | –2619842 | –3437094 | –10812 | –14555 | –716494 | –1070 | –3226 |
| Jiangxi | –12677049 | –41203 | –4124340 | –4255753 | –15214 | –35740 | –1006705 | –12185 | –9114 |
| Shandong | –27251414 | –1091884 | –2747776 | –11705877 | –26339 | –11509 | –2442583 | –1982 | –5844 |
| Henan | –28839177 | –2270985 | –8054756 | –9256718 | –68910 | –91449 | –923616 | –15075 | –23508 |
| Hubei | –19439097 | –338275 | –3463478 | –7818672 | –38933 | –161279 | –1482162 | –2832 | –23287 |
| Hunan | –20459246 | –239611 | –5030633 | –7594501 | –55429 | –44057 | –1784722 | –31877 | –29641 |
| Guangdong | –29484344 | –1318699 | –7334593 | –10415526 | –20578 | –88955 | –5356594 | –13395 | –19891 |
| Guangxi | –14219725 | –778232 | –2886929 | –5277282 | –62237 | –109782 | –545451 | –60799 | –5055 |
| Hainan | –2034331 | –8737 | –549960 | –737817 | –1399 | –2738 | –115334 | –1111 | –1169 |
| Chongqing | –7317828 | –202998 | –167640 | –3473595 | –18148 | –111044 | –564306 | –11106 | –5185 |
| Sichuan | –28695603 | –1036794 | –855115 | –13401847 | –111218 | –460664 | –1539933 | –21670 | –200853 |
| Guizhou | –8102833 | –750438 | –3227255 | –2062570 | –4897 | –11577 | –104973 | –595 | –5297 |
| Yunnan | –13187481 | –238311 | –2045274 | –5451948 | –38388 | –142490 | –386688 | –16078 | –19431 |
| Tibet | | | | | | | | | |
| Shaanxi | –10173664 | –168146 | –2645896 | –3678963 | –55490 | –98948 | –409993 | –13615 | –2430 |
| Gansu | –6101504 | –15112 | –2390364 | –1848014 | –11832 | –39036 | –209969 | –932 | –5827 |
| Qinghai | –1671433 | –14521 | –404200 | –626356 | –13808 | –41407 | –64619 | –8033 | –3590 |
| Ningxia | –1952512 | –4897 | –379459 | –784078 | –4640 | –49165 | –199367 | –2403 | –21495 |
| Xinjiang | –7773597 | –34962 | –217695 | –3760470 | –25958 | –45078 | –626738 | –19762 | –16839 |

## All Contraception Distribution at the End of Statistical Year of 2016

Unit: %

| Region | Male Sterilization | Female Sterilization | Intrauterine Device | Subcutaneous Implant | Oral And Injected Contraceptives | Condom | Externally Applied Drug | Others |
|---|---|---|---|---|---|---|---|---|
| **Whole Country** | **3.45** | **25.83** | **53.03** | **0.23** | **0.80** | **16.16** | **0.15** | **0.34** |
| Beijing | 0.02 | 0.51 | 18.53 | 0.06 | 1.47 | 78.89 | 0.10 | 0.41 |
| Tianjin | 0.12 | 4.15 | 44.79 | 0.09 | 1.14 | 48.09 | 0.28 | 1.34 |
| Hebei | 2.73 | 19.79 | 66.33 | 0.09 | 0.46 | 9.21 | 0.03 | 1.36 |
| Shanxi | 0.32 | 27.88 | 68.52 | 0.06 | 0.30 | 2.59 | 0.00 | 0.33 |
| Inner Mongolia | 0.06 | 12.09 | 66.32 | 0.19 | 0.59 | 20.62 | 0.01 | 0.12 |
| Liaoning | 0.00 | 2.07 | 79.98 | 0.10 | 0.99 | 16.52 | 0.21 | 0.14 |
| Jilin | 0.02 | 4.04 | 79.07 | 1.95 | 0.38 | 14.47 | 0.05 | 0.02 |
| Heilongjiang | 0.01 | 6.36 | 81.15 | 0.25 | 1.26 | 10.55 | 0.09 | 0.32 |
| Shanghai | 0.21 | 2.71 | 41.03 | 0.14 | 2.59 | 51.05 | 0.56 | 1.71 |
| Jiangsu | 0.78 | 8.21 | 66.20 | 0.06 | 0.76 | 23.40 | 0.27 | 0.32 |
| Zhejiang | 0.22 | 19.61 | 47.16 | 0.10 | 0.50 | 31.98 | 0.13 | 0.29 |
| Anhui | 1.24 | 37.32 | 48.07 | 0.19 | 0.83 | 12.20 | 0.01 | 0.13 |
| Fujian | 4.78 | 40.18 | 41.25 | 0.15 | 0.20 | 13.36 | 0.02 | 0.06 |
| Jiangxi | 0.11 | 46.69 | 35.69 | 0.05 | 0.29 | 16.82 | 0.14 | 0.21 |
| Shandong | 6.13 | 17.88 | 56.01 | 0.14 | 0.03 | 19.78 | 0.01 | 0.02 |
| Henan | 10.54 | 40.63 | 42.88 | 0.27 | 0.36 | 5.09 | 0.07 | 0.16 |
| Hubei | 2.48 | 27.65 | 53.45 | 0.33 | 1.18 | 14.70 | 0.03 | 0.19 |
| Hunan | 1.15 | 37.80 | 44.92 | 0.18 | 0.10 | 15.28 | 0.25 | 0.32 |
| Guangdong | 6.29 | 36.72 | 24.63 | 0.04 | 0.38 | 31.77 | 0.08 | 0.09 |
| Guangxi | 7.83 | 30.39 | 53.30 | 0.01 | 1.01 | 6.73 | 0.65 | 0.07 |
| Hainan | 0.49 | 39.32 | 48.35 | 0.02 | 0.16 | 11.48 | 0.09 | 0.09 |
| Chongqing | 4.74 | 1.38 | 74.31 | 0.18 | 3.11 | 15.76 | 0.37 | 0.14 |
| Sichuan | 3.68 | 2.49 | 76.33 | 0.69 | 2.04 | 13.08 | 0.08 | 1.61 |
| Guizhou | 11.58 | 52.85 | 31.49 | 0.06 | 0.12 | 3.74 | 0.02 | 0.14 |
| Yunnan | 2.53 | 24.26 | 64.67 | 0.26 | 1.81 | 5.97 | 0.23 | 0.27 |
| Tibet | 0.01 | 7.57 | 14.38 | 9.48 | 18.97 | 43.62 | 5.35 | 0.63 |
| Shaanxi | 1.79 | 37.30 | 50.58 | 0.65 | 1.47 | 7.93 | 0.23 | 0.05 |
| Gansu | 0.08 | 52.44 | 39.70 | 0.16 | 0.93 | 6.52 | 0.03 | 0.15 |
| Qinghai | 0.07 | 33.80 | 54.23 | 0.56 | 3.68 | 6.34 | 0.99 | 0.33 |
| Ningxia | 0.02 | 26.83 | 49.22 | 0.16 | 2.21 | 20.51 | 0.26 | 0.79 |
| Xinjiang | 0.20 | 4.08 | 77.14 | 0.13 | 0.71 | 16.84 | 0.49 | 0.41 |

## Comparison of All Contraception Distribution at the End of Statistical Year of 2016 with the Same Period of Last Year

Unit: %

| Region | Male Sterilization | Female Sterilization | Intrauterine Device | Subcutaneous Implant | Oral And Injected Contraceptives | Condom | Externally Applied Drug | Others |
|---|---|---|---|---|---|---|---|---|
| **Whole Country** | **−0.40** | **−0.41** | **−1.53** | **0.04** | **−0.10** | **2.36** | **0.01** | **0.02** |
| Beijing | 0.00 | −0.13 | −2.17 | −0.01 | −0.17 | 2.44 | −0.01 | 0.04 |
| Tianjin | 0.03 | −1.05 | −5.15 | −0.03 | −0.21 | 6.08 | −0.25 | 0.59 |
| Hebei | −0.31 | −2.00 | 0.89 | 0.00 | −0.03 | 1.32 | 0.00 | 0.12 |
| Shanxi | −0.03 | −1.43 | 0.88 | −0.01 | 0.02 | 0.46 | 0.00 | 0.10 |
| Inner Mongolia | −0.01 | −1.41 | −0.04 | −0.01 | −0.05 | 1.49 | 0.00 | 0.04 |
| Liaoning | 0.00 | −0.44 | −0.63 | −0.01 | −0.01 | 0.99 | 0.04 | 0.07 |
| Jilin | 0.01 | −0.45 | −1.36 | 1.59 | 0.17 | 0.00 | 0.00 | 0.02 |
| Heilongjiang | 0.00 | −0.71 | −0.71 | 0.14 | 0.02 | 1.22 | 0.00 | 0.05 |
| Shanghai | 0.00 | 0.01 | 0.07 | 0.00 | 0.04 | −0.14 | 0.03 | −0.01 |
| Jiangsu | −0.18 | −0.66 | 0.61 | 0.00 | −2.36 | 2.47 | 0.01 | 0.11 |
| Zhejiang | −0.01 | −0.99 | −1.81 | −0.01 | −0.07 | 2.86 | −0.01 | 0.05 |
| Anhui | −0.20 | −1.84 | −2.69 | −0.03 | 0.10 | 4.60 | 0.01 | 0.05 |
| Fujian | −0.13 | −0.65 | −1.39 | −0.01 | 0.03 | 2.14 | 0.00 | 0.01 |
| Jiangxi | −0.20 | −1.86 | −2.89 | 0.01 | −0.03 | 4.87 | 0.00 | 0.10 |
| Shandong | −0.72 | 0.28 | −3.58 | −0.02 | −0.01 | 4.06 | 0.00 | −0.02 |
| Henan | −0.70 | −0.04 | 0.33 | 0.00 | 0.02 | 0.37 | −0.01 | 0.04 |
| Hubei | −0.10 | −0.77 | −1.08 | 0.02 | −0.01 | 1.94 | 0.01 | −0.01 |
| Hunan | −0.29 | −0.96 | −0.24 | −0.01 | −0.01 | 1.40 | 0.00 | 0.09 |
| Guangdong | −0.52 | −1.28 | −1.90 | 0.00 | 0.02 | 3.68 | 0.01 | −0.01 |
| Guangxi | −0.18 | −0.67 | 0.39 | −0.01 | −0.16 | 0.63 | −0.03 | 0.02 |
| Hainan | −0.08 | −2.88 | 0.34 | 0.00 | 0.04 | 2.59 | 0.00 | 0.00 |
| Chongqing | −0.07 | −0.10 | −1.37 | 0.00 | 0.36 | 1.08 | 0.09 | 0.00 |
| Sichuan | −2.37 | −0.09 | −1.23 | 0.10 | 0.34 | 3.01 | −0.06 | 0.30 |
| Guizhou | −0.77 | −0.39 | −0.92 | −0.01 | 0.02 | 2.01 | 0.01 | 0.06 |
| Yunnan | −0.05 | −0.34 | −0.81 | −0.03 | 0.22 | 0.97 | 0.02 | 0.02 |
| Tibet | | | | | | | | |
| Shaanxi | 0.06 | −1.92 | 0.25 | 0.00 | −0.02 | 1.62 | 0.03 | 0.01 |
| Gansu | 0.00 | −2.84 | 1.19 | −0.10 | 0.15 | 1.58 | 0.01 | 0.01 |
| Qinghai | 0.00 | −0.91 | 0.48 | 0.01 | 0.06 | 0.15 | 0.23 | −0.02 |
| Ningxia | −0.01 | −1.43 | −0.82 | −0.03 | −0.16 | 3.45 | 0.05 | −1.05 |
| Xinjiang | −0.02 | −0.23 | −0.94 | −0.02 | 0.01 | 1.22 | 0.00 | −0.01 |

**(Wang Ruisi)**

# Relevant Statistical Data

## Marriage Registration Service

Unit: Couple person

| Region | Marriage Registration Number | Marriage Registration Population | Classification by Residence Place | | |
|---|---|---|---|---|---|
| | | | Mainland Resident Marriage Registration Number | Mainland Resident Marriage Registration Population | Number of Marriage Registration Concerning Foreign Affairs, and Overseas Chinese and Hong Kong, Macao and Taiwan Resident |
| **Whole Country** | **11428216** | **22856432** | **11386050** | **22770310** | **42166** |
| Central Level | | | | | |
| Beijing | 166207 | 332414 | 165195 | 330390 | 1012 |
| Tianjin | 98164 | 196328 | 97848 | 195696 | 316 |
| Hebei | 551896 | 1103792 | 550919 | 1101838 | 977 |
| Shanxi | 300121 | 600242 | 299966 | 599932 | 155 |
| Inner Mongolia | 198392 | 396784 | 198191 | 396382 | 201 |
| Liaoning | 312562 | 625124 | 310900 | 621800 | 1662 |
| Jilin | 221505 | 443010 | 220749 | 441498 | 756 |
| Heilongjiang | 306307 | 612614 | 304778 | 609556 | 1529 |
| Shanghai | 125215 | 250430 | 123531 | 247062 | 1684 |
| Jiangsu | 716111 | 1432222 | 714705 | 1429410 | 1406 |
| Zhejiang | 366823 | 733646 | 363896 | 727792 | 2927 |
| Anhui | 713361 | 1426722 | 711977 | 1423954 | 1384 |
| Fujian | 314648 | 629296 | 309569 | 619138 | 5079 |
| Jiangxi | 302014 | 604028 | 300907 | 601814 | 1107 |
| Shandong | 670678 | 1341356 | 669587 | 1339174 | 1091 |
| Henan | 968979 | 1937858 | 968087 | 1936174 | 892 |
| Hubei | 513823 | 1027646 | 512629 | 1025258 | 1194 |
| Hunan | 499373 | 998746 | 497770 | 995540 | 1603 |
| Guangdong | 786123 | 1572246 | 777990 | 1556826 | 8133 |
| Guangxi | 393951 | 787902 | 391762 | 783524 | 2189 |
| Hainan | 78255 | 156510 | 77730 | 155460 | 525 |
| Chongqing | 278527 | 557054 | 277882 | 555764 | 645 |
| Sichuan | 727118 | 1454236 | 725628 | 1451256 | 1490 |
| Guizhou | 453162 | 906324 | 452777 | 905554 | 385 |
| Yunnan | 446076 | 892152 | 443130 | 886268 | 2946 |
| Tibet | 30055 | 60110 | 30044 | 57650 | 11 |
| Shaanxi | 332406 | 664812 | 331860 | 663720 | 546 |
| Gansu | 219095 | 438190 | 218951 | 437902 | 144 |
| Qinghai | 61187 | 122374 | 61167 | 122334 | 20 |
| Ningxia | 62028 | 124056 | 61983 | 123760 | 45 |
| Xinjiang | 214054 | 428108 | 213942 | 427884 | 112 |

Note: The statistical data in This Column are from 2017 Volume of China Civil Affairs Statistical Yearbook

*Continued*
Unit: Couple, Person

| Region | Classification by Residence Place | | | | | | |
| --- | --- | --- | --- | --- | --- | --- | --- |
| | Mainland Resident | #Female | Hong Kong Resident | Macao Resident | Taiwan Resident | Overseas Chinese | Foreigner |
| **Whole Country** | **40809** | **26367** | **5364** | **1305** | **7177** | **5127** | **24550** |
| Central Level | | | | | | | |
| Beijing | 919 | 645 | 57 | 6 | 125 | 18 | 899 |
| Tianjin | 308 | 226 | 10 | | 45 | 5 | 264 |
| Hebei | 976 | 276 | 10 | 7 | 71 | 10 | 880 |
| Shanxi | 154 | 2306 | 45 | 35 | 49 | 17 | 10 |
| Inner Mongolia | 200 | 124 | 5 | 2 | 32 | 4 | 159 |
| Liaoning | 1653 | 1249 | 37 | 12 | 177 | 88 | 1357 |
| Jilin | 747 | 509 | 14 | 14 | 102 | 31 | 604 |
| Heilongjiang | 1527 | 978 | 26 | 14 | 183 | 312 | 996 |
| Shanghai | 1533 | 1100 | 95 | 16 | 312 | 36 | 1376 |
| Jiangsu | 1390 | 1056 | 54 | 14 | 420 | 20 | 914 |
| Zhejiang | 2071 | 1146 | 39 | 9 | 218 | 2288 | 1229 |
| Anhui | 1383 | 505 | 25 | 7 | 220 | 21 | 1112 |
| Fujian | 5023 | 3036 | 1182 | 108 | 1368 | 770 | 1707 |
| Jiangxi | 1107 | 414 | 45 | 13 | 218 | 23 | 808 |
| Shandong | 1024 | 663 | 82 | 9 | 138 | 24 | 905 |
| Henan | 891 | 559 | 26 | 18 | 248 | 14 | 587 |
| Hubei | 1193 | 873 | 113 | 31 | 340 | 13 | 698 |
| Hunan | 1600 | 1211 | 144 | 58 | 625 | 32 | 747 |
| Guangdong | 8077 | 5368 | 2802 | 809 | 780 | 1272 | 2526 |
| Guangxi | 2189 | 566 | 136 | 40 | 308 | 45 | 1660 |
| Hainan | 523 | 409 | 167 | 11 | 218 | 12 | 119 |
| Chongqing | 643 | 517 | 61 | 16 | 203 | 1 | 356 |
| Sichuan | 1485 | 1057 | 100 | 30 | 402 | 33 | 930 |
| Guizhou | 385 | 282 | 34 | 12 | 125 | 11 | 202 |
| Yunnan | 2944 | 427 | 22 | 4 | 83 | 5 | 2834 |
| Tibet | 11 | 5 | 1 | 1 | | 2 | 7 |
| Shaanxi | 543 | 310 | 18 | 4 | 116 | 7 | 404 |
| Gansu | 143 | 95 | 8 | 2 | 34 | 2 | 99 |
| Qinghai | 20 | 6 | 1 | | 3 | 1 | 15 |
| Ningxia | 35 | 21 | 3 | 1 | 7 | | 44 |
| Xinjiang | 112 | 83 | 2 | 1 | 7 | | 102 |

*Continued*
Unit: Couple, Person

| Region | Classification by Marital Status | | | |
|---|---|---|---|---|
| | First Marriage Number | Remarriage Number | | |
| | | | #Female | #Marriage Resumption Number |
| **Whole Country** | **19132566** | **3723866** | **1950215** | **473905** |
| Central Level | | | | |
| Beijing | 200750 | 131664 | 64185 | 22282 |
| Tianjin | 161474 | 34854 | 17357 | 16023 |
| Hebei | 851411 | 252381 | 137026 | 313 |
| Shanxi | 530845 | 69397 | 37974 | 6943 |
| Inner Mongolia | 280929 | 115855 | 63865 | 17159 |
| Liaoning | 554958 | 70166 | 35715 | 27482 |
| Jilin | 395931 | 47079 | 23706 | 20978 |
| Heilongjiang | 522071 | 90543 | 46531 | 28564 |
| Shanghai | 159162 | 91268 | 45320 | 20340 |
| Jiangsu | 1162847 | 269375 | 139073 | 46357 |
| Zhejiang | 605781 | 127865 | 65408 | 13195 |
| Anhui | 1141695 | 285027 | 149119 | 39537 |
| Fujian | 539946 | 89350 | 46971 | 501 |
| Jiangxi | 508278 | 95750 | 50732 | 13401 |
| Shandong | 995075 | 346281 | 183520 | 1610 |
| Henan | 1850977 | 86981 | 44042 | 41399 |
| Hubei | 971991 | 55655 | 28727 | 6914 |
| Hunan | 786720 | 212026 | 114854 | 16702 |
| Guangdong | 1365312 | 206934 | 99589 | 33170 |
| Guangxi | 674702 | 113200 | 64054 | 8841 |
| Hainan | 140883 | 15627 | 7942 | 1688 |
| Chongqing | 380608 | 176446 | 92677 | 15586 |
| Sichuan | 1093585 | 360651 | 194176 | 33747 |
| Guizhou | 866973 | 39351 | 19877 | 11368 |
| Yunnan | 744088 | 148064 | 74314 | 1329 |
| Tibet | 57556 | 2554 | 757 | 6 |
| Shaanxi | 544943 | 119869 | 66039 | 12670 |
| Gansu | 425510 | 12680 | 6541 | 3121 |
| Qinghai | 108285 | 14089 | 7408 | 32 |
| Ningxia | 102977 | 21079 | 11346 | 2453 |
| Xinjiang | 406303 | 21805 | 11370 | 10194 |

*Continued*
Unit: Couple, Person

| Classification by Age | | | | |
|---|---|---|---|---|
| 20-24 | 25-29 | 30-34 | 35-39 | 40 and above |
| **5523560** | **8722990** | **2930063** | **1606326** | **4073493** |
| | | | | |
| 21823 | 131703 | 71047 | 40945 | 66896 |
| 31602 | 78295 | 37983 | 19448 | 29000 |
| 354407 | 417655 | 125335 | 66690 | 139705 |
| 166794 | 233317 | 60024 | 33021 | 107086 |
| 73790 | 162569 | 57319 | 29918 | 73188 |
| | | | | |
| 94733 | 241673 | 98548 | 56149 | 134021 |
| 70461 | 155955 | 65334 | 39863 | 111397 |
| 91744 | 183161 | 85482 | 57385 | 194842 |
| | | | | |
| 18272 | 90749 | 49426 | 28144 | 63839 |
| 312668 | 523310 | 133374 | 83723 | 379147 |
| 131708 | 318670 | 100190 | 48857 | 134221 |
| 408540 | 479682 | 126145 | 89677 | 322678 |
| 136169 | 281545 | 83570 | 35030 | 92982 |
| 175245 | 233559 | 68429 | 40093 | 86702 |
| 280593 | 633220 | 179906 | 87953 | 159684 |
| | | | | |
| 522989 | 749452 | 210709 | 145827 | 308981 |
| 230535 | 420687 | 125568 | 62473 | 188383 |
| 220364 | 436726 | 144355 | 680268 | 129233 |
| 431319 | 655385 | 228708 | 99803 | 157031 |
| 191565 | 291790 | 142970 | 63607 | 97970 |
| 37945 | 54474 | 23676 | 11063 | 29352 |
| | | | | |
| 157671 | 180705 | 69499 | 34164 | 115015 |
| 406453 | 486418 | 176593 | 100575 | 284197 |
| 241104 | 268869 | 118078 | 79376 | 198897 |
| 230713 | 267523 | 115157 | 74329 | 204430 |
| 17326 | 21565 | 10189 | 5546 | 5393 |
| | | | | |
| 157114 | 305958 | 85223 | 35728 | 80789 |
| 131162 | 183729 | 48289 | 20120 | 54890 |
| 28371 | 46894 | 16325 | 9541 | 21243 |
| 34874 | 43015 | 13550 | 8670 | 23947 |
| 115506 | 144646 | 59062 | 30540 | 78354 |

## Divorce Registration Service

| Region | Total | Department of Civil Affairs Totaling | | | |
| --- | --- | --- | --- | --- | --- |
| | | | Mainland Resident Divorce Registration | Divorce Registration Concerning Foreign Affairs, and Overseas Chinese and Hong Kong, Macao and Taiwan Resident | #Foreigner |
| **Whole Country** | **4158211** | **3486257** | **3479942** | **6315** | **2894** |
| Beijing | 105805 | 97583 | 97327 | 256 | 190 |
| Tianjin | 65220 | 60164 | 60087 | 77 | 60 |
| Hebei | 220153 | 179332 | 179260 | 72 | 49 |
| Shanxi | 76520 | 58962 | 58945 | 17 | 0 |
| Inner Mongolia | 98364 | 79024 | 78990 | 28 | 14 |
| Liaoning | 160101 | 136114 | 135865 | 249 | 179 |
| Jilin | 129229 | 116755 | 116648 | 107 | 73 |
| Heilongjiang | 187192 | 164660 | 164468 | 192 | 103 |
| Shanghai | 82558 | 74350 | 73845 | 505 | 307 |
| Jiangsu | 261305 | 219687 | 219427 | 260 | 139 |
| Zhejiang | 147096 | 122870 | 122483 | 387 | 192 |
| Anhui | 217237 | 185039 | 184915 | 124 | 74 |
| Fujian | 96338 | 80169 | 79323 | 846 | 244 |
| Jiangxi | 102139 | 86405 | 86290 | 115 | 57 |
| Shandong | 254506 | 201101 | 200958 | 143 | 87 |
| Henan | 277458 | 239324 | 239210 | 114 | 48 |
| Hubei | 183118 | 160236 | 160041 | 195 | 78 |
| Hunan | 193452 | 164083 | 163844 | 239 | 79 |
| Guangdong | 211858 | 186406 | 185025 | 1381 | 403 |
| Guangxi | 112768 | 92691 | 92514 | 177 | 82 |
| Hainan | 16631 | 13139 | 13050 | 89 | 15 |
| Chongqing | 139029 | 122072 | 121931 | 141 | 61 |
| Sichuan | 296234 | 255173 | 254928 | 245 | 107 |
| Guizhou | 121041 | 92896 | 92836 | 60 | 21 |
| Yunnan | 119305 | 95481 | 95285 | 196 | 168 |
| Tibet | 3484 | 2848 | 2848 | 0 | 0 |
| Shaanxi | 101433 | 78588 | 78526 | 62 | 38 |
| Gansu | 50325 | 33451 | 33433 | 18 | 9 |
| Qinghai | 15164 | 9939 | 9937 | 2 | 2 |
| Ningxia | 19544 | 14641 | 14634 | 7 | 6 |
| Xinjiang | 93575 | 63074 | 63063 | 11 | 9 |

Note: The number of whole country divorce registration service includes the military divorces.

*Continued*
Unit: Couple, Person

| Department of Court Totaling | | | Divorce Cognizance | Judicial No Divorce | Regulated No Divorce |
| --- | --- | --- | --- | --- | --- |
| | Judicial Divorce | Regulated Divorce | | | |
| **671954** | **218735** | **453219** | **1381673** | **297673** | **53593** |
| 8222 | 2779 | 5443 | 18299 | 3639 | 145 |
| 5056 | 1658 | 3398 | 13225 | 3395 | 903 |
| 40821 | 12964 | 27857 | 84864 | 19220 | 1081 |
| 17558 | 6220 | 11338 | 38401 | 7583 | 3416 |
| 19340 | 2774 | 12566 | 36153 | 2847 | 1260 |
| 23987 | 8300 | 15687 | 50029 | 9597 | 1133 |
| 12474 | 5405 | 7069 | 24147 | 3803 | 434 |
| 22532 | 6410 | 16122 | 37153 | 2392 | 432 |
| 8208 | 2537 | 5671 | 17662 | 4082 | 234 |
| 41618 | 10796 | 30822 | 97089 | 25530 | 4079 |
| 24226 | 7621 | 16605 | 51199 | 13271 | 1588 |
| 32198 | 8977 | 23221 | 71696 | 18599 | 1461 |
| 16169 | 7477 | 8692 | 34518 | 8920 | 477 |
| 15734 | 6106 | 9628 | 37190 | 9703 | 1843 |
| 53405 | 20078 | 33327 | 117863 | 29645 | 6616 |
| 38134 | 13767 | 24367 | 87411 | 24307 | 1597 |
| 22882 | 7180 | 15702 | 47994 | 13804 | 857 |
| 29369 | 10773 | 18596 | 62038 | 17878 | 1632 |
| 25452 | 10960 | 14492 | 51265 | 12070 | 702 |
| 20077 | 8294 | 11783 | 37632 | 8798 | 1104 |
| 3492 | 1292 | 2200 | 6279 | 1009 | 725 |
| 16957 | 5971 | 10986 | 33519 | 7854 | 744 |
| 41061 | 12193 | 28868 | 78152 | 16800 | 3215 |
| 28145 | 7993 | 20152 | 49237 | 7032 | 1500 |
| 23824 | 6925 | 16899 | 43826 | 5767 | 2875 |
| 636 | 90 | 546 | 915 | 28 | 79 |
| 22845 | 6319 | 16526 | 49716 | 7576 | 5555 |
| 16874 | 5388 | 11486 | 37357 | 7220 | 2283 |
| 5225 | 1276 | 3949 | 10425 | 957 | 861 |
| 4903 | 1525 | 3378 | 11804 | 2279 | 778 |
| 30501 | 4681 | 25820 | 44548 | 2117 | 3984 |

## Orphan and Children Adoption

| Region | Orphan Number | Concentrated Raised Orphan | Social Scattered Orphan | Adoption Registration Totaling | Chinese Citizen Adoption Registration |
|---|---|---|---|---|---|
| **Whole Country** | **460450** | **87502** | **372948** | **18736** | **15965** |
| Central Level | | | | | |
| Beijing | 2071 | 1660 | 411 | 140 | 96 |
| Tianjin | 805 | 552 | 253 | 62 | 20 |
| Hebei | 16479 | 2163 | 14316 | 255 | 219 |
| Shanxi | 12850 | 2688 | 10162 | 244 | 102 |
| Inner Mongolia | 5185 | 1182 | 4003 | 197 | 102 |
| Liaoning | 7233 | 3165 | 4068 | 183 | 160 |
| Jilin | 5106 | 1491 | 3615 | 23 | 7 |
| Heilongjiang | 7286 | 1369 | 5917 | 69 | 45 |
| Shanghai | 1827 | 1726 | 98 | 306 | 246 |
| Jiangsu | 16510 | 3269 | 13241 | 1721 | 1561 |
| Zhejiang | 4235 | 2196 | 2039 | 2483 | 2403 |
| Anhui | 27250 | 3216 | 24034 | 737 | 654 |
| Fujian | 5504 | 1871 | 3633 | 1076 | 1008 |
| Jiangxi | 21358 | 5342 | 16016 | 284 | 167 |
| Shandong | 17360 | 2862 | 14498 | 1982 | 1841 |
| Henan | 34032 | 4855 | 29177 | 717 | 259 |
| Hubei | 19284 | 3067 | 16217 | 695 | 614 |
| Hunan | 37274 | 4950 | 32324 | 706 | 630 |
| Guangdong | 35807 | 8860 | 26947 | 1436 | 1080 |
| Guangxi | 21888 | 2385 | 19503 | 1757 | 1594 |
| Hainan | 1548 | 336 | 1212 | 86 | 86 |
| Chongqing | 5404 | 1374 | 4030 | 247 | 208 |
| Sichuan | 28878 | 3991 | 24887 | 1001 | 949 |
| Guizhou | 20232 | 2801 | 17431 | 253 | 168 |
| Yunnan | 24176 | 1820 | 22356 | 1255 | 1171 |
| Tibet | 5967 | 5967 | | 13 | 13 |
| Shaanxi | 11569 | 2569 | 9000 | 387 | 207 |
| Gansu | 18828 | 2593 | 16235 | 86 | 48 |
| Qinghai | 15771 | 1778 | 13993 | 49 | 45 |
| Ningxia | 6646 | 439 | 6207 | 37 | 26 |
| Xinjiang | 22090 | 4965 | 17125 | 249 | 236 |

| Hong Kong Resident | Macao Resident | Taiwan Resident | Overseas Chinese | Adaptation Registration of Foreigner | Registration of Agreed Recission of Adoption | #Chinese Citizen |
|---|---|---|---|---|---|---|
| 77 | 3 | 26 | 25 | 2771 | 562 | 531 |
| | | | 1 | 44 | 1 | 1 |
| 2 | | | | 42 | 5 | 5 |
| | | | | 36 | 10 | 10 |
| 1 | | | | 142 | | |
| | | | | 95 | 1 | 1 |
| | | | 1 | 23 | 1 | 1 |
| | | | | 16 | | |
| 1 | | 2 | | 24 | 6 | 6 |
| | | 1 | 2 | 60 | 5 | 5 |
| 1 | | | | 160 | 45 | 45 |
| | | 1 | 14 | 80 | 72 | 72 |
| | | | | 83 | | |
| 8 | | 7 | | 68 | 6 | 5 |
| | | | | 117 | 34 | 34 |
| 3 | | 1 | 1 | 141 | 4 | 4 |
| | | | 2 | 458 | 30 | 30 |
| 3 | | 1 | | 81 | 6 | 6 |
| | | | | 76 | 40 | 40 |
| 50 | 3 | 3 | 3 | 356 | 12 | 11 |
| 2 | | 7 | | 163 | 117 | 117 |
| 2 | | | | | | |
| 3 | | 1 | | 39 | 20 | 20 |
| 1 | | 1 | 1 | 52 | 72 | 72 |
| | | | | 85 | 4 | 4 |
| | | | | 84 | 1 | 1 |
| | | 1 | | 180 | 45 | 17 |
| | | | | 38 | | |
| | | | | 4 | 3 | 3 |
| | | | | 11 | | |
| | | | | 13 | 22 | 21 |

## Adopted Children

| Region | Adopted | | | | |
|--------|---------|--------|-------------------|--------------------------------------------|------------------------------|
| | Total | Female | Disabled Children | Adopted Orphan in Social Welfare Institution | #Adopted by Foreign People |
| **Whole Country** | **18736** | **12586** | **2554** | **8884** | **2490** |
| Central Level | | | | | |
| Beijing | 140 | 70 | 49 | 49 | 43 |
| Tianjin | 62 | 30 | 36 | 59 | 41 |
| Hebei | 255 | 139 | 52 | 124 | 36 |
| Shanxi | 244 | 113 | 34 | 192 | 140 |
| Inner Mongolia | 197 | 97 | 22 | 111 | 95 |
| Liaoning | 183 | 96 | 21 | 65 | 22 |
| Jilin | 23 | 4 | | 22 | 16 |
| Heilongjiang | 69 | 26 | 15 | 22 | 14 |
| Shanghai | 306 | 242 | 61 | 175 | 59 |
| Jiangsu | 1721 | 1153 | 274 | 877 | 160 |
| Zhejiang | 2483 | 1933 | 27 | 1501 | |
| Anhui | 737 | 481 | 9 | 312 | 83 |
| Fujian | 1076 | 833 | 68 | 467 | 66 |
| Jiangxi | 284 | 207 | 110 | 184 | 115 |
| Shandong | 1982 | 1187 | 164 | 675 | 141 |
| Henan | 717 | 343 | 474 | 565 | 458 |
| Hubei | 695 | 457 | 85 | 220 | |
| Hunan | 706 | 471 | 76 | 305 | 76 |
| Guangdong | 1436 | 1016 | 339 | 1019 | 356 |
| Guangxi | 1757 | 1438 | 162 | 818 | 151 |
| Hainan | 86 | 69 | | 49 | |
| Chongqing | 247 | 153 | 36 | 68 | 38 |
| Sichuan | 1001 | 560 | 56 | 394 | 50 |
| Guizhou | 253 | 185 | 71 | 123 | 84 |
| Yunnan | 1255 | 847 | 64 | 129 | |
| Tibet | 13 | | | 12 | |
| Shaanxi | 387 | 198 | 174 | 220 | 180 |
| Gansu | 86 | 46 | 37 | 55 | 38 |
| Qinghai | 49 | 23 | 6 | 4 | 4 |
| Ningxia | 37 | 25 | 11 | 17 | 11 |
| Xinjiang | 249 | 144 | 21 | 51 | 13 |

*Continued*
Unit: Person

| Orphan Number in Social Orphanage | | Adopted Number by immediate Relatives | | Number with Parents of Special | | Others | |
|---|---|---|---|---|---|---|---|
| | #Adopted by Foreigner | | #Adopted by Foreigner | Difficulties | #Adopted by Foreigner | | #Adopted by Foreigner |
| **4696** | **244** | **1076** | **7** | **601** | **8** | **3479** | **22** |
| 64 | | 3 | | 3 | | 21 | 1 |
| | | 1 | 1 | 1 | | 1 | |
| 57 | | 26 | | 4 | | 44 | |
| 13 | | 18 | | 7 | 2 | 14 | |
| 9 | | 20 | | 39 | | 18 | |
| 81 | | 13 | | 2 | 1 | 22 | |
| | | | | | | 1 | |
| 10 | | 14 | 2 | 8 | 3 | 15 | 5 |
| 80 | | 14 | | 1 | | 36 | 1 |
| 298 | | 125 | | 19 | | 402 | |
| 692 | 68 | 86 | | 3 | | 201 | 12 |
| 281 | | 32 | | 16 | | 96 | |
| 326 | | 44 | 2 | 7 | | 232 | |
| 50 | | 12 | 2 | 1 | | 37 | |
| 604 | | 21 | | 14 | | 668 | |
| 31 | | 62 | | 29 | | 30 | |
| 217 | 80 | 70 | | 62 | | 126 | 1 |
| 175 | | 71 | | 27 | | 128 | |
| 186 | | 108 | | 20 | | 103 | |
| 458 | 12 | 70 | | 49 | | 362 | |
| 17 | | 2 | | 9 | | 9 | |
| 78 | | 21 | | 11 | | 69 | 1 |
| 220 | | 116 | | 143 | 1 | 128 | 1 |
| 36 | 1 | 3 | | 16 | | 75 | |
| 573 | 83 | 38 | | 56 | 1 | 459 | |
| 1 | | | | | | | |
| 45 | | 20 | | 36 | | 66 | |
| 18 | | 7 | | | | 6 | |
| 8 | | 22 | | 2 | | 13 | |
| 11 | | | | | | 9 | |
| 57 | | 37 | | 16 | | 88 | |

**(Wang Ruisi)**

图书在版编目（CIP）数据

2017 卷中国卫生和计划生育年鉴 =2017 Health in
China：英文 / 中国卫生和计划生育委员会编著；陈迎，
曲杨主译. —北京：人民卫生出版社，2019
　ISBN 978-7-117-27985-7

　Ⅰ.①2… 　Ⅱ.①中…②陈…③曲… 　Ⅲ.①卫生工
作 – 中国 –2017– 年鉴 – 英文②计划生育 – 中国 –2017–
年鉴 – 英文　Ⅳ.①R199.2-54②C924.25-54

中国版本图书馆 CIP 数据核字（2019）第 021045 号

| | | |
|---|---|---|
| 人卫智网　www.ipmph.com | 医学教育、学术、考试、健康，购书智慧智能综合服务平台 | |
| 人卫官网　www.pmph.com | 人卫官方资讯发布平台 | |

2017 卷中国卫生和计划生育年鉴（英文版）

主　　译：陈　迎　曲　杨
出版发行：人民卫生出版社（中继线 010-59780011）
地　　址：北京市朝阳区潘家园南里 19 号
邮　　编：100021
E - mail：pmph @ pmph.com
购书热线：010-59787592　010-59787584　010-65264830
印　　刷：北京建宏印刷有限公司
经　　销：新华书店
开　　本：787×1092　1/16　印张：35　插页：12
字　　数：809 千字
版　　次：2019 年 8 月第 1 版　2019 年 8 月第 1 版第 1 次印刷
标准书号：ISBN 978-7-117-27985-7
定　　价：330.00元
打击盗版举报电话：010-59787491　E-mail：WQ @ pmph.com
（凡属印装质量问题请与本社市场营销中心联系退换）